MW00709922

Pediatric Environmental Health

3rd Edition

Author: Council on Environmental Health
American Academy of Pediatrics

Ruth A. Etzel, MD, PhD; Editor
Sophie J. Balk, MD; Associate Editor

Suggested Citation: American Academy of Pediatrics Council
on Environmental Health. [chapter title]. In: Etzel, RA, ed.
Pediatric Environmental Health, 3rd Edition Elk Grove Village, IL:
American Academy of Pediatrics; 2012:[page number]

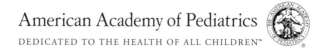

American Academy of Pediatrics
DEDICATED TO THE HEALTH OF ALL CHILDREN™

3rd Edition
2nd Edition – 2003
1st Edition – 1999

Library of Congress Control Number: 2011937340
ISBN: 978-1-58110-313-7
MA0457

The recommendations in this publication do not indicate an exclusive course of treatment or serve as a standard of medical care. Variations, taking into account individual circumstances, may be appropriate.

Inclusion in this publication does not imply an endorsement by the American Academy of Pediatrics (AAP). The AAP is not responsible for the content of the resources mentioned. Addresses, phone numbers, and Web site addresses are as current as possible, but may change at any time.

3-209/1011

1 2 3 4 5 6 7 8 9 10

Table of Contents

■ ■ ■ ■ ■ ■

III. Food and Water

IV. Chemical and Physical Exposures

V. Special Topics

VI. Public Health Aspects of Environmental Health

VII. Appendices

Council on Environmental Health Executive Committee

■ ■ ■ ■ ■ ■

Helen J. Binns, MD, MPH,
  Chairperson
Heather L. Brumberg, MD, MPH
Joel A. Forman, MD
Catherine J. Karr, MD, PhD
Kevin C. Osterhoudt, MD, MSCE
Jerome A. Paulson, MD
Megan T. Sandel, MD, MPH
James M. Seltzer, MD
Robert O. Wright, MD, MPH

Michael W. Shannon, MD, MPH†
  Former Chair

Dana Best, MD, MPH
Christine L. Johnson, MD
Lynnette J. Mazur, MD, MPH
James R. Roberts, MD, MPH
  Former Committee Members

---

†Deceased

Liaison Representatives

Mary E. Mortensen, MD, MS
Centers for Disease Control and Prevention/National Center for Environmental Health
Peter Grevatt, PhD
US Environmental Protection Agency
Sharon Savage, MD
National Cancer Institute
Walter J. Rogan, MD
National Institute of Environmental Health Sciences

AAP Staff

Paul Spire

Preface

■ ■ ■ ■ ■ ■

The publication of *Pediatric Environmental Health*, 3rd Edition, reflects many advances in our understanding of the etiology, identification, management, and prevention of diseases and conditions linked to the environment. The field of environmental health is growing rapidly and new information becomes available almost daily. Hardly a week goes by in which parents don't read an article or hear a news story about the effects of the environment on health, and they may ask their pediatrician for advice about this topic. Since March, stories about the massive earthquake in Japan and the subsequent nuclear crisis have dominated the news. Dramatic events such as these offer an opportunity to bring focus to environmental issues, to teach children about them, and to bring attention to prevention and remediation. They also highlight the many different "environments" in which a child lives: the bedroom, the home, the family, the school, the neighborhood, the community or town, the state, the country, the world—in some ways these are concentric circles. Although large scale events such as the disastrous earthquake and tsunami in Japan heighten our awareness that environmental crises have important physical and psychological effects on children and their families, it is easy to overlook the fact that less visible (or invisible) environmental threats can also have profound physical and psychological effects on children and their families. We as pediatricians must attend to both. This book provides a foundation for understanding where to begin.

First published in 1999, this book is intended for pediatricians and others who are interested in preventing children's exposures to environmental hazards during infancy, childhood, and adolescence. In this edition, we present updated summaries of the evidence that has been published in the scientific literature about environmental hazards to children. Twenty-two new chapters have been introduced in this edition, including topics such as birth defects, global climate change, plasticizers, and the precautionary principle. Major modifications have been made to all 43 chapters from the second edition. Knowledge, research, and information relevant to pediatric practice started growing at an exponential rate after the children's environmental health and disease prevention research programs were established by the US Environmental Protection Agency and the National Institute of Environmental Health Sciences. New associations are being discovered and our knowledge of existing ones is constantly being refined and expanded. As the field of pediatric environmental health evolves, appropriate guidance may change with the publication of additional research findings.

Although all of the 65 contributors to this book are from North America, most of the information presented here should be useful to those in other parts of the world. Children's exposures to some contaminants may be higher in less industrialized countries than in North America; nonetheless, the book can be expected to provide reliable background information for clinicians who are faced with providing practical advice to parents and communities. A chapter about environmental health considerations for children in developing nations gives pediatricians in North America a glimpse of the array of problems facing children growing-up in a variety of international settings.

The book is meant to be practical, containing information that is useful in office practice, but that could also be helpful to a clinician preparing a grand rounds presentation for colleagues or testimony before a group of state legislators. Throughout the book, we have taken the liberty of combining the contributions of multiple authors in each chapter. Though the third edition is more than double the size of the first, there are still many aspects of environmental health that could not be covered. The Council gave priority to those topics that appeared to have the greatest effect on child health, or to be of concern to parents. I hope that the information presented in the handbook will foster an informed understanding of environmental health among those who care for children.

Parents of young children are intensely interested in the impact of the environment on their children's health. They may look to their pediatrician for guidance about how to evaluate news reports about potential hazards in the air, water, and food. Yet the history of such well-established hazards as the exposure of children to secondhand smoke shows many years of epidemiologic and laboratory research before the weight of the evidence compels a consensus. While the evidence is accumulating, what should a worried parent do? Prudently avoid exposure after the first study suggesting problems is published? At what point should the pediatrician advocate a specific action? Obviously, there are no easy answers to these questions. Issues of value, scientific understanding, and cost are involved. Each hazardous exposure must be considered in the context of other problems facing the child and the financial, emotional, and intellectual resources available to surmount them. After fully understanding the facts and uncertainties, reasonable pediatricians may choose different ways to respond to the accumulating evidence.

I have many people to thank for their contributions to this book. First, I am grateful to those who contributed the 33 chapters to the first edition and the 43 chapters to the second edition because their outstanding work provided an excellent foundation for this revised and expanded third edition. Forty one councils, committees and sections of the American Academy of Pediatrics (AAP) reviewed and provided comments on new and revised chapters of this edition. I owe special thanks to Paul Spire, who managed to juggle requests from multiple authors with unflagging good cheer and worked tremendously hard to keep this book on track, and to Jennifer Shaw, senior medical copy editor, and Theresa Weiner, Manager, Division of Publishing and Production Services, for their invaluable help in its preparation. I am immensely grateful to the associate editor, Sophie J. Balk, MD, for her careful attention to ensuring that complex topics were clearly explained and that key action steps for the clinician were provided. Thanks also to Helen Binns, MD, MPH, Chair of the Council on Environmental Health for her strong leadership and to the hardworking members of the Council, who provided many new chapters and reviewed and updated the existing chapters of the book. I owe special thanks to Carole E. Allen, MD, District I Chair and member of the AAP Board of Directors for her painstaking (because she had a broken arm) yet thoughtful and comprehensive review of the book for consistency with AAP policy.

Special credit is due to two esteemed pediatrician scholars who made enormous contributions to the field of pediatric environmental health: Robert W. Miller, MD, DrPH and Michael W. Shannon, MD, MPH. Dr Miller, a world-renowned epidemiologist at the National Cancer Institute, served on the Committee from 1970 to 2004 and chaired it from 1973 until 1979. He was among the first scholars to emphasize the need to consider the special vulnerability of the fetus and child to chemicals in the environment. In 1973, he was instrumental in organizing the Conference on the Susceptibility of the Fetus and Child to Chemical Pollutants, held in Brown's Lake, WI. The Conference uncovered a serious problem: no federal health agency had the responsibility for research into the special exposures and susceptibility of the fetus and child. Throughout his life, Dr Miller worked to ensure that pediatricians knowledgeable about child health and the environment were appointed to leadership roles in government agencies and had a place at the table when key decisions affecting children's health were deliberated. He is fondly remembered as the father of pediatric environmental health because of his vision in articulating the need for special consideration of children's exposures to chemicals and his role as the mentor for many past and present pediatric environmental health leaders.

Dr Shannon, an internationally-recognized pediatrician, toxicologist, and emergency physician at the Harvard Medical School, served on the Committee from 1997 to 2007 and chaired it from 2003 until 2007. He also played a pivotal role in the AAP efforts in disaster preparedness and was a prolific writer, inspired educator, and trusted mentor to fellows and students interested in the effects of drugs and chemicals on children. His role as an Associate Editor of the 3rd edition of *Pediatric Environmental Health* was cut short by his sudden death in March 2009. This book is dedicated to the memory of these treasured colleagues.

Ruth A. Etzel, MD, PhD
Editor

Contributors

■ ■ ■ ■ ■ ■

The American Academy of Pediatrics (AAP) gratefully acknowledges the invaluable assistance provided by the following individuals who contributed to the preparation of this edition of *Pediatric Environmental Health*. Their expertise, critical review, and cooperation were essential to the development of this manual.

Every attempt has been made to recognize all those who contributed to this effort; the AAP regrets any omissions that may have occurred.

Organizational affiliations are provided for identification purposes only.

Kelly J. Ace, PhD, JD; *Institute for the Study of Disadvantage and Disability; Atlanta GA*

Terry Adirim, MD, MPH; *Health Resources and Services Administration; Rockville, MD*

Carole E. Allen, MD; *Arlington, MA*

Mark A. Anderson, MD, MPH; *Centers for Disease Control and Prevention, National Center for Environmental Health; Atlanta, GA*

Sophie J. Balk, MD; *Children's Hospital at Montefiore, Albert Einstein College of Medicine; Bronx, NY*

Cynthia F. Bearer, MD, PhD; *University of Maryland School of Medicine; Baltimore, MD*

Nancy Beaudet, MS, CIH; *University of Washington; Seattle, WA*

Dana Best, MD, MPH; *Silver Spring, MD*

Helen J. Binns, MD, MPH; *Northwestern University Feinberg School of Medicine; Chicago, IL*

Elizabeth Blackburn, RN; *US Environmental Protection Agency; Washington, DC*

Alice Brock-Utne, MD; *Marin Community Clinics; Novato, CA*

Heather L. Brumberg, MD, MPH; *New York Medical College; Valhalla, NY*

Irena Buka, MB, ChB, FRCPC; *University of Alberta; Edmonton, AB, Canada*

Evan R. Buxbaum, MD, MPH; *Redwood Pediatric Group; Fortuna, CA*

Aimin Chen, MD, PhD; *University of Cincinnati College of Medicine; Cincinnati, OH*

Molly Droge, MD; *Parkville, MO*

Ruth A. Etzel, MD, PhD; *George Washington University School of Public Health and Health Services; Washington, DC*

Joel A. Forman, MD; *Mount Sinai School of Medicine; New York, NY*

Laurence J. Fuortes, MD, MS; *University of Iowa Carver College of Medicine; Iowa City, IA*

Robert J. Geller, MD; *Emory University School of Medicine; Atlanta, GA*

George P. Giacoia, MD; *Eunice Kennedy Shriver National Institute of Child Health and Human Development; Bethesda, MD*

Lynn R. Goldman, MD, MPH; *George Washington University School of Public Health and Health Services; Washington, DC*

Penny Grant, MD; *Children's Hospital at Montefiore; Bronx, NY*

Peter Grevatt, PhD; *US Environmental Protection Agency; Washington, DC*

Harold E. Hoffman, MD, FRCPC; *University of Alberta; Edmonton, AB, Canada*

Olson Huff, MD; *Asheville, NC*

Christine Johnson, MD; *Naval Medical Center San Diego; San Diego, CA*

Catherine J. Karr, MD, PhD, MS; *University of Washington School of Medicine; Seattle, WA*

Neha Kaul, MSc; *New York University; New York, NY*

Janice J. Kim, MD, MPH; *California Department of Public Health; Richmond, CA*

Kathy King, MSc, MPhil; *New York University; New York, NY*

Steven E. Krug, MD; *Northwestern University Feinberg School of Medicine; Chicago, IL*

Philip J. Landrigan, MD, MSc; *Mount Sinai School of Medicine; New York, NY*

Martha Linet, MD; *National Cancer Institute; Bethesda, MD*

Kathleen MacKinnon; *US Environmental Protection Agency; Washington, DC*

Donald R. Mattison, MD, MS; *Eunice Kennedy Shriver National Institute of Child Health and Human Development; Bethesda, MD*

Lynnette Mazur, MD, MPH; *Shriners Hospitals for Children; Houston, TX*

Mary Anne McCaffree, MD; *University of Oklahoma Health Sciences Center; Oklahoma City, OK*

Siobhan McNally, MD, MPH; *Community Health Programs – Berkshires; Pittsfield, MA*

Mark D. Miller, MD, MPH; *California Environmental Protection Agency; Oakland, CA*

Mary Mortensen, MD, MS; *Centers for Disease Control and Prevention, National Center for Environmental Health; Atlanta, GA*

Liam R. O'Fallon, MA; *National Institute of Environmental Health Sciences; Research Triangle Park, NC*

Kevin Osterhoudt, MD, MSCE; *The Children's Hospital of Philadelphia; Philadelphia, PA*

Jerome A. Paulson, MD; *Children's National Medical Center; Washington, DC*

Devon C. Payne-Sturges, DrPH; *US Environmental Protection Agency; Washington, DC*

Cynthia Pellegrini; *March of Dimes; Washington, DC*

Susan H. Pollack, MD; *Kentucky Injury Prevention and Research Center, University of Kentucky; Lexington, KY*

Travis Riddell, MD, MPH; *University of Washington School of Medicine; Jackson, WY*

James R. Roberts, MD, MPH; *Medical University of South Carolina; Charleston, SC*

Walter J. Rogan, MD; *National Institute of Environmental Health Sciences; Research Triangle Park, NC*

I. Leslie Rubin, MD, MPH; *Morehouse School of Medicine; Institute for the Study of Disadvantage and Disability; Atlanta, GA*

Megan T. Sandel, MD; *Boston University School of Medicine; Boston, MA*

Sharon A. Savage, MD; *National Cancer Institute; Bethesda, MD*

David J Schonfeld, MD; *Cincinnati Children's Hospital Medical Center; Cincinnati, OH*

James M. Seltzer, MD; *Fallon Clinic; Worcester, MA*

Michael Shannon, MD, MPH; *Harvard Medical School; Boston, MA*

Katherine M. Shea, MD, MPH; *University of North Carolina Gillings School of Global Public Health, Chapel Hill, NC*

Perry E. Sheffield, MD, MPH; *Mount Sinai School of Medicine; New York, NY*

Gina Solomon, MD, MPH; *University of California San Francisco Medical Center; San Francisco, CA*

Paul Spire; *American Academy of Pediatrics; Elk Grove Village, IL*

June Tester, MD, MPH; *Children's Hospital & Research Center Oakland; Oakland, CA*

David A. Turcotte, ScD, MS; *University of Massachusetts, Lowell; Lowell, MA*

Ian Van Dinther; *American Academy of Pediatrics; Elk Grove Village, IL*

Alvaro Osornio Vargas, MD, PhD; *University of Alberta; Edmonton, AB, Canada*

David Wallinga, MD, MPA; *Institute for Agriculture and Trade Policy; Minneapolis, MN*

Michael L. Weitzman, MD; *New York University Langone Medical Center; New York, NY*

Nsedu Obot Witherspoon, MPH; *Children's Environmental Health Network; Washington, DC*

Tracey J. Woodruff, PhD, MPH; *Program on Reproductive Health and the Environment, University of California, San Francisco; San Francisco, CA*

Alan D. Woolf, MD, MPH; *Harvard Medical School; Boston, MA*

Robert O. Wright, MD, MPH; *Harvard Medical School; Boston, MA*

Chapter 1

Introduction

■ ■ ■ ■ ■ ■

Environmental hazards are among the top health concerns many parents have for their children.[1,2] Little time is spent during medical school and pediatric residency training on environmental hazards and their relationship to illness among children,[3-5] and many pediatricians report that they are not fully prepared or comfortable taking an environmental history or addressing parents' concerns about the environment in clinical practice.[6-9] General medical and pediatric textbooks devote scant attention to illness as a result of environmental factors. Information pertinent to pediatric environmental health is widely scattered in epidemiologic, toxicologic, and environmental health journals that may not regularly be read by pediatricians.[10]

Fifty-four years have passed since the American Academy of Pediatrics (AAP) formed its first committee on environmental health. In that time, substantial progress has been made in understanding the role of the environment in the illnesses of childhood and adolescence. Consideration of illnesses traditionally associated with the environment, such as waterborne and foodborne diseases, has expanded to include study of toxic chemicals and other environmental hazards that derive from the rapid expansion of industry and technology.[11]

This is the third edition of *Pediatric Environmental Health*, a book written by the AAP Council on Environmental Health and intended to be useful to practicing pediatricians and other clinicians. The first edition was published by the AAP in 1999; the second in 2003.[12,13] This book is organized into 7 sections. The first section gives background information. The second, third, and fourth sections focus on specific environments, food and water, and chemical and physical hazards. The fifth section addresses a variety of special topics. The sixth section provides information about public health aspects of environmental health, and the seventh section describes resources for pediatricians and others.

Most chapters on chemical and physical hazards are organized in sections that describe the pollutant, routes of exposure, systems affected, clinical effects, diagnostic methods, treatment, and prevention of exposure and include suggested responses to questions that pediatricians may have or that parents may ask. The Resources section refers readers to additional resources to be considered when further information is needed.

The AAP Council on Environmental Health recognizes that pediatric environmental health is a specialty field in the early stages of development. Knowledge in some areas has evolved rapidly, whereas in other areas, there may be more questions than answers. The council and the editors have attempted to make readers aware of the controversial areas and gaps in scientific information. The goal of this book is to provide clinicians with the most accurate information needed to prudently advise parents and children about specific pollutants and situations commonly encountered in 21st century life.

References

1. Stickler GB, Simmons PS. Pediatricians' preferences for anticipatory guidance topics compared with parental anxieties. *Clin Pediatr (Phila)*. 1995;34(7):384–387

2. US Environmental Protection Agency. *Public Knowledge and Perceptions of Chemical Risks in Six Communities: Analysis of a Baseline Survey*. Washington, DC: US Environmental Protection Agency; 1990. Publication No. EPA 230-01-90-074

3. Pope AM, Rall DP, eds. *Environmental Medicine: Integrating a Missing Element into Medical Education*. Washington, DC: National Academies Press; 1995

4. Roberts JR, Gitterman BA. Pediatric environmental health education: a survey of US pediatric residency programs. *Ambul Pediatr*. 2003;3(1):57–59

5. Roberts JR, Balk SJ, Forman J, Shannon M. Teaching about pediatric environmental health. *Acad Pediatr*. 2009;9(2):129–30

6. Kilpatrick N, Frumkin H, Trowbridge J, et al. The environmental history in pediatric practice: a study of pediatricians' attitudes, beliefs, and practices. *Environ Health Perspect*. 2002;110(8): 823–871

7. Trasande L, Schapiro ML, Falk R, et al. Pediatrician attitudes, clinical activities, and knowledge of environmental health in Wisconsin. *WMJ*. 2006;105(2):45-49

8. Trasande L, Boscarino J, Graber N, et al. The environment in pediatric practice: a study of New York pediatricians' attitudes, beliefs, and practices towards children's environmental health. *J Urban Health*. 2006;83(4):760-772

9. Trasande L, Ziebold C, Schiff JS, Wallinga D, McGovern P, Oberg CN. The role of the environment in pediatric practice in Minnesota: attitudes, beliefs, and practices. *Minn Med*. 2008;91(9):36-39

10. Etzel RA. Introduction. In: *Environmental Health: Report of the 27th Ross Roundtable on Critical Approaches to Common Pediatric Problems*. Columbus, OH: Ross Products Division, Abbott Laboratories; 1996:1

11. Chance GW, Harmsen E. Children are different: environmental contaminants and children's health. *Can J Public Health*. 1998;89(Suppl 1):S9–S13

12. American Academy of Pediatrics, Committee on Environmental Health. *Handbook of Pediatric Environmental Health*. Etzel RA, Balk SJ, eds. Elk Grove Village, IL: American Academy of Pediatrics; 1999

13. American Academy of Pediatrics, Committee on Environmental Health. *Pediatric Environmental Health*. 2nd ed. Etzel RA, Balk SJ, eds. Elk Grove Village, IL: American Academy of Pediatrics; 2003

Chapter 2

History and Growth of Pediatric Environmental Health

■ ■ ■ ■ ■ ■

HISTORY OF PEDIATRIC ENVIRONMENTAL HEALTH
IN THE AMERICAN ACADEMY OF PEDIATRICS

In 1954, errant fallout from a nuclear weapons test on Bikini Island, an atoll of the Marshall Islands, caused the development of acute burns from beta radiation on neighboring islanders. Subsequently, 2 children exposed to fallout prior to 1 year of age developed severe hypothyroidism. Of 18 children exposed before 10 years of age, 14 developed thyroid neoplasia (13 benign and 1 malignant), and 1 developed leukemia.[1] At about the same time, fallout in southwestern Utah from weapons tests in Nevada apparently caused sickness in sheep, and people who were exposed worried about later effects. In 1956, expert committees of the National Academy of Sciences and the British Medical Research Council reported on the biological effects of ionizing radiation in humans. These reports led to a marked reduction in unnecessary exposures from the use of radiotherapy for benign disorders and from fluoroscopy. Therefore, in 1957, because of concerns about fallout from weapons testing and fears of nuclear war, the American Academy of Pediatrics (AAP), in keeping with its tradition of promoting research and advocacy for child health, established the Committee on Radiation Hazards and Congenital Malformations to develop policy on exposure of children to ionizing radiation. This was the forerunner of the current-day Council on Environmental Health.

In 1961, as the interests of the committee broadened, its name was changed to the Committee on Environmental Hazards. In 1966, an expert overview of the effects of radiation on children was organized by the Committee on Environmental Hazards—the Conference on the Pediatric Significance of Peacetime Radioactive Fallout.[2] The participants included pediatricians, radio-biologists, scientists from relevant government health agencies, and Dr Benjamin Spock, who spoke about the psychological effects of radioactive fallout in children.

The committee, recognizing that man-made chemicals were increasingly permeating the environment, organized the Conference on the Susceptibility of the Fetus and Child to Chemical Pollutants, held in 1973 in Brown's Lake, WI.[3] Fresh thinking was sought by bringing together scientists knowledgeable about the effects of chemicals on the environment but not about child health and pediatricians who knew about child health but had not given much thought to environmental effects. This meeting led to more interaction between pediatric experts and federal agencies concerned with the environment to discuss the possible effects of the environment on the health of children.

The Conference on Chemical and Radiation Hazards to Children, held in 1981 and chaired by Drs. Laurence Finberg and Robert W. Miller, was an expert consultation on the topic that enabled the exchange of concerns and information with the pediatric community[4] and led to further interactions between the committee and federal environmental health agencies. The Council on Pediatric Research called for including pediatricians in meetings of government agencies and on other committees that make policy or deliberate on environmental matters of national importance. To foster relations with other groups, the AAP Committee on Environmental Hazards, which met twice a year, held every other meeting at an organization concerned with environmental research, such as the US Environmental Protection Agency (EPA), the National Institute of Environmental Health Sciences (NIEHS), the Kettering Laboratories, and the National Institute of Child Health and Development.

In 1991, the name of the Committee on Environmental Hazards was changed to the Committee on Environmental Health to emphasize prevention. In 2009, the Committee was renamed the Council on Environmental Health, with responsibility for advising the Board of Directors on policy issues involving child health and the environment and also developing educational materials for pediatricians.

GROWTH OF PEDIATRIC ENVIRONMENTAL HEALTH IN THE UNITED STATES

Over the period of 1981 to 1993, academic and health organizations became more interested in studying the impact of the environment on infant and child health. In 1992, a special interest group on pediatric environmental health was organized in the Ambulatory Pediatric Association, reflecting growing interest in this topic among academic pediatricians. In 1993, the publication of a report by the National Academy of Sciences, titled *Pesticides in the Diets of Infants and Children*,[5] was instrumental in highlighting environmental hazards unique to children and the relative paucity of information relating environmental exposures and child health outcomes. In October 1995, EPA Administrator Carol Browner directed the agency to formulate a new national policy requiring, for the first time, that the health risks to children and infants from environmental hazards be considered when conducting environmental risk assessments.[6]

In 1996, the Food Quality Protection Act became law. One requirement of this act was that the EPA use an additional safety factor in risk assessments when risks for children are uncertain.

On April 21, 1997, President Clinton issued Executive Order 13045, Protection of Children from Environmental Health Risks and Safety Risks, which directed agencies to ensure that policies, programs, activities, and standards address disproportionate risks to children that result from environmental health risks or safety risks. In 1997, the EPA established the Office of Children's Health Protection to make the protection of children's health a fundamental goal of public health and environmental protection in the United States. A task force, cochaired by the secretary of the US Department of Health and Human Services and the administrator of the EPA, was established to recommend federal environmental health and safety policies, priorities, and activities to protect children.

Since 1998, many Centers for Children's Environmental Health and Disease Prevention Research have been funded by the EPA and NIEHS. Combining research and outreach, these Centers form a national network to address a range of childhood diseases and outcomes that may result from environmental exposures, including impairments in overall growth and development, impairments in nervous system development, and respiratory dysfunction. Center investigators work closely with communities, health care providers, researchers, and government officials to conduct research with the goal of preventing and reducing childhood diseases in these areas.

Pediatric Environmental Health Specialty Units, established in 1998 and funded by the Agency for Toxic Substances and Disease Registry (ATSDR) and the EPA through the Association of Occupational and Environmental Clinics, have increased awareness and knowledge of health care providers and health agency officials about pediatric environmental health. They are an important resource for information about children's environmental health issues and for assistance in clinical evaluations such as guidance on the utility of biological or environmental testing or interpreting test results.

The first edition of the AAP *Handbook of Pediatric Environmental Health* was published in October 1999.[7] It was distributed to more than 27 000 pediatricians and pediatric residents and was widely used in the United States and other countries to teach about the health effects to children of exposures to contaminants in the environment.

In 2000, the Committee on Environmental Health initiated the first in a series of 4 annual workshops on pediatric environmental health for incoming pediatric chief residents held at the annual meeting of the Pediatric Academic Societies. This effort was funded by the Office of Children's Health Protection at the EPA. That year, the AAP also launched the Environmental Health Nexus, an AAP section open to pediatricians with an interest in environmental health that designed and planned educational programming for the AAP. The Nexus was incorporated into the Council on Environmental Health in 2009. In many state AAP chapters, committees on environmental health developed educational activities and programming for chapter meetings.

In March 2001, the Committee on Environmental Health held a workshop, with funding from the ATSDR, to bring together pediatricians from each chapter of the AAP with experts in pediatric environmental health from the regional offices of federal agencies (including the ATSDR and EPA). The proceedings of this conference were published in a special supplement to *Pediatrics*.[8] In 2002, through the Ambulatory Pediatric Association (later renamed the Academic Pediatric Association), the first formal fellowship training programs in pediatric environmental health were initiated. These 3-year training programs are designed to provide pediatricians with specific competencies[9] to enable them to undertake environmental health research, teaching, and advocacy. Fellowship training in pediatric environmental health[10] is available in Boston, New York, Cincinnati, Pittsburgh, Vancouver, San Francisco, and Seattle.

The second edition of *Pediatric Environmental Health* was published in October 2003.[11] It was distributed to more than 24 000 pediatricians and pediatric residents in the United States and abroad. The first textbook to focus on environmental threats to child health also was published in 2003.[12]

In 2000, the US Congress authorized the planning and implementation of a National Children's Study. This study is led by a consortium of federal partners, including the US Department of Health and Human Services (including the *Eunice Kennedy Shriver* National Institute of Child Health and Human Development, the NIEHS, Centers for Disease Control and Prevention), EPA, and US Department of Education.[13]

The National Children's Study is designed to examine the effects of environmental influences on the health and development of more than 100 000 children across the United States, following them from before birth until 21 years of age. The goal of the study is to improve the health and well-being of children. Researchers will analyze how environmental exposures, genetic influences, and psychosocial experiences interact with each other and what helpful and/or harmful effects they might have on children's health. By studying children across phases of growth and development, researchers will be better able to understand the role of these factors on health and disease.

The seven initial National Children's Study research sites, known as Vanguard Centers, began recruitment of families into the National Children's Study in 2009.[14] Eventually, the study is expected to have approximately 40 study centers recruiting volunteers from the planned 105 study locations throughout the United States.

GROWTH OF INTERNATIONAL PEDIATRIC ENVIRONMENTAL HEALTH

In 1999, the World Health Organization (WHO) set up a Task Force for the Protection of Children's Environmental Health. Its objectives were to prevent disease and disability associated with chemical and physical threats to children, taking into consideration biological risks in the environment and acknowledging the importance of social and psychosocial factors. The Task Force promoted the development of training materials about children's health and the environment and advocated for environmental policies to protect children.[15,16]

In 2002, the 1st WHO International Conference on Environmental Threats to the Health of Children: Hazards and Vulnerability was held in Bangkok, Thailand. The conference focused on science-oriented issues, research needs, and capacity building while addressing the concrete needs for action and policies at the community, country, regional, and international levels. The major outcome of this conference was the Bangkok Statement, which set priorities for action and a commitment to national and international activities in the area of children's health and the environment.[17] In 2005, the WHO published a book titled *Children's Health and the Environment: A Global Perspective*.[18] The 2nd WHO International Conference on Children's Environmental Health, Healthy Environments Healthy Children: Increasing Knowledge and Taking Action, was held in Buenos Aires, Argentina in November 2005. This conference responded to calls for action concerning children's health and the environment that were made by the preceding Health and Environment Ministerial of the Americas (June 2005) and the Summit of the Americas (November 2005). In June 2009, the 3rd WHO International Conference on Children's Health and the Environment, From Research to Policy and Action, was held in Busan, Republic of Korea. Table 2.1 lists international conventions and resolutions related to children's health and the environment.

In 2007, the International Pediatric Association, in collaboration with the WHO, launched the International Pediatric Environmental Health Leadership Institute, with funding from the EPA Office of Children's Health Protection. As part of this Institute, training courses on children's health and the environment were held in Nairobi, Kenya; New Delhi, India; and Port au Prince, Haiti.[19] The training used the WHO Training Package for Health Care Providers,

Table 2.1: Conventions and Resolutions Relating to Children's Health and the Environment	
1989	**UN Convention on the Rights of the Child** http://www.unicef.org/crc
1990	**Declaration on the Survival, Protection and Development of Children** (World Summit for Children) www.unicef.org/wsc/declare.htm
1992	**Agenda 21, Chapter 25** (United Nations Conference on Environment and Development) www.un.org/esa/sustdev/documents/agenda21/index.htm
1997	**Declaration of the Environment Leaders of the Eight on Children's Environmental Health** http://www.g7.utoronto.ca/environment/1997miami/children.html
1999	**Declaration of the Third European Ministerial Conference on Environment and Health** www.euro.who.int/document/e69046.pdf
2001	**UN Millennium Development Goals** www.who.int/mdg
2002	**United Nations General Assembly Special Session on Children** www.unicef.org/specialsession **The Bangkok Statement (WHO International Conference)** www.who.int/docstore/peh/ceh/Bangkok/bangkstatement.htm **World Summit on Sustainable Development:** Launch of the Healthy Environments for Children Alliance and the Global Initiative of Children's Environmental Health Indicators www.who.int/heca/en www.who.int/ceh/publications/924159188_9/en/index.html
2003	**IFCS Forum IV Recommendations on Children and Chemicals** www.who.int/ifcs/en
2004	**Fourth Ministerial Conference on Environment and Health (Europe):** Adoption of the Children's Environment and Health Action Plan for Europe (CEHAPE) http://www.euro.who.int/__data/assets/pdf_file/0006/78639/E83338.pdf

Table 2.1: Conventions and Resolutions Relating to Children's Health and the Environment, *continued*	
2005	**International Conference on Children's Environmental Health: The Buenos Aires Commitment** www.who.int/ceh/news/pastevents/buenosairesdecleng/en/index.html
2006	**Strategic Approach to International Chemicals Management (SAICM)** www.saicm.org
2007	**Declaration of the Commemorative High-Level Plenary Meeting Devoted to the Follow-up to the Outcome of the Special Session on Children** www.un.org/ga/62/plenary/children/highlevel.shtml
2009	**G8 Environmental Ministers' Meeting in Siracusa, Italy, April, 2009** http://www.g8ambiente.it/?costante_pagina=programma&id_lingua=3 **3rd WHO International Conference on Children's Health and the Environment: Busan, Republic of Korea, June, 2009** www.who.int/ceh/3rd conference/en/index.html

a set of modules covering the major environmental issues for children.[20] The trainees were expected to complete a community project, give a presentation at their home hospital, and document children's environmental diseases using a "green sheet" in the medical record. Those who did so were eligible to take an examination for special certification. The first qualifying examination in pediatric environmental health was held in Athens, Greece, in August 2007 and the second in Johannesburg, South Africa in 2010.

These and other activities should further enhance pediatricians' understanding of the effects of environmental hazards on children's health throughout the world.

References

1. Merke DP, Miller RW. Age differences in the effects of ionizing radiation. In: Guzelian PS, Henry CJ, Olin SS, eds. *Similarities and Differences Between Children and Adults: Implications for Risk Assessment.* Washington, DC: International Life Sciences Institute; 1992:139–149
2. American Academy of Pediatrics, Committee on Environmental Hazards. Conference on the Pediatric Significance of Peacetime Radioactive Fallout. *Pediatrics.* 1968;41(1):165–378
3. American Academy of Pediatrics, Committee on Environmental Hazards. The susceptibility of the fetus and child to chemical pollutants (special issue). *Pediatrics.* 1974;53(5 Spec Issue):777–862

4. Finberg L. *Chemical and Radiation Hazards to Children: Report of the Eighty-fourth Ross Conference on Pediatric Research.* Columbus, OH: Ross Laboratories; 1982

5. National Research Council. *Pesticides in the Diets of Infants and Children.* Washington, DC: National Academies Press; 1993

6. US Environmental Protection Agency. *Environmental Health Threats to Children.* Washington, DC: US Environmental Protection Agency; 1996. Publication No. EPA 175-F-96-001

7. American Academy of Pediatrics, Committee on Environmental Health. *Handbook of Pediatric Environmental Health.* Etzel RA, Balk SJ, eds. Elk Grove Village, IL: American Academy of Pediatrics; 1999

8. Balk SJ, ed. A partnership to establish an environmental safety net for children. *Pediatrics.* 2003;112(Suppl):209–264

9. Etzel RA, Crain EF, Gitterman BA, Oberg C, Scheidt P, Landrigan PJ. Pediatric environmental health competencies for specialists. *Ambul Pediatr.* 2003;3(1):60–63

10. Landrigan PJ, Woolf AD, Gitterman B, et al. The Ambulatory Pediatric Association fellowship in pediatric environmental health: a 5-year assessment. *Environ Health Perspect.* 2007;115(10):1383-1387

11. American Academy of Pediatrics, Committee on Environmental Health. *Pediatric Environmental Health.* 2nd ed. Etzel RA, Balk SJ, eds. Elk Grove Village, IL: American Academy of Pediatrics; 2003

12. Wigle DT. *Child Health and the Environment.* New York, NY: Oxford; 2003

13. Branum AM, Collman GW, Correa A, et al. The National Children's Study of environmental effects on child health and development. *Environ Health Perspect.* 2003;111(4):642-646

14. Scheidt P, Dellarco M, Dearry A. A major milestone for the National Children's Study. *Environ Health Perspect.* 2009;117(1):A13

15. European Environment Agency. *Children's Health and Environment: A Review of Evidence. A Joint Report From the European Environment Agency and the WHO Regional Office for Europe.* Echternach, Luxembourg: Luxembourg Office for Official Publications of the European Communities; 2002. Environmental Issue Report No. 29

16. United Nations Environment Programme, United Nations Children's Fund, World Health Organization. *Children in the New Millenium: Environmental Impact on Health.* Nairobi, Kenya: United Nations Environment Programme; New York, NY: United Nations Children's Fund; and Geneva, Switzerland: World Health Organization; 2002

17. The Bangkok Statement. A Pledge to Promote the Protection of Children's Environmental Health. International Conference on Environmental Threats to the Health of Children: Hazards and Vulnerability, Bangkok, Thailand, 3-7 March 2002. Available at: http://ehp.niehs.nih.gov/bangkok/. Accessed August 2, 2010

18. World Health Organization. *Children's Health and the Environment: A Global Perspective. A Resource Manual for the Health Sector.* Pronczuk-Garbino J, ed. Geneva, Switzerland: World Health Organization; 2005

19. International Pediatric Association. Available at: http://www.ipa-world.org/Program_Areas/Children_Environmental_Health/Pages/Internationalhealth.aspx. Accessed August 2, 2010

20. World Health Organization. Training Package for Health Care Providers. Available at: http://www.ipa-world.org/Program_Areas/Children_Environmental_Health/Pages/TrainingPackageHealthCareProviders.aspx. Accessed August 2, 2010

Chapter 3

Children's Unique Vulnerabilities to Environmental Hazards

■ ■ ■ ■ ■ ■

This chapter discusses the scientific basis for children's unique vulnerabilities to environmental hazards. It describes differences between adults and children and among children in different life stages, in physical, biological, and social environments. It explains why children should not be treated as "little adults." Six developmental stages are considered: fetus (although there are multiple stages of fetal development), newborn (birth–2 months of age), infant/toddler (2 months–2 years of age), preschool child (2–6 years of age), school-aged child (6–12 years of age), and adolescent (12–18 years of age).

CRITICAL WINDOWS OF VULNERABILITY

The developing fetus and child are uniquely susceptible to toxicities of certain drugs and environmental toxicants (a "toxicant" refers to a chemical agent; "toxin" is appropriately used for a biological agent). Extensive epidemiologic evidence supports a causal relationship between prenatal and early childhood exposure to environmental toxicants with a variety of resulting health effects on the fetus and child.[1] Well-known adverse outcomes for the developing fetus attributable to transplacental exposure include the effects of thalidomide on limb development, ethanol on brain development, and diethylstilbestrol on the reproductive system. The neurotoxic effects of lead have been demonstrated repeatedly with prenatal exposure as well as during early childhood.[2] Fetal and childhood development occur rapidly and may be easily deranged. The timing of exposures with regard to developmental outcome is an important concept. In embryonic or fetal stages, some narrow "critical windows of exposure"—highly susceptible periods of organogenesis—have been defined.[3] In contrast, there are very few actual "critical windows" known in childhood. Because data are lacking, there is significant uncertainty about many of the effects of environmental toxicants on children. This area is the subject of intense investigation. Some of the work on "critical windows" was published in a supplement to *Environmental Health Perspectives* (http://ehpnet1.niehs.nih.gov/docs/2000/suppl-3/toc.html).

HUMAN ENVIRONMENTS

A child's environment can be divided into physical and social components. Both components interact with each individual's unique biology to influence that individual's health. The manner in which a child's body absorbs, distributes, and metabolizes environmental toxicants not only is determined by that child's genetic code but also is heavily affected by developmental stage. The physical environment consists of anything that comes in contact with the body. Air, for example, which is in constant contact with lungs and skin, is a large part of the physical environment. To define the physical environment more precisely, it may be necessary to divide a large environment (a "macro" environment) into smaller units ("micro" environments). For example, the macro environment may be Detroit; a micro environment may be the floor of the kitchen of a house in Detroit. Micro environments can differ enormously between adults and children. For example, in a room in which the air is contaminated with mercury, the mercury vapor may not be evenly dispersed—air near the floor may have a higher concentration of mercury than air near the ceiling.[4] The environment of an infant lying on the floor, therefore, would be different from that of a standing adult. The social environment includes the day-to-day circumstances of living as well as regulations that may affect day-to-day living.

EXPOSURE: THE PHYSICAL ENVIRONMENT

A child's exposure is the sum of the exposures in several environments during the course of a day, including the home, school, child care setting, and play areas. Estimates of exposure often are made retrospectively, because it is difficult to study the activities and exposures of young children. Even if the total amount of exposure to a toxicant is the same for 2 children, different patterns of exposure may have different health effects. For example, ingestion of nitrates in well water may cause hemoglobin to become reduced to methemoglobin.[5] However, if the nitrates are ingested at a slow enough rate for enzymes to oxidize the methemoglobin back to hemoglobin, no deleterious health effects occur. This is an example of a threshold effect; the health problem will not occur until the toxicant reaches a particular level in the body.

EXPOSURE FROM CONCEPTION TO ADOLESCENCE

In most instances, fetal exposures come from the pregnant woman. Preterm infants who spend months in the neonatal intensive care unit have very different exposures compared with healthy full-term infants (exposure to noise, light, compressed gases, intravenous solutions, plasticizers, diagnostic radiation, etc).[6,7] Exposures of newborns, infants, toddlers, preschool children, school-aged children, and adolescents differ with changes in physical location, breathing zones, oxygen consumption, types of foods consumed, amount of food consumed, and normal behavioral development.[8,9]

PHYSICAL LOCATION

Physical location changes with development. Newborn exposures usually are similar to those experienced by the mother. A newborn, however, frequently spends prolonged periods in a single environment, such as a crib. Because infants and toddlers often are placed on the floor, carpet, or grass, they have greater exposures to chemicals associated with these surfaces, such as pesticide residues. Biomonitoring data often demonstrate greater body burdens of chemicals in young children. For example, residues of metabolites of the pesticide chlorpyrifos were nearly twice as high in the 6- to 11-year-old group as in adults.[10] In addition, infants who are unable to walk or crawl may experience sustained exposure to some agents, because they cannot remove themselves from their environment (eg, prolonged exposure to the sun). Preschool-aged children may spend part of their day in child care settings with varied environments, including some time outdoors. School-aged children may be exposed to toxicants when schools are built near highways (resulting in exposure to motor vehicle emissions). Adolescents have a school environment and also are beginning to select other physical environments, often misjudging or ignoring risks. For example, listening to loud music may result in permanent hearing loss. Adolescents may work part-time in hazardous physical environments.[11,12] Children may participate in after-school sports that often occur outdoors in the mid to late afternoon, when levels of ozone peak.[13] This situation poses an increased risk to children with asthma.

BREATHING ZONES

The breathing zone for an adult is typically 4 to 6 ft above the floor. For a child, it is closer to the floor, depending on the height and mobility of the child. Within lower breathing zones, chemicals heavier than air, such as mercury, may concentrate.[14] Chemicals vaporizing from carpet or flooring will also have higher concentrations near the floor.

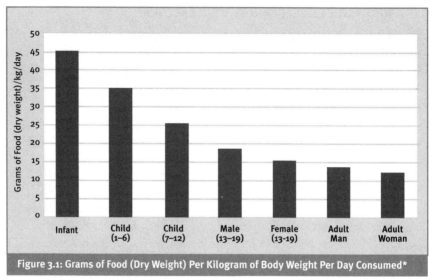

Figure 3.1: Grams of Food (Dry Weight) Per Kilogram of Body Weight Per Day Consumed*

*From Plunkett LM, Turnbull D. Rodricks JV[16]

OXYGEN CONSUMPTION

Children are smaller than adults, and their metabolic rates are higher relative to their size. Thus, children consume more oxygen than adults and produce more carbon dioxide (CO_2) per kg of body weight. This increased CO_2 production requires higher minute ventilation. Minute ventilation for a newborn and adult are approximately 400 mL/min per kg and 150 mL/min per kg, respectively.[15,16] Thus, a child's dose of air pollutants is greater than that of an adult when adjusted for body mass.

QUANTITY AND QUALITY OF FOOD CONSUMED

The amount of food that children consume per kg of body weight is higher than that of adults, not only because children need more calories to maintain homeostasis than adults do, but also because children are growing. Fig 3.1 shows grams of food consumed daily per kilogram of body weight. The difference is threefold between a child younger than 1 year and an adult. Unfortunately, data do not exist for further subdivisions of children (eg, a newborn vs a 6-month-old infant).

In addition, children consume different types of food, and the diversity of the foods they eat is much smaller than it is for adults. The diet of newborn infants is generally limited to human milk or infant formula. The diet of a typical child contains more milk products and certain fruits and vegetables compared with a typical adult diet.[16] Fig 3.2 shows differences in consumption of apples, beef, and potatoes for different age groups.

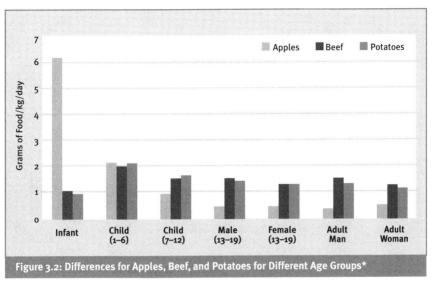

Figure 3.2: Differences for Apples, Beef, and Potatoes for Different Age Groups*

*From Plunkett LM, Turnbull D. Rodricks JV[16]

WATER

An average newborn consumes 6 oz (180 mL/kg/day) of human milk or formula per kg of body weight (for an average male adult, this is equivalent to drinking 35 twelve-oz cans of a beverage per day). If a newborn drinks reconstituted formula and the water used to reconstitute the formula comes from a single tap water source, the newborn may be exposed to any contaminants in the water. Differences in water consumption for different age groups are shown in Fig 3.3. If the water or liquid contains a contaminant, children may receive more of it relative to their size compared with adults.[16]

LARGER RATIO OF SURFACE AREA TO BODY MASS

A newborn's surface area-to-body mass ratio is 3 times larger than an adult's; a child's surface area-to-body mass ratio is 2 times larger than an adult's. Thus, children absorb more, kg for kg, than do adults.[9,16]

NORMAL BEHAVIORAL DEVELOPMENT

Infants and young children pass through a developmental stage of intense oral exploratory behavior. This normal oral exploration may place children at risk, such as in environments with high levels of lead dust. Wood used in some playground equipment is treated with arsenic (as chromated copper arsenate [CCA]; see Chapter 22) and creosote, potentially exposing children when they place their mouths directly on these materials or when they place their hands in their mouths after playing on these materials. Additionally, children often lack the experience or cognitive ability to recognize hazardous situations.

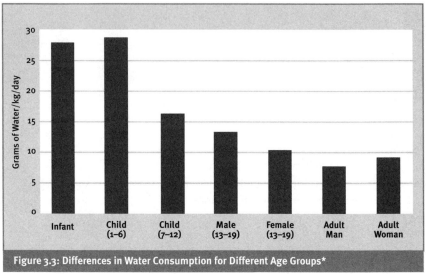

Figure 3.3: Differences in Water Consumption for Different Age Groups*

*From Plunkett LM, Turnbull D. Rodricks JV[16]
Note: The citation of grams of water consumed per kilogram per day in this table is considerably underestimated because water consumed as breast milk was not included in the analysis. Thus for total water consumption per kilogram per day, the values in the text are accurate.

Ambulatory children may be exposed to excessive ultraviolet radiation from sunlight, because they may not recognize the hazard. Adolescents, as they gain freedom from parental authority, may be less protected from some exposures. Although adolescents are at a stage of development at which physical strength and stamina are at a peak, they are still acquiring abstract reasoning skills and often fail to consider cause and effect, particularly delayed effects. Thus, adolescents may place themselves in situations with greater risk than would adults.

ABSORPTION, DISTRIBUTION, METABOLISM, AND TARGET ORGAN SUSCEPTIBILITY: THE BIOLOGICAL ENVIRONMENT

Absorption

Absorption generally occurs by 1 of 4 routes: transplacental, percutaneous, respiratory, and gastrointestinal. Absorption also may occur via the intravenous route. Absorption through mucosal surfaces, including through the eye, also may occur.

Transplacental

Many toxicants readily cross the placenta. These include compounds with low molecular weight, such as carbon monoxide; those that are fat soluble; and specific elements, such as calcium and lead. Because carbon monoxide has a higher affinity for fetal hemoglobin than for adult hemoglobin, the concentration of carboxyhemoglobin is higher in the fetus than in the pregnant woman.[17,18] Therefore, the infant may have a reduced level of oxygen delivered to tissues. Lipophilic compounds, such as polycyclic aromatic hydrocarbons (found in cigarette smoke), methylmercury, and ethanol, also readily gain access to the fetal circulation; levels of methylmercury are higher in the fetus than in the mother.[19]

Percutaneous

The skin undergoes enormous changes during development, resulting in changes in absorptive and other properties. Pathways of absorption through the skin are particularly important for fat-soluble compounds. Chemicals such as nicotine and cotinine have been described in amniotic fluid,[20,21] but absorption through the fetal skin has not been studied. The skin of a fetus lacks the exterior dead keratin layer, one of the major barriers of fully developed skin. The acquisition of keratin occurs over 3 to 5 days following birth. Therefore, a newborn's skin remains particularly absorptive up to about 2 to 3 weeks of life.[22] Epidemics involving absorption of chemicals through the skin in newborns include hypothyroidism from iodine in Betadine scrub solutions,[23] neurotoxicity from hexachlorophene,[24] and hyperbilirubinemia from a phenolic disinfectant used to clean hospital equipment.[25] The absorptive and other properties of children's skin may differ from those of adult skin until at least 2 years of age.[26,27] An additional factor with regard to absorption is the larger surface area-to-body mass ratio of newborns and infants compared with older children and adults.

Respiratory

Lung development proceeds through proliferation of pulmonary alveoli and capillaries until 5 to 8 years of age. Thereafter, the lungs grow through alveolar expansion.[28] Lung function continues to increase through adolescence and is vulnerable to exposure to air pollutants. Exposure to hazardous air pollutants at currently observed concentrations has been associated with statistically significant deficits in forced expiratory volume in 1 second (FEV_1) attained at 18 years of age.[29]

Gastrointestinal

The gastrointestinal tract undergoes numerous changes during development. Certain pesticides as well as chemicals from tobacco smoke are present in amniotic fluid,[21] but it is not known whether the fetus, which actively swallows amniotic fluid, absorbs them. Following birth, stomach acid secretion is relatively low, but adult levels are achieved by several months of age, markedly affecting absorption of chemicals from the stomach. If acidity levels are too low, bacterial overgrowth in the small bowel and stomach may result in the formation of chemicals that can be absorbed. For example, several cases of methemoglobin-emia in infants in Iowa were traced to well water contaminated with nitrate that was converted to nitrite by intestinal bacteria.[5]

The small intestine transports certain chemicals to the blood and may respond to increased nutritional needs by increasing absorption of that particular nutrient. For example, the intestines of infants and children absorb more calcium from food sources compared to adults. Lead, which may be absorbed in place of calcium, also may be absorbed to a greater extent: an adult absorbs 5% to 10% of ingested lead, whereas a 1- to 2-year-old can absorb up to 50%.[30]

Distribution

The distribution of chemicals varies with body composition, such as fat and water content, which vary with developmental stage. For example, animal models show that lead is retained to a larger degree in the infant animal brain than in the adult animal brain.[31] Lead also may accumulate more rapidly in children's bones.[32]

Metabolism

Metabolism of a chemical may result in its activation or deactivation.[33] The activity in each step of these metabolic pathways is determined by the child's developmental stage and genetic susceptibility. Therefore, some children are genetically more susceptible to adverse effects from certain exposures. For example, children (and adults) with glucose-6-phosphate dehydrogenase (G6PD) deficiency are at risk of hemolytic anemia if exposed to chemicals such as naph-thalene. Large differences also exist in the activity of enzymes at various develop-mental stages. The same enzyme may be more or less active depending on the age of the child. Two examples are the enzymes involved in the P450 cytochrome family, which metabolize such xenobiotics as theophylline and caffeine,[34] and alcohol dehydrogenase, which converts ethanol to acetaldehyde.[35]

The differences between metabolism in children and adults may harm or protect children from environmental hazards or drugs. Such is the case for acetaminophen. In the adult, high levels of acetaminophen are metabolized to products that may cause hepatic failure. Infants born to women with high blood acetaminophen levels have similar acetaminophen levels but do not sustain liver damage, because their metabolic pathways have not yet developed enough to break down acetaminophen into harmful metabolites.[36-40]

Target Organ Susceptibility

During growth and maturation, children's organs may be affected by exposure to harmful chemicals.[40] Following cellular proliferation, individual cells undergo 2 further processes to become adult cells: differentiation and migration. Differentiation occurs when cells take on specific tasks within the body.

The trigger for differentiation may be hormonal, so chemicals that mimic hormones may alter the differentiation of some tissues. Because children's organ systems, including the reproductive system, continue to differentiate, chemicals that mimic hormones may have effects on the development of those organ systems. For example, a growing body of evidence documents such endocrine-disrupting effects from phthalate exposure in animals and humans.[41]

Cell migration is necessary for certain cells to reach their destination. Neurons, for example, originate in a structure near the center of the brain and then migrate to predestined locations in one of the many layers of the brain. Chemicals may have a profound effect on this process (eg, ethanol exposure resulting in fetal alcohol syndrome).

Synaptogenesis occurs rapidly during the first 2 years.[42] Waves of synapses are formed as learning continues to occur throughout life. Dendritic trimming is the active removal of synapses. A 2-year-old's brain contains more synapses than at any other age. These synapses are trimmed back to allow more specificity of the resulting neural network. Data suggest that low-dose lead may interfere with this synapse trimming.[43]

Some organs continue developing for several years, increasing the vulnerability of these organs. For example, brain tumors frequently are treated by radiation therapy in adults with uncomfortable but reversible adverse effects. However, in infants, radiation therapy generally is avoided because of the profound and permanent effects on the developing central nervous system. Similarly, lead and mercury affect the brain and nervous system of children. The brain attains four fifths of its adult size by the end of the second year of life.[44] By adolescence, there are no gross changes in brain morphology.[44] However, electroencephalographic and other studies demonstrate continued neurodevelopmental maturation.[44] Magnetic resonance imaging data confirm that the brain changes until the late teens and early 20s, with higher-order association cortices maturing after lower-order somatosensory and visual cortices.[45]

Exposure to secondhand smoke compromises lung development. The rate of growth of lung function in children exposed to secondhand smoke is slower than that of nonexposed children. FEV_1 values of children exposed to secondhand smoke are measurably lower than those of children without exposure.[46] Adolescents' increased susceptibility to tobacco dependence (Chapter 40) illustrates an example of the "critical windows" concept. Studies suggest that the adolescent central nervous system is more vulnerable to nicotine dependence compared with that of adults. Adolescents may become dependent easily, often before the onset of daily smoking.[47,48]

Tissues undergoing growth and differentiation are particularly susceptible to cancer because of the shortened period for DNA repair and the changes occurring within the DNA during cell growth. The epidemic of scrotal cancer among adolescent chimney sweeps of Victorian England illustrates the likelihood that the scrotum at this developmental stage has increased susceptibility to the chemicals in soot.[49] Although occupational exposure at that time to cancer-causing chemicals such as soot was common in many occupations, scrotal tumors were uncommon except in young male chimney sweeps. Children and adolescents are more susceptible to the effects of ionizing radiation, as was demonstrated by the effects of the 1986 meltdown of the nuclear reactor in Chernobyl, Ukraine. This event resulted in heavy contamination of the area with plutonium, cesium, and radioactive iodine; almost 17 million people were exposed to excess radiation. Four years after exposure, a large excess of cases of thyroid cancers in adolescents and in children began to emerge, underscoring the special vulnerability at young ages to the effects of radioactive iodine.[50]

REGULATIONS AND LAWS: THE SOCIAL ENVIRONMENT

Regulatory policies usually do not take into account the unique combinations of developmental characteristics, physical environment, and biological environment that place children at risk. Most laws and regulations are based on studies using adult men weighing an average of 70 kg and, hence, are intended to protect adult men. However, advances have been made to change regulations to protect children. For example, the Food Quality Protection Act of 1996 stated that pesticide "tolerances" (the amount of pesticide legally allowed to be left in or on a harvested crop) must be set to protect the health of infants and children. In the United States, rules eliminating cigarette vending machines made cigarettes less available to children as compared with countries where these machines are ubiquitous, allowing unfettered access by children. A ban on flavored cigarettes in the United States that took effect in September 2009 is another example of legislation specifically aimed at protecting children from exposure to environmental toxicants. The Consumer Product Safety Improvement Act of 2008 focused specifically on the unique vulnerabilities of children by applying special limitations on toxicants, such as lead, in products intended for children's use.

How can a clinician integrate information about children's developmental susceptibility into his or her daily practice? The roles of educator, investigator, and advocate are extremely important. The most important intervention is educating parents, children, and others about exposures. Prevention efforts have the most impact when developmentally appropriate. Parents, children, teachers, community leaders, and policy makers will benefit from additional education from clinicians about the unique vulnerabilities of children to environmental pollution. The role of the clinician as investigator also is important. Most diseases caused by environmental factors have been diagnosed by an alert clinician, and publication of case studies has enabled further description of these illnesses. Finally, clinicians must advocate for children. In addition to the day-to-day, office-based work advocating for the safety and health of individual patients, clinicians may also have opportunities to ensure that regulatory policies take into account children's unique vulnerabilities.

References

1. Wigle D, Arbuckle T, Turner M, et al. Epidemiologic evidence of relationships between reproductive and child health outcomes and environmental chemical contaminants. *J Toxicol Environ Health B Crit Rev.* 2008;11(5-6):373–517

2. Bellinger D. Teratogen update: lead and pregnancy. *Birth Defects Res A Clin Mol Teratol.* 2005;73(6):409–420

3. Selevan SG, Kimmel CA, Mendola P. Identifying critical windows of exposure for children's health. *Environ Health Perspect.* 2000;108(Suppl 3):451–455

4. Agocs MM, Etzel RA, Parrish RG, et al. Mercury exposure from interior latex paint. *N Engl J Med.* 1990;323(16):1096–1101

5. Lukens JN. Landmark perspective: the legacy of well-water methemoglobinemia. *JAMA.* 1987;257(20):2793–2795

6. Lai TT, Bearer CF. Iatrogenic environmental hazards in the neonatal intensive care unit. *Clin Perinatol.* 2008;35(1):163-181

7. Calafat A, Needham L, Silva M, Lambert G. Exposure to di-(2-ethylhexyl) phthalate among premature neonates in a neonatal intensive care unit. *Pediatrics.* 2004;113(5):e429-e434

8. Moya J, Bearer CF, Etzel RA. Children's behavior and physiology and how it affects exposure to environmental contaminants. *Pediatrics.* 2004;113(4 Suppl):996-1006

9. US Environmental Protection Agency. *Child-Specific Exposure Factors Handbook (Final Report) 2008.* Washington, DC: US Environmental Protection Agency; 2008. Publication No. EPA/600/R-06/096F

10. Centers for Disease Control and Prevention. *Fourth National Report on Human Exposure to Environmental Chemicals.* Atlanta, GA: Centers for Disease Control and Prevention; 2009. Available at: http://www.cdc.gov/exposurereport. Accessed February 16, 2011

11. Runyan CW, Schulman M, Dal Santo J, Bowling JM, Agans R, Ta M. Work-related hazards and workplace safety of US adolescents employed in the retail and service sectors. *Pediatrics.* 2007;119(3):526-534

12. Runyan CW, Dal Santo J, Schulman M, Lipscomb HJ, Harris TA. Work hazards and workplace safety violations experienced by adolescent construction workers. *Arch Pediatr Adolesc Med.* 2006;160(7):721-727

13. McConnell R, Berhane K, Gillialand F, et al. Asthma in exercising children exposed to ozone: a cohort study. *Lancet.* 2002;359(9304):386-391

14. Foote RS. Mercury vapor concentrations inside buildings. *Science.* 1972;177(48):513–514

15. Snodgrasss WR. Physiological and biochemical differences between children and adults as determinants of toxic response to environmental pollutants. In: Guzelian PS, Henry CJ, Olin SS, eds. *Similarities and Differences Between Children and Adults: Implications for Risk Assessment.* Washington, DC: ILSI Press; 1992:35–42

16. Plunkett LM, Turnbull D, Rodricks JV. Differences between adults and children affecting exposure assessment. In: Guzelian PS, Henry CJ, Olin SS, eds. *Similarities and Differences Between Children and Adults: Implications for Risk Assessment.* Washington, DC: ILSI Press; 1992:79–94

17. Longo LD, Hill EP. Carbon monoxide uptake and elimination in fetal and maternal sheep. *Am J Physiol.* 1977;232(3):H324–H330

18. Longo LD. Carbon monoxide in the pregnant mother and fetus and its exchange across the placenta. *Ann NY Acad Sci.* 1970;174(1):312–341

19. Sakamoto M, Murata K, Kubota M, Nakai K, Satoh H. Mercury and heavy metal profiles of maternal and umbilical cord RBCs in Japanese population. *Ecotoxicol Environ Saf.* 2010; 73(1):1-6

20. Jauniaux E, Gulbis B, Acharya G, Thiry P, Rodeck C. Maternal tobacco exposure and cotinine levels in fetal fluids in the first half of pregnancy. *Obstet Gynecol.* 1999;93(1):25-29

21. VanVunakis H, Langone JJ, Milunsky A. Nicotine and cotinine in the amniotic fluid of smokers in the second trimester of pregnancy. *Am J Obstet Gynecol.* 1974;120(1):64–66

22. Holbrook KA. Structure and biochemical organogenesis of skin and cutaneous appendages in the fetus and newborn. In: Polin RA, Fox WW, eds. *Fetal and Neonatal Physiology.* Philadelphia, PA: WB Saunders; 1998:729–752

23. Clemens PC, Neumann RS. The Wolff-Chaikoff effect: hypothyroidism due to iodine application. *Arch Dermatol.* 1989;125(5):705

24. Shuman RM, Leech RW, Alvord EC Jr. Neurotoxicity of hexachlorophene in the human: I. A clinicopathologic study of 248 children. *Pediatrics.* 1974;54(6):689–695

25. Wysowski DK, Flynt JW Jr, Goldfield M, Altman R, Davis AT. Epidemic neonatal hyperbilirubinemia and use of a phenolic disinfectant detergent. *Pediatrics.* 1978;61(2):165–170

26. Nikolovski J, Stamatas G, Kollias N, Wiegand B. Barrier function and water-holding and transport properties of infant stratum corneum are different from adult and continue to develop through the first year of life. *J Invest Dermatol.* 2008;128(7):1728–1736

27. Giusti F, Martella A, Bertoni L, Seidenari S. Skin barrier, hydration, ph of skin of infants under two years of age. *Pediatr Dermatol.* 2001;18(2):93–96

28. Dietert RR, Etzel RA, Chen D, et al. Workshop to identify critical windows of exposure for children's health: immune and respiratory systems work group summary. *Environ Health Perspect.* 2000;108(Suppl 3):483–490

29. Gauderman W, Avol E, Gilliland F, et al. The effect of air pollution on lung development from 10 to 18 years of age. *N Engl J Med.* 2004;351(11):1057-1067

30. US Environmental Protection Agency. *Review of the National Ambient Air Quality Standards for Lead: Exposure Analysis Methodology and Validation.* Washington, DC: Air Quality Management Division, Office of Air Quality Planning and Standards, US Environmental Protection Agency; 1989

31. Momcilovic B, Kostial K. Kinetics of lead retention and distribution in suckling and adult rats. *Environ Res.* 1974;8(2):214–220

32. Barry PS. A comparison of concentrations of lead in human tissues. *Br J Ind Med.* 1975;32: 119–139

33. Faustman EM, Silbernagel SM, Fenske RA, Burbacher TM, Ponce RA. Mechanisms underlying children's susceptibility to environmental toxicants. *Environ Health Perspect.* 2000;108(Suppl 1):13–21

34. Nebert DW, Gonzalez FJ. P450 genes: structure, evolution, and regulation. *Annu Rev Biochem.* 1987;56:945–993

35. Card SE, Tompkins SF, Brien JF. Ontogeny of the activity of alcohol dehydrogenase and aldehyde dehydrogenases in the liver and placenta of the guinea pig. *Biochem Pharmacol.* 1989;38(15):2535–2541

36. Byer AJ, Traylor TR, Semmer JR. Acetaminophen overdose in the third trimester of pregnancy. *JAMA.* 1982;247(22):3114–3115

37. Kurzel RB. Can acetaminophen excess result in maternal and fetal toxicity? *South Med J.* 1990;83(8):953–955

38. Rosevear SK, Hope PL. Favourable neonatal outcome following maternal paracetamol overdose and severe fetal distress. Case report. *Br J Obstet Gynaecol.* 1989;96(4):491–493

39. Stokes IM. Paracetamol overdose in the second trimester of pregnancy. Case report. *Br J Obstet Gynaecol.* 1984;91(3):286–288

40. World Health Organization. Environmental Health Criteria 237: *Principles for Evaluating Health Risks in Children Associated with Exposure to Chemicals.* Geneva, Switzerland: World Health Organization; 2006. Available at: http://www.who.int/ipcs/publications/ehc/ehc237.pdf. Accessed February 16, 2011

41. Swan S. Environmental phthalate exposure in relation to reproductive outcomes and other health endpoints in humans. *Environ Res.* 2008;108(2):177–184

42. Adams J, Barone S Jr, LaMantia A, et al. Workshop to identify critical windows of exposure for children's health: neurobehavioral work group summary. *Environ Health Perspect.* 2000;108(Suppl 3):535–544

43. Goldstein GW. Developmental neurobiology of lead toxicity. In: Needleman HL, ed. *Human Lead Exposure.* Boca Raton, FL: CRC Press; 1992:125–135

44. Behrman RE, Kleigman RM, Jenson HB. *Nelson Textbook of Pediatrics.* 18th ed. Philadelphia, PA: WB Saunders; 2007

45. Gogtay N, Giedd JN, Lusk L, et al. Dynamic mapping of human cortical development during childhood through early adulthood. *Proc Natl Acad Sci U S A.* 2004;101(21):8175–8179

46. Tager IB, Weiss ST, Munoz A, Rosner B, Speizer FE. Longitudinal study of the effects of maternal smoking on pulmonary function in children. *N Engl J Med.* 1983;309(12):699–703

47. DiFranza JR, Savageau JA, Rigotti NA, et al. Development of symptoms of tobacco dependence in youths: 30 month follow up data from the DANDY study. *Tob Control.* 2002;11(3):228-235

48. DiFranza JR, Rigotti NA, McNeill AD, et al. Initial symptoms of nicotine dependence in adolescents. Tob Control. 2000;9(3):313-319

49. Nethercott JR. Occupational skin disorders. In: LaDou J, ed. *Occupational Medicine.* Norwalk, CT: Appleton & Lange; 1990

50. American Academy of Pediatrics, Committee on Environmental Health. Radiation disasters and children. *Pediatrics.* 2003;111(6 Pt 1):1455-1466

Chapter 4

Individual Susceptibility To Environmental Toxicants

■ ■ ■ ■ ■ ■

There is substantial variation among individuals in the effects of a given dose of any environmental toxicant. That variation tends to take on the distribution of a bell-shaped curve. The location of a particular individual on the bell curve is not random; it is determined largely by the factors that constitute that individual's susceptibility. In recent years, the environmental health community has paid increasing attention to the causes of variation in susceptibility. A better understanding of this variation allows us to appreciate which patients may be at increased risk of a toxicant's ill effects and suggests mitigating factors (ie, potential treatments) that may lessen the burden of a given toxic exposure.

This chapter discusses the concepts essential to understanding variation in susceptibility to chemicals and explores 3 important realms: genetic, social, and nutritional variants that have been shown to specifically modify the relationship between environmental toxicant exposure and health outcomes. An individual's age and developmental stage also are important factors in determining susceptibility (see Chapter 3). Fetuses and young children are often, but not always, considered to be at increased risk of environmental hazards, compared with older children, adolescents, and adults.

Although these concepts apply to many environmental diseases, the chapter focuses on 2 widely studied and prototypical pediatric environmental health issues: asthma and lead poisoning.

CONCEPTS AND DEFINITIONS

Susceptibility is the condition of having one of 2 or more interacting causes (ie, risk factors) and, therefore, being either predisposed to, or at enhanced vulnerability to, the effects of another. Susceptibility results in variation in the effect of a given exposure within a population when the dose is held constant. Epidemiologists use the term "effect modification" to describe this phenomenon, and when statistically modeled, it is often referred to as "interaction." Physicians may be most familiar with the term "synergy," which is conceptually the same.

Effect modification is similar to the biological concepts of synergism and antagonism. For example, in patients with chronic infections (such as those with cystic fibrosis), a pathogen may be resistant to 2 individual antibiotics, but when exposed to the 2 antibiotics simultaneously, the pathogen is effectively treated. Together, the effect of the 2 antibiotics is multiplicative or synergistic— ie, it is greater than the sum of the individual effects of each antibiotic. Effect modification can also work antagonistically. For example, the herbal remedy St John's wort induces the metabolism of oral contraceptives, decreasing their action and sometimes resulting in breakthrough bleeding and contraceptive inefficacy.[1] When taken together, oral contraceptives are less effective than if taken without St John's wort. The disorder glucose-6-phosphate dehydrogenase (G6PD) deficiency is fundamentally an example of genetic susceptibility to chemicals— in this case, oxidants. A drug with mild oxidant properties would not produce hemolysis in a male who did not carry the allele for this x-linked disorder, but in someone who does carry this allele, this same drug can cause severe hemolysis.

There is a critical difference between effect modification and the more familiar epidemiologic concept of *confounding*. Confounding occurs when 2 factors independently affect an outcome and people exposed to one of the factors are also disproportionately associated with the other. For example, a study might find that drinking coffee was associated with attention problems. Smoking is also associated with attention problems, and people who smoke tend to drink more coffee. If smoking caused the attention problem but was not measured, one might think that coffee consumption caused the attention problem when in fact, coffee consumption was a surrogate measure of smoking, the true cause. In our example, the *combination* of coffee and smoking was not needed to produce attention problems. There is no intrinsic biological link between coffee and attention problems, other than the observation that they happen to occur together. Effect modifiers, however, are intrinsically (ie, biologically) interrelated in producing the outcome of interest. For example, one must have both the genotype for G6PD deficiency and take an oxidant drug to produce hemolysis. As such, effect modifiers have tremendous importance and potential. Understanding the factors that modify the relationship between environmental exposures and the end toxic effect can lead to new insights into mechanisms, can identify individuals who are most severely affected by environmental toxicants, and can suggest interventions to mitigate the effects of exposures.

GENETIC SUSCEPTIBILITY

Interaction between genes and the environment is an extremely common occurrence. In fact, virtually all "genetic diseases" have significant environmental components and vice versa. To bring this concept into clinical perspective, phenylketonuria (PKU) is defined as a genetic disease. Specifically, it is an autosomal recessive trait; nearly all cases are associated with mutations in the gene encoding phenylalanine hydroxylase, which has been mapped to human chromosome 12q24.1.[2] The devastating neurodevelopmental effects of PKU are caused by excessive accumulation of phenylalanine, an essential amino acid usually metabolized by phenylalanine hydroxylase. Children with PKU who are identified early and treated with restrictive diets develop normally.[3] In this example, there are 2 factors (one genetic and one environmental) necessary for the development of PKU. To develop the disease, one must have both the genetic disposition and unrestricted exposure to phenylalanine. PKU is viewed as a genetic disease, because exposure to phenylalanine is universal, and PKU mutations are rare. Consider, however, if the converse were true—ie, if a population evolved in which PKU mutations were common, and that population did not consume unrestricted amounts of phenylalanine. New unrestricted exposures to this amino acid would be devastating to this population. In this scenario, phenylalanine would be considered a neurotoxicant (like lead) and excessive ingestion of foods containing it to be poisonous. In other words, PKU would be thought of as an environmental disease.

Similarly, diseases with strong environmental triggers are being shown increasingly to have genetic components. These genetic components are different from the more traditional concept of genetics. Genetic factors do not "cause" disease, unlike, for example, the alleles for cystic fibrosis. Instead, genetic components confer increased *risk* of developing the disease. The best known of such genetic risk factors is the E4 allele, a variant in the apolipoprotein E gene. This allele is associated with developing Alzheimer disease. Individuals with 1 copy of this allele have a two- to fivefold increased risk of developing Alzheimer disease. If a person has 2 copies of the E4 allele, the risk is increased by approximately 10-fold. However, more than half of people homozygous for this allele will never develop Alzheimer disease.[4] The allele is a risk factor and should not be thought of as causal in the way of Mendelian genetic diseases, such as cystic fibrosis. A more appropriate view is that E4 is a risk factor, similar to, for example, risk factors for heart attacks, such as smoking or dietary cholesterol.

Genetic risk factors also exist for childhood diseases, and many of these genetic factors modify the effects of environmental risk factors. There is strong evidence that genes and the environment interact in the pathogenesis of asthma. As of 2006, at least 10 genes were associated with asthma or atopy, each described in at least 10 studies.[5]

The relationship between genes and environmental exposure can be quite complex, as demonstrated by the CD14/-159 polymorphism and exposure to house dust endotoxin. Individuals with the T-allele of CD14/-159 have higher atopic response (as measured by serum immunoglobulin [Ig]E concentrations) when exposed to high levels of house dust, but individuals with the C-allele have higher IgE concentrations when exposed to low levels of house dust.[6] Therefore, depending on one's genetic makeup, endotoxins in house dust may predispose a child to asthma and allergies, or paradoxically, exposure to house dust may actually be *protective*. This finding, developed by multiple investigators over the past several years,[7-10] may provide the key to understanding the complex relationship between genes and environment in atopic disease. The protective effect of endotoxins in some individuals is direct evidence in support of the "hygiene hypothesis," which proposes that microbial exposure during early life protects against later development of atopic disease. This may be the case among individuals with the appropriate genetic makeup.[11-12] Nonetheless, there are still individuals in whom early life exposure is not protective, and this difference may be attributable to genetic susceptibility. This may explain why the hygiene hypothesis, a theory of environmental risk, has been so difficult to validate. It may only apply to individuals with a particular genetic background.

There is an additional layer of complexity in the relationship between genetics, environment, and disease; environmental toxicants, such as metals, may act to alter gene expression through *epigenetic* mechanisms. Epigenetics (literally "on genes") is a field that investigates heritable changes in gene expression that occur without changes in genetic sequence.[13] The term has also grown to include effects on gene expression that are "programmed" but not necessarily heritable.

Environmental factors can alter epigenetic "marks" (chemical additions to the gene sequence that regulate gene expression and alter the function of a gene without altering the DNA sequence). Gene expression is, in part, controlled by multiple epigenetic marks that can occur either on DNA itself or on DNA binding proteins (histones).

The most studied of epigenetic marks is DNA methylation. Cytosine methylation in the DNA sequence is overrepresented in cytosine-guanine repeat sequences. Such repeats are very common in promoter regions that regulate gene expression. This methylation pattern can alter the 3-dimensional structure of DNA. Methylated cytosines lead to a tightly wound 3-dimensional structure that hides the promoter region of a gene within a coil. "Unmethylated" cytosines lead to a more open structure that allows transcription factors to bind to DNA and initiate gene expression.

The extent to which specific DNA sequences are bound to methyl groups is a principal determinant of cell differentiation. The clinical consequences of altered DNA methylation patterns are becoming more apparent. Altered DNA methylation systems in the brain may lead to clinical syndromes, such as mental retardation and autism spectrum disorders.[14] DNA methylation patterns altered by environmental chemicals may be inherited by offspring if these altered methylation patterns occur in gamete cells.

There is widespread interest in DNA methylation and other epigenetic marks as mechanisms of environmental diseases. Several studies have demonstrated an association between DNA methylation and environmental metals, including nickel, cadmium, arsenic, and lead.[15-17] The effect may be because of metal-induced oxidative stress. Exposure to specific metals has been shown to result in global DNA hypomethylation and/or gene-specific DNA hypermethylation.[18] In animal models, DNA hypomethylation alters the function and survival of neurons.[19]

Together, these findings suggest a novel pathway by which environmental chemicals modify the expression of DNA to result in toxicity. There is also the potential that by altering such marks in a targeted fashion, environmentally induced diseases, including certain cancers, could be treated.

SOCIAL SUSCEPTIBILITY

Social factors, particularly socioeconomic status, are widely known to affect many health outcomes; they are implicated in the prevalence of many diseases and have repeatedly been associated with overall morbidity and mortality. Social factors play a major role in neurodevelopment, which is also an outcome relevant to many toxic exposures of childhood. Individuals of lower socioeconomic status are at increased risk of exposure to several environmental toxicants (see Chapter 52). More than simply acting as confounders, however, social factors may also modify the relationship between environmental exposures and outcomes.

Low income, or poverty, is itself not toxic but is a marker of factors that coincide with poverty (chemical exposure, social stress, exposure to violence, social isolation, etc). It is these factors, usually unmeasured, that cause the health effects of poverty. Traditionally, poverty has been believed to be a potential "confounder" of chemical toxicants, such as lead, with measures of poverty included in evaluations to account for its independent effects on developmental outcomes. A new paradigm has arisen in the last several years, and investigators are now studying whether poverty is not a confounder but is, instead, a modifier of lead toxicity. In this paradigm, there is synergism between environmental toxicants and factors that coincide with poverty. Fig 4.1 outlines the many factors to consider when unraveling the effects of lead exposure on cognitive function.

For example, Rauh et al[20] demonstrated an interaction between secondhand smoke (SHS) and maternal hardship on cognitive development among minority 24-month-old children in New York City. In their study, children with prenatal secondhand smoke exposure were twice as likely to be significantly delayed, and

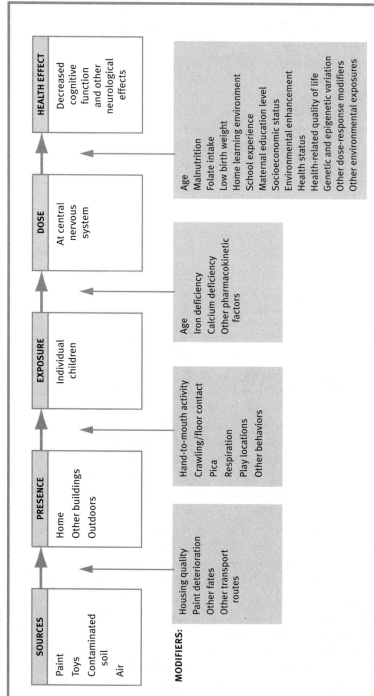

For the prototypical example of lead poisoning, this diagram illustrates the many factors that may modify an individual's susceptibility.

Figure 4.1: Biologic Impact Pathway of Lead on Cognitive Function

among children of mothers who reported significant unmet basic needs, the effect of secondhand smoke on cognitive function was significantly exacerbated. The reason for this interaction is uncertain, but several theories emerge. Mothers with fewer unmet needs may be better able to compensate for the toxic effect of secondhand smoke by providing positive developmental support for their children in the form of increased social interaction, an enhanced developmental environment, improved prenatal and postnatal nutrition, or reduced exposure to other developmental neurotoxicants also associated with poverty.

The cognitive effect of childhood exposure to lead, the most thoroughly studied developmental neurotoxicant, is also modified by social factors. In a cohort of children in Mexico City, increased maternal self-esteem attenuated the negative effect of lead exposure on cognitive development of 24-month-old children.[21]

In a striking animal model, environmental enhancement was demonstrated to reverse the neurological effects of lead exposure. Guilarte et al[22] exposed rats to neurotoxic levels of lead and then randomized them to standard cages or enriched environments with shared cages, greater space allowance per rat, and interactive objects. Rats in enriched environments showed better spatial learning and recovery of gene expression in the hippocampus, specifically associated with lead-related neurotoxicity. In effect, the social environment served as an effective "treatment" for lead poisoning.

The effects of lead poisoning on neurodevelopment have been considered by many experts to be irreversible. Adults with history of childhood lead exposure tend to have smaller brain volume,[23] and higher childhood lead concentrations are associated with increased criminal arrests in early adulthood.[24] Chelation therapy, the mainstay of treatment for acute childhood lead poisoning, was shown in a multicenter study to have no significant effect in reversing lead-induced cognitive deficits caused by chronic lead exposure.[25] Chelation therapy clearly remains the treatment of choice for acute severe systemic lead poisoning. However, the findings of Guilarte et al, which need to be validated in human populations, open the door to the possibility that some of the developmental effects associated with chronic "low level" lead poisoning could be remediated, in part, through social interventions. This is a promising finding for a disease process with otherwise dim treatment prospects.

NUTRITIONAL SUSCEPTIBILITY

Nutritional factors may affect both the absorption and the in vivo effects of environmental toxicants. This has been demonstrated particularly with heavy metals. Iron deficiency anemia, which is independently known to negatively affect early development,[26] is also associated with subsequent lead poisoning.[27] Iron-deficient individuals absorb a greater proportion of ingested lead, thought to be because a common iron receptor in the gastrointestinal epithelium is up-regulated in the setting of iron deficiency.[28] Similarly, increased calcium intake has been associated with lower blood lead concentration.[29,30] Low dietary calcium, likewise, will increase lead absorption and also perhaps mobilize lead for deposit in bone cortex.[31]

A study of children in the rural Philippines showed an interaction between lead and folate concentrations on cognitive function.[32] Among these generally poor and undernourished children, higher folate concentrations appeared to have a protective effect against lead's neurotoxic effects. The pathophysiology of this relationship is unclear, but folate is known to play a major role in neurodevelopment and also influences DNA expression because of its indispensable role in DNA methylation. DNA methylation is known to regulate gene expression, and the study findings might be explained by lead-induced changes in gene expression modified, in turn, by folate metabolism.

Together, these findings suggest multiple potential roles for nutritional supplementation in mitigating the effects of lead exposure. In one trial of this hypothesis in India, supplementing the diets of school children with iron-fortified rice decreased blood lead concentration,[33] but the cognitive effects of such interventions have not been established. A randomized trial in the United States of calcium supplementation among lead-exposed children failed to find a benefit in reducing the risk of lead poisoning.[34]

Nutrition plays a very important independent role in child health, particularly in neurodevelopment. These findings suggest that improved nutrition, in the form of specific micronutrients, may provide additional benefits in protection from environmental toxicants. Other elements of nutrition may also help protect against the effects of toxic exposures. For example, breastfeeding has been shown in multiple studies of fetal polychlorinated biphenyl (PCB) exposure to protect against adverse neurodevelopmental outcomes.[35-38] It is unclear whether this effect is attributable to the nutritional benefits of breastfeeding as compared with cow milk-based infant formula or to the enhanced social interaction between mother and infant that may be inherent to breastfeeding.

CONCLUSION

Genetic predisposition, social milieu, and nutritional quality are likely contributors to an individual child's susceptibility to environmental toxicants. The relationship between environmental exposure and outcome is not linear; rather, it is a complex web of interconnecting and interdependent factors likely to be unique for each exposed individual.

These determinants of susceptibility are of tremendous clinical importance to the clinician caring for children exposed to environmental toxicants. The most effective way to address environmental health threats will always be primary prevention through avoidance of exposure. Accordingly, primary prevention should be particularly emphasized among susceptible individuals, whether attributable to genetic, social, or nutritional risk factors.

When primary prevention is not possible and exposure has already occurred, treatment becomes the next best option. Although genetic predisposition may not (yet) be modifiable, nutritional status and social environment may well be. The data above suggest that social and nutritional interventions may have real effects on environmental health outcomes. In our lead poisoning example, chelation therapy, the treatment of choice for acute high-dose lead poisoning, has not been associated with improved developmental outcomes after lead exposure. Social interventions, such as Early Intervention programs, and nutritional supplementation may be effective in improving these outcomes.

Social and nutritional interventions need not necessarily be complex to be effective. Pediatricians are confronted daily with concerned parents worried about the myriad of toxicants in the modern environment to which their children are constantly exposed. What a powerful message it could be to say that one might ameliorate some of the effects of these exposures by providing a rich social environment and a complete and nutritious diet. Such a message does not mean that lead or other environmental poisons are not worrisome, nor is it meant to shift the blame for toxicity away from the chemical (or polluters causing the exposure) to the parents. Such a message instead conveys to parents that, while it may require significant effort, children may be able to overcome some or many of the toxic effects of chemical exposures and lead a long and fruitful life. Given that environmental toxicants frequently occur in disadvantaged communities, many of these issues, particularly with regard to the nutritional and social environments, can be seen as environmental justice issues. Addressing environmental contaminants should always include addressing the social and nutritional problems that are commonly experienced by children.

References

1. Hall SD, Zaiqui W, Huang S, et al. The interaction between St John's wort and an oral contraceptive. *Clin Pharamacol Ther.* 2003;74(6):525-535
2. Erlandsen H, Stevens RC. The structural basis of phenylketonuria. *Mol Genet Metab.* 1999;68(2):103-125
3. Koch R, Azen C, Friedman EG, Williamson ML. Paired comparisons between early treated PKU children and their matched sibling controls on intelligence and school achievement test results at eight years of age. *J Inherit Metab Dis.* 1984;7(2):86-90
4. Myers RH, Schaefer EJ, Wilson PW, et al. Apolipoprotein E epsilon4 association with dementia in a population-based study: The Framingham study. *Neurology.* 1996;46(3):673-677
5. Ober C, Hoffjan S. Asthma genetics 2006: the long and winding road to gene discovery. *Genes Immun.* 2006;7(2):95-100
6. Martinez FD. CD14, endotoxins, and asthma risk: actions and interactions. *Proc Am Thorac Soc.* 2007;4(3):221-225

7. Baldini M, Lohman AC, Halonen M, et al. A polymorphism in the 5' flanking region of the CD14 gene is associated with circulating soluble CD14 levels and with total serum immunoglobulin E. *Am J Respir Cell Mil Biol.* 1999;20(5):976-983

8. Eder W, Klimecki W, Yu L, et al. Opposite effects of CD14/-260 on serum IgE levels in children raised in different environments. *J Allergy Clin Immunol.* 2005;116(3):601-607

9. Martinez FD. Gene-environment interactions in asthma and allergies: a new paradigm to understand disease causation. *Immunol Allergy Clin North Am.* 2005;25(4):709-721

10. Simpson A, John SL, Jury F, et al. Endotoxin exposure, CD14, and allergic disease: an interaction between genes and the environment. *Am J Respir Crit Care Med.* 2006;174(4): 386-392

11. Liu AH, Leung DY. Renaissance of the hygiene hypothesis. *J Allergy Clin Imunol.* 2006;117(5):1063-1066

12. Schaub B, Lauener R, van Mutius E. The many faces of the hygiene hypothesis. *J Allergy Clin Imunol.* 2006;117(5):969-977

13. Bollati V, Baccarelli A. Environmental epigenetics. *Heredity.* 2010; 105: 105-112

14. Shahbazain MD, Zoghbi HY. Rett syndrome and MeCP2: linking epigenetics and neuronal function. *Am J Hum Genet.* 2002;71(6):1259-1272

15. McVeigh GE, Allen PB, Morgan DR, et al. Nitric oxide modulation of blood vessel tone identified by waveform analysis. *Clin Sci.* 2001;100(4):387-393

16. Dolinoy DC, Weidman JR, Jirtle RL. Epigenetic gene regulation: linking early developmental environment to adult disease. *Reprod Toxicol.* 2007;23(3):297-307

17. Bleich S, Lenz B, Ziegenbein M, et al. Epigenetic DNA hypermethylation of the HERP gene promoter induces down-regulation of its MRNA expression in patients with alcohol dependence. *Alcohol Clin Exp Res.* 2006;30(4):587-591

18. Wright RO, Baccarelli A. Metals and neurotoxicology. *J Nutr.* 2007;137(12):2809-2813

19. Jacob RA, Gretz DM, Taylor PC, et al. Moderate folate depletion increases plasma homocysteine and decreases lymphocyte DNA methylation in postmenopausal women. *J Nutr.* 1998;128(7):1204-1212

20. Rauh VA, Whyatt RM, Garfinkel R, et al. Developmental effects of exposure to environmental tobacco smoke and maternal hardship among inner-city children. *Neurotoxicol Teratol.* 2004;26(3):373-385

21. Surkan PJ, Schnaas L, Wright RJ, et al. Maternal self-esteem, exposure to lead, and child neurodevelopment. *Neurotoxicology.* 2008;29(2):278-285

22. Guilarte TR, Toscano CD, McGlothan JL, Weaver SA. Environmental enrichment reverses cognitive and molecular deficits induced by developmental lead exposure. *Ann Neurol.* 2003;53(1):50-56

23. Cecil KM, Brubaker CJ, Adler CM, et al. Decreased brain volume in adults with childhood lead exposure. *PLoS Med.* 2008;5(5):e112

24. Wright RO, Dietrich KN, Ris MD, et al. Association of prenatal and childhood blood lead concentrations with criminal arrests in early adulthood. *PLoS Med.* 2008;5(5):e101

25. Rogan WJ, Dietrich KN, Brody DJ, et al. The effect on chelation therapy with succimer on neurophychological development in children exposed to lead. *New Engl J Med.* 2001;344(19): 1421-1426

26. Lozoff B, Jimenez E, Wolf AW. Long-term developmental outcome of infants with iron deficiency. *N Engl J Med.* 1991;325(10):687-694

27. Wright RO, Tsaih SW, Schwartz J, et al. Association between iron deficiency and blood lead level in a longitudinal analysis of children followed in an urban primary care clinic. *J Pediatr.* 2003;142(1):9-14

28. Barton JC, Conrad ME, Nuby S, Harrison I. Effects of iron in the absorption and retention of lead. *J Lab Clin Med.* 1978;92(4):536-547

29. Mahaffey KR, Gartside PS, Gluek CJ. Blood lead levels and dietary calcium intake in 1 to 11 year old children: the Second National Health and Nutrition Examination Survey, 1976 to 1980. *Pediatrics.* 1986;78(2):257-262

30. Lacasaña M, Romieu I, Sanin LH et al. Blood lead levels and calcium intake in Mexico City children under five years of age. *Int J Health Res.* 2000;10(4):331-340

31. Morris C, McCarron DA, Bennett WM. Low-level lead exposure, blood pressure, and calcium metabolism. *Am J Kidney Dis.* 1990;15(6):568-574

32. Solon O, Riddell TJ, Quimbo SA, et al. Associations between cognitive function, blood lead concentration, and nutrition among children in the central Philippines. *J Pediatr.* 2008;152(2): 237-243

33. Zimmerman MB, Muthayya S, Moretti D, et al. Iron fortification reduces blood lead levels in children in Bangalore, India. *Pediatrics.* 2006;117(6):2014-2021

34. Sargent JD, Dalton MA, O'Connor GT, Olmstead EM, Klein RZ. Randomized trial of calcium glycerophosphate-supplemented infant formula to prevent lead absorption. *Am J Clin Nutr.* 1999;69(6):1224-1230

35. Jacobson JL, Jacobson SW. Intellectual impairment in children exposed to polychlorinated biphenyls in utero. *N Engl J Med.* 1996;335(11):783-789

36. Patantin S, Lanting C, Mulder PGH, Boersma ER, Sauer PJJ, Weisglas-Kuperus N. Effects of environmental exposure to PCBs and dioxins on cognitive abilities in Dutch children at 42 months of age. *J Pediatr.* 1999;134(1):33-41

37. Walkowiak J, Wiener J, Fastabend A, et al. Environmental exposure to polychlorinated biphenyls and quality of the home environment: effects on psychodevelopment in early childhood. *Lancet.* 2001;358(9293):1602-1607

38. Jacobson JL, Jacobson SW. Prenatal exposure to polychlorinated biphenyls and attention at school age. *J Pediatr.* 2003;143(6):780-788

Chapter 5

Taking An Environmental History and Giving Anticipatory Guidance

■ ■ ■ ■ ■ ■

During much of the 20th century, when it was routine for doctors to make house calls, doctors could observe the home environment of a child or adolescent. Making house calls is no longer part of standard practice. Today's pediatricians, therefore, must ask questions to find out about the home environment and other places where the child or adolescent lives or spends time, learns, and plays. Questions about these environments are basic to a comprehensive health history. The answers can help pediatricians to understand a child's physical surroundings and to offer appropriate guidance to prevent some and mitigate other possibly hazardous exposures. Questions can be incorporated into health supervision (well child and adolescent) visits and visits for illnesses with known environmental causes. Questions about the environment also are appropriate when symptoms are unusual, persistent, or when multiple people in the home (or child care setting, school, etc) have similar symptoms.

When taking histories, it is important to keep in mind that parents may face important challenges in modifying their home environments. For example, renters may not know the age of the home or may be unable to undertake mold investigations. When offering advice, pediatricians should recognize that recommendations may be difficult or impossible to implement because of factors such as cost or lack of influence on a landlord. There may be discomfort with "raising a fuss" as in situations when one parent is advised to ask another parent to stop smoking inside the home. Additionally, recommendations may not be followed, because families' cultural beliefs and practices may differ from those of the pediatrician.

Keeping these caveats in mind, this chapter reviews important areas in a pediatric environmental history and provides advice that may prevent or mitigate exposures. Because there are many items in the complete history, it is unlikely that busy practitioners will have the time to ask about everything. At minimum, it seems prudent to suggest that pediatricians inquire about the age and condition of the home, secondhand smoke (SHS) exposure, dietary exposure to mercury in fish, exposure to ultraviolet radiation, and parental occupation. Other questions may be asked depending on the situations of individual patients taking into account factors such as the child's age, socioeconomic status, geographic location, and known hazards in the community. Children who were adopted from or who have visited developing nations may be at higher risk for certain environmental exposures compared with children who have not traveled to these areas.

Laboratory testing of biological samples (such as blood or urine [Chapter 6]) and/or of environmental samples (including air, water, soil, or dust [Chapter 7]) may help clinicians to evaluate children with potential environmental exposures or environmentally related disorders.

HEALTH SUPERVISION VISITS

Health supervision visits are key elements in the care of infants, children, and adolescents in the United States.[1] Many areas must be reviewed during well visits; however, and time constraints are a common challenge for most practitioners. Environmental health history screening forms have been developed to facilitate the history-taking process.[2] Pediatric practices that use electronic health records (EHRs) may chose to customize their electronic health records to include questions about children's and adolescents' environments.

The following are basic areas of questioning about the child's and adolescent's environment[3]:

1. Physical surroundings;
2. Tobacco smoke exposure and tobacco use by household members;
3. Water sources;
4. Exposures from food;
5. Sun and other exposure to ultraviolet radiation (UVR); and
6. Exposures resulting from household member occupations and hobby activities.

The patient's developmental stage is an important consideration during history taking. Table 5.1 suggests when to introduce environmental questions. Table 5.2 gives a summary of questions and where in the book to find additional information.

Table 5.1: When to Introduce Environmental Questions*	
TOPIC	SUGGESTED TIME
Home environment including carbon monoxide, renovation, mold; secondhand smoke (SHS); water source; consumption of fish; occupational exposures	Prenatal visit; newborn visit; new patient
SHS, sun exposure, mold	When the child is 2 months old
Risk of poisoning from chemicals and pesticides; lead poisoning	When the child is 6 months old
Wooden playsets and picnic tables, arts and crafts exposures	Preschool period
Occupational exposures, exposures from hobbies, tanning parlors	When the patient is a teenager
Lawn and garden products, lawn services, scheduled chemical applications, sun exposure	Spring and summer
Wood stoves and fireplaces, gas stoves	Fall and winter

* This table is adapted from Balk SJ et al.[3]

1. Physical Surroundings

At Home

Young children spend 80% to 90% of their time indoors—in their own home or in a relative's home or child care setting. These environments may contain environmental hazards.

Important questions related to the home include:

- What type of building environments does your child live in or spend time in?
- What are the age and condition of your home? Is there lead, mold, or asbestos?
- Is there ongoing or planned renovation?
- Do you have carbon monoxide (CO) detectors?
- What type of heating/air system does your home have?
- Where and how do you store chemicals and pesticides?
- Do you use chemicals in the garden or spray the lawn with pesticides?
- Have you tested your home for radon?
- Do you live in an area where elevated levels of lead in the soil could be a concern?
- Do your children play on a wooden playset or use a wooden picnic table?

Table 5.2: Summary of Environmental Health Questions for Health Supervision Visits*

AREA	QUESTIONS	FOR MORE INFORMATION, SEE CHAPTER ON
Surroundings — At home	What type of home does your child live in or spend time in?	Child Care Settings, Indoor Air Pollutants, Lead
	What are the age and condition of your home? Is there lead, mold or asbestos?	Asbestos, Indoor Air Pollutants, Lead
	Is there ongoing or planned renovation?	Asbestos, Lead
	Do you have carbon monoxide (CO) detectors?	Carbon Monoxide
	What type of heating/air system does your home have?	Indoor Air Pollutants
	Where and how do you store chemicals and pesticides?	Pesticides
	Do you use chemicals in the garden or spray the lawn with pesticides?	Pesticides
	Have you tested your home for radon?	Radon
	Do you think there is lead in your soil?	Lead
	Do you have a playset or picnic table made of treated wood?	Arsenic
— At school	Are there concerns about your child's school environment?	Schools
— In the community	Is there a source of pollution in your community?	Environmental Equity, Indoor Air Pollutants, Outdoor Air Pollutants, Waste Sites
Tobacco smoke exposure	Do you smoke? Do you allow smoking in your car? Do other household members or child's caregivers smoke or allow smoking in the home or car?	Asthma, Tobacco Use and Secondhand Tobacco Smoke Exposure

Table 5.2: Summary of Environmental Health Questions for Health Supervision Visits*, *continued*		
AREA	**QUESTIONS**	**FOR MORE INFORMATION, SEE CHAPTER ON**
Water sources	Do you use tap water? Well water?	Lead, Nitrates, Water, Arsenic
Exposures from food	Do you eat fish? Does your child eat fish? What kinds and how often?	Mercury, PCBs
Sun and other exposure to ultraviolet radiation (UVR)	Is your child protected from excessive sun exposure? Do you visit tanning parlors?	Ultraviolet Radiation
Exposures resulting from parents' and teens' occupations and hobby activity	What jobs do household members hold? What are the hobbies of household members?	Arts and Crafts, Schools, Lead

*This table is adapted from Balk SJ et al.[3]

What type of building environments does your child live in or spend time in?
Is it a single-family home, apartment, mobile home, or temporary shelter?
Single-family homes or apartments may have high levels of radon in basements
or lower floors, or friable asbestos. Mobile homes may be constructed using
materials such as particle board and pressed-wood products containing formaldehyde, a respiratory and dermal irritant.

What are the age and condition of your home? Is there lead, mold, or asbestos?
Lead: Lead paint could be used in home construction until the late 1970s.
Buildings constructed before 1950 are most likely to have leaded paint that may
peel, chip, or chalk. Lead dust can be released from poorly maintained surfaces,
and by friction, such as occurs at windows.

Recommendations: Federal law requires testing of Medicaid-eligible children
at 1 and 2 years of age. Other children should be tested according to state or
local guidelines.[4]
Mold and Dampness: Homes that have flooded or that have leaky plumbing
or roofs may have mold growth; exposure often results in respiratory symptoms.
A damp or musty smell indicates the presence of mold. Ineffective and unused
ventilation contributes to mold or dampness. Mold can cause allergies; it can
trigger, and possibly cause, asthma. Exposure to the mold *Stachybotrys atra*

(also known as *Stachybotrys chartarum*) has been associated with the development of acute pulmonary hemorrhage in young infants, although a causal relationship between acute pulmonary hemorrhage and damp, moldy indoor environments has not been firmly established. Exposure to secondhand smoke in the presence of mold increases the infant's risk of developing acute pulmonary hemorrhage.[5]

Recommendations: Water leaks and other sources of water intrusion should be repaired, and all reservoirs of mold should be removed. Areas of visible mold measuring ≤9 square feet can be removed using a dilute solution of chlorine bleach (1 part chlorine to 10 parts water)[6] or household detergent. It is important to use an adequately ventilated space if bleach is used. Infants, young children, and anyone with respiratory tract disease should stay away from the area until it has been cleaned. Professional removal by a trained mold remediation company is recommended for moldy areas >9 square feet or if removal of building materials is required.[6] Mold present on hard surfaces can be wiped clean. Dry cleaning may be attempted for visible mold growth on clothing. Permeable and semipermeable materials, such as upholstered furniture and carpeting, should be discarded if there is mold growth. Surfaces in the cleaned area should then be vacuumed with a high-efficiency particulate air (HEPA) vacuum before resuming use of the area. Mold is ubiquitous, and the expectation of creating an entirely "mold-free" environment is unrealistic. However, a healthy environment is dry and free of visible mold growth beyond that which normally occurs (eg, bathroom mold). Children (especially infants) and others should not be exposed to moldy environments.

Information about cleaning homes that have been flooded is available from the US Environmental Protection Agency (EPA; http://www.epa.gov/iaq/flood/flood_booklet_en.pdf).

Asbestos: Asbestos was commonly used decades ago as insulation around boilers and pipes, in ceiling and floor tiles, and other areas. Asbestos coverings can deteriorate, or if disturbed, asbestos can be released into the air during renovation or other work. Airborne asbestos may be inhaled into the lungs, possibly resulting in mesothelioma or lung cancer years after exposure.

Recommendations: Asbestos can be identified by calling a certified inspector or by contacting the manufacturer of the product. Undamaged asbestos is best left alone. Asbestos in poor condition (more than a very small amount) must be removed by a certified asbestos contractor.[7]

Is there ongoing or planned renovation?

Renovation of a bedroom is common to prepare for the birth of a baby or to update the room decor as the child grows. Improper renovation procedures may expose a pregnant woman, her fetus, or child to lead or other dusts, asbestos, and molds. Newly installed carpets may release irritating or toxic vapors.

Recommendations: Pregnant women and young children should vacate their premises during renovation if there is the possibility of exposure to lead and other contaminants. Only certified contractors should conduct renovation activities that involve removal of lead or asbestos. Ventilation is advised to limit exposure to irritating or toxic vapors.

Do you have CO detectors?

Unintentional CO poisoning causes hundreds of deaths in the United States each year.

Recommendations: Chimneys should be inspected and cleaned each year. Combustion appliances must be properly installed, maintained, and vented according to manufacturers' instructions. The Consumer Product Safety Commission recommends that parents install CO detectors that meet the most recent standards of the Underwriters Laboratories (UL) in every sleeping area and should never ignore an alarming CO detector. Note: children may already be symptomatic from excess CO when a CO monitor alarm sounds.

What type of heating/air system does your home have?

Wood stoves and fireplaces emit respiratory irritants (nitrogen dioxide [NO_2], respirable particulates, and polycyclic aromatic hydrocarbons), especially when they are not properly vented and maintained. Gas stoves, which may produce NO_2, are used in more than half of US homes. Respiratory symptoms may occur when gas stoves are used as supplemental heat. Wood stoves, fireplaces, and other fuel-burning appliances may be sources of CO.

Recommendations: Parents should be advised to properly maintain and clean heating systems. Use of wood-burning appliances should be discouraged when children have asthma or other chronic respiratory conditions. Information about wood stoves, including health effects of exposure, and installing cleaner and more efficient stoves, is available from the EPA.[8]

Where and how do you store chemicals and pesticides?

Pesticides and other chemicals can cause acute poisoning and death as well as subacute and chronic poisoning.

Recommendations: Parents can be encouraged to use the least toxic options for pest control. Integrated pest management (IPM) is an approach that integrates chemical and nonchemical methods to provide the least toxic alternative for pest control. IPM uses regular monitoring (rather than predetermined chemical applications) to determine whether and when treatments are needed. If toxic chemicals are used, they should be placed of children's reach. Chemicals should be stored in original containers and never in containers such as soda or juice bottles.

Do you use chemicals in the garden or spray the lawn with pesticides?
Children may inhale and absorb pesticide residues as they crawl or play on
freshly sprayed outdoor surfaces, such as lawns and gardens, or on indoor
surfaces, such as upholstery or rugs. Pesticide residues may adhere to plush toys.

Recommendations: Spraying or "bombing" with pesticides is hazardous,
especially while children are young or when a woman is pregnant. Pediatricians
should discourage using pesticides in the home or garden for ornamental
purposes. There is no clearly established length of time that parents must
prohibit children from playing in freshly sprayed lawns and gardens. If a parent
has applied an herbicide, it is reasonable to advise that at least 24 to 48 hours
pass before a child has contact with the lawn. Insecticides are generally more
toxic to animals than are compounds designed to kill plants. It is, therefore,
reasonable to advise avoiding contact for a longer time period, such as 48 to
72 hours, after insecticide application.[3]

Have you tested your home for radon?
Approximately 10% of lung cancer in the United States is attributable to radon,
a preventable exposure.

Recommendations: The EPA and the US Surgeon General recommend testing
homes below the 3rd floor for radon.[9] The EPA recommends that radon testing
be performed before buying or selling a home.[9]

**Do you live in an area where elevated levels of lead in the soil could
be a concern?**
Lead contaminates soil when paint chips from old buildings mixes with the soil.
Lead was present in gasoline in the United States until the 1970s. Because lead
moves little once deposited, lead that originated from auto emissions or deteriorating paint can be present in soil. In urban areas, soil lead levels are highest
around building foundations.

Recommendations: If high levels of lead in soil are suspected and there are
young children who play there, parents are encouraged to have the soil tested.
High lead levels in soil may be reduced by mixing or covering the high-lead
soil with low-lead soil and by landscape treatments or by physically removing
the soil.[10,11]

Do your children play on a wooden playset or use a wooden picnic table?
Outdoor wooden playsets and picnic tables may have been treated with the
preservative chromated copper arsenate (CCA) to protect wood from decay.
Children's hand-mouth behavior may result in exposure to arsenic leaching from
the chromated copper arsenate. Manufacturers reached a voluntary agreement
with the EPA to end the manufacture of chromated copper arsenate-treated
wood for most consumer applications by December 31, 2003. Some stocks of

wood treated before then were expected to be found on shelves until mid-2004. Hundreds of thousands of play structures, decks, and tables were built before the ban and are still in use.

Recommendations: If there is a wooden playset, deck, or picnic table manufactured before 2003, parents can call the manufacturer to determine whether it contains chromated copper arsenate. Chromated copper arsenate in decks, play structures, or picnic tables should be treated with a clear sealant every 6 months to 1 year to decrease the amount of arsenic leaching out of the wood. Alternatively, parents can choose to have the set or table safely dismantled. Chromated copper arsenate-treated wood should not be burned or sawed, because this will increase the amount of arsenic released. If parents keep a playset, they should wash children's hands with soap and water immediately after outdoor play, and especially before eating. Children should not eat while playing on chromated copper arsenate-treated playground equipment. It is prudent to cover a treated picnic table with a cloth before eating.

At School

Are there concerns about your child's school environment?

Many hazards found in school environments are similar to those in homes. In addition, children engaging in arts and crafts activities may encounter potential hazards, such as felt-tip markers (containing aromatic hydrocarbons) and oil-based paints. Children with certain disabilities may be at more risk of toxic exposures. Visually impaired children working close to a project or children with asthma may be affected by fumes. Children unable to follow safety precautions may contaminate their skin or place art materials in their mouths. Emotionally disturbed children may abuse art materials, endangering themselves and others.

Recommendations: Parents concerned about possible exposures in the school should be encouraged to act as advocates for their child. Pediatricians may sometimes be helpful in the advocacy process.

In the Community

Is there a source of pollution in your community? Do you live near a major roadway or highway?

Toxic hazards may exist in the neighborhood or community. Sources of exposure include polluted lakes and streams, industrial plants, and dump sites. Children can be exposed to lead if they live downwind from a lead smelter or to pesticides or other chemicals if they live on farms or at the urban-rural interface. Air quality is often poorer around homes and buildings located within 300 meters of a major highway. Low-income communities and racial/ethnic minority communities are more likely to face toxic hazards, termed "environmental disparities" or "environmental injustice" (see Chapter 52).

A child or teenager may have been exposed to a one-time disaster, such as Hurricane Katrina or the World Trade Center disaster. Exposure to such dramatic environmental occurrences may have long-term effects on physical and mental health.

Other aspects of "community" may affect health—for example, health is often influenced by the presence or absence of safe places to walk and exercise.

Recommendations: Parents concerned about possible exposures in their community should be encouraged to act as advocates for their family. Pediatricians can be helpful in the advocacy process. If the family is planning a move, it may be relevant to consider proximity of the new home to traffic pollution, because air quality is affected near major highways. This is especially relevant if the child has a respiratory condition.

2. Tobacco Smoke Exposure

- Do you smoke? Are you interested in quitting?
- Do other family members of your household or the child's caregivers smoke?
- Is your home and the caregiver's home smoke free, even when the child is not present?
- Are your cars/motor vehicles smoke free, even when the child is not present?

Exposure to secondhand smoke (also known as environmental tobacco smoke) places exposed individuals at risk of significant morbidity and mortality. "Third-hand smoke" is the term used to describe the mixture of gases and particles clinging to smokers' hair and clothing and to furniture and carpeting in a room. Third-hand smoke may linger long after secondhand smoke has cleared from a room.[12]

Recommendations: If parents or other caregivers smoke, pediatricians should advise them to quit and offer help in doing so. Educating parents about the associations between secondhand smoke and their child's illness may help them to quit. Parents can also be informed that their children are more likely to begin smoking if parents smoke. The US Public Health Service recommends that clinicians ask about smoking at every clinical encounter and offer smokers at least a brief (1- to 3-minute) intervention at each visit.[13] Quit-smoking telephone counseling, available throughout the nation, is effective in helping smokers to quit. Whether or not parents choose to quit, they should, nevertheless introduce and enforce strict no-smoking bans in the home and car. If they have been smoking, parents and others should wash hands and change clothes before interacting with their child. Parents should strive to avoid exposing children to any environment that contains tobacco smoke. Pediatricians should discuss the hazards of cigarette smoking with school-aged children and teenagers.

Teenagers who smoke should be advised to quit. Even if they are not smokers, teenagers should be asked about secondhand smoke exposure, as they may be exposed by family or friends who do smoke.

3. Water Sources

- Do you use tap water? Well water?

Water contaminants of particular concern for US infants and children are lead and nitrates.

Lead: Tap water used to reconstitute infant formula may be contaminated with lead.[14] Most large municipal water supplies maintain lead levels less than the EPA standard of 15 parts per billion. Most systems have acceptable lead levels. Until the late 1980s, lead solder was widely used to connect copper pipes; plumbing fixtures also may contain lead. It is possible for lead to leach from lead-containing components of water systems.[15] Changes in water additives may increase lead leaching.[16]

Recommendations: To decrease the possibility of contamination from leaded pipes and solder, water that has been standing in pipes overnight should be run until it becomes as cold as it can get, before it is used. Parents should be advised to use only water from the cold-water tap for drinking, cooking, and especially for making baby formula. Hot water is likely to contain higher levels of lead.[17] Depending on the child's age, housing situation, and other risk factors, children should be tested with a blood lead test. Parents can also choose to test their water for lead. Bottled water may be an acceptable, although expensive, alternative. Certain countertop filters and certain filters applied to the tap can remove lead.

Nitrates and Coliforms: Infants exposed to high levels of nitrates in well water may develop methemoglobinemia, which may result in death. Well water may also contain coliform bacteria. High levels of nitrates or coliforms in the water may indicate the presence of pesticides.

Recommendations: When buying or purchasing a home, parents should test private wells for nitrates, coliforms, inorganic compounds (total dissolved solids, iron, magnesium, calcium, chloride), and lead. Testing for nitrates and coliforms should be performed annually. Repeat testing for other contaminants should be considered if a new source of contamination becomes known (for example, if a neighbor discovers a new contaminant in his or her well).[18] Local health or environmental departments can advise about testing.[19]

Well water should be tested for nitrates and coliforms before being offered to an infant. Water high in nitrates or coliforms should not be given to infants. Boiling water for infant formula is rarely necessary. Overboiling water for infant formula preparation concentrates lead and nitrates. Water brought to a rolling boil for 1 minute kills microorganisms such as *Cryptosporidium* species without concentrating lead or nitrates.[20]

4. Exposures from Food

- Do you eat fish?
- Does your child eat fish?
- What kinds and how often?

Although fish is an excellent source of protein and can contain omega-3 fatty acids, certain fish may be contaminated with excessive amounts of mercury or polychlorinated biphenyls (PCBs). Exposure to these contaminants may have adverse effects, especially on fetuses and young children.

Recommendations: Families eating commercially caught fish should choose fish low in mercury and other pollutants. Pregnant women, women of child-bearing age, nursing mothers, and young children should completely avoid fish with high mercury content (king mackerel, shark, swordfish and tilefish) and limit consumption of other fish. Families catching their own fish should be instructed to follow fish advisories issued by state and local health departments to determine which fish are safe to eat.

5. Sun and Other Exposure to Ultraviolet Radiation (UVR)

- Is your child protected from excessive sun exposure?
- Do you visit tanning parlors?

About one quarter of a person's exposure to the sun occurs before 18 years of age. Early exposure to UVR increases skin cancer risk. Teenagers increasingly visit tanning parlors, thereby also raising their skin cancer risk.

Recommendations: Advice about sun protection includes covering up with clothing and hats, timing children's activities to avoid peak sun exposure, consulting the Ultraviolet Index, using sunscreen and reapplying frequently as needed, and wearing sunglasses. Teenagers should not visit tanning parlors.

6. Exposures Resulting From Parents' Occupations and Hobbies

- What are parents' and teenagers' jobs?
- What are parents' and teenagers' hobbies?

Parental occupations may produce hazards for a child. Workplace contaminants may be transported to the home on clothes, shoes, and skin surfaces.[21] Lead poisoning has been described in children of lead storage battery workers,[22] asbestos-related lung diseases have been found in families of shipyard workers,[23] and elevated mercury concentrations have been reported in children whose parents worked in a mercury thermometer plant.[24] Parents who work with art materials at home may expose children to toxicants, such as lead used in solder, pottery glazes, or stained glass.

Employment may help teenagers develop skills and responsibility and earn money, but work activities may carry the risk of toxic exposure or injury.

Environmental exposures include UVR with outdoor work, secondhand smoke encountered in restaurants and bars, pesticides from lawn-care and farm work, and noise from operating equipment. Work may also interfere with an adolescent's education, sleep, and social behavior. Federal and state child labor laws regulate employment of children younger than 18 years. These laws address the minimum ages for general and specific types of employment, maximum daily and weekly number of hours of work permitted, prohibition of work during night hours, prohibition of certain types of employment, and the registration of minors for employment.[25]

Hobby activity may pose a risk to school-aged children and adolescents. Shooting at an indoor firing range may result in lead exposure.[26] Toluene and other solvents may be encountered in glues used in model-building. Adolescents may be especially at risk of huffing (inhaling) if glue is present in their environments, resulting in easy access.

Recommendations: An occupational history may be obtained when information about family composition and the family history is obtained. Workers exposed to toxic substances are legally entitled to be notified of this exposure under federal "right-to-know" and "hazard communication" laws. Parents who work with toxic substances should shower, if possible, and change clothes and shoes before leaving work. At home, children should not be allowed in rooms where parents work with toxic substances.

VISITS FOR ILLNESS: CONSIDERING ENVIRONMENTAL ETIOLOGIES IN THE DIFFERENTIAL DIAGNOSIS

Secondhand tobacco smoke is the most common toxicant associated with respiratory diseases, such as asthma; recurrent lower and upper airway disease; and persistent middle ear effusion. Lead poisoning may present with symptoms of recurrent abdominal pain, constipation, irritability, developmental delay, seizures, or unexplained coma. Foods and medications brought from other countries may be sources of lead and other heavy metals. Headaches may be caused by acute and chronic exposure to CO from improperly vented heating sources, formaldehyde, and chemicals used on the job. Pediatricians should ask about mold and water damage in the home when they treat infants with acute pulmonary hemorrhage.

Environmental causes of illness may not always be apparent.[27] Because most environmental or occupational illnesses present as common medical problems or have nonspecific symptoms, the diagnosis may be missed unless a history of exposure is obtained. This is especially important if the illness is atypical or unresponsive to treatment. The following questions may provide information about whether an illness is related to the environment.

1. Do symptoms subside or worsen in a particular location (eg, home, child care, school, or certain room)?
2. Do symptoms subside or worsen during a particular time? At a particular time of day? On weekdays or weekends? During a particular week or season?
3. Do symptoms worsen during a particular activity? While the child is playing outside, or engaging in hobby activities, such as working with arts and crafts?
4. Are siblings or other children experiencing similar symptoms?
5. What are parents' thoughts about why symptoms are occurring?

Three case examples illustrate integrating environmental health etiologies into the differential diagnosis:

Case 1: Asthma

A 5 year-old boy comes to your office for follow-up. He has had mild intermittent asthma for most of his life. His known triggers for wheezing episodes are cold weather and upper respiratory tract infections. What else do you need to know?

Environmental triggers that may precipitate asthma include:
- Secondhand smoke
- Molds
- Dust mites
- Cockroaches
- Animal allergens
- Nitrogen oxides
- Odors
- Volatile organic compounds, such as formaldehyde

Most of these triggers are amenable to environmental interventions. Asking about environmental exposures and suggesting ways to decrease exposures may result in improved symptoms.

Case 2: Fever and Rash

A 3 year-old boy comes in with a 1-week history of fever, rash, and difficulty walking. His past medical history is unremarkable. Physical examination reveals an irritable child with temperature of 40 C; there is conjunctival injection, pharyngeal erythema, swelling of hands and feet, and a macular rash. What is in your differential diagnosis?

The differential diagnosis includes:
- Kawasaki disease
- Measles
- Scarlet fever
- Juvenile rheumatoid arthritis
- Acrodynia

Although the child described in this case turns out to have Kawasaki disease, the differential diagnosis includes acrodynia ("pink disease"), a rare hypersensitivity reaction to mercury that occurs mainly in children. In the past, acrodynia was described after exposure to mercury-containing teething powders, and in more recent times after exposure to mercury-containing diaper rinses and latex paints. Prominent symptoms are anorexia, generalized pain, paresthesias, and apathy. Physical examination reveals an acral rash that is predominantly pink, papular, and pruritic and may progress to desquamation and hypotonia. Other features include irritability, tremors, diaphoresis, hypertension, and tachycardia.[1]

Case 3: Seizure (adapted from Khine et al[28])

A 3 year-old Hispanic girl with a history of seizures presents to the emergency department (ED) after a generalized tonic-clonic seizure. She received rectal diazepam at home before her arrival in the ED. She is awake but tired. She is afebrile and her physical examination is normal. The child's past medical history is significant for a seizure disorder of unknown etiology diagnosed at 3 months of age. An MRA/MRI of the brain and electroencephalogram (EEG) done 2 years previously were normal. What is in the differential diagnosis?

The differential diagnosis includes:

- Seizure disorder of unknown etiology
- Infection
- Brain tumor
- Toxic ingestion
- Other toxic exposure

Alcohol, acetaminophen, aspirin and iron are not detected on serum toxicology screening. The results of urine toxicology screening for drugs of abuse are negative.

A recent report has called attention to seizures occurring in children exposed to camphor, a known cause of seizures and reported after camphor ingestion, inhalation, and dermal absorption.[28] Camphor (alcanfor in Spanish) is commonly used as a natural remedy in certain populations. When questioned specifically about camphor, the mother reveals that she was rubbing a properly labeled camphor ointment over the child's upper chest, forehead, and back hourly for several hours before the onset of the seizure, to relieve her cold symptoms. The mother used camphor-containing products in various other ways, such as putting it in the vaporizer, placing it in a bowl with water under the crib, hanging camphor tablets in a meshed cloth on the posts of the crib, and spreading crushed tablets around the house to control roaches. Two of the mother's other children had seizure disorders; all had evaluations and normal imaging studies. The other siblings did not suffer seizures when they previously lived in the grand-mother's apartment for 1 year. The grandmother did not allow the use of camphor during that time. Use of camphor products in the home was discontinued, and anticonvulsant medications were discontinued for the children. On follow-up 10 weeks after this seizure, no further episodes of seizures were reported in any of the children.

The US Food and Drug Administration (FDA) restricts the camphor content to less than 11% in some products intended for medicinal use. Camphor products intended for use as pesticides must be registered with the EPA. Nevertheless, many imported camphor-containing products fail to meet FDA and EPA requirements for labeling and content. This case illustrates the importance of asking about camphor use when a child has a seizure and of educating families about the risks of using camphor.

Resources

National Environmental Education Foundation (NEEF)

http://www.neefusa.org/health

NEEF is a national nonprofit organization with several educational initiatives related to pediatric environmental health, including a Pediatric Environmental History Initiative. Resources include history forms for taking a general environmental history and for a child with asthma.

Canadian Association of Physicians for the Environment (CAPE)

http://www.cape.ca/children/history.html

Contains detailed information about the pediatric environmental health history.

Agency for Toxic Substances and Disease Registry (ATSDR)

http://www.atsdr.cdc.gov/csem/exphistory/ehcover_page.html

Elements of an environmental history are reviewed in "Taking an Exposure History," one of many monographs in the Case Studies in Environmental Medicine series available from the ATSDR. The history is geared to adults in the workplace but the examples used and principles illustrated can be helpful to pediatricians.

http://www.atsdr.cdc.gov/emes/subtopic/pediatrics.html

ATSDR–PSR Environmental Health Toolkit. ATSDR's Division of Toxicology and Environmental Medicine (DTEM), the Greater Boston Physicians for Social Responsibility (PSR), and the University of California-San Francisco Pediatric Environmental Health Specialty Unit (PEHSU) teamed up to develop an environmental health anticipatory guidance training module with downloadable tools for use in clinical practice.

References

1. Kliegman RM, Behrman RE, Jenson HB, Stanton BF, eds. *Nelson's Textbook of Pediatrics.* 18th ed. Philadelphia, PA: Saunders Elsevier; 2007
2. National Environmental Education Foundation. Pediatric Environmental History Forms. Available at: http://www.neefusa.org/health/PEHI/HistoryForm.htm. Accessed September 22, 2010
3. Balk SJ, Forman JA, Johnson CL, Roberts JR. Safeguarding kids from environmental hazards. *Contemp Pediatr.* March 2007;64–81
4. American Academy of Pediatrics, Committee on Environmental Health. Lead exposure in children: prevention, detection, and management. *Pediatrics.* 2005;116(4):1036-1046
5. American Academy of Pediatrics, Committee on Environmental Health. Spectrum of noninfectious health effects from molds. *Pediatrics.* 2006;118(6):2582-2586
6. National Environmental Education Foundation. Mold/mildew and asthma. In: *Environmental Management of Pediatric Asthma: Guidelines for Health Care Providers.* Washington, DC: National Environmental Education Foundation; 2005:23. Available at: http://www.neefusa.org/pdf/AsthmaDoc.pdf. Accessed September 22, 2010
7. US Environmental Protection Agency. An Introduction to Indoor Air Quality. Available at: www.epa.gov/iaq/asbestos.html#Steps%20to%20Reduce%20Exposure. Accessed September 22, 2010
8. US Environmental Protection Agency. Choosing Appliances. Available at: http://www.epa.gov/burnwise/appliances.html. Accessed September 22, 2010
9. US Environmental Protection Agency. A Citizen's Guide to Radon: The Guide to Protecting Yourself and Your Family From Radon. Available at: http://www.epa.gov/radon/pubs/citguide.html. Accessed September 22, 2010
10. GreenNet Chicago. Information for Community Gardeners on Lead Contamination. Available at: http://www.greennetchicago.org/pdf/GreenNet_Lead_Feb_2005.pdf. Accessed September 22, 2010
11. Children's Memorial Research Center. *A Field Guide to Safer Yards: Protecting Your Children.* Chicago, IL: Children's Memorial Research Center, Safer Yards Project; 2002. Available at: http://www.childrensmrc.org/uploadedFiles/Research/Pediatric_Practice_Research_Group_ (PPRG)/Resources/lead/SY_Brochure_6-3.pdf?n=6191. Accessed September 22, 2010
12. Winickoff JP, Friebely J, Tanski SE, et al. Beliefs about the health effects of "thirdhand" smoke and home smoking bans. *Pediatrics.* 2009;123(1):e74-e79
13. Agency for Healthcare Research and Quality. Treating Tobacco Use and Dependence: 2008 Update. Available at: http://www.ahrq.gov/path/tobacco.htm. Accessed September 22, 2010
14. Baum CR, Shannon MW. The lead concentration of reconstituted infant formula. *J Toxicol Clin Toxicol.* 1997;35(4):371-375
15. National Safety Council. Lead in Water. Available at: http://www.nsc.org/resources/issues/articles/lead_in_water.aspx. Accessed September 22, 2010
16. Edwards M, Triantafyllidou S, Best D. Elevated blood lead in young children due to lead-contaminated drinking water: Washington, DC: 2001-2004. *Environ Sci Technol.* 2009;43(5):1618-1623
17. US Environmental Protection Agency. Lead in Drinking Water. Available at: http://water.epa.gov/drink/info/lead/index.cfm. Accessed September 22, 2010
18. American Academy of Pediatrics, Committee on Environmental Health and Committee on Infectious Diseases. Drinking water from private wells and risks to children. *Pediatrics.* 2009;123(6):1599–1605

19. Centers for Disease Control and Prevention, Division of Parasitic Diseases. Well Water Testing Frequently Asked Questions. Available at: http://www.cdc.gov/ncidod/dpd/healthywater/factsheets/wellwater.htm. Accessed September 22, 2010

20. US Environmental Protection Agency. Office of Ground Water and Drinking Water. Guidance for people with severely weakened immune systems. Internet: http://water.epa.gov/aboutow/ogwdw/upload/2001_11_15_consumer_crypto.pdf. Accessed September 22, 2010

21. Chisolm JJ. Fouling one's own nest. *Pediatrics.* 1978;62(4):614-617

22. Whelan EA, Piacitelli GM, Gerwel B, et al. Elevated blood lead levels in children of construction workers. *Am J Public Health.* 1997;87(8):1352-1355

23. Kilburn KH, Lilis R, Anderson HA, et al. Asbestos disease in family contacts of shipyard workers. *Am J Public Health.* 1985;75(6):615-617

24. Hudson PJ, Vogt RL, Brondum J, Witherell L, Myers G, Pascal DC. Elemental mercury exposure among children of thermometer plant workers. *Pediatrics.* 1987;79(6):935-938

25. Pollack SH. Adolescent occupational exposures and pediatric take-home exposures. *Pediatr Clin North Am.* 2001;48(5):1267-1289

26. Goldberg RL, Hicks AM, O'Leary LM, London S. Lead exposure at uncovered outdoor firing ranges. *J Occup Med.* 1991;33(6):718-719

27. Goldman LR. The clinical presentation of environmental health problems and the role of the pediatric provider. What do I do when I see children who might have an environmentally related illness? *Pediatr Clin North Am.* 2001;48(5):1085-1098

28. Khine H, Weiss D, Graber N, Hoffman RS, Esteban-Cruciani N, Avner JR. A cluster of children with seizures caused by camphor poisoning. *Pediatrics.* 2009;123(5):1269-1272

Chapter 6

Medical Laboratory Testing
of Body Fluids and Tissues

■ ■ ■ ■ ■ ■

Medical laboratory testing is an important tool to help clinicians evaluate children with potential environmental exposures or environmentally related disorders. Interpretation of results of toxicologic tests of body fluids and tissues requires meticulous consideration in the clinical assessment and environmental evaluation of each case. Parents may make specific requests for medical laboratory testing of body fluids or body tissues because of perceived exposures or to explore the etiology of observed symptoms in their children. Often, these requests cannot be accommodated because of limitations in clinical laboratory capability. Although medical laboratory testing often serves as an important tool to help clinicians to assess, manage, and prevent environmentally related disorders in children, such testing frequently has significant limitations. Growing numbers of laboratory tests are being developed in research institutions, but few are appropriate for use in clinical practice.

WHAT TO CONSIDER BEFORE ORDERING A CLINICAL LABORATORY TEST
Children may present to a pediatrician with symptoms of an environmentally related disorder or following a potential exposure. In all cases, a detailed exposure history should be taken, as described in Chapter 5.

Children are exposed to chemical contaminants as they breathe, eat, drink, and play. Very few of these potential exposures can be accurately quantified or even identified. Because children often present for assessment and management of environmentally related disorders long after a potential exposure, it is not usually possible to identify the specific contribution that a chemical environmental contaminant may have made to the etiology of their disorder. The utility and validity of laboratory testing in relation to concerns about the effect of environmental chemicals on the health of children is extremely limited. Shotgun approaches that involve testing for multiple possible contaminants are not useful. Testing, where possible, should only be performed if an exposure history is suggestive and if the laboratory result will influence the treatment of the patient.

Chemical contaminants may affect children concurrently with exposure, sequentially, and/or synergistically. The effects of exposure will depend on many factors, including the dose, the child's age, genetic predisposition (eg, genetic polymorphisms for metabolizing [detoxifying] enzymes and predisposition to cancer[1] or polymorphisms for cytokines such as tumor necrosis factor-alpha [TNF-α] and predisposition to asthma[2]), and other environmental influences, including psychosocial, socioeconomic, ethnic, cultural, dietary, and other factors[3] (see Chapter 4).

There are several important factors to consider when assessing a child's potential exposure. Relevant information regarding exposure may include the physical state of the chemical (ie, gas, liquid, solid, dust, or vapor), the route of exposure (ie, inhalation, ingestion, or dermal), dates of exposure, any concurrent exposures, and doses of specific exposures. Dosing requires knowledge of quantity, frequency, and duration of exposure that may arise from more than one source. It is also helpful to know about the specific chemical contaminant's behavior in the environment and in the body. All are important factors when taking an exposure history and considering medical laboratory testing.

Consumer products often have Material Safety Data Sheets that provide valuable basic product information, including the following:
1. Product name, chemical name, and common name
2. Physical properties and chemical characteristics
3. Physical hazards (eg, flammability)
4. Health concerns and all carcinogenic properties
5. Routes of entry (eg, inhalation, ingestion, skin contact, eye contact)
6. Exposure limits
7. Precautions for handling and control measures, emergency measures
8. Contact information for a responsible party

It is sometimes helpful to obtain testing of environmental media (eg, air, water, and soil). Clinicians may sometimes collaborate with industrial hygienists, professionals who identify and evaluate exposures and exposure pathways in various media. Although industrial hygienists are traditionally focused on occupational settings, finding an industrial hygienist who has experience in nonoccupational settings may be helpful when evaluating an affected child (see Chapter 7). An industrial hygienist may initiate sampling of environmental media and will advise on timing and collecting environmental samples. Although many chemical contaminants can be measured in various environmental media, very few of these are actually measured in body fluids or tissues in a clinical service laboratory. Some of these chemical contaminants are, however, measured from body fluids and tissues in environmental health research laboratories, such as the one at the National Center for Environmental Health at the Centers for Disease Control and Prevention in Atlanta.[4]

ASSESSMENT OF A CHILD WITH AN ENVIRONMENTALLY RELATED DISORDER BEFORE ORDERING LABORATORY TESTS

It is important to take an environmental history when assessing children with problems including headaches, recurrent abdominal pain, sleep disturbance, asthma, allergies, and neurodevelopmental issues. This history will help the pediatrician to decide whether to request a laboratory test or tests related to an environmental exposure. Questions include:

- What is the health problem?
- Could the problem be related an environmental exposure?
- If so, what is the potential exposure?
- Did the potential exposure occur before the health problem appeared?
- Are laboratory tests available that will help to document the exposure?
- Will the laboratory measurements correlate with toxicity?
- Are there concurrent exposures or concurrent health conditions that may be related to the identified health problem?

WHEN SHOULD A LABORATORY TEST BE ORDERED IN THE INVESTIGATION OF A POTENTIAL EXPOSURE?

The pediatrician should pursue laboratory testing if the clinical picture suggests an environmental exposure and a relevant standardized laboratory test is available that will help to determine appropriate therapy. When a child presents with headache, carbon monoxide exposure should be considered in the differential diagnosis, for example, if the headaches occur in the morning and the child sleeps in a basement bedroom near the furnace. A carboxyhemoglobin level (COHb) should be measured if carbon monoxide poisoning is suspected. Clinicians who evaluate children for neurodevelopmental disorders should consider having the blood lead concentration measured.[5]

Laboratory test selection and results are influenced by absorption (through all routes), metabolism, and elimination of the environmental agent or chemical; the duration of the exposure; and the timeframe since exposure ceased, if it has. Some toxic chemicals can be measured directly in body fluids; however, the total amount of the substance that may be present in the child is not necessarily determined by testing certain body fluids. For example, a blood lead concentration determines the amount of lead circulating in the child's blood following an exposure and may remain elevated for a few weeks or years once the child is removed from the exposure, depending on the cumulative exposure dose. Following an acute exposure, a child's blood lead is redistributed to achieve equilibrium with lead in bones and soft tissues. Most of the body stores of lead are in bones (70%), where it is difficult to measure. Bone x-ray fluorescence measurements, if available, would be a more accurate reflection of the true body burden or internal dose of the substance but have no clinical utility. Arsenic, which is cleared from the blood in a few hours, can be measured in the urine as it is excreted within 1 to 2 days following absorption through the respiratory or gastrointestinal systems. Urine arsenic is considered a reliable indicator of recent exposures; however, interpretation for low-dose exposure is currently not established.

Before ordering any test, it is wise for the pediatrician to communicate with a laboratory clinical consultant or an environmental health expert to discuss test selection, specimen collection, laboratory analysis, and interpretation.

THE CLINICAL SERVICE LABORATORY

Laboratories that conduct tests used for clinical purposes require ongoing quality control and formal accreditation. Research laboratories may have the capability to measure a large number of chemicals, but most research laboratories are not accredited to perform clinical tests or to interpret them. Medical laboratories must have reliable processing and quality control, certification, and efficient reporting of results. All laboratories in the United States (including research laboratories) that perform diagnostic testing on human materials must have government certifications. For Clinical Laboratory Improvement Amendments (CLIA)[6] certification (the minimum requirement for laboratory operation), trace elemental laboratories must comply with regulations for proficiency testing, quality control, quality assurance, patient test management, personnel, certification, and inspections. Many laboratories seek additional accreditation from laboratory professional accrediting organizations, such as the College of American Pathologists.[7]

Reliable toxicologic evaluation of body fluids requires planning. Correct specimens need to be taken (eg, spot urine, 24-hour urine, blood test). The collection facility and staff need to be ready and aware of special containers and appropriate timing of special specimen collection after exposure to allow for adequate processing time in the laboratory (eg, reliable COHb assessment requires collection of blood immediately after exposure, because concentrations within the body fall very quickly once a patient is exposed to oxygen or air). Accurate collection of specimens as well as their immediate processing is necessary if valid results are expected. Collected samples may undergo changes in the specimen container or deteriorate overnight. If testing is not available locally, correct transportation of specimens needs to be ensured. Certain metals (eg, mercury, arsenic, cadmium, aluminum, copper, selenium) can be measured through their excretion in the urine and results are more accurate if a 24-hour urine collection, rather than a single urine sample, is analyzed. For arsenic testing, seafood should be avoided for 3 days before testing, because seafood may contain organic arsenic, which is nontoxic but may contribute to the total arsenic concentration.

PARENTS MAY REQUEST INTERPRETATION OF UNUSUAL TESTS

Parents may bring to the pediatrician's office results of laboratory testing performed at great cost in an accredited laboratory. Interpretation of these results is difficult, because there are many laboratories performing tests without accreditation, and the results often cannot be validated. Reference ranges for certain chemical substances may not be available. In this case, laboratories may set their own reference ranges, which may vary between laboratories depending on the standards used—for example, laboratory detection limit, which is lowest amount measured; normal range, which is the range in which 95% of healthy subjects fall; or population reference range, which indicates the test value expected from the usual exposure in daily life or background level in the population. Some laboratories may use the toxic threshold (ie, the lowest level at which adverse health effects are expected). Hence, significant room for confusion exists when interpreting the test results. If test results are not consistent with the clinical assessment, the pediatrician needs to review and assess the child again.

Assessing and interpreting body burdens of chemical contaminants in children's bodies is difficult and currently very limited.

HAIR TESTING

Although certain substances (eg, methyl mercury) can be tested in hair,[8] this testing is primarily a research procedure and currently cannot be used reliably when clinically assessing individual patients. Potential external contamination (eg, shampoo, hair coloring agents, or airborne pollutants) may alter test results.

Frequently Asked Questions

Q *Chemical X was measured in my child's blood, and I have been given a result. I am told that chemical X is a carcinogen. Does this mean my child will get cancer?*

A No. More than 300 environmental chemicals can be measured in human body fluids. These environmental chemicals may cause certain toxic effects, including cancer. The human body has many mechanisms to prevent cancer. The process of cancer development in the body involves many complex steps that occur over many years. Certain substances, such as antioxidants that are present in many fruits and vegetables, can protect the body from developing cancers. Only a small percentage of people exposed to carcinogens will get cancer. Employing healthy eating habits and avoidance of known carcinogens, especially from tobacco, will help to protect people from cancer.

Q *I paid a lot of money to have blood tests carried out on my child to identify the presence of harmful chemicals. The results showed that my child does have harmful chemicals in his body. How can I get these harmful chemicals out of my child's body?*

A In most cases, it is not necessary to take special steps to get them out. The body has methods to deactivate and remove chemicals from the body by metabolism and excretion. Furthermore, identifying and removing sources of the child's exposure to hazardous chemicals are important. You should consult with your pediatrician and, if needed, with a pediatric environmental health specialist, to determine whether your child has any health problems that might be related to the chemicals identified by laboratory testing. Be aware that many such tests are not carried out in an accredited laboratory, and reference ranges are not available. They are, therefore, not interpretable.

Q *I have heard that laboratories will measure many harmful chemicals in my child's blood. Can you order all the possible tests for him?*

A No. It is not good clinical practice to orders such tests, because we do not yet know what the results mean. Interpretation of the results is not possible because of lack of available information on reference values and levels that may be linked with harmful effects. Very few chemicals can be measured and interpreted accurately.

References

1. Dong LM, Potter JD, White E, Ulrich CM, Cardon LR, Peters U. Genetic susceptibility to cancer: The role of polymorphisms in candidate genes. *JAMA*. 2008;299(20):2423-2436

2. Gao J, Shan G, Sun B, Thompson PJ, Gao X. Association between polymorphism of tumour necrosis factor alpha-308 gene promoter and asthma: a meta-analysis. *Thorax*. 2006;61(6): 466-471

3. Irigaray P, Newby JA, Clapp R, et al. Lifestyle-related factors and environmental agents causing cancer: an overview. *Biomed Pharmacother*. 2007;61(10):640-658

4. Centers for Disease Control and Prevention. *Fourth National Report on Human Exposure to Environmental Chemicals*. Atlanta (GA): Centers for Disease Control and Prevention; 2009. Available at: http://www.cdc.gov/exposurereport/. Accessed February 17, 2011

5. Hussain J, Woolf AD, Sandel M, Shannon MW. Environmental evaluation of a child with developmental disability. *Pediatr Clin North Am*. 2007;54(1):47-62

6. Hoffman HE, Buka I, Phillips S. Medical laboratory investigation of children's environmental health. *Pediatr Clin North Am*. 2007;54(2):399-415

7. College of American Pathologists. Available at www.cap.org. Accessed February 17, 2011

8. Agency for Toxic Substances and Disease Registry. *Hair Analysis Panel Discussion. Summary report: hair analysis panel discussion: exploring the state of the science*. Atlanta, GA: Agency for Toxic Substances and Disease Registry; December 2001. Page VII. Available at: http://www.atsdr.cdc. gov/HEC/CSEM/pcb/lab_tests.html. Accessed February 17, 2011

Chapter 7

Environmental Measurements

■ ■ ■ ■ ■ ■

This chapter provides an overview of evaluation tools used to measure environmental exposures—including contaminants in air, water, soil, and dust—to better equip pediatricians to address environmental exposure questions, request exposure characterization surveys, and evaluate exposure monitoring results. A basic understanding of environmental measurements helps clinicians to understand when and how exposure monitoring is important to case management, including prevention of future exposure. Examples include measuring formaldehyde that volatilizes ("off-gasses") in a mobile home, heating oil that contaminates rural drinking well water, and lead dust that results from home renovation.

Although a clinician may suspect that a patient's diagnosis is attributable to an environmental exposure, acting on this assumption may be hampered by insufficient exposure information. In some cases, an exposure of concern may be identified through the environmental exposure history (Chapter 5). In other cases, the exposure information is vague because of lack of understanding of the complex array of potential environmental exposures, such as chemicals with no odor or other warning properties. In addition, a physician/patient/parent may be influenced by his or her belief system, media reports, or anxiety. The absence of exposure monitoring data limits the pediatrician's ability to attribute an illness to an environmental exposure. Testing of the home, child care setting, school, or other sites can identify important exposures and enhance clinical care.

Biological monitoring tests, such as measurements in urine or blood, which characterize absorbed dose, may confirm an exposure suspicion (see Chapter 6). Biological tests are useful, because they integrate all routes of exposure (ingestion, inhalation, dermal absorption, transplacental). Unfortunately, biological monitoring tests are available for only a limited number of environmental toxicants, reference values frequently do not exist for children, and adult reference values are difficult to extrapolate to children. In addition, a biological test result does not provide insight into the relative importance of different sources of exposure when multiple sources are present. For example, an elevated blood lead level could result from exposure to sources including household paint dust, drinking water, or "take-home" exposure resulting from a parent's occupation. Identifying the significant sources of exposure is important for intervention and prevention efforts.

A clinician may be asked to comment on exposure monitoring results. Parents may expect their pediatrician to understand environmental exposure assessment reports, to interpret results, and to assess the child health risks associated with measured exposures. A clinician may also be asked to comment on the need for costly exposure mitigation interventions or postremediation clearance sampling. Parents may seek guidance about when it is safe for a child to return to a remediated environment. In some instances, however, insufficient exposure information may limit the development of an exposure reduction plan to prevent future exposures.

ENVIRONMENTAL EXPOSURE EVALUATION

Several methods are available to measure chemical exposures in the environment.

Environmental Monitoring and Reference Values

Collecting, analyzing, and interpreting environmental measurements in the absence of standardized exposure evaluation methods and health-based reference values are frequently problematic and not recommended in the clinical setting. Published research protocols may describe sample collection and analysis methods. Without standardization, however, results from one laboratory may not be comparable to results from another. Further, the accuracy of the results may vary from batch to batch even at the same laboratory. Once exposure data exist, there may be significant momentum to interpret the data and provide a health risk message. In the absence of established reference values, interpretation of sample results is fraught with difficulty. The interpretation may vary from expert to expert, and the published literature may provide a limited framework for developing an interpretation. Even when health reference values exist, emerging research may modify the exposure interpretation framework.

The Toxicological Profiles produced by the Agency for Toxic Substances and Disease Registry (ATSDR) include a comprehensive list of regulations and advisories in each substance-specific profile (http://www.atsdr.cdc.gov/toxprofiles/index.asp). Profiles exist for approximately 175 common environmental contaminants. The regulations section includes a listing of regulations and guidelines for contaminants in air, water, soil, and food from a variety of organizations including the World Health Organization (WHO), the International Agency for Research on Cancer (IARC), the Occupational Safety and Health Administration (OSHA), the US Environmental Protection Agency (EPA), the US Food and Drug Administration (FDA), and the American Conference of Governmental Industrial Hygienists. Reference values and exposure results may be reported in mass or parts per million units. Table 7.1 provides information about units used to measure liquid, solid, and air concentrations.

Material Safety Data Sheets

For products used in work settings, chemical manufacturers are required by the Occupational Safety and Health Administration to create material safety data sheets (MSDSs). Material safety data sheets are health and safety information sheets that identify the hazardous chemical ingredients present at ≥1% of the formulation (except carcinogens that must be identified if present at ≥0.1%). Material safety data sheets also describe health hazard information, including signs and symptoms of exposure and health problems associated with exposure, routes of exposure, regulatory limits, and other information. Asthma triggers, such as fragrance chemicals, however, may not be listed on the material safety data sheets if they are present in concentrations <1%. In addition, manufacturers may classify some ingredients as proprietary; disclosure of these ingredients is only possible through a regulatory mechanism of the Occupational Safety and Health Administration.

Material safety data sheets are frequently available for household products, including cleaning agents, paints, stains, adhesives, and pesticides. The National Library of Medicine Household Products Database (see resource list) provides material safety data sheet information for hundreds of household products. Material safety data sheets are also frequently available online at the product manufacturer's Web page or by directly contacting the product manufacturer or a local supplier.

Environmental Consultants

Interpreting environmental monitoring data may require involving a knowledgeable and experienced professional who can help to correctly identify the exposure, select the correct monitoring method and sampling plan, ensure correct timing of the sampling, and interpret results. Industrial hygienists are trained in the anticipation, identification, evaluation, and control of chemical, physical, and biological hazards in work, residential, or other settings. Industrial hygienists incorporate all potential routes of exposure in an exposure evaluation. They have expertise in sample collection and analytical methods, interpretation of results, and exposure control, reduction, and remediation strategies. During environmental health investigations, hygienists use visual, olfactory, and other sensory clues

Table 7.1: Units Used for Environmental Samples

MATRIX	PARTS PER MILLION (ppm)	PARTS PER BILLION (ppb)
Soil, house dust, or other solid	ppm = mg of contaminant/kg of solid matrix 1 ppm = 1 mg/kg = 1 µg/g 1000 ppm = 1 mg/g 1% = 10 000 ppm 1 ppm = 1000 ppb	ppb = µg/kg of solid matrix 1 ppb = 1 µg/kg = 1 nanogram (ng)/g 1000 ppb = 1 µg/g 1 ppb = 1000 ppt (parts per trillion)
Water or liquid	ppm = mg of contaminant/L of liquid matrix 1 ppm = 1 mg/L = 1 µg/mL 1% = 10 000 ppm 1 ppm = 1000 ppb	ppb = µg/L of matrix 1 ppb = 1 µg/L 1 ppb = 1000 ppt
Air	ppm = one part of the chemical in one million parts of air ppm to mg/m³ conversion: Y mg/m³ = (X ppm) (molecular weight of substance) ÷ 24.45 mg/m³ to ppm conversion: X ppm = (Y mg/m³) (24.45) ÷ (molecular weight) 1% = 10 000 ppm 0.001 ppm = 1 ppb = 1000 parts per trillion (ppt)	ppb = one part of the chemical in one billion parts of air ppb to µg/m³ conversion: Y µg/m³ = (X ppb) (molecular weight) ÷ 24.45 µg/m³ to ppb conversion: X ppb = (Y µg/m³) (24.45) ÷ (molecular weight) 1% = 10 000 ppm 0.001 ppm = 1 ppb = 1000 ppt

as well as occupants' symptoms. Although the field of industrial hygiene historically has focused on occupational settings, the exposure evaluation framework also applies to environmental exposures relevant to children. Other environmental science professionals may also have the qualifications necessary to effectively evaluate pediatric environmental exposures.

OUTDOOR POLLUTANTS

Outdoor (ambient) air pollution is monitored by the EPA in partnership with state governments. As described in Chapter 21, air pollutants that are monitored include: ozone, particulate matter, lead, sulfur oxide compounds (SO_x), nitrogen oxide compounds (NO_x), carbon monoxide (CO), and approximately 185 other toxic chemicals associated with small and large industrial facilities, vehicle emissions, and other sources. Using these data in the context of individual patient care can be difficult, because the patient may live some distance from the nearest monitoring station, and local factors, such as prevailing winds and geography, may limit the applicability of the data to an individual. When industrial site emissions are of interest, it may be useful to contact the state agency responsible for air quality to learn whether monitoring data are available.

Although the EPA Emergency Planning and Community Right-to-Know Act requires the EPA's Toxics Release Inventory (TRI) Program to disclose toxic chemicals that are stored and/or released to the air, water, and land, the law is primarily designed to aid response planning in the event of a chemical spill or release. As such, disclosure is based on quantities stored or released and not on ambient air concentrations, so the utility and specificity of the data for health care are limited. It is difficult to use the Toxics Release Inventory to address concerns regarding chronic, low-dose exposures associated with industrial emissions. Although a chemical release report can be generated by zip code (http://www.epa.gov/triexplorer), the information is not specific enough for use in patient care, except under extreme release circumstances. The EPA National Air Toxics Assessments program used the Toxics Release Inventory, state and local pollution inventories, and other databases to model median outdoor concentrations of approximately 90 toxic air pollutants in 1999 (http://www.epa. gov/ttn/atw/nata1999/mapconc99.html).

It is possible to characterize chemicals associated with industrial or other pollution sources when the chemicals have established analytical methods and reference standards for community exposures. Methods used to measure industrial chemical pollutants may not be applicable to measure community exposures that are typically orders of magnitude lower than occupational exposures. In addition, there are only a limited number of community exposure standards. Occupational standards are set to protect typical adults working 8 hours a day and 40 hours a week for 30 years, whereas community exposure standards are set to protect the most sensitive members of society and assume a 24-hour-a-day, 7-days-a-week, lifetime exposure pattern. In the absence of rigorous sample collection or analytical methods for contaminants found in the community at low concentrations, or in the absence of regulatory reference values, community exposure characterization is not recommended, because it is extremely difficult to interpret results in the context of individual patient care.

INDOOR POLLUTANTS

Unlike outdoor air pollution, indoor air pollution is not monitored. Indoor air pollutants include secondhand tobacco smoke (see Chapter 40), CO from combustion sources, fungal spores from mold growth, and off-gassing from construction materials and furnishings (see Chapter 20). Industrial air or groundwater pollutants may also affect indoor air quality by infiltration of outdoor air pollutants indoors and by infiltration of toxicants from contaminated plumes located below structures in which children spend time. Commonly used methods to characterize airborne chemical exposures include using meters with digital displays ("direct-read instruments"), colorimetric chemical detector tubes, or sampling pumps with specialized sample media. Table 7.2 summarizes the approach to measuring airborne contaminants and the approximate costs.

Direct-read instruments are available for a variety of contaminants and provide immediate information about contaminant concentration. For example, CO meters are commonly used by fire departments to evaluate furnaces and other combustion sources. Some instruments "datalog" or can measure and record contaminant concentrations for selected averaging windows (seconds, minutes, or hours) over an extended period of time (days to weeks). Datalogging provides average, maximum, and minimum exposure data and provides an opportunity to correlate events (eg, window cleaning) in time with contaminant "spikes" (eg, ammonia, butyl Cellosolve [a chemical used in cleaning agents]) in the recorded data, which may be useful in identifying contaminant sources. Although typically rented by trained professionals, these instruments are available to the public and generally include instruction manuals. Rental costs vary depending on type of equipment and duration of the rental.

Color diffusion or dosimeter tubes are available for some chemicals (gases and vapors) and a box of ten tubes generally costs less than $100. Passive color tubes, the size of a small pen, rely on air diffusion to move the contaminant of interest through the medium. As the contaminant reacts with the material inside the tube, a color change occurs and the length of the colored stain is read using the scale printed on the outside of the glass tube. The user must carefully follow directions because the calibrated scale is based on the duration of sampling. With an error margin of ±25%, passive colorimetric tubes are useful screening tools for contaminants. Care must be taken when selecting a

Table 7.2: Airborne Contaminants Measurement Approach and Cost

AIRBORNE CONTAMINANT	RECOMMENDED METHODS AND COMMENTS	APPROXIMATE COST
Carbon monoxide (furnace or other combustion source)	If carbon monoxide exposure is suspected, vacate the premises immediately and contact the local fire department Passive or active (with hand pump) colorimetric tube with level of detection <5 ppm	<$100/box of 10 passive or active tubes Pump $425 (rental <$60/wk) Consultant $300+
Mercury (elemental)	Direct read instrument needed Contact local fire department, local health department, or hire a professional A single CFL or mercury thermometer break usually does not require testing as long as proper clean-up guidelines are followed	Local government resources, if available, likely no cost Consultant $1000+
Radon	Work with state or local health department or private laboratory Use a radon air test kit	<$30
Lead or asbestos clearance samples	Hire a professional	>$200
Indoor mold and mold-related concerns	Hire a professional	>$1200 (depends on number of samples collected)
Gasoline vapor fingerprint, heating oil vapor	Hire a professional and/or contact local department of ecology or department of health Passive thermal desorption tube Summa canister	Professional >$1000 Passive tube >$400 Summa canister $250

continued on page 70

continued from page 69

Table 7.2: Airborne Contaminants Measurement Approach and Cost, *continued*

AIRBORNE CONTAMINANT	RECOMMENDED METHODS AND COMMENTS	APPROXIMATE COST
Fungal mycotoxins	Sampling not recommended Sample collection and analysis methods not standardized Consensus reference levels not established Research method — not readily available commercially	NA
Allergens (dust mites, cat, dog, bird, insects, rodent, etc.)	Sampling not recommended Sample collection and analysis methods not standardized Consensus reference levels not established Research method — not readily available commercially	NA

ppm indicates parts per million; CFL, compact fluorescent light; NA, not applicable.

specific tube, as many colorimetric tubes are designed for industrial settings with higher contaminant concentrations. To select a tube, the contaminant concentration should first be estimated by reviewing community air standards or results in published papers and then carefully checking the tube concentration ranges available to determine whether the detection range is appropriate for the situation. Ozone and CO are 2 examples of chemicals for which concentrations may be measured using colorimetric tubes.

Characterizing formaldehyde or organic vapors in indoor air requires using passive samplers. Samples are passively collected and then must be submitted to a laboratory for analysis. Passive sampler costs are higher, starting at $50/sampler (not including laboratory costs) for formaldehyde and higher for other organic vapors.

Active color diffusion tube samples are collected by using a calibrated hand pump ($425 purchase cost or <$60/wk rental) in conjunction with a colorimetric tube (<$100/box of 10). Because a higher volume of air is sampled, active sampling colorimetric tubes are available with lower levels of detection than passive colorimetric systems.

Colorimetric tubes, passive samplers, or direct-read instruments are not available for many environmental contaminants. In these cases, an industrial hygienist or another environmental specialist is needed to measure contaminant levels. Sample collection involves using a small air pump that pulls air at a defined rate through filters or sorbent tubes in which the contaminant of interest is concentrated for analysis. When validated methods exist, this approach provides very accurate measurements in the lower concentration ranges expected in residential, school, or other environments in which children spend time. Evaluation costs typically start at $1000 and include the consultant's time, sampling equipment, laboratory costs for sample analysis, and a written report including an interpretation of the results.

Mold

Environmental evaluation for molds is common and typically includes a careful indoor and outdoor inspection for visible mold growth, water damage, conditions conducive to water intrusion, and the presence of musty odors. Although visual inspection is often sufficient to identify problematic mold growth contributing to poor indoor air quality, air, wipe, tape-lift, and/or bulk samples are frequently collected and analyzed for molds and related indoor pollutants. If an inspection reveals extensive visible mold growth and/or damp indoor spaces, the water infiltration and/or moisture problems require correction and mold remediation is recommended. Extensive sampling to identify specific mold species or count spores is usually not required, except in the context of a research investigation.

Characterization of mold exposure and interpretation of results generally require the assistance of a trained professional, such as a certified industrial hygienist. The cost of a residential or building evaluation starts at approximately $1200 and increases significantly depending on the number of samples collected. Home test kits, such as "settle plates," are not recommended, because the sample results are highly variable, difficult to interpret, and often inaccurate. Sampling in extremely contaminated areas may require use of respiratory protection and adherence to other safety precautions and may present a hazard to building occupants if not performed appropriately.

Air Sample Collection

Two common air sample collection methods are the culturable or "viable" method and the spore trap method that counts both viable and nonviable spores. With viable samples, a known volume of air is directed toward a nutrient medium that is then incubated for a specified period of time. Mold colonies are identified and enumerated by a skilled microscopist. Results are reported in colony-forming units per cubic meter of air sampled (CFU/m^3). The main advantage of viable sampling is the enhanced ability to identify some mold colonies. However, viable sampling underrepresents the airborne mold population, because it does not detect nonviable spores, which may have toxic or allergenic properties.

With nonviable or spore-trap methodology, spores and other particulates are collected by directing a known volume of air onto a sticky surface, which is then analyzed. The spores, fibers, pollen, dander, skin cells, and other particulates are identified and enumerated by a skilled microscopist. Results are reported as the number of spores, fibers, or other particulates per m^3 of air sampled. Important spore-trap advantages are: (1) both fresh viable and old, nonviable spores are counted providing a more accurate representation of total exposure; (2) nonfungal particles (eg, skin cells, fiberglass, and pollens) that can contribute to poor indoor environment quality can be identified and counted; and (3) spore chains, which indicate an active growth site nearby, can be identified. Nonviable sampling identifies mold spores by their morphology; because some molds have similar appearances, identification is less precise than with the viable method. For example, *Penicillium* and *Aspergillus* molds can not be differentiated by this method.

Air samples are collected in problem indoor locations and, as a comparison location, outdoors. Sometimes samples are also collected in nonproblem indoor locations to provide additional comparison information. Comparison samples should be collected within hours of the samples collected in problem locations. Use of an accredited environmental microbiology laboratory is recommended to analyze all mold samples. Environmental Microbiology Laboratory Accreditation Program (EMLAP) laboratories have met rigorous performance standards as defined by the American Industrial Hygiene Association.

Bulk, Swab, and Tape-Lift Samples

Bulk, swab, and tape-lift samples provide surface mold information. Bulk samples are collected from areas with visible mold growth. A sample the size of a dime or smaller of moldy drywall or other material, or a chunk of the mold, is submitted and identified via microscopy. Swab samples are collected by wiping a surface with a moistened, sterile swab. The material is then cultured and identified. Clear adhesive tape is gently pushed against the surface of interest in tape-lift sample collection. The tape is then placed on a standard glass microscope slide for direct microscopic examination.

Mold Results Interpretation

Interpreting mold monitoring data is challenging. There are no state or federal regulatory levels or consensus guidelines that define mold counts indicative of indoor mold growth (or "amplification") or mold exposure problems. Thus, experienced professionals may arrive at different conclusions regarding the likelihood of an indoor mold source when interpreting the same data.[1] The most common "rule" of air sample interpretation is to compare specific mold colony or spore counts in problem indoor locations to the mold colony or spore counts outdoors and/or to the counts in nonproblem indoor locations. Outdoor counts generally are higher than indoor counts and typically reflect the same mix of molds. Generally, as the indoor count exceeds and dwarfs the outdoor count for a specific mold, the likelihood of a mold amplification problem increases. However, mold growth is also possible if the problem area count is higher than expected for that type of mold, or if a specific mold dominates the indoor sample count but does not dominate the comparison location(s) count. Because of the complexities of mold monitoring, exceptions to the rule are common. Interpretation is aided by knowledge of the unique characteristics of each mold identified, such as how frequently it is identified and typical concentrations outdoors and in damp environments, moisture requirements for growth, common growth substrates, and ease of spore generation.

Mold spore release is highly variable.[2] Repeated fungal bioaerosol measurements can vary by orders of magnitude over the course of one day.[3] This is compounded by the fact that sample collection duration is ≤15 minutes. This is in sharp contrast to the 8- or 24-hour (or longer) sampling approach used to characterize chemical concentrations in the environment. In addition, 1 or, at most, 2 samples are collected at each location during a typical survey, which is insufficient to capture within- and between-day mold spore variability. Seasonal spore release variability is also important.[4] In addition, certain genera of mold spores or bacteria may be present in the air but not compete well on the nutrient media selected for the survey, which is why they may be found infrequently despite their presence.[5]

Bulk Sample Interpretation

The utility of bulk, swab, and tape-lift samples is limited, as there are no regulatory reference values or comparison sample locations (such as an outdoor air sample). Swab and tape-lift samples may be collected on surfaces cleaned frequently, reflecting recent spore deposition, and are useful for clearance sampling. Swabs and tape lifts from rarely cleaned reservoirs, such as the tops of door jambs, reflect deposition over an unknown period of time (months, years), which limits the utility of the information. Samples collected in ducted heating, air conditioning, and ventilation systems can be very useful, as these systems can be effective collectors as well as disseminators of bioaerosols associated with indoor environment contamination.

Radon

The EPA recommends that all homes be tested for radon using an air test kit; more information can be found in Chapter 39.

Lead in Paint, Dust, and Soil

Potential residential lead hazards, described in Chapter 31, include interior and exterior paint, household dust, outdoor soil, lead-glazed pottery, toys and other household items, drinking water (addressed below), spices, and herbal remedies. Soil, water, paint chips, household dust, and other materials can be tested for lead for less than $50 per sample by a lead-accredited analytical laboratory. Some states offer lead programs to aid sample collection and analysis for homeowners.

Paint samples are relatively easy to collect if the paint is chipping, peeling, or damaged. Samples must contain all paint layers down to the wood, because lead is often found in the older layers and not in the top layers. As an alternative, a direct-reading x-ray fluorescence (XRF) analyzer can be used. Portable x-ray fluorescence scanners use nondestructive methods to detect lead in paint independent of the thickness or composition of the various layers of paint. They can also be used to test toys and other surfaces; accuracy of x-ray fluorescence use for these purposes is under examination. X-ray fluorescence scanners require use by trained and experienced technicians, as the instruments contain a radioactive source.

Surface wipe samples are used to characterize the lead content in settled household dust and also to verify that lead containment or lead dust clean-up efforts were effective. Wipe samples should be collected and analyzed by parties independent of the renovation or remediation contractors who did the work. Sample collection involves donning gloves, wiping a 4 inch^2 (10 cm^2) area (using tape or a template to delineate the area) with a wipe moistened with distilled water, and placing the wipe in the sealed container provided by an analytical laboratory (see National Institute of Occupational Safety and Health, lead in

surface wipe sampling method at http://www.cdc.gov/Niosh/nmam/pdfs/9100.
pdf). Settled dust samples may be collected from floors and window sills and
troughs, as reference values exist for those locations (Table 7.3). Lead surface test
kits, which include wipes, sealed containers, distilled water, and gloves, are available from some lead-accredited laboratories.

Soil testing methods are described in detail (http://player-care.com/lead_
handbk-2a.pdf). To reduce costs, individual samples can be combined into a
composite sample. Comparison values are included in Table 7.3.

To better ensure that laboratory test results are accurate, it is essential to
use a lead-accredited laboratory. The EPA maintains a list by state of currently
accredited laboratories (http://www.epa.gov/lead/pubs/nllaplist.pdf), which
includes those participating in the National Lead Laboratory Accreditation
Program. Accredited laboratories participate in periodic performance evaluations, including proficiency testing. Some states also operate parallel lead and
other laboratory accreditation programs, so additional accredited laboratories
may be available in a particular region. Some states operate an environmental
laboratory that accepts samples from the public. Sample collection kits are available from many laboratories and include sample collection directions, sample
containers and sample handling procedures.

Home lead test kits to detect lead in paint, dust, soil, jewelry, vinyl and other
surfaces are not recommended for use by lay people. Although readily available in hardware stores, research has shown these test kit results are inaccurate, because interfering substances can cause false-negative and false-positive
results.[6,7] The EPA has, however, recognized 3 lead paint test kits when used by
professionals. The EPA maintains a list of these recognized kits and describes
test kit limitations (http://www.epa.gov/lead/pubs/testkit.htm).

DRINKING WATER

Drinking water testing requires collection of a water sample for submission to
an accredited laboratory for analysis. The EPA Web portal (http://water.epa.gov/
scitech/drinkingwater/labcert/index.cfm) lists accredited laboratories in specific
areas. In some states, this search tool can be used to identify all laboratories
accredited to analyze environmental samples. Accredited laboratories must meet
performance standards, including proficiency testing, which help to ensure that
test results are accurate. People interested in testing water are advised to choose
an analytical laboratory that provides sample collection kits, which include
sample collection directions, containers (including pretreated containers and/or
sample preservatives), sample storage and transport guidelines, and other information to ensure the accuracy of analytical results. For example, lead testing requires
acid-washed containers, and nitrate testing requires a preservative. Except for
postage, sample collection kits are typically included in the analysis cost.

Table 7.3: Lead Standards

LEADED MATERIAL	STANDARD	REFERENCE
Lead-based paint definition	> 1.0 mg lead/cm² (XRF) or > 0.5% lead by weight (lab analysis of paint chip)	EPA TSCA 403[a]
Dust-lead hazard definition	40 µg/ft² of floor (wipe samples) 250 µg/ft² interior window sills (wipe samples)	EPA TSCA 403 40 CFR Part 745[a] HUD 35-1320
Lead abatement clearance requirements	40 µg/ft² of floor (wipe samples) 250 µg/ft² interior window sills 400 µg/ft² window wells	EPA TSCA 403 40 CFR Part 745[a]
Outside soil	400 ppm lead in bare soil in a child's play area 1200 ppm lead in bare soil in the rest of the yard	EPA TSCA 403 40 CFR Part 745[a]
Residential drinking water	Standing and running water sample Action level: 0.015 mg/L = 15 ppb	Safe Drinking Water Act Lead and Copper Rule, 56 FR 26460b
School drinking water (local standards may be lower)	Standing and running water sample Action level: 0.020 mg/L = 20 ppb	Safe Drinking Water Act Lead and Copper Rule, 56 FR 26460b

XRF indicates x-ray fluorescence; TSCA, Toxic Substances Control Act; ppm, parts per million; ppb, parts per billion.
[a] http://www.epa.gov/lead/pubs/leadhaz.htm
[b] http://www.epa.gov/safewater/standard/index.html

If local plumbing-related contaminants are the concern, standing and running water samples are collected at a high-use location, such as the kitchen sink. Drinking water contaminant reference values are available at http://www.epa.gov/safewater/contaminants/index.html.

Public utilities must test sources of drinking water for a wide variety of contaminants. Well and source water contaminants also can be characterized by an analytical laboratory. Analytical costs for inorganic and other contaminants such as nitrate, nitrite, fluoride, metals, and bacteria are less than $50/test. Costs to characterize individual organic compounds ("fingerprinting") are higher, ranging from $60 to $200 per chemical to quantify trihalomethanes, gasoline, heating oil, synthetic organic compounds, or pesticides; costs are potentially higher for other compounds. Tests for radon in drinking water are approximately $50 per test. Table 7.4 summarizes the approach to measuring drinking water contaminants as well as the approximate costs.

TESTING OF DIETARY SUPPLEMENTS, SPICES, COSMETICS, AND FOOD PESTICIDES

Herbal remedies, dietary supplements, spices, candy, other food items, and cosmetics can be tested for metals such as lead or mercury, pesticides, and other contaminants. A local accredited laboratory will be able to provide guidance regarding pricing, sample collection, and submission. Table 7.5 summarizes the approach to measuring contaminants in dietary supplements, spices, etc, and lists approaches to measuring other contaminants as well as the approximate costs.

Frequently Asked Questions

Q   *Our home is being remodeled and the contractor is in the final steps of finishing the project. We recently learned that homes like ours, built before 1978, are likely to contain lead-based paint. What should we do before we move our children back into our home?*

A   Discuss your lead dust exposure concern with your renovation contractor. Starting in April 2010, the EPA required certification of contractors in lead-safe work practices to prevent lead dust contamination during renovation, repair, or painting activities in homes, schools, and child care facilities built before 1978. The rule requires the contractor to apply methods to limit the dispersal of dust during work and leave a work site that has passed a visually clean reference standard comparing a wipe sample to a picture of a reference standard. Evaluations of the sensitivity of this method are underway. Individual states may apply more stringent standards that require surface dust wipe samples to be collected and analyzed in a laboratory. If wipe samples results exceed the EPA 40 $\mu g/ft^2$ floor or 250 $\mu g/ft^2$ interior window sill standards, further cleaning is necessary using a high-efficiency

Table 7.4: Drinking Water Contaminants Measurement Approach and Cost

CONTAMINANT	RECOMMENDED ACTION AND COMMENTS	APPROXIMATE COST
Lead, cadmium, copper, iron, other heavy metals Arsenic (well water) Nitrates	Work with county, state, or private lab to obtain sampling kit to include sample collection instructions, container, and storage/shipping instructions	<$50
Radon	Work with county, state, or private lab to obtain sampling kit to include sample collection instructions, container, and storage/shipping instructions	<$50
Microbiological	Work with county, state, or private lab to obtain sampling kit to include sample collection instructions, container, and storage/shipping instructions	$20
Organic chemicals: Gasoline fingerprint Heating oil fingerprint Trihalomethanes Chloramines	Work with county, state, or private lab to obtain sampling kit to include sample collection instructions, container, and storage/shipping information	>$60 depending on organic compound
Pesticides	Work with county, state, or private lab to obtain sampling kit to include sample collection instructions, container, and storage/shipping information	$70–$200 for common pesticides

Table 7.5: Miscellaneous Contaminants Measurement Approach and Cost

CONTAMINANT	RECOMMENDED ACTION	APPROXIMATE COST
Lead, mercury, other heavy metals in spices, alternative medicines, teas, or herbal remedies	Work with county, state, or private lab to obtain sampling kit to include sample collection instructions, container, and storage/shipping information	<$50
Suspected asbestos-containing material	Hire a professional	>$200
Pesticide residues on food, grass, play equipment, toys	Work with county, state, or private lab to obtain sampling kit to include sample collection instructions, container, and storage/shipping information	$150
Contaminants in fish: mercury, PCBs, DDT	Sampling not recommended Check for local fish advisories For patients frequently consuming fish meals, check EPA and other fish testing databases for contaminant levels in relevant waterways	NA
PCBs, dioxin, PBDEs in human milk	Sampling generally not recommended except for exceptional exposures Laboratory methods not standardized Consensus reference levels not established Research method—not readily available commercially.	NA

continued on page 80

continued from page 79

Table 7.5: Miscellaneous Contaminants Measurement Approach and Cost, *continued*

CONTAMINANT	RECOMMENDED ACTION	APPROXIMATE COST
Fungal mycotoxins in dust	Sampling not recommended Sample collection and analysis methods not standardized Consensus reference levels not established Research method—not readily available commercially	NA
Allergens (dust mites, cat, dog, bird, insects, rodent) in dust	Sampling not recommended Sample collection and analysis methods not standardized Consensus reference levels not established Research method—not readily available commercially	NA
Endocrine disrupters: bisphenol A, phthalates in food or water from plastic storage containers	Sampling not recommended Sample collection and analysis methods not standardized Consensus reference levels not established Research method—not readily available commercially	NA

PCBs indicates polychlorinated biphenyls; NA, not applicable; DDT, dichlorodiphenyltrichloroethane; PBDEs, polybrominated diphenyl ethers

particulate air (HEPA) filter vacuum and by damp wiping all surfaces. When clean, additional sampling should be performed by a qualified and experienced independent contractor to verify effectiveness of the remediation and clean up. If the home has a forced-air heating system, it may be necessary to damp wipe the furnace interior and ducts. Carpet, soft furnishings, and ducts with internal duct liners can be difficult to evaluate and decontaminate and may require disposal.

Homeowners with limited financial resources could collect samples for analysis in lieu of hiring a certified professional, but should be warned that lead contamination may be unevenly distributed, so finding low concentrations in one area does not ensure low concentrations in others. The EPA Lead Renovation, Repair and Painting Web page describes the program in detail (http://www.epa.gov/lead/pubs/renovation.htm).

Asbestos may also be present in homes built before 1986 in ceiling tiles, roll vinyl or tile floor coverings, insulation, and other materials. If asbestos-containing materials are disturbed, exposure control procedures are required to prevent asbestos contamination of the home. Contact a local EPA office for more information.

Q *A compact fluorescent light (CFL) broke on a carpeted floor in our daughter's nursery 2 weeks ago. We used a vacuum to clean the mess. Should we have the air tested to determine whether there is still a mercury air problem in the nursery?*

A Air testing following breakage of CFLs is not currently recommended. Instructions on strategies to minimize mercury exposures are outlined at http://www.epa.gov/mercury/spills/#fluorescent.

Resources

Agency for Toxic Substances and Disease Registry (ATSDR) Toxicological Profiles
   http://www.atsdr.cdc.gov/toxprofiles/index.asp

EPA Accredited Laboratories
   http://www.epa.gov/lead/pubs/nllaplist.pdf

EPA Ambient PM and Ozone Web portal AIRNow
   http://airnow.gov

EPA Emergency Planning and Community Right-to-Know Act (EPCRA) Web Portal
   http://www.epa.gov/oem/content/lawsregs/epcraover.htm

EPA Fish Advisories Web page
   http://www.epa.gov/waterscience/fish/states.htm

EPA Lead Paint Test Kits for Use by Professionals
http://www.epa.gov/lead/pubs/testkit.htm

EPA Lead in Paint, Dust and Soil Web Portal
http://www.epa.gov/lead/index.html

EPA Mercury Releases and Spills
http://www.epa.gov/mercury/spills/#fluorescent

EPA Mold Site
http://www.epa.gov/mold

**EPA Mold Remediation in Schools and Commercial Buildings
(also applies to residences)**
http://www.epa.gov/mold/publications.html

EPA National Air Toxics Assessments Program
http://www.epa.gov/ttn/atw/nata1999/mapconc99.html

EPA Toxic Air Pollutants Web Portal
http://www.epa.gov/air/toxicair/newtoxics.html

**EPA Toxics Release Inventory (TRI) Program Chemical Release
Report queries**
http://www.epa.gov/triexplorer

**Maine Department of Environmental Protection Compact Fluorescent
Lamp Study**
http://www.maine.gov/dep/rwm/homeowner/cflreport.htm

**Maine Department of Environmental Protection CFL breakage clean-up
guidelines**
http://www.maine.gov/dep/rwm/homeowner/cflreport/appendixe.pdf

National Library of Medicine Household Products Database
http://householdproducts.nlm.nih.gov

SKC Comprehensive Catalog and Sampling Guide 2009
http://skcinternational.com/products/product_page_3a.asp

References

1. Johnson D, Thompson D, Clinkenbeard R, Redus J. Professional judgment and the interpretation of viable mold air sampling data. *J Occup Environ Hyg.* 2008;5(10):656-663

2. McCartney HA, Fitt BDL, Schmechel D. Sampling bioaerosols in plant pathology. *J Aerosol Sci.* 1997;28(3):349–364

3. Flannigan B. Air sampling for fungi in indoor environments. *J Aerosol Sci.* 1997;28(3):381-392

4. Chao HJ, Schwartz J, Milton DK, Burge HA. Populations and determinants of airborne fungi in large office buildings. *Environ Health Perspect.* 2002;110(8):777-782

5. Hugenholtz P, Goebel BM, Pace NR Impact of culture-independent studies on the emerging phylogenetic view of bacterial diversity. *J Bacteriol.* 1998;180(18):4765-4774

6. Cobb D, Hatlelid K, Jain B, Recht J, Saltzman LE. *Evaluation of Lead Test Kits.* Washington, DC: US Consumer Product Safety Commission; 2007

7. Rossiter WJ Jr, Vangel MG, McKnight ME, Dewalt G. *Spot Test Kits for Detecting Lead in Household Paint: A Laboratory Evaluation.* National Institute of Standards and Technology; 2000. Publication No. NISTIR 6398. Available at: http://www.fire.nist.gov/bfrlpubs/build00/PDF/b00034.pdf. Accessed February 17, 2011

Chapter 8

Preconceptional and Prenatal Exposures

■ ■ ■ ■ ■ ■

Harmful environmental exposures associated with poor health outcomes may occur to ova and sperm before fertilization (preconceptional exposures) and also in utero. Occupational and environmental risks to the fetus are becoming increasingly important as more women have entered the workforce. According to the US Department of Labor Bureau of Labor Statistics, 56.2% of women (approximately 68 million women) were employed in 2008, and 65.1% of women of reproductive age (16-44 years [approximately 39 million women]) were employed (http://www.bls.gov/cps/wlf-databook-2009.pdf). The Bureau of Labor Statistics released data demonstrating that 51.7% of mothers (1.7 million women) with children younger than 1 year were employed in 2008 (http://www.bls.gov/news.release/pdf/famee.pdf). With so many women of reproductive age employed in the workforce, preconceptional and prenatal exposures are increasingly relevant.

Preconceptional exposures of ova or sperm to environmental contaminants may lead to the development of an abnormal fetus. Additionally, a woman's exposure to contaminants may result in a delayed exposure to the developing fetus by the ongoing elimination of the chemical from the mother's body (secondary fetal exposure). Because the initial exposure is before conception, these exposures are nonconcurrent with the pregnancy. For some chemicals, such as organohalogens (eg, polychlorinated biphenyls [PCBs], which accumulate and persist in the body for many years), the fetus can be affected by nonconcurrent and concurrent maternal exposures.

Concern with prenatal exposures is based on the knowledge that there are certain periods during development—"critical windows"—when the fetus is much more vulnerable to the effects of exposures than at other times. A well-known example is the exposure to thalidomide resulting in limb-reduction defects. In addition, thalidomide exposure has been associated with a slightly higher incidence of autism spectrum disorders than expected for the general population in a retrospective observational study.[1] A period of extreme vulnerability to ionizing radiation exists from gestational age 10 to 17 weeks; exposure during this period may result in microcephaly.[2] Critical windows have not been clearly defined for most exposures. Effects (such as neurodevelopmental effects or cancer) arising from preconceptional and prenatal exposures may be latent until later in childhood, adolescence, or adulthood.

This chapter describes preconceptional and prenatal exposures and the spectrum of adverse outcomes known to be associated with parental occupational and environmental exposures. For more detail on specific agents, refer to the corresponding chapter.

PRECONCEPTIONAL EXPOSURES

Exposures to the Ovum

The ovum from which the fetus is derived develops during the early fetal life of the mother and arrests in the prophase of the cell cycle until ovulation, which may occur up to 50 years later. The notion of the vulnerability of the oocyte to environmental exposures is supported by the increasing incidence of nondisjunctional events, such as trisomy 21, with increasing maternal age,[3] suggesting that prolonged environmental exposure may be a contributing factor. Environmental contaminants that may affect the oocyte have been measured in samples of human follicular fluid (and in seminal plasma).[4]

The easiest outcome to measure is loss of fertility. Scientific evidence is sufficient to causally link maternal active smoking with delayed conception.[5] Few outcome studies on environmental exposures resulting in fertility loss or other adverse effects have been reported, however, because such transgenerational studies require a lengthy period of observation between exposure and outcome. One exception is the population of children whose mothers took diethylstilbestrol (DES) during pregnancy, because maternal DES exposure was well documented. Compared with unexposed fetuses, girls exposed to DES in utero were more likely to develop clear cell adenocarcinoma of the vagina and other adverse genital and reproductive effects. Boys were more likely to develop nonmalignant epididymal cysts. Transgenerational effects from DES exposure (effects in individuals whose grandmothers took DES during pregnancy [ie, DES grandchildren]) have also been documented. These include an increased incidence of hypospadias in DES grandsons and ovarian cancer in granddaughters.[6]

Exposures to the Sperm

In contrast to effects on ova, effects on sperm can be measured relatively easily in the next generation. There is, therefore, more scientific evidence to suggest that paternal occupational exposures before conception may constitute a risk to the fetus. Medical conditions such as obesity, exposures to ionizing radiation, and exposures to tobacco and alcohol have been related to decreased sperm counts or male infertility.[7,8] The sperm itself is vulnerable to the effects of mutagens; in its final form, the sperm has no DNA repair mechanisms. It has, therefore, been suggested that the sperm may be a vulnerable target for carcinogenesis. The association of paternal occupation with cancer risk in offspring has been extensively researched with studies reaching varying conclusions. A 2008 review of paternal exposures and childhood cancers found inconsistencies from study to study attributed, in part, to imprecision in exposure assessment, making it difficult to directly link paternal exposures with childhood cancers.[9]

Studies on the association of birth defects with paternal occupation were also reviewed and found to have many of the same limitations as studies of paternal occupation and cancer.[5,7,8] Limited evidence, however, shows associations of certain birth defects with paternal occupational exposures (eg, neural tube defects are associated with exposure to phenoxy herbicides potentially contaminated by 2,3,7,8-tetrachlorodibenzo-p-dioxin or unspecified solvents).[4,5] A 2008 study found that older fathers had a slightly increased chance of having babies with certain birth defects (eg, heart defects and tracheoesophageal fistula/esophageal atresia).[9] The same study found that paternal age younger than 25 years was also associated with a slightly increased risk of several selected birth defects in offspring; thus, the relationship of paternal age and birth defects remains unclear. The strongest association between advanced paternal age and health outcome is for achondroplasia.[10]

Secondary Fetal Exposure: Maternal Body Burden

Fetal exposure may result from ongoing excretion or mobilization of chemicals stored in the mother's body. This mobilization is sometimes termed "nonconcurrent" fetal exposure. Adipose tissue and skeletal tissue are known storage sites for various chemicals. For example, polychlorinated biphenyls (PCBs) are persistent pollutants stored in adipose tissue. Following a Taiwanese poisoning episode with PCBs, children born up to 6 years after maternal exposure had similar developmental abnormalities (developmental delays, mildly disordered behavior, and increased activity levels) as those found in children born within 1 year of maternal exposure.[11,12] The developmental delays persisted in these children at all times measured. Thus, these children had significant effects from maternal exposure to PCBs that occurred up to 6 years before their birth.

The major repository for lead is bone, where the half-life of lead is years to decades.[13] Chronic lead exposure may result in significant accumulation of lead in the skeleton. During pregnancy, calcium turnover is greatly increased, which increases mobilization of lead stores from bone.[13,14] Congenital lead poisoning because of an elevated maternal body burden was illustrated in 2 case reports of children born to women inadequately treated for childhood plumbism.[15,16] Maternal skeletal mobilization of lead is a major source of fetal exposure[14] and negatively affects a child's neurologic development.[17]

Concurrent Maternal Prenatal Exposures

Prenatal exposures to the mother arise from sources including maternal occupation, paraoccupational (exposure through a third party, such as a spouse or family member), air, water, and diet. Internet resources for estimating the risk of exposures to pregnant women are contained on the Toxicology Data Network (TOXNET http://toxnet.nlm.nih.gov), which includes the Developmental and Reproductive Toxicology Database (DART [http://toxnet.nlm.nih.gov/cgi-bin/sis/htmlgen?DARTETIC]).

Maternal Occupational Exposures

Several maternal occupations increase the risk of a poor pregnancy outcome. Associations between workplace exposures and poor reproductive outcome (eg, spontaneous abortion, miscarriage, and birth defects) have been found for lead, mercury, organic solvents, ethylene oxide, and ionizing radiation.[5] More information is found in Chapter 44. The US Department of Labor Occupational Safety and Health Administration Web site on reproductive hazards (http://www.osha.gov/SLTC/reproductivehazards/index.html) provides many relevant resources.

Concerns have focused on maternal exposure to solvents and birth defects, primarily because of the large number of women involved in computer chip manufacture and the working conditions in such plants. A large multicenter case-control study showed that mothers of children with congenital malformations were 44% more likely to have reported exposure to glycol ether than were mothers of children without congenital malformations (odds ratio, 1.44; 95% confidence interval [CI], 1.10–1.90).[18] In another study, 32 infants born to women occupationally exposed to organic solvents were compared with 28 nonexposed infants on their performance of color vision and visual acuity.[19] Solvent-exposed children had significantly higher error scores on red-green and blue-yellow color discrimination and poorer visual acuity compared with the unexposed group. Clinical red-green color vision loss was found in 3 of the 32 in the exposed group, compared with none in the unexposed group.

Occupational exposure to radiation is common in the fields of aviation and medical technology. Recommendations for pregnant aircrew members regarding acceptable exposure to galactic radiation related to length of time of flight as well as altitudes in flight is available at http://www.faa.gov/library/reports/medical/oamtechreports/2000s/media/00_33.pdf.

Paraoccupational Exposure

A paraoccupational exposure occurs when the father or another household member brings or tracks home occupational chemicals, when the home itself is in an occupational setting, or when industrial chemicals are purposely brought home for home use.

Air

Air pollution is an important source of exposure to the pregnant woman and fetus. For example, exposure of the mother to secondhand tobacco smoke (also known as environmental tobacco smoke) has been linked to preterm birth, decreased birth weight, and increased risk of sudden infant death syndrome[4,20,21] and obesity in the offspring.[22] A 2008 review determined that limited evidence exists to support the association of maternal exposure to outdoor air pollution with preterm birth, decreased birth weight, and cardiac defects.[5] However, studies of pregnant women exposed to the World Trade Center disaster found significant associations between maternal exposure to certain air pollutants and increased risks of intrauterine growth restriction,[23] decreased birth weight and head circumference, and decreased gestational length.[24] An interaction between secondhand tobacco smoke and polycyclic aromatic hydrocarbons (PAHs, as measured by benzo[a]pyrene [BAP]-DNA adducts in cord blood) was associated with decreasing Bayley Mental Development Index scores in exposed infants.[25]

Water

Because the fetus develops through multiple short critical periods, the quality of water consumed by a pregnant woman is a daily concern; a yearly average of contaminants is not sufficient to protect the developing fetus. Public and well water supplies can vary greatly over the course of a year. A 2008 review of prenatal chemical exposures and reproductive and pregnancy outcomes examined the relationship of drinking water contaminants to adverse pregnancy outcomes.[5] It concluded that limited evidence exists to support an association between exposure to byproducts of chlorinated water disinfectants (such as trihalomethane) and increased risk of spontaneous abortions, stillbirths, or having an infant who is small for gestational age or who has a neural tube defect.[5]

Diet

Contaminants in the diet may result in important exposures. In Minamata Bay, Japan, methylmercury from an acetaldehyde-producing plant contaminated the food chain in the 1950s.[26] Pregnant women from a fishing village on that bay gave birth to severely neurologically damaged infants, whereas the women had only mild transient paresthesias or no symptoms at all. Current recommendations suggest that pregnant women avoid consumption of shark, swordfish, king mackerel, and tile fish and limit their intake of other fish, such as tuna, because of mercury content (see Chapter 32).[27]

Nutritional status is important in pregnancy outcome. For example, folic acid taken before and during pregnancy reduces the risk of neural tube defects. Most women of reproductive age, however, do not consume the daily requisite 400 µg of folic acid.[28] During pregnancy, daily intake of folic acid should increase to 600 µg.[28] Obesity in pregnancy is associated with diabetes, hypertension, infertility, stillbirth, congenital anomalies such as neural tube defects, macrosomia, birth injury, and increased risk of Cesarean delivery.[28] It is difficult, however, to isolate the effects of obesity versus diabetes on pregnancy outcomes, because the 2 conditions are often linked.

Maternal medications and dietary supplements are other possible sources of exposure. One well-known example of a medication with adverse effects on the fetus is the class of angiotensin-converting enzyme (ACE) inhibitors. When taken in the second and third trimesters, angiotensin-converting enzyme inhibitors can adversely affect kidney development.[29] Many other prescription and over-the-counter medications have very little information on the risks of use during pregnancy or lactation.[29]

PATHWAYS OF FETAL EXPOSURE

Placenta-Dependent Pathways

For a placenta-dependent chemical to reach the fetus, it must first enter the mother's bloodstream and then cross the placenta in significant amounts. Not all environmental toxicants meet these criteria. Three properties that enable chemicals to cross the placenta are low molecular weight, fat solubility, and resemblance to nutrients that are specifically transported. Information about an individual chemical's ability to cross the placenta may be found by using the Toxicology Data Network (TOXNET http://toxnet.nlm.nih.gov), which includes the Developmental and Reproductive Toxicology Database (http://toxnet.nlm.nih.gov/cgi-bin/sis/htmlgen?DARTETIC), or by reviewing its Material Safety Data Sheet.

An example of a low molecular weight compound is carbon monoxide (CO). Carbon monoxide is an asphyxiant, because it displaces oxygen from hemoglobin, forming carboxyhemoglobin (COHb). If enough COHb accumulates in the circulation, cellular metabolism is impaired by the inhibition of oxygen transport, delivery, and use. Fetal COHb accumulates more slowly than maternal COHb but increases to a steady state approximately 10% greater than in the maternal circulation. Thus, nonfatal CO poisoning of the mother may prove fatal to the fetus.

Examples of fat-soluble chemicals that readily cross the placenta are ethanol and polycyclic aromatic hydrocarbons (PAHs), including benzo(a)pyrene, a carcinogen present in secondhand tobacco smoke. Alcohol causes fetal alcohol spectrum disorders; the most severe end of the spectrum is fetal alcohol syndrome. Alcohol use during pregnancy is considered the main preventable cause of mental retardation (http://www.cdc.gov/ncbddd/fasd/documents/SurgeonGenbookmark.pdf, http://www.cdc.gov/ncbddd/fasd/documents/FAS_guidelines_accessible.pdf). In pregnant ewes, intravenous infusion of ethanol results in identical maternal and fetal blood alcohol concentrations.[30] PCBs have been measured in equal concentrations in fetal and maternal blood.[31]

Calcium is a nutrient that is actively transported across the placenta to provide the fetus with 100 to 140 mg/kg of calcium per day during the third trimester. It is thought that lead is transported by the calcium transporter. The average contribution of maternal skeletal lead mobilized to the infant's cord blood lead has been calculated to be 79%.[14] Calcium supplementation decreases maternal bone resorption, thereby lowering the amount of lead mobilized from maternal bone that would then become available to the fetus.[14] A randomized controlled trial conducted in Mexico City showed that women who received 1200 mg daily of calcium carbonate had moderately lower lead concentrations during pregnancy.[32] This effect was greater in compliant mothers, in mothers with higher baseline lead concentrations, and during the second trimester.

Placenta-Independent Pathways

Placenta-independent hazards to the fetus include ionizing radiation, heat, noise, and possibly electromagnetic fields. Ionizing radiation is a well-characterized teratogen (see Chapter 30). Much of our knowledge about the effects of radiation comes from studies of the survivors of the atomic bombs in Hiroshima and Nagasaki.[33]

Ionizing radiation is associated with birth defects such as microcephaly or cancers.[34] Exposure to low-dose Cobalt-60 ionizing radiation was associated with increased time to pregnancy.[35] Not all forms of radiation are hazardous to the fetus. Neither radon nor ultraviolet radiation reaches the fetus.

Heat may directly penetrate to the fetus; exposure to heat in the first trimester has been associated with neural tube defects.[36] Noise has a waveform, which may be transmitted to the fetus. Noise has been associated with certain birth defects, preterm birth, and low birth weight.[37]

There is increasing attention to intrauterine programming and epigenetic phenomena. This occurs when environmental factors change the gene expression through DNA methylation and chromatin remodeling; such alterations may continue to affect future generations.[38] One example is the association between

Table 8.1: Spectrum of Phenotypic Effects

- Infertility
- Spontaneous abortion/miscarriage
- Preterm birth
- Intrauterine growth retardation
- Microcephaly
- Major and minor malformations
- Deformations
- Metabolic dysfunction
- Cognitive dysfunction
- Behavioral dysfunction
- Pulmonary dysfunction
- Hearing loss
- Endocrine dysfunction
- Effects on vision
- Cancer

maternal smoking during pregnancy and increased risk of childhood obesity.[39] Another is concern about early exposure to endocrine-disrupting chemicals such as bisphenol A and the development of adult chronic diseases such as obesity.[38,39]

SPECTRUM OF OUTCOMES

Developmental processes—from the fertilization of an egg to the birth of baby through the completion of adult development—are highly intricate. The sites of action of chemicals and radiation are numerous. An intrauterine exposure to radiation or chemicals may result in a broad array of phenotypic effects that often are not thought of as teratogenic effects. Table 8.1 lists some phenotypes that may be seen.

The environment has been strongly linked to birth defects. A study of 371 933 women investigated the relative risk of a child's being born with a birth defect similar to the birth defect affecting the preceding sibling[40]; the relative risk of a similar birth defect was 11.6 (95% confidence interval, 9.3–14.0) and decreased by more than 50% when the mother changed her living environment between the 2 pregnancies.

Developmental neurotoxicity deserves special mention. The development of the central nervous system requires expression of unique proteins in specific cell populations during specific critical windows. There is concern that injury to these populations may result in neurodevelopmental disorders, such as mental retardation, autism spectrum disorders, dyslexia, and attention-deficit/hyperactivity disorder. It is estimated that 3% to 8% of the 4 million children born each year in the United States are affected by a neurodevelopmental disability.[41] Some are caused by genetic aberrations (eg, Down syndrome, fragile X syndrome), some by perinatal anoxia or meningitis, and some by exposure to drugs (eg, alcohol, cocaine). For most neurodevelopmental disabilities, however, the cause is unknown. Environmental chemicals such as lead, tobacco, PCBs, and mercury, are known developmental neurotoxicants. Of the chemicals produced in or imported into the United States at more than 1 million pounds a year, fewer than 10% have been tested to determine whether they have the potential to cause developmental damage.[42] As of 2006, of all chemicals regulated by the US Environmental Protection Agency (EPA), only 112 had any developmental neurotoxicity testing.[43] Thus, it is possible that neurodevelopmental disabilities seen after birth are linked to in utero exposure to one or multiple chemicals.

PREVENTION OF EXPOSURE

For women who are planning pregnancies, an occupational and environmental exposure history may be obtained during preconception or interconception health visits. Because half of all pregnancies are unplanned,[44] it is important to obtain an exposure history for every woman of reproductive age. It is not enough to know the woman's occupation. The clinician must ask about the nature of her work, the nature of her partner's work, their hobbies and home activities, secondhand smoke exposure at home and elsewhere, and the characteristics of their residence and neighborhood.[27] Additional areas of inquiry include the composition of the diet and use of tobacco, alcohol, or street drugs.[28,29] The clinician should inquire about medicines (prescribed, over-the-counter, or natural/alternative/herbal) used during the pregnancy. The Select Panel for Preconception Health and Health Care of the US Centers for Disease Control and Prevention created the Web site "Before, Between & Beyond Pregnancy," which includes a preconception curriculum for health care providers (http://www.beforeandbeyond.org).

Women who work have a right to know about the chemicals with which they work, and they have a right to be protected from harmful exposures. Material safety data sheets are available to any employee who requests them. These sheets supply information about potential reproductive hazards. Personal protective gear should be available, and increased monitoring of potential exposures should be instituted. In certain instances, temporary job shifting may prevent exposure.

Frequently Asked Questions

Q *What can I do to improve the likelihood of having a healthy, full-term baby?*

A The first step in having a healthy baby is ensuring that the mother is healthy. The mother's health begins before conception. If you are a woman of childbearing age, take a folic acid supplement every day. Ingesting 0.4 mg (400 µg) of folic acid per day will prevent certain kinds of birth defects, particularly defects of the nervous system. Pregnant women should increase their folic acid intake to 0.6 mg (600 µg) per day. Because many pregnancies are not planned and women may not know they are pregnant until the first trimester is well under way, folic acid should be taken by all women of childbearing age. Folic acid is available as part of many multivitamin supplements. Make sure that any medications you take are safe during pregnancy.

Do not drink alcohol, do not smoke, and try not to be around others who smoke. Avoid eating the 4 large, predatory fish that contain high amounts of mercury (swordfish, shark, tilefish, and king mackerel) and limit your intake of white (albacore) tuna. It is important to continue to consume regularly (at least two 3-oz servings a week) other seafood before and during pregnancy, especially seafood rich in fatty acids and low in mercury (eg, salmon, pollock, scallops), to ensure that sufficient amounts of the essential fatty acids docosa-hexaenoic acid (DHA) and eicosapentaenoic acid (EPA) are available for the development of the fetal brain.[45] If you work with chemicals, become as informed as possible about the possible risks those chemicals could pose to your fetus, and take necessary precautions. Remember that environmental hazards can exist not only at work but at home or even as a result of other household members' exposures. It is important to be aware of potential environmental exposures that might occur during preparation for the baby's arrival such as nursery renovations.

Q   *Is there any information about chemical exposures and risks to women who work in hair or nail salons?*

A   Exposures at nail and hair salons involve multiple substances. Hair salons may use chemicals such as aromatic amines (hair dye) or formaldehyde-based disinfectants. Nail salons use solvents, such as acetone or toluene, and acrylates. Because of the presence of these multiple substances as well as differences in ventilation and time of exposure, true reproductive health risks are difficult to determine. Furthermore, very few human studies examine multiple substance exposures and associated health risks. Current recommendations for hairdressers include working fewer than 35 hours per week, wearing gloves, avoiding standing for long periods of time, ensuring good ventilation, covering products and garbage when not in use, and maintaining separate areas to eat. Nail salons have similar issues. Recommendations for nail salon workers include ensuring good ventilation, keeping products and garbage closed if not in use, removing garbage frequently, using appropriate dust masks for grinding nails, using gloves, and having separate places to eat. It is also recommended that products containing liquid methyl methacrylate (MMA) be avoided, mainly because studies in animals exposed to MMA show adverse respiratory and liver effects. Information about protecting nail salon workers may be found at the Nail Salons Project of the US EPA (http://www.epa.gov/opptintr/dfe/pubs/projects/salon/index. htm). Additional information may be found through The Organization of Teratology Information Specialists (http://www.otispregnancy.org/other-education-materials-and-links-s13109) and Tox Town (http://toxtown.nlm. nih.gov/text_version/locations.php?id=28).

Resources

The March of Dimes
www.marchofdimes.com/professionals/19640.asp
Offers education for professionals about preconception issues.

Toxicology Data Network (TOXNET)
http://toxnet.nlm.nih.gov
A cluster of databases covering toxicology, hazardous chemicals, environmental health, and related areas. It is managed by the Toxicology and Environmental Health Information Program (TEHIP) in the Division of Specialized Information Services (SIS) of the National Library of Medicine (NLM). *One such database on TOXNET is Developmental and Reproductive Toxicology Database (DART)*—References to developmental and reproductive toxicology literature—http://toxnet.nlm.nih.gov/cgi-bin/sis/htmlgen?DARTETIC.

Organization of Teratology Information Specialists (OTIS)
www.otispregnancy.org
Provides fact sheets on different hazards and links to medical providers in the United States and Canada.

Occupational Safety and Health Administration (OSHA) Reproductive Hazards
www.osha.gov/SLTC/reproductivehazards
Information relevant to reproductive hazards in the workplace.

Center for the Evaluation of Risks to Human Reproduction, National Toxicology Program, Department of Health and Human Services
http://cerhr.niehs.nih.gov/index.html
Information about risk of exposure to individual chemicals.

National Institute for Occupational Safety and Health, Reproductive Health
www.cdc.gov/niosh/topics/repro

References

1. Miller MT, Strömland K, Ventura L, Johansson M, Bandim JM, Gillberg C. Autism associated with conditions characterized by developmental errors in early embryogenesis: a mini review. *Int J Dev Neurosci.* 2005;23(2-3):201-219
2. Yamazaki JN, Schull WJ. Perinatal loss and neurological abnormalities among children of the atomic bomb. Nagasaki and Hiroshima revisited, 1949 to 1989. *JAMA.* 1990;264(5):605-609
3. Sherman SL, Lamb NE, Feingold E. Relationship of recombination patterns and maternal age among non-disjoined chromosomes 21. *Biochem Soc Trans.* 2006;34(Pt 4):578-580
4. Younglai EV, Foster WG, Hughes EG, Trim K, Jarrell JF. Levels of environmental contaminants in human follicular fluid, serum, and seminal plasma of couples undergoing in vitro fertilization. *Arch Environ Contam Toxicol.* 2002;43(1):121–126

5. Wigle DT, Arbuckle TE, Turner MC, et al. Epidemiologic evidence of relationships between reproductive and child health outcomes and environmental chemical contaminants. *J Toxicol Environ Health, Part B.* 2008;11(5-6):373-517

6. Newbold RR. Prenatal exposure to diethylstilbestrol (DES). *Fertil Steril.* 2008;89 (Suppl 1):e55-e56

7. Frey KA, Navarro SM, Kotelchuck M, et al. The clinical content of preconception care: preconception care for men. *Am J Obstet Gynecol.* 2008;199(Suppl 2):S389-S395

8. Cordier S. Evidence for a role of paternal exposures in developmental toxicity. *Basic Clin Pharmacol Toxicol.* 2008;102(2):176-181

9. Yang Q, Wen SW, Leader A, et al. Paternal age and birth defects: how strong is the association? *Hum Reprod.* 2007;22(3):696-701

10. Rousseau F, Bonaventure J, Legeai-Mallet L, et al. Mutations in the gene encoding fibroblast growth factor receptor-3 in achondroplasia. *Nature.* 1994;371(6494):252-254

11. Chen YC, Guo YL, Hsu CC, Rogan WJ. Cognitive development of Yu-Cheng ("oil disease") children prenatally exposed to heat-degraded PCBs. *JAMA.* 1992;268(22):3213-3218

12. Chen YC, Yu ML, Rogan WJ, Gladen BC, Hsu CC. A 6-year follow-up of behavior and activity disorders in the Taiwan Yu-Cheng children. *Am J Public Health.* 1994;84(3):415-421

13. Hu H, Shih R, Rothenberg S, et al. The epidemiology of lead toxicity in adults: measuring dose and consideration of other methodologic issues. *Environ Health Perspect* 2007;115(3):455-462

14. Gulson BL, Mizon KJ, Korsch MJ, et al. Mobilization of lead from human bone tissue during pregnancy and lactation—a summary of long-term research. *Sci Total Environ.* 2003;303(1-2): 79-104

15. Shannon MW, Graef JW. Lead intoxication in infancy. *Pediatrics.* 1992;89(1):87-90

16. Thompson GN, Robertson EF, Fitzgerald S. Lead mobilization during pregnancy. *Med J Aust.* 1985;143(3):131

17. Hu H, Téllez-Rojo MM, Bellinger D, et al. Fetal lead exposure at each stage of pregnancy as a predictor of infant mental development. *Environ Health Perspect.* 2006;114(11):1730-1735

18. Cordier S, Bergeret A, Goujard J, et al. Congenital malformation and maternal occupational exposure to glycol ethers. Occupational Exposure and Congenital Malformations Working Group. *Epidemiology.* 1997;8(4):355-363

19. Till C, Westall CA, Rovet JF, Koren G. Effects of maternal occupational exposure to organic solvents on offspring visual functioning: a prospective controlled study. *Teratology.* 2001;64(3):134-141

20. American Academy of Pediatrics, Committee on Environmental Health, Committee on Substance Abuse, and Committee on Native American Child Health. Policy statement— tobacco use: a pediatric disease. *Pediatrics.* 2009;124(5):1474-1487

21. American Academy of Pediatrics, Committee on Environmental Health, Committee on Native American Child Health, Committee on Adolescence. Secondhand and prenatal tobacco smoke exposure. *Pediatrics.* 2009;124(5):e1017-e1044

22. Oken E, Levitan EB, Gillman MW. Maternal smoking during pregnancy and child overweight: systematic review and meta-analysis. *Int J Obes.* 2008;32(2):201-210

23. Berkowitz GS, Wolff MS, Janevic TM, Holzman IR, Yehuda R, Landrigan PJ. The World Trade Center disaster and intrauterine growth restriction. *JAMA.* 2003;290(5):595-596

24. Lederman SA, Rauh V, Weiss L, et al. The effects of the World Trade Center event on birth outcomes among term deliveries at three lower Manhattan hospitals. *Environ Health Perspect.* 2004;112(17):1772-1778

25. Perera F, Deliang T, Rauh V, et al. Relationship between polycyclic aromatic hydrocarbon-DNA adducts, environmental tobacco smoke, and child development in the World Trade Center cohort. *Environ Health Perspect.* 2007;115(10):1497-1502

26. Harada M. Methyl mercury poisoning due to environmental contamination ("Minamata disease"). In: Oehme FW, ed. *Toxicity of Heavy Metals in the Environment.* New York, NY: Marcel Dekker; 1978:261

27. McDiarmid MA, Gardiner PM, Jack BW. The clinical content of preconception care: environmental exposures. *Am J Obstet Gynecol.* 2008;199(Suppl 2):S357-S361

28. Gardiner PM, Nelson L, Shellhaas CS, et al. The clinical content of preconception care: nutrition and dietary supplements. *Am J Obstet Gynecol.* 2008;199(Suppl 2):S345-S356

29. Dunlop AL, Gardiner PM, Shellhaas CS, et al. The clinical content of preconception care: the use of medications and supplements among women of reproductive age. *Am J Obstet Gynecol.* 2008;199(Suppl 2):S367-S372

30. Clarke DW, Smith GN, Patrick J, Richardson B, Brien JF. Activity of alcohol dehydrogenase and aldehyde dehydrogenase in maternal liver, fetal liver and placenta of the near-term pregnant ewe. *Dev Pharmacol Ther.* 1989;12(1):35–41

31. Bush B, Snow J, Koblintz R. Polychlorobyphenyl (PCB) congeners, p,p'-DDE, and hexachlorobenzene in maternal and fetal cord blood from mothers in upstate New York. *Arch Environ Contam Toxicol.* 1984;13(5):517–527

32. Ettinger AS, Lamadrid-Figueroa H, Téllez-Rojo MM, et al. Effect of calcium supplementation on blood lead levels in pregnancy: a randomized placebo-controlled trial. *Environ Health Perspect.* 2009;117(1):26-31

33. Blot WJ. Growth and development following prenatal and childhood exposure to atom radiation. *J Radiat Res (Tokyo).* 1975;16(Suppl):82–88

34. Brent RL. Saving lives and changing family histories: appropriate counseling of pregnant women and men and women of reproductive age, concerning the risk of diagnostic radiation exposures during and before pregnancy. *Am J Obstet Gynecol.* 2009;200(1):4-24

35. Lin CM, Chang WP, Doyle P, et al. Prolonged time to pregnancy in residents exposed to ionising radiation in Co-60 contaminated buildings. *Occup Environ Med.* 2010;67(3):187-195

36. Milunsky A, Ulcickas M, Rothman KJ, Willett W, Jick SS, Jick H. Maternal heat exposure and neural tube defects. *JAMA.* 1992;268(7):882–885

37. American Academy of Pediatrics, Committee on Environmental Health. Noise: a hazard for the fetus and newborn. *Pediatrics.* 1997;100(4):724–727

38. Grandjean P, Bellinger D, Bergman Å, et al. The Faroes statement: human health effects of developmental exposure to chemicals in our environment. *Basic Clin Pharmacol Toxicol* 2008;102(2):73-75

39. Trasande L, Cronk C, Durkin M, et al. Environment and obesity in the National Children's Study. *Environ Health Perspect.* 2009;117(2):159-166

40. Lie RT, Wilcox AJ, Skjaerven R. A population-based study of the risk of recurrence of birth defects. *N Engl J Med.* 1994;331(1):1–4

41. Weiss B, Landrigan PJ. The developing brain and the environment: an introduction. *Environ Health Perspect.* 2000;108(Suppl 3):373–374

42. Goldman LR, Koduru S. Chemicals in the environment and developmental toxicity to children: a public health and policy perspective. *Environ Health Perspect.* 2000;108(Suppl 3):443–448

43. Makris SL, Raffaele K, Allen S, et al. A retrospective performance assessment of the developmental neurotoxicity study in support of OECD test guideline 426. *Environ Health Perspect.* 2009;117(1):17-25

44. Finer LB, Henshaw SK. Disparities in rates of unintended pregnancy in the United States, 1994 and 2001. *Perspect on Sex Reprod Health.* 2006;38(2):90–96

45. Institute of Medicine. *Seafood Choices: Balancing Benefits and Risks, 2006.* Available at: http://www.iom.edu/Reports/2006/Seafood-Choices-Balancing-Benefits-and-Risks.aspx. Accessed February 24, 2011

Chapter 9

Built Environment

■ ■ ■ ■ ■ ■

The term "built environment" refers to both the physical structure and socio-cultural characteristics of the home, neighborhood, school, and community. Pediatricians are in a unique position to collaborate with urban planners and policy makers in designing communities and neighborhoods that promote children's health.[1]

The 20th century exodus of many families from cities to suburbs and the modern dependence on the car for transportation fundamentally changed how many American children live.[2] Because of zoning laws originally designed to separate people from the noxious fumes of industry, the reign of the single-family unit dwelling, and the extra land that this urban design strategy demands, commercial areas are often far removed from residential areas, and more time is spent in the car during long commutes. Shopping areas are designed around parking lots rather than connected to pedestrian causeways. Land area is not sufficiently prioritized for parks and playing fields, and consequently, many parks are too far for children to reach easily by biking or walking. Acreage requirements in school siting regulations have led to a large-scale shift from neighborhood schools to schools located on the fringes of a community, where land is less expensive. These design shifts have affected children's health by influencing their ability to play and be active, increasing hours they are sedentary, and potentially affecting their mental health.

The direction of this past century's shift in the design of built environments is set against the backdrop of alarming increases in pediatric chronic diseases, such as obesity, asthma, and mental health disorders. The obesity epidemic, in particular, leads us to consider what has changed in our 21st century lives that has led a third of American children to become overweight or obese and, thus, more likely to develop "adult diseases," including diabetes and hypertension. With regard to mental health disorders, the built environment can affect children's opportunities for interactions with nature, and this may have important effects on mental health. Mental health may also be affected by the way in which school and community design can foster (or inhibit) a community's social interconnectedness.

THE BUILT ENVIRONMENT AND PHYSICAL ACTIVITY

A century ago, the link between the built environment and health was more intuitively obvious. Living in dark, poorly ventilated, crowded housing increased the risk of tuberculosis and other diseases. Contaminated water supplies put people at risk of waterborne diseases, such as cholera. Housing codes and sanitation infrastructure evolved to separate (and protect) people from toxic elements in their environments, and as conditions improved, health improved.[3] We face different health challenges in the early years of the new millennium. Today, people are much less likely to succumb to a single infectious disease than they are to develop chronic diseases, such as coronary artery disease, diabetes, and cancer, or stress-related conditions. Over time, children have become increasingly at risk of many of these adverse health outcomes, largely because of the drastic increase in obesity.[4] In light of this, in the past decade there has been a resurgence of interest from the health professions regarding the built environment, largely sparked by the ways in which our built environment has contributed to physical inactivity.

In theory, children have opportunities for physical activity at home, in centers of recreation, in neighborhood parks and play areas, and on the way to school. Physical activity includes free play, sports, walking or cycling with friends, or walking or cycling to get to school. However, features of the built environment, such as how neighborhoods are designed, where schools are located, and access to centers of recreation, all affect children's opportunities for physical activity. Unfortunately, all American children do not share the same access to opportunities for physical activity, and for many, the built environment discourages physical activity.

Active Commuting to School

Active commuting to school, defined as either walking or biking, can be an important source of regular physical activity. In the last half century, there has been a decline in this form of physical activity. Between 1969 and 2001, national rates of elementary school students' active transportation to school declined from 41% to 13%.[5] Both boys and girls are actively commuting to school less. Although there are some variations in trends by ethnicity (overall, more Hispanic and black children walk to school), the overall downward trend is striking. School policy, community safety programs, and school siting have had important and sometimes unintended adverse effects on health promotion.

The significant decline in active commuting to school is partly explained by proximity to schools. The closer children live to the school, the more likely they are to actively commute. In 1969, 66% of students lived within 3 miles of school. In 2001, only 49% did. Proximity does not, however, fully explain the decline of walking. Over the past 30 years, proximity between home and school seems to be playing a declining role in whether children actively commute. In 1977, if a child lived 1.9 miles from school versus 1 mile, the odds of active commuting were decreased by a factor of 50. In 2001, the odds only decreased by a factor of 21,[5] highlighting the importance of considering other factors that influence how much children actively commute.

The location of schools in relationship to residential communities can also affect active commuting. Historically, small neighborhood schools served as "anchors" within the community and places for after-school programs, for social and recreational gathering, and as disaster shelters.[6] However, after the 1950s, many states established policies on the size and location of school buildings that influenced school siting. According to those guidelines, to receive state funding, schools required a minimum acreage (eg, elementary schools needed to be on at least 10 acres), and more students translated to larger required school grounds size (eg, an extra acre for every 100 students).[7] Because untapped acreage sufficient to meet these standards is most often at the edge of an urban area, neighborhood schools (typically only 2 to 8 acres in size) were frequently demolished or closed in favor of larger schools at the outskirts of communities. Recommendations on school size from the Council of Education Facilities Planners International (CEFPI) were revised in 2004[8] and no longer recommend minimum acreage. There is increasing interest in supporting smaller schools, but change to policies on school land size occurs slowly.

When schools are far from where students live, students walk to school less and ride more in cars or on buses. The increase in vehicle miles traveled can affect not only physical activity levels but also local air pollution. "School sprawl," thus, not only affects "calories burned" but also contributes to exacerbations of respiratory conditions, such as asthma. Pediatricians' understanding of the communities they work in and the health risks posed to children therein places them in a unique position to counsel policy makers, city planners, and developers.[9]

Safety

Parents' perceptions of crime and traffic safety may influence whether or not children actively commute to school. In a study of Australian children, 81% of parents of 10- to 12-year-olds reported a strong concern about strangers, and

78% expressed a strong concern about road safety. Forty-seven percent reported
no lights or crossings, and 42% reported their children needed to cross several
roads to get to their school.[10] Road safety concern was the factor most strongly
associated with the likelihood that 10- to 12-year-olds walked or biked to
school. Lack of a road barrier on a busy road, no lights or crossings, a steep road
without a barrier, and a school distance greater than 800 meters were associated
with less active transport. Lack of other children in the area also decreased active
commuting. When parents of American children were asked which of 6 possible
barriers exist for children walking to school, long distance was identified by
50% of respondents; traffic danger by 40%; adverse weather conditions by 24%;
crime danger by 18%; and opposing school policy by 7%. Sixteen percent of
parents reported no barriers. Their children were 6 times more likely to walk
or bike to school.[11]

The relationship between safety and physical activity is complex. Although
road safety plays a role in active transportation to school, the role of safety
from crime is less well understood. Perceptions and the presence of neighborhood crime may affect physical activity. However, crime prevention strategies,
themselves, may unintentionally decrease physical activity, whether with a
physical barrier such as a fence that limits access to a recreation area or playground after hours, or with the increased validation of parental fears of crime.[12]

Walkability

The principle of walkability is used to describe how the built environment
relates to walking behavior. Just as walking to school is influenced by the built
environment, walking for other utilitarian reasons, and for recreation, is also
affected. Residential density, proximity and ease of access to nonresidential
land uses, street connectivity, walking or cycling facilities, aesthetics, pedestrian
traffic safety, and crime safety all play a role in walkability.[13] Hills, sidewalks, and
proximity to destinations affect walkability.[14] Increased neighborhood walkability
increases how much children walk to school.[15]

When looking at how a neighborhood is designed, one salient feature is the
proximity of one residence to another. For example, some suburban neighborhoods are built with large lots with a single family home on each lot. Homes
may each be on as much as a third of an acre. In more urban neighborhoods,
there are often multifamily dwellings built close together with smaller lot sizes.
When homes are located more closely together, children walk more.[16]

Geographic features of a neighborhood can have a positive or negative influence on walking, depending on whether the individual is walking for utilitarian
or recreational reasons. For example, although the presence of hills decreases
walking for transportation to a destination, hills (and also the presence of
sidewalks) seem to increase rates of walking for recreation. Having destinations
like a grocery store or park nearby can also increase walking.

For adolescents, walkability can be affected by social features of their neighborhood. When adolescents are more likely to talk or wave to neighbors, they are also more likely to walk as a means of transportation.[17]

Centers of Recreation

Parks, gyms, playgrounds, and sports fields offer important recreational (outside the school day) opportunities for physical activity and are increasingly important as fewer children participate in physical activity at school. From 1991 to 2001, participation in daily physical education class decreased from 41.6% to 32.2%.[2]

For 4- to 7-year-olds and nonoverweight 8- to 12-year-olds, increased park area per capita is associated with increased physical activity.[18] Particularly in minority populations, access to parks predicts physical activity.[19] Yet, there are significantly fewer centers of physical activity available in poor neighborhoods and in neighborhoods with more ethnic minorities. In a study of 20 000 7th to 12th graders, children from neighborhoods characterized by low education levels and high proportions of ethnic minorities were half as likely to have access to a physical activity center (school, public park, gym, or YMCA).[20] The more physical activity centers in a neighborhood, the fewer children who were overweight.

Access to Healthy Foods

The built environment can affect nutrition through the availability and convenience of fruits and vegetables. This, in turn, is associated with whether healthful or unhealthful food is consumed.

Access to large grocery stores increases fruit and vegetable intake, whereas access to convenience stores decreases intake. Low income, minority, and rural neighborhoods have less access to supermarkets and healthful food but have increased access to convenience stores and the nutrient-poor, high-calorie foods that are often found in these food outlets.[21] In a study of neighborhoods in Detroit, increased access to supermarkets increased adult fruit and vegetable servings by 0.69 servings per day. White, black, and Hispanic adults all consumed more servings of fruits and vegetables when a large grocery store was present in their neighborhood, with the highest increase for Hispanic adults. Convenience stores significantly decreased fruit and vegetable intake among Hispanic adults.[22]

As the importance of access to healthy food is increasingly recognized, innovative food programs are gaining in popularity. Community gardens, urban farms, and collaborations between backyard vegetable gardens and local food banks all offer ideas for solutions for inadequate access to fresh fruits and vegetables. City and state land use policies can affect the success of these types of programs. The ultimate effect of these programs on children's health, particularly in vulnerable populations, remains to be seen.

BUILT ENVIRONMENT AND MENTAL HEALTH

Researchers have begun to explore the potential relationships of the built environment to mental health outcomes in children and adults. However, the literature base is still nascent. One pathway through which the built environment may influence mental health is through restoration, the ability to recover from stress and regain attention and focus. Exposure to acute and chronic stress has documented effects on physical health, such as reduced immune function and fatigue. Once fatigue sets in, it is increasingly difficult for an individual to pay attention and inhibit impulses. In people with no underlying disorders of inattention, these symptoms of inattention and impulsivity are reduced after exposure to natural settings and natural views.[23,24] Thus, the built environment may exert influence in its ability to assist with recovery from stress.

In a regional study[25] and a national study,[26] parents of children with attention-deficit/hyperactivity disorder (ADHD) reported that their children's attention and behavioral symptoms improved more after activities in green outdoor settings when compared with activities in built outdoor settings (eg, parking lots, downtown areas) or indoor settings. This suggests a potential therapeutic benefit of exposure to natural settings for children with ADHD.

Personal Control

Personal control is the theoretical concept describing beliefs about the amount of control or influence people have over their environment. People have a better sense of well-being when they can control their surroundings.[27,28]

Exposure to acute noise, crowding, and malodorous pollutants in laboratory settings leads participants to behave with learned helplessness. Even when the insulting influence is removed, the adverse behavior continues as if the insult is still present. Exposure to noise from airports adversely affects the ability of schoolchildren to perform tasks such as jigsaw completion.[29,30] Additional studies examined how other aspects of one's residential environment such as crowding[31,32] and design of corridors[33,34] create the same manifestations of helpless behavior.

Living in neighborhoods characterized by a poor-quality built environment (eg, housing with internal plumbing leaks, nonfunctioning kitchen facilities, toilet breakdowns, poor street sidewalks, building exteriors in dilapidated condition) was associated with greater reporting of lifetime depression and depression in the past 6 months.[35]

Social Support

The built environment can alter the degree and nature of social contact that people have with one another.

The only study thus far to look at sprawl and mental health found that, although the degree of urban sprawl was associated with chronic medical conditions and a low score on an index of health-related quality of life, it was not significantly associated with mental health disorders.[36]

Social Capital

"Social capital" refers to the interconnectedness of a community on levels of social networks, social participation, trust, and reciprocity. Trust and reciprocity between neighbors may explain some of the discrepancies in health from one neighborhood to another.[36] A study of 342 neighborhoods in Chicago found that the degree to which neighbors trusted one another was correlated with health outcomes, such as total mortality, death from heart disease, and "other" causes of death for white and black men and women.[38]

CONCLUSION

Policies and programs that promote active transport to school, improve access to park space and green space, improve access to nutritious foods, improve social connectedness, promote neighborhood walking, and improve neighborhood trust can be designed with children's health in mind. There is great potential for innovative design and programming through collaboration among pediatricians, policy makers, developers, and designers.

Frequently Asked Questions

Q *What can a pediatrician recommend to parents who want information about what to look for when selecting a neighborhood in which to live?*

A Consider whether children will be able to walk or bike to school. Look for the nearest source of fresh fruits and vegetables. Look at distance to shops and activities and consider whether these locations are close enough to walk or bike to. Ask potential neighbors how friendly and connected the neighbors are to each other. Ask potential neighbors whether they see children in the neighborhood walking or biking to school. Find the nearest park and consider whether it is within walking distance.

Q *How can a pediatrician get involved in the community to promote a healthy built environment?*

A Examples of community service are serving on community boards with the goal of improving access to healthy food, working with community organizations that build trust and connectedness among members of the community, working with schools to promote walking and biking to school, and working with schools to promote community gardens.

Resource

The Children and Nature Initiative of the National Environmental Education Foundation (NEEF)

Phone: (202) 833-2933

Web site: http://www.neefusa.org/health/children_nature.htm

NEEF's Children and Nature Initiative addresses preventing serious health conditions, including obesity and diabetes, and reconnecting children to nature. The Initiative educates pediatric health care providers about prescribing outdoor activities to children. The program also connects health care providers with local nature sites so that they can refer families to safe and easily accessible outdoor areas.

References

1. Allender S, Cavill N, Parker M, Foster C. 'Tell us something we don't already know or do!' – The response of planning and transport professionals to public health guidance on the built environment and physical activity. *J Public Health Policy.* 2009;30(1):102-116

2. Brownson R, Boehmer T, Luke D. Declining rates of physical activity in the United States: What are the contributors? *Ann Rev Public Health.* 2005;26:421-443

3. Buck C, Liopis A, Najera E, Terris M, eds. *The Challenge of Epidemiology: Issues and Selected Readings.* Washington, DC: Pan American Health Organization; 1988

4. Ogden C, Carroll M, Flegal K. High body mass index for age among US children and adolescents, 2003–2006. *JAMA.* 2008;299(20):2401-240

5. McDonald N. Active transportation to school: trends among U.S. schoolchildren, 1969–2001. *Am J Prev Med.* 2007;32(6):509-516

6. Passmore S. *Education and Smart Growth: Reversing School Sprawl for Better Schools and Communities: Translation Paper.* Coral Gables, FL: Funder's Network for Smart Growth and Livable Communities; 2002

7. Beaumont CE, Pianca EG. *Why Johnny Can't Walk to School.* Washington, DC: National Trust for Historic Preservation; 2002

8. *Creating Connections: The CEFPI Guide for Educational Facility Planning.* Scottsdale, AZ: Council of Educational Facility Planners International; 2004

9. Tester JM. The built environment: designing communities to promote physical activity in children. *Pediatrics.* 2009;123(6):1591-1598

10. Timperio A, Crawford D, Telford A, Salmon J. Perceptions about the local neighborhood and walking and cycling among children. *Prev Med.* 2004;38:39-47

11. Centers for Disease Control and Prevention. Barriers to children walking to or from school— United States, 2004. *MMWR Morb Mortal Wkly Rep.* 2005;54(38):949-952

12. Foster S, Giles-Corti B. The built environment, neighborhood crime and constrained physical activity: an exploration of inconsistent findings. *Prev Med.* 2008;47(3):241-251

13. Moudon AV, Lee C, Cheadle AD, et al. Operational definitions of walkable neighborhood: theoretical and empirical insights. *J Phys Activity Health.* 2006;3(Suppl 1):S99-S117

14. Lee C, Moudon AV. Correlates of walking for transportation or recreation purposes. *J Phys Activity Health.* 2006;3(Suppl 1):S77-S98

15. Kerr J, Rosenberg D, Sallis JF, Saelens BE, Frank LD, Conway T. Active commuting to school: associations with environment and parental concerns. *Med Sci Sports Exerc.* 2006;38(4):787-793

16. Roemmich JN, Epstein LH, Raja S, Yin L. The neighborhood and home environments: disparate effects on physical activity and sedentary behaviors in youth. *Ann Behav Med.* 2007;33(1):29-38

17. Carver A, Timperio AF, Crawford DA. Neighborhood road environments and physical activity among youth: the CLAN study. *J Urban Health.* 2008;85(4):532-544

18. Roemmich JN, Epstein LH, Raja S, Yin L, Robinson J, Winiewicz D. Association of access to parks and recreational facilities with the physical activity of young children. *Prev Med.* 2006;43(6):437-441

19. Cohen D, McKenzie TL, Sehgal A, Williamson S, Golinelli D, Lurie N. Contribution of public parks to physical activity. *Am J Public Health.* 2007;97(3):509-514

20. Gordon-Larsen P, Nelson MC, Page P, Popkin B. Inequality in the built environment underlies key health disparities in physical activity and obesity. *Pediatrics.* 2006;117(2):417-424

21. Larson NI, Story MT, Nelson MC. Neighborhood environments: disparities in access to healthy foods in the U.S. *Am J Prev Med.* 2009;36(1):74-81

22. Zenk SN, Lachance LL, Schulz AJ, Mentz G, Kannan S, Ridella W. Neighborhood retail food environment and fruit and vegetable intake in a multiethnic urban population. *Am J Health Promot.* 2009;23(4):255-264

23. Kaplan S. The restorative benefits of nature: toward an integrative framework. *J Environ Psychol.* 1995;15:169-182

24. Kaplan R, Kaplan S. *The Experience of Nature.* New York, NY: Cambridge University Press; 1989

25. Faber Taylor A, Kuo FE, Sullivan WC. Coping with ADD: the surprising connection to green play settings. *Environ Behav.* 2001;33(1):54-77

26. Kuo FE, Faber Taylor A. A potential natural treatment for attention-deficit/hyperactivity disorder: evidence from a national study. *Am J Public Health.* 2004;94(9):1580-1586

27. Bandura A. *Self Efficacy.* San Francisco, CA: W. H. Freeman; 1987

28. Taylor SE, Brown JD. Illusions and well-being: a social psychological perspective on mental health. *Psychol Bull.* 1988;103(2):193-210

29. Cohen S, Evans G, Stokols D, Krantz D. *Behavior, Health, and Environmental Stress.* New York, NY: Plenum; 1986

30. Bullinger M, Hygge S, Evans G, Meis M, van Mackensen S. The psychological cost of aircraft noise for children. *Zentralblatt Hygiene Umweltmedizin.* 1999;202(2-4):127-138

31. Fleming I, Baum A, Weiss L. Social density and perceived control as mediators of crowding stress in high density neighborhoods. *J Pers Soc Psychol.* 1987;52:899-906

32. Evans GW, Lepore SJ, Sejwal B, Palsane MN. Chronic residential crowding and children's well-being: an ecological perspective. *Child Dev.* 1998;69(6):1514–1523

33. Baum A, Valins S. Architectural mediation of residential density and control: crowding and the regulation of social contact. In: Berkowitz L, ed. *Advances in Experimental Social Psychology.* New York, NY: Academic; 1979:131-175

34. Baum A, Gatchel R, Aiello J, Thompson, D. Cognitive mediation of environmental stress. In: Harvey J, ed. *Cognition, Social Behavior, and the Environment.* Hillsdale, NJ: Erlbaum; 1981:513-533

35. Galea S, Ahern J, Rudenstine S, Wallace Z, Vlahov D. Urban built environment and depression: a multilevel analysis. *J Epidemiol Community Health.* 2005;59(10):822-827

36. Sturm R, Cohen D. Suburban sprawl and physical and mental health. *Public Health.* 2004;118(7):488-496

37. Chavez R, Kemp L, Harris E. The social capital: health relationship in two disadvantaged neighbourhoods. *J Health Serv Res Policy.* 2004;9(Suppl 2):29-34

38. Lochner KA, Kawachi I, Brennan RT, Buka SL. Social capital and neighborhood mortality rates in Chicago. *Soc Sci Med.* 2003;56(8):1797-805

Chapter 10

Child Care Settings

■ ■ ■ ■ ■ ■

Every day, 12 million preschoolers—including 6 million infants and toddlers, regardless of their parents' work status—are in some form of nonparental care.[1] This accounts for approximately half of children younger than 6 years. Typical child care arrangements for young children when parents work are child care centers (22%), family child care homes (17%), parents (22%), relatives (29%), and in-home caregivers other than the parent or relative (3%).[1] Children enter care as early as 6 weeks of age and can be in care for 40 or more hours per week until they reach school age.[1] Millions of school-aged children are in after-school and summer activities, and more than 6 million children are home alone on a regular basis.[1]

Child care settings are located in single-family homes or buildings specifically designed for child care or within office buildings, schools, churches, malls, health clubs, and other sites. The American Public Health Association and American Academy of Pediatrics (AAP) recommend that these child care settings be designed or modified to meet current standards published in *Caring for Our Children: National Health and Safety Performance Standards—Guidelines for Out-of-Home Child Care Programs*.[2] These standards, which apply to all aspects of child care settings, including environmental health aspects, should be met regardless of the setting or whether the care provided is full time or part time.

States establish and enforce child care licensing regulations that include health and safety requirements. The scope and intensity of state enforcement activities differ among the provider types within states as well as among states overall. For example, most states do not regulate some types of providers, such as relatives or in-home nannies and au pairs.[3] Child care centers typically have more health and safety regulations and oversight compared with family child care homes, hourly drop-off care, and parochial and preschool programs (particularly if they operate on a part–time basis). Compliance with regulations often depends on the degree to which child care providers agree with the rationale for the regulations as well as the quality and frequency of inspection. The licensing and enforcement activities most commonly considered to be critical are background checks, monitoring visits, sanctions, training for licensing staff, and caseload of licensing staff.[3]

The occurrence of environmental hazards in child care varies widely and is influenced by the following:

- Type of setting;
- Licensing requirements;
- Location, age, and condition of the structure;
- Past use of the land or structure;
- Current use of other parts of the structure;
- Behaviors and practices of adults in the setting; and
- Prevalence of hazards in the community.

Hazards in child care settings include those related to food and food sharing, with risks of food contamination and allergic reactions. These are covered in Chapter 18. Hazards related to using toxic arts and crafts materials are covered in Chapter 42. Information about the importance of handwashing, safety in the use of toys, selection and maintenance of equipment, and playground design to avoid choking, falling, and strangulation hazards is presented in *Caring for our Children: National Health and Safety Performance Standards—Guidelines for Out-of-Home Child Care Programs.*[2]

Hazards in a child care setting can adversely affect a group of children. On the other hand, children may benefit when hazards are reduced or controlled. For example, children exposed to secondhand tobacco smoke (SHS), radon, or lead paint at home may reduce their total daily exposure by spending time in child care if the child care setting is free of these hazards.

Environmental hazards in child care settings are similar to those found in other environments (see Table 10.1). Of the few studies that document environmental hazards in child care, indoor air quality, secondhand smoke, lead, and pesticides are of primary concern (see Chapters 20, 40, 31, and 37, respectively).

INDOOR AIR QUALITY

Children spend 80% to 90% of their time indoors (home, child care, school, after-school care, etc), and indoor air quality is an important health concern (see Chapter 20) stimulating federal initiatives such as *Indoor Air Quality: Tools for Schools,*[4] *Home*A*Syst/Farm*A*Syst,*[5] and *HealthySEAT.*[6] Pollutants that contribute to poor indoor air quality include secondhand smoke, molds and other biological products, lead and heavy metals, pesticides, sanitizers,

Table 10.1: Possible Environmental Hazards in Child Care Settings

ENVIRONMENTAL HAZARD	INDOOR SOURCES	OUTDOOR SOURCES
Carbon monoxide (CO)	▪ Malfunctioning or improperly vented fuel-burning appliances such as stoves, furnaces, fireplaces, clothes dryers, water heaters, and space heaters ▪ Poorly maintained home heating systems such as dirty furnaces filter or blocked flues	▪ Playground located near high-traffic area or near the exhaust outlet of a building ▪ Auto, truck, or bus exhaust from attached garages, nearby roads, or parking areas
Secondhand tobacco smoke	▪ Smoking in the child care area ▪ Smoking allowed when children are not present ▪ A multiple-use building with a smoking area that is not properly ventilated and exhausted to the outside	▪ Fresh air intake (eg, doorway) located near an outside smoking area or an exhaust outlet that emits tobacco smoke in an area where children play
Molds and other biological pollutants	▪ Plumbing leaks, roof leaks, and flooding provide moisture for molds and other biological pollutants	▪ Water from river or sewer overflows
Volatile organic compounds (VOCs)	▪ Building materials and furnishings (eg, formaldehyde), paints, cleaning supplies, and coverings on floors	
Lead and other heavy metals	▪ Leaded dust or paint chips, particularly on floors, windowsills, and window wells, and during renovation of pre-1978 structures ▪ Leaded paint on furniture or toys, leaded ceramic dishware, plumbing, remedies, and other sources ▪ Certain toys, arts and crafts supplies, paints, dishware, and lead plumbing	▪ Leaded soil or leaded paint on the building's exterior, fences, sheds, or playground equipment ▪ Improperly contained materials from renovations in the vicinity of the setting ▪ Soil contamination at the site from prior industrial use or geological mineral deposits ▪ Toxic clays and play structures or contents of storage areas accessible to children

continued on page 112

continued from page 111

Table 10.1: Possible Environmental Hazards in Child Care Settings, *continued*

ENVIRONMENTAL HAZARD	INDOOR SOURCES	OUTDOOR SOURCES
Pesticides including lawn and garden chemicals, herbicides, insecticides, rodenticides; sanitizers; and disinfectants	■ Improper storage, labeling, handling, or use of pesticides in any child care area, particularly in the following high-risk areas: diaper changing areas, food preparation and storage, carpeted areas, laundry, maintenance and custodial supply rooms, rooms where children eat and play, other areas prone to pest infestation ■ Pest-infested food and storage areas, bedding, laundry rooms, spaces under sinks due to preventable problems such as poor sanitation, water leaks, and unprotected openings to the outside ■ Industrial strength cleaning products and room deodorizers used indoors	■ Improper storage, labeling, handling, or use of chemical products in any area accessible to children, particularly unsecured storage sheds ■ Infested playgrounds and storage sheds, space under sheds, debris, and clutter or dense foliage near the foundation
OTHER HAZARDS		
Medications	■ Improper storage, labeling, handling, or use of medications.	
Cleaners, other chemicals	■ Improperly storage, labeling, handling or using chemical products in any area accessible to children, particularly unsecured storage sheds	
Asbestos	■ Friable, nonintact asbestos in exposed insulation, ceilings, floors, or duct work ■ Renovation without appropriate asbestos containment	■ Disasters (eg, collapse of the World Trade Center towers)

Table 10.1: Possible Environmental Hazards in Child Care Settings, *continued*

OTHER HAZARDS

Bisphenol A (BPA)	■ Consumer products such as baby bottles, sippy cups, toys, protective coating on food cans, personal care products	
Mercury	■ Ingestion of certain fish; broken fluorescent light bulbs, thermostats	■ Release from industrial processes such as mining and coal burning
Noise	■ Room design or materials that amplify sounds	■ Adjacent roadways, airports, or industrial sources of sound
Radon	■ Cracks and openings in foundations resulting in radon leakage from the ground into buildings	
Phthalates	■ Vinyl flooring, plastic clothing (eg, rain coats), detergents, adhesives, personal-care products (eg, fragrances, nail polish, soap), vinyl (eg, poly-vinyl chloride [PVC]) and plastic products (eg, toys, plastic bags)	
Ultraviolet radiation		■ Excessive sun exposure because of inadequate shade in the playground, and inadequate use of sun-protective clothing, hats, and sunscreen

disinfectants, combustion byproducts, and volatile organic compounds (VOCs). One study of indoor air quality investigated carbon dioxide (CO_2) levels in 91 child care centers in Quebec, Canada. Ninety percent had CO_2 levels that exceeded the office building standard.[7] Increased CO_2 levels were associated with the number of children in a given area. A high CO_2 level (>1000 parts per million [ppm]) can be used as a rough indicator of the effectiveness of ventilation and can serve as a marker for other indoor air pollutants.[7] Airflow in child care settings should be between 15 and 20 cubic feet/minute per person and result in more than 4 air changes per hour. Carbon dioxide levels, which are useful in determining the adequacy of ventilation, should be less than 1000 parts per million when a room has been occupied for 4 to 6 hours (see Chapter 11 and Ventilation for Acceptable Indoor Air Quality [www.ashrae.org]). A study in 2 North Carolina counties looked for 7 indoor air allergens in 89 child care facilities and found each allergen in the majority of facilities.[8] The report indicates that children and child care professionals may be exposed to indoor allergens through their facilities. Another study in Singapore assessed indoor air quality measurements among 346 classrooms in 104 randomly selected child care centers. The types of ventilation systems were identified. When compared with air-conditioned buildings, naturally ventilated buildings had lower concentrations of indoor pollutants and CO_2 levels and were associated with the lowest occurrence of respiratory problems among children.[9] The negative effects that indoor air pollution has on children have been well documented.[10] In rural counties of New York State, an indoor air quality study of child care facilities observed high levels of pollutants such as lead, radon, carbon monoxide, asbestos, and mold.[11] As a result, recommendations were made to lower exposure levels in low-income child care facilities.[11]

SECONDHAND TOBACCO SMOKE

The American Academy of Pediatrics strongly supports smoke-free child care environments. Some states have enacted laws to protect children from secondhand smoke exposure in commercial and home-based child care centers. As of December 31, 2007, 34 states had enacted laws prohibiting smoking in commercial child care centers. As of that date, smoking in both commercial and home-based child care centers was banned in only 8 states. Eleven states did not have any laws to address smoking in commercial and home-based child care centers. Smoking in home-based child care centers was banned in 33 states. Some states allowed smoking in designated areas of commercial child care centers, and others permitted smoking in designated areas of home-based child care centers. Certain states placed time restrictions on smoking in child care centers including restricting smoking to nonbusiness hours. Toxicants in secondhand smoke, however, remain on surfaces and then revolatilize and resuspend, resulting in exposure from "thirdhand smoke." Children may, therefore, be exposed if employees are allowed to smoke when children are not present. Data suggest that state laws are more lenient toward home-based child care centers than commercial child care centers in allowing smoking when children are no longer present.[12] Children may additionally be exposed when there is smoking in another part of the building that shares a common ventilation system with the center. They can also be exposed when a person who smokes transports children to or from the child care setting in a car, school bus, or van. These vehicles should be smoke free at all times. Custodial staff or drivers must never smoke. Child care workers who smoke outside the child care setting or on breaks should be asked to change clothes or wear a cover-up before working with children. Eliminating smoking at all times and implementing a total ban on smoking in child care centers is the only way to ensure that children avoid secondhand smoke exposure.

LEAD

There are few studies of lead hazards in child care. The prevalence of lead in family child care homes is probably similar to the prevalence among homes in the community. A survey of schools, preschools, and child care centers conducted in Washington state found that 62% of 75 facilities built before 1979 contained leaded paint, and 31% contained elevated leaded soil or dust.[13] The First National Environmental Health Survey of Child Care Centers, published in 2005, surveyed 168 licensed randomly selected child care facilities to measure lead in soil and dust samples.[14] Twenty-eight percent of the surveyed facilities contained lead-based paint, and 14% contained one or more significant lead-based hazards.[14] Significant lead-based paint hazards were 4 times as likely to be found in facilities in which the majority of children were black, compared with those in which the majority of children were white.[14]

Exposure to lead in child care settings may be underestimated by routine surveillance systems. When a child has been poisoned by lead, sources in the home, such as lead-based paint, are tested for and identified. Sources of lead away from the home (such as child care settings) are more likely to be overlooked. Two studies of children attending child care centers with high environmental lead levels (in paint, dust, or soil)[13,15] found only one child who had a confirmed blood lead concentration exceeding 10 µg/dL (12 µg/dL).[15] These results, however, cannot be generalized to all child care settings. In both studies, the average age of the participants was approximately 5 years, and in 1 study, the rate of participation was low.[13] Children in these 2 studies may have been protected from lead exposure by continual supervision, a high frequency of hand washing (averaging once per hour), and standard cleaning practices, including daily wet mopping of floors. The risk of exposure is higher for younger children, when children have poor hygiene, when maintenance practices are inadequate, or when housing renovations occur without appropriate testing and containment measures.

Another potential source of lead exposure is drinking water. In 2004, the US Environmental Protection Agency (EPA) requested that state environmental and health agencies provide information about how they monitor and protect children from exposure to lead, particularly in schools and child care facilities.[16] Actions taken to reduce children's exposures to lead in drinking water and recommendations for future collaboration were provided by 49 states, Puerto Rico, and the Navajo Nation.[16] Because there is no federal law requiring sampling of drinking water in schools and child care facilities, periodic water testing at facilities is an important preventive step.

Federal regulations address the problem of lead only in the child's home. Federal funding for remediation of lead hazards can be applied to homes, but not to child care settings.

PESTICIDES AND OTHER POTENTIALLY TOXIC PRODUCTS

Pesticides

Children are highly vulnerable to the adverse effects of pesticides (see Chapter 37). The first national survey of pesticide exposures in child care facilities demonstrated that among 63% of surveyed centers, the number of pesticides used in each ranged from 1 to 10.[17] Frequency of pesticide use ranged from 1 to 107 times annually.[17] The most commonly used pesticides were pyrethroids, followed by organophosphates.[17] In another survey of 89 child care providers in North Carolina, the majority responded that they use high-risk pesticide application methods.[18] A quarter of the respondents indicated using Integrated Pest Management (IPM) (see Chapter 37); those using pest-control contractors were less likely to use integrated pest management for pest control.[18]

Communities in which children are at increased risk of exposure include agricultural areas as well as urban settings where pesticides are used extensively in schools, homes, and child care centers for control of cockroaches, rats, and other pests. Pesticide use in child care settings is common, because young children spill food that attracts pests, and many of the buildings used for child care are old and poorly maintained for control of pests by other means. In some cases, facilities use regular pesticide application for prevention even when there is not an obvious problem, rather than increasing best practices, such as integrated pest management, and reducing the opportunity to attract pests. Children may be exposed through sources such as:

- Residues from indoor or outdoor pesticide use (from the indoor air, surfaces, household dust, and soil/drift);
- Pets treated with flea dips;
- Residues on food;
- Playground structures made of wood treated with wood-preserving pesticides, such as chromated copper arsenate;

- Lawn and garden products; and/or
- Insect repellents.

The incidence of poisoning by pesticides and other products (such as medications, arts and crafts materials, toxic plants, and petroleum products) was higher when children were in their own homes.[19] Children in child care centers may be protected somewhat, because they usually are supervised by an adult, the facility and equipment are designed for children, and licensing procedures and public health inspections help to eliminate hazards. However, the potential for poisonings is real. In Colorado, health inspectors visiting child care settings 2 weeks after licensing inspections found that toxic chemicals were accessible to children in 68% of settings.[20] Products such as pesticides may be used as directed but still are not safe to use in child care settings.[21] Pediatricians should encourage parents to inquire about the type of pesticides and other chemicals used and any known or potential health implications for children.

Cleaning Products

Sanitizing and disinfecting are important processes that help to promote clean and healthy child care facilities. The terms cleaning, sanitizing, and disinfecting are sometimes used interchangeably, possibly resulting in confusion and using cleaning procedures that are not effective.[2]

The purpose of *cleaning* is to physically remove all visible dirt and contamination with a household soap or mild detergent.[2] *Sanitizing* is the process used after visible dirt is removed from a surface. Sanitizing is designed to greatly reduce the number of pathogens that are likely to cause disease. Sanitizing refers to applying heat or a chemical, such as household bleach, to clean surfaces that is sufficient to yield a 99.9% reduction in representative (but not all) disease-causing microorganisms of public health importance. An example of cumulative heat treatment is found in the operation of some household dishwashers. Household dishwashers that effectively sanitize dishes and utensils using hot water may be used to clean and sanitize the outer surfaces of plastic toys. However, dishwashers that use a heating element to dry dishes should be used with caution to avoid melting soft plastic toys. Some dishwashers may permit the heating element used for drying to be deactivated while retaining the sanitizing process. Child care staff can consult the manufacturer's user's guide for instructions. Surfaces that have contact with children's mouths and with food (eg, crib railings, mouthing toys, dishes, high chair trays) should be sanitized. *Disinfecting* is more rigorous than sanitizing. Disinfecting refers to applying cumulative heat or a chemical to result in the elimination of almost all microorganisms from inanimate surfaces. Pathogens of public health importance and nearly all other microorganisms are eliminated, but not to the degree achieved by sterilization. Surfaces such as changing tables and counter tops should be disinfected. *Caring for Our Children: National Health and Safety Performance Standards—Guidelines for Out-of-Home Child Care Programs* contains more details.[2] Although it is common for child care facilities to perform all 3 of these tasks, it is important to avoid using harsh and irritating products whenever possible. There are a variety of alternatives for facilities to consider. If a bleach solution is used to sanitize or disinfect a surface, providers must be sure to adhere to the suggested water-to-bleach formula.

Plastics

In 2008, the National Toxicology Program of the National Institutes of Health raised concerns about exposure to bisphenol A (BPA) during pregnancy and childhood because of a potential effect on human growth and development.[22] In January 2010, the US Food and Drug Administration expressed concern about the possible effects of bisphenol A on the brain and prostate gland of the fetus, infant, and child and also raised concerns about effects on behavior.[23] More research was recommended. Existing research has suggested connections between low-dose bisphenol A exposure and conditions such as cancer, obesity, early puberty, hyperactivity, and diabetes.[22] Bisphenol A is used in products including some baby bottles, sippy cups, reusable water bottles, and microwave-able plastic containers.[22] Parents and child care providers should be encouraged to purchase and use bisphenol A-free bottles, sippy cups, and other containers.[22] Bisphenol A can leak from scratches, so scratched or worn bisphenol A-containing bottles and cups should be discarded. Very hot liquids should not be placed into containers made with bisphenol A, and labels should be checked to ensure microwave safety before microwaving foods and liquids. In response to consumer preferences, the 6 largest manufacturers of baby bottles are already producing baby bottles without bisphenol A. Canada has banned bisphenol A from children's products.[24]

Medications

Adhering to the "five rights of medication administration"—right child, right time, right medication, right dose, and right route—may help to prevent accidental poisoning through a medication error. Providers should have clear guidelines to govern administration of medication in the child care setting. Guidelines include having clear instructions, ensuring that medications are placed in child-resistant containers, and obtaining permission from the parent or guardian to administer the medication. Storage procedures include assessing the need for refrigeration of medication and ensuring that an emergency medication will be readily accessible. Unused medications should be returned to parents for safe disposal.

CHARACTERISTICS OF CHILD CARE SETTINGS THAT MAY EXACERBATE HAZARDS

Characteristics of child care facilities may affect environmental quality. First, low salaries (the average salary of a child care worker ranges from $14 100 to $22 780 per year, depending on the state)[25] and lack of benefits result in a high turnover rate among child care providers. Because approximately one third of child care providers leave their centers each year, child care service operators need to continually educate new employees.[26] Keeping staff training current is a significant challenge for child care centers. Approximately 2.3 million individuals provide child care and education for children younger than 5 years. Of those, an estimated 1.2 million are working within a formal child care setting, and the remaining 1.1 million providers are paid relatives, friends, or neighbors.[27] In addition, 36 states require no training in early childhood care and education, intensifying the need for voluntary continuing education.[28] Research reports indicate that provider education, retention, and compensation are the best indicators for child care quality.[29] Second, child care businesses usually operate with a low profit margin. The largest portion of a family child care home or center budget is dedicated to staff salaries. Tuition funded by public assistance often is at low, fixed dollar amounts. These conditions result in limited funds for preventive measures, such as ventilation maintenance, lead hazard abatement, remodeling, or renovation. It is difficult for centers to close temporarily to implement measures to reduce or eliminate environmental hazards. Finally, when a center is located within a larger facility, such as a church or office building, hazards may arise as a result of practices that occur in other parts of the facility.

MEASURES TO PREVENT OR CONTROL ENVIRONMENTAL HAZARDS IN CHILD CARE SETTINGS

Caring for Our Children: The National Health and Safety Performance Standards— Guidelines for Out-of-Home Child Care Programs identifies measures for prevention and control of environmental hazards.[2] Some of these are discussed here. The standards should be consulted for details on the features of the facility and the operational activities that reduce environmental risks. An important aspect of prevention is frequent handwashing; children should be encouraged to wash their hands or use hand sanitizer throughout the day, especially after toileting and outdoor play and before eating meals or snacks.

Primary Prevention

Site Selection

An environmental audit, conducted from both a child's and adult's perspective, should be performed before selecting a child care site and before new construction begins or an existing building is renovated. The audit should at least include assessments of (1) historical land use to determine the potential for soil contamination with toxic or hazardous waste, such as old gasoline storage; (2) mold, lead, and asbestos in older buildings; (3) potential sources of infestation, noise, air pollution, and toxic exposures; (4) location of the playground in relation to stagnant water, roadways, industrial emissions, and building exhaust outlets; and (5) access to a safe drinking water supply (public or private), a public sewer or approved septic tank system, and other utilities such as electricity. Although geologic factors may suggest potential radon exposure, there are no reliable methods of testing for radon prior to construction.

Architectural Design and Building Materials

Modern homes and buildings are more tightly sealed, and mechanical cooling and heating systems are common in all climate zones. Thousands of new materials used as goods, finishes, and furnishings have resulted in increased indoor pollution.[30] From the perspective of architectural design and building materials, indoor air quality depends on (1) the absence of pollutants (source management—includes removal, substitution, and encapsulation); (2) the power of ventilation systems to supply fresh indoor air; (3) the ability of local exhaust systems and air filters to remove pollutants; and (4) controlling exposure to pollutants, such as cleaning products, through the principles of time of use and location of use.[31] Prevention and control measures include ensuring frequent air exchanges and sufficient ventilation of air to the outside; having some windows that open, preferably offering cross-ventilation, especially in bathrooms, diapering areas, and kitchens; and properly placing fresh-air intakes, which prevent exhaust from automobiles and the building systems from reaching hazardous levels indoors. Pesticide use can be reduced by sealing openings and using screens on the doors and windows. Less toxic building materials, paints, cleaners, and other products can be selected to minimize levels of toxic substances.[30]

Child Care Regulation and Monitoring

To prevent environmental hazards, it is essential to consult an environmental health specialist (such as one located in a local health department) before construction or remodeling begin to review construction or remodeling plans. Child care settings should be monitored by trained licensers who visit during construction or remodeling, inspect them before the center opens and routinely during operation, and investigate complaints. All parts of the child care setting, not only the food service area, must be inspected to identify potential environmental hazards so preventive actions can be implemented. Table 10.2 provides key environmental health questions to include in a routine health and safety inspection of a child care facility. Providers may refer to *Caring for Our Children: National Health and Safety Performance Standards—Guidelines for Out-of-Home Child Care Programs* for a comprehensive listing of standards and rationale.[2]

Table 10.2: Some Key Questions to Assess Potential Environmental Hazards in a Child Care Setting

- Is the setting smoke-free? Is there a smoke-free policy? Is smoking allowed when children are not present? Is smoking allowed in other parts of the building?

- Does the facility appear clean, in good repair, and without water-marked areas or areas of peeling and chipping paint?

- Is there evidence of water damage or mold? Have flooding or plumbing problems occurred? Are there musty odors?

- Are the rooms adequately ventilated?

- Has the child care center or home been tested for radon?

- Are fuel-burning furnaces, stoves, or other equipment in use?

- Are medications and chemical products properly labeled and stored in areas inaccessible to children and in a manner so as not to contaminate food? Are staff members trained in the safe use of chemical products and administration of medications?

- Are arts and crafts supplies free of hazardous substances and labeled in compliance with the American Society for Testing and Materials?

- Are the kitchen and bathroom areas operated in compliance with health department regulations?

- Are hand-washing policies followed and monitored? Are soap and clean towels always available? Paper towels, rather than cloth towels, generally are preferred in child care settings. Individual cloth towels may be used for each child but must be changed frequently.

- Are indoor and outdoor storage closets and sheds locked so their contents are inaccessible to children? All maintenance, lawn care and other hazardous equipment, and chemical products (such as gasoline, paints, pesticides, and cleaning products) must be inaccessible to children.

- Is a carbon monoxide detector present and in working order?

- If the building was constructed before 1978, has the building been assessed for lead paint, dust, and soil hazards? Homes and other buildings built before 1978 may contain lead, and those built before 1950 have the most lead. If remodeling or renovation work is under way, have lead and asbestos hazards been assessed, and have children been protected from the release of these potentially hazardous toxicants?

- Is there standing water?

- Is integrated pest management used?

- Are there adequate shady areas for play outside?

State or local health departments may need to develop additional environmental health regulations that specifically address child care facilities.

Education

In Sweden, continued education of child care providers was shown to be a strong predictor of having few safety hazards in child care centers.[32] Providers with specialized training are more likely to be nurturing, reinforce early literacy skills, and enhance early learning.[33] Through Healthy Child Care America (a national campaign initiated in 1995 by the US Department of Health and Human Services' Maternal and Child Health Bureau and Child Care Bureau and coordinated by the AAP), many states have established a health consultation system that responds to the needs of child care providers for health and safety education. Often, this system includes personnel from local health departments who have expertise in environmental hazards, communicable diseases, injury control, nutrition, sanitation, and/or safety. Health professionals who provide child care consultation can assist child care providers to identify environmental hazards, understand health risks, and implement preventive actions. Many times, child care providers seek consultation directly from their community's pediatricians and other health professionals. More information for health professionals, including strategies for advocacy, training, consultation, and policy making, may be obtained in *The Pediatrician's Role in Promoting Health and Safety in Child Care* (http://www.healthychildcare.org/PedsRole.html).

To prevent environmental health hazards, all employees, including maintenance personnel, should be included in continuing education. Janitorial and custodial staff should be regularly monitored to ensure the safest practices. The Occupational Safety and Health Administration requires that material safety data sheets (MSDSs) be kept on file to explain health hazards from chemicals that are used, proper use and storage procedures, and emergency procedures in case of toxic chemical exposure. Staff also may use material safety data sheets to choose nontoxic chemicals. Parents have a right to ask for the material safety data sheets for chemicals used at child care facilities.

Child care providers may not have knowledge about, or experience or supervisory support in, administering medications. To avoid having child care providers administer medications to children, pediatricians may consider prescribing formulations that require fewer dosages or altering the time of administration. When medications must be given while a child is in child care, specific written instructions should be on the bottle and on a separate piece of paper. Instructions are especially important for medications that are used on an as-needed basis. Instructions are needed for prescription and nonprescription medications and topical preparations, including sunscreen.

Child Care Program Policies and Procedures

Child care providers are well positioned to respond quickly and appropriately to environmental hazards. By developing child care policies, safer practices can become part of everyday routine. For example, (1) smoking should be prohibited (even among noncaregivers in a family child care home) while children are present and at all other times; (2) plumbing leaks, roof leaks, and flooding should be cleaned up within 24 hours and wet areas should be cleansed with detergent and water to prevent growth of molds and other biological pollutants; (3) emergency preparedness plans should include procedures for responding to hazardous material incidents and chemical/biological/radiologic threats; and (4) staff should receive education in administration of medications and use of chemicals. Some states have specific regulations and trainings that conform to those regulations. A medication administration training module can be found at http://www.healthychildcare.org/HealthyFutures.html.

Secondary Prevention

It is possible to avoid some hazardous situations by educating providers and others working in child care settings to recognize and appropriately control hazards (eg, by properly storing or using chemicals). Other hazards may require more costly and complex measures. For example, when extensive mold is found, interim control measures may be needed before full remediation is possible. Remediation procedures should meet applicable standards and regulations. If conditions are potentially hazardous, the center may need to be shut down. When the facility has limited financial resources, environmental health regulators play an important role in ensuring that children's health is not jeopardized. This may require community collaboration to offset the burden of cost.

ILLNESS OR DEATH OCCURRING IN A CHILD WHO ATTENDS OUT-OF-HOME CHILD CARE

When a child's illness or symptoms may have an environmental etiology, parents, health care personnel, and public health investigators should evaluate potential exposures in the child's home environment and out-of-home settings. An increased risk of SIDS has been documented in out-of-home child care settings, but the reason is not understood.[34] Environmental exposures in the child care setting should be considered as part of the death scene investigation.

Frequently Asked Questions

Q *How can I make my child care facility safer for children with asthma?*

A The 2 most important steps that a child care facility can take to prevent asthma attacks in children are to prohibit smoking and to keep the facility free of molds and other biological pollutants. Of the 13 million children

5 years and younger enrolled in child care in the United States, an estimated
1.4 million have asthma (approximately 1 child in 11).[35] Child care programs
need specific information on file (provided by the parent or guardian and
the child's physician) for every child with asthma. The information should
explain known triggers for the child's asthma, medications and how to use
them, symptoms indicating when the asthma is worsening, and what to do
in an emergency. The Asthma and Allergy Foundation of America, New
England Chapter, has an "Asthma-Friendly Child Care Checklist" available
in English, Spanish, Haitian Creole, and Portuguese, with information for
making child care environments safe for children with asthma and allergies. It can be ordered through http://www.asthmaandallergies.org/Articles/
Asthma%20Friendly%20Child%20Care.pdf or by calling 877-2-ASTHMA.
The National Heart, Lung, and Blood Institute has a similar but shorter
checklist—"How Asthma-Friendly Is Your Child-Care Setting?"— available in English and Spanish, which includes an extensive list of resources for
child care providers, available at: http://www.nhlbi.nih.gov/health/public/
lung/asthma/child_ca.htm.

Q *Are sandboxes and sand safe for children?*

A Sandboxes are safe if constructed and filled with appropriate materials
and properly maintained. Sandbox frames are sometimes made with
inexpensive railroad ties, which may cause splinters and may be saturated
with creosote, a carcinogen. Nontoxic landscaping timbers or nonwood
containers are preferred.

In 1986, concern was first expressed that some types of commercially
available play sand contained tremolite, a fibrous substance found in some
crushed limestone and crushed marble (see Chapter 23). It was hypothesized
that the long-term effects of exposure to tremolite would be identical to
those of asbestos. Despite these concerns, the US Consumer Product Safety
Commission denied a petition prohibiting marketing of play sand containing
significant levels of tremolite. The Consumer Product Safety Commission
currently has no standards or labeling requirements regarding the source or
content of sand.

Parents and directors of facilities may have difficulty determining
which sand is safe. They should attempt to buy only natural river sand
or beach sand. They should avoid products that are made from crushed
limestone, crushed marble, crushed crystalline silica (quartz) or those that
are obviously dusty. When there is doubt, parents may send a sample to a
laboratory to determine whether the sand contains tremolite or crystalline
silica. Information about reliable laboratories can be obtained from the
EPA Regional Asbestos Coordinators (see Resources, Chapter 23).

Table 10.3: Diluting Bleach		
TYPE OF OBJECT OR SURFACE	**AMOUNT OF HOUSEHOLD BLEACH TO ADD TO WATER**	**CONCENTRATION IN PARTS PER MILLION (ppm)**
To **sanitize** mouth and food contact surfaces, such as crib railings, mouthing toys, dishes, utensils, and high chair trays	1 tablespoon in 1 gallon of water	100
To **disinfect** environmental surfaces, such as door knobs, counter tops, changing areas, and toilet areas	1/4 cup in 1 gallon of water 1 tablespoon in 1 quart of water	500–800

Once installed, the sandbox should be covered to prevent contamination with animal feces and parasites. Sand should be raked regularly to remove debris and dry it out. A sand rake does a better job than a garden rake.

Q   *Which chemical disinfectants and sanitizers are recommended in child care settings?*

A   Although chemical disinfectants and sanitizers are essential to control communicable diseases in the child care setting, they are potentially hazardous to children, particularly if the products are in concentrated form. Products must be stored in their original labeled containers and in places inaccessible to children. Diluted disinfectants and sanitizers in spray bottles must be labeled and stored out of the reach of children. Solutions should not be sprayed when children are nearby to avoid inhalation and exposing skin and eyes.

Before using any chemical, child care providers should read the product label and manufacturer's material safety data sheet. They should consult public health personnel with questions. It is important to follow label instructions. Questions to consider when selecting a disinfectant are: Is it inactivated by organic matter? Is it affected by hard water? Does it leave a residue? Is it corrosive? Is it a skin, eye, or respiratory irritant? Is it toxic (by skin absorption, ingestion, or inhalation)? What is its effective shelf life after dilution? Household bleach (chlorine as sodium hypochlorite) is active against most microorganisms, including bacterial spores and can be used as a disinfectant or sanitizer, depending on its concentration. Bleach is available at various strengths. Household or laundry bleach is a solution of 5.25%, or 52 500 parts per million (ppm), of sodium hypochlorite. The "ultra" form is only slightly more concentrated and should be diluted and used in the same fashion as ordinary strength household bleach. Higher-strength industrial bleach solutions are not appropriate to use in child care settings. See Table 10.3 for instructions on diluting bleach with water.

Household bleach is effective, economical, convenient, and available at grocery stores. It can be corrosive to some metal, rubber, and plastic materials. Bleach solutions gradually lose their strength, so fresh solutions must be prepared daily, and stock solutions must be replaced every few months. In child care settings, a bleach solution is typically applied using spray bottles. Spray bottles should be labeled with the name of the solution and the dilution. Contact time is important. What is typically observed in a child care setting is "spray and wipe." Bleach solution should be left on for at least 2 minutes before being wiped off. It can be allowed to dry, because it leaves no residue.

Household bleach can be used to sanitize dishes and eating utensils. The concentration of chlorine used in the process is much less than that used for disinfecting other objects. One rationale for sanitizing (as opposed to disinfecting) dishes and eating utensils is that these objects are typically contaminated by only one person and are washed and rinsed thoroughly before being treated with the sanitizing agent. Other objects typically are contaminated by more than one person and less thoroughly washed, resulting in a potentially greater microbial load and diversity of microorganisms.

Q *Is it beneficial to use cleaners that contain disinfectants?*

A By separating out the cleaning and disinfecting processes, you will reduce the amount of disinfectant chemicals used. Soiled objects or surfaces will block the effects of a disinfectant or sanitizer. Therefore, proper disinfection or sanitizing of a surface requires that the surface be cleaned (using soap or detergent and a water rinse) before disinfecting or sanitizing.[2] Bleach (the sanitizer/disinfectant) and ammonia (the cleaner) should never be mixed, because the mixture produces a poisonous gas. Not all items and surfaces require sanitizing or disinfecting. Guidelines for cleaning, sanitizing, and disinfecting can be found in *Caring for Our Children: National Health and Safety Performance Standards—Guidelines for Out-of-Home Child Care Programs.*[2]

Q *What are alternative or less toxic homemade cleaning products? Are they safe?*

A Alternative or less toxic cleaners are made from ingredients such as baking soda, liquid soap, and vinegar. For example, an all-purpose floor cleaner might consist of 2 tablespoons of liquid soap or detergent and 1 gallon of hot water. Many of the ingredients are inexpensive, so you may save money over time. They also may require more "elbow grease"; you may have to scrub harder. Although the ingredients in homemade cleaners (eg, baking soda for scrubbing, vinegar for cutting grease) are safer, not all are nontoxic. Treat them as you would any other cleaner, with caution.

Q *Should I place my child in child care if there isn't a "no smoking" policy in place?*

A No. The American Academy of Pediatrics states that in schools, child care programs, and other venues for children, there should be no tobacco use in or around the premises, regardless of whether children are present.[36] Children should not be exposed to secondhand smoke, and smoke-free policies should be written or stated, enforced, and monitored by the director of the center and parents.

Q *I know that there are health concerns related to carpeting. What precautions should I take?*

A The ideal floor is warm to the touch, skid-proof, easily cleanable, moisture resistant, nontoxic, and does not generate static electricity.[30] This can best be achieved by using hard flooring materials. Carpets are an easy gathering place for biological pollutants, such as molds and dust mites, as well as lead dust and pesticide residues. Instead of wall-to-wall carpeting, consider using area rugs (that are secured to avoid slipping) on hard surfaces; these tend to be easier to clean than installed carpeting. Carpets, pads, and adhesives emit ("off-gas") volatile organic compounds. For children, the elderly, and people with lung conditions, allergies, and allergic-type sensitivities, exposure to fairly low amounts of volatile organic compounds may result in problems such as headaches; nausea; irritation to eyes, nose, and throat; and difficulty breathing. If installing new carpet, look for low–volatile organic compound-emitting carpets and nontoxic adhesives and pads. Ask the carpet store or installer to air out the carpet for at least 24 to 48 hours in the store or warehouse. During installation, make sure the room is well ventilated. After the carpet is installed, continue to ventilate and wait at least 72 hours before using the room. Other preventive measures include: vacuum daily using a good filtering vacuum cleaner; leave shoes worn out-of-doors at the entry way; choose carpet that cleans easily; do not saturate the carpet when wet-cleaning, and ensure the carpet is dry within 24 hours; and use low- or no-solvent cleaning products. Thoroughly clean and dry water-damaged carpets within 24 hours or remove and replace them. Be aware that some carpet comes already treated with antimicrobial products. When possible, avoid the use of pesticides on carpeting.[37]

Q *Are air cleaners that generate ozone safe and effective to use in my child care program?*

A No. Ozone generators that are sold as air cleaners intentionally produce the gas ozone. Manufacturers and vendors of ozone devices often use terms such as "energized oxygen" or "pure air" to suggest that ozone is a healthy kind of oxygen.[38] Ozone is a toxic gas. For more information, see the EPA indoor air quality publications at http://www.epa.gov/iaq/pubs/ozonegen.html.

Q   *Should pets be allowed in child care settings?*

A   Many child care providers who care for children in their homes have pets, and many centers include pets as part of their educational program. Other than service dogs, animals should be avoided or limited in schools and child care settings.[39]

   If a pet is in the child care setting, guidelines to protect health and safety and to avoid risks should be followed. Health and safety concerns for children include allergies, injuries (eg, dog and cat bites), and infections (eg, salmonellosis caused by common bacteria carried by such animals as chickens, iguanas, and turtles). Healthy Child Care Washington in developed a concise handout, "Animals and Domestic Pets" (2007), available at: http://www.healthychildcare-wa.org/Health Risks from Animals.pdf

Q   *I just got a call from my neighbor, who would like to donate her home playground equipment to my child care program. I have a copy of the Consumer Product Safety Commission (CPSC)'s Handbook for Public Playground Safety (http://www.cpsc.gov/cpscpub/pubs/playpubs.html), and her playground equipment doesn't seem to meet their guidelines, but I'm not sure. What should I do?*

A   Playground equipment is a leading source of childhood injury. Many deaths and injuries have occurred on home playgrounds.[40] Since 1981, the Consumer Product Safety Commission has worked to strengthen playground safety guidelines and standards. If you are uncertain whether the playground equipment meets Consumer Product Safety Commission guidelines, get professional advice. Contact your local parks and recreation office or the National Recreation and Park Association (http://www.nrpa.org), and they will connect you with a certified playground inspector in the area. This person can determine the safety of the equipment, provide advice about the types of equipment to best suit the ages of the children in your care and your physical space, and the type and amount of shock-absorbing surfacing needed around play equipment.

Resources

American Academy of Pediatrics and American Public Health Association.
Caring for Our Children: National Health and Safety Performance Standards— Guidelines for Out-of-Home Child Care Programs, 2nd ed. This resource is available in electronic format at the National Resource Center for Health and Safety in Child Care's Web site at http://nrc.uchsc.edu and in hard copy through the American Academy of Pediatrics and the American Public Health Association. Child care regulations for every state are posted on the federally funded National Resource Center for Health and Safety in Child Care's Web site at http://nrc.uchsc.edu. This site also has a search engine for accessing specific child care topics by state. The 3rd edition of *Caring for Our Children* is scheduled for release in 2011.

Healthy Child Care America Campaign, American Academy of Pediatrics

http://www.aap.org/advocacy/hcca/network.htm

This includes a list of state contacts and resource materials and links.

The Eco-Healthy Child Care Program

http://www.cehn.org/ehcc

This national program for child care providers throughout the United States works with child care professionals to eliminate or reduce environmental health hazards found in and around child care facilities. The Eco-Healthy Child Care Program was created in 2010 through a merger of the Oregon Environmental Council's eco-healthy child care program, which began as an Oregon-based initiative in 2005 and the Healthy Environments for Child Care Facilities and Preschools program, created by the Washington, DC-based Children's Environmental Health Network.

References

1. Children's Defense Fund. *Child Care Basics. Children's Defense Fund Issue Basics: April 2005.* Washington, DC: Children's Defense Fund; 2005. Available at: http://www.childrensdefense. org/child-research-data-publications/data/child-care-basics.pdf. Accessed February 28, 2011

2. American Public Health Association, American Academy of Pediatrics. *Caring for Our Children: National Health and Safety Performance Standards. Guidelines for Out-of-Home Child Care Programs.* 2nd ed. Washington, DC: American Public Health Association; and Elk Grove Village, IL: American Academy of Pediatrics; 2002

3. General Accounting Office. *Child Care: State Efforts to Enforce Safety and Health Requirements.* Washington, DC: General Accounting Office; 2000. Available at: http://www.gao.gov/new. items/he00028.pdf

4. US Environmental Protection Agency, Indoor Environments Division. *IAQ Tools for Schools Action Kit.* IAQ Coordinator's Guide. Available at: http://www.epa.gov/iaq/schools/tools4s2. html. Accessed February 28, 2011

5. Home*A*Syst. *Help Yourself to a Healthy Home: Protect Your Children's Health.* Available at: http://www.uwex.edu/homeasyst/text.html. Accessed February 28, 2011

6. US Environmental Protection Agency, Healthy School Environments. *Healthy School Environments Assessment Tool (HealthySEAT).* Available at: http://www.epa.gov/schools/. Accessed February 28, 2011

7. Daneault S, Beausoleil M, Messing K. Air quality during the winter in Quebec day-care centers. *Am J Public Health.* 1992;82(3):432-434

8. Arbes Jr S, Sever M, Mehta J, Collette N, Thomas B, Zeldin D. Exposure to indoor allergens in day-care facilities: results from 2 North Carolina counties. *J Allergy Clin Immunol.* 2005;116(1):133-139

9. Zauraimi MS, Tham KW, Chew FT, Ooi PL. The effect of ventilation strategies of child care centers on indoor air quality and respiratory health of children in Singapore. *Indoor Air.* 2007;17(4):317-327

10. Roberts JW, Dickey P. Exposure of children to pollutants in house dust and indoor air. *Rev Environ Contam Toxicol.* 1995;143:59-79

11. Laquatra J, Maxwell LE, Pierce M. Indoor air pollutants: limited-resource households and child care facilities. *J Environ Health.* 2005;67(7):39-43

12. Centers for Disease Control and Prevention. National Center for Chronic Disease Prevention and Health Promotion. State Smoke-Free Indoor Air Fact Sheet: Day Care Centers. Available at: http://www.portal.state.pa.us/portal/server.pt?open=18&objID=446198&mode=2. Accessed February 28, 2011

13. Washington State Department of Health. *Environmental Lead Survey in Public and Private School Preschools and Day Care Centers.* Olympia, WA: Washington State Department of Health; 1995:1–20

14. Fraser A, Marker D, Rogers J, Viet SM. First National Environmental Health Survey of Child Care Centers, Final Report, July 15, 2003. Volume I: Analysis of Lead Hazards. Washington, DC: U.S. Department of Housing and Urban Development, Office of Healthy Homes and Lead Hazard Control; 2003

15. Weismann DN, Dusdieker LB, Cherryholmes KL, Hausler W Jr, Dungy CI. Elevated environmental lead levels in a day care setting. *Arch Pediatr Adolesc Med.* 1995;149(8):878-881

16. US Environmental Protection Agency. *Controlling Lead in Drinking Water for Schools and Day Care Facilities: A Summary of State Programs.* Washington, DC: US Environmental Protection Agency; 2004. Available at: http://www.epa.gov/safewater/lcrmr/pdfs/report_lcmr_schoolssummary.pdf. Accessed February 28, 2011

17. Tulve NS, Jones PA, Nishioka MG, et al. Pesticide measurements from the first national environmental health survey of child care centers using a multi-residue GC/MS analysis method. *Environ Sci Technol.* 2006;40(20):6269-6274

18. Strandberg J, Karel B, Mills K. Toxic Free North Carolina. *Avoiding Big Risks for Small Kids. Results of the 2008 NC Child Care Pest Control Survey.* Available at: http://www.toxicfreenc.org/informed/pdfs/avoidingbigrisksforsmallkids-web.pdf. Accessed February 28, 2011

19. Gunn WJ, Pinsky PF, Sacks JJ, Schonberger LB. Injuries and poisoning in out-of-home child care and home care. *Am J Dis Child.* 1991;145(7):779-781

20. Aronson SS. Role of the pediatrician in setting and using standards for child care. *Pediatrics.* 1993;91(1 Pt 2):239-243

21. Fenske RA, Black KG, Elkner KP, Lee CL, Methner MM, Soto R. Potential exposure and health risks of infants following indoor residential pesticide applications. *Am J Public Health.* 1990;80(6):689-693

22. California Childcare Health Program. Risks Associated with Bisphenol A in baby bottles. San Francisco, CA: California Childcare Health Program; September 2008. Available at: http://www.ucsfchildcarehealth.org/pdfs/factsheets/BisphenolEn0908.pdf. Accessed February 28, 2011

23. US Food and Drug Administration. Bisphenol A (BPA). Update on Bisphenol A (BPA) for Use in Food: January 2010. Available at: http://www.fda.gov/newsevents/publichealthfocus/ucm064437.htm. Accessed January 28, 2011

24. Heightened Concern Over BPA [editorial]. *New York Times.* January 21, 2010:A38. Available at: http://www.nytimes.com/2010/01/21/opinion/21thur2.html. Accessed January 28, 2011

25. National Association of Child Care Resource and Referral Agencies. What Child Care Providers Earn. 2006 Annual Mean Wage. Available at: http://www.naccrra.org/randd/child-care-workforce/provider_income.php. Accessed February 28, 2011

26. Bank H, Behr A, Schulman K. *State Developments in Child Care, Early Education, and School-Age Care.* Washington, DC: Children's Defense Fund; 2000:57. Available at: http://www.childrensdefense.org/pdf/2000_state_dev.pdf. Accessed February 28, 2011

27. Center for the Child Care Workforce. Estimating the Size and Components of the U.S. Child Care Workforce and Caregiving Population. May 2002. Available at: http://www.naccrra.org/randd/child-care-workforce/cc_workforce.php. Accessed March 28, 2011

28. National Child Care Information Center. Center Child Care Licensing Requirements. August 2004. Available at: http://www.naralicensing.org/associations/4734/files/1005_2008_Child%20 Care%20Licensing%20Study_Full_Report.pdf. Accessed March 28, 2011

29. National Association of Child Care Resource and Referral Agencies. Child Care Workforce. 2006. Available at http://www.naccrra.org/randd/child-care-workforce/cc_workforce.php. Accessed February 28, 2011

30. Olds AR. *Child Care Design Guide.* New York, NY: McGraw-Hill; 2001

31. US Environmental Protection Agency. *IAQ Design Tools for Schools.* Washington, DC: US Environmental Protection Agency; 2001. Available at: http://www.epa.gov/iaq/schooldesign. Accessed February 28, 2011

32. Sellstrom E, Bremberg S. Education of staff—a key factor for a safe environment in day care. *Acta Paediatr.* 2000;89(5):601-607

33. National Association of Child Care Resource and Referral Agencies. *Building a National Community-Based Training System for Child Care Resource and Referral.* Arlington, VA: National Association of Child Care Resource and Referral Agencies; 2005:7

34. Kiechl-Kohlendorfer U, Moon RY. Sudden infant death syndrome (SIDS) and child care centres (CCC). *Acta Paediatr.* 2008;97(7):844-845

35. Asthma and Allergy Foundation of America, New England Chapter. *For Child Care Providers.* Available at: http://www.asthmaandallergies.org/N_Childcare%20Providers.htm. Accessed January 28, 2011

36. American Academy of Pediatrics Committee on Environmental Health, Committee on Substance Abuse, Committee on Adolescence, and Committee on Native American Child Health. Policy statement—tobacco use: a pediatric disease. *Pediatrics.* 2009;124(5):1474–1487

37. Vermont Department of Health. *An Air Quality Fact Sheet on Carpet.* Burlington, VT: Vermont Department of Health. Available at: http://www.state.vt.us/health/_hp/airquality/carpet/carpet. htm. Accessed February 28, 2011

38. US Environmental Protection Agency. *Ozone Generators that are Sold as Air Cleaners: An Assessment of Effectiveness and Health Consequences.* Washington, DC: US Environmental Protection Agency. Available at: http://www.epa.gov/iaq/pubs/ozonegen.html. Accessed February 28, 2011

39. American Academy of Pediatrics Committee on School Health, National Association of School Nurses. *Health, Mental Health, and Safety Guidelines for Schools.* Taras H, Duncan P, Luckenbill D, et al, eds. Elk Grove Village, IL: American Academy of Pediatrics; 2004

40. US Consumer Product Safety Commission. *Home Playground Equipment-Related Deaths and Injuries.* Washington, DC: US Consumer Product Safety Commission; 2001. Available at: http://www.cpsc.gov/library/playground.pdf. Accessed January 28, 2011

Chapter 11

Schools

■ ■ ■ ■ ■ ■

The typical school-aged child spends approximately 1170 hours per year at school—which translates into more than 2300 days during the 13 years between kindergarten and 12th grade.[1] That figure can increase by thousands of hours if children also participate in after-school programs or extracurricular activities. This chapter describes how physical, nutritional, and psychosocial aspects of the school environment can affect a child's health and well-being. It discusses the importance of the environmental health history in identifying school-related adverse health factors, and work to promote improved safety, health, and wellness in schools. Additional specific guidance is available in the *Health, Mental Health and Safety Guidelines for Schools* (available at http://www.nationalguidelines.org*)*.

PHYSICAL DIMENSIONS OF THE SCHOOL ENVIRONMENT

School Buildings

Most schools in the United States were built before 1984 and have not undergone major renovation since that time.[2] Because of this, they are likely to contain materials such as asbestos (see Chapter 23) and lead (see Chapter 31). Children's risk of exposure to such substances is greatest when buildings are being renovated or fall into disrepair—a common state in inner cities and poorly resourced rural areas. Routine inspection of school buildings and construction sites to identify hazards is critical.

High-Performance Schools

High-performance school buildings are efficient in their use of energy, water, and materials and are also safe, secure, stimulating, and healthy. They require careful attention to site selection and design. They also require commissioning, a systematic process of ensuring that the buildings perform interactively and in a way consistent with design intent and operational needs. The Collaborative for High-Performance Schools (www.chps.net) and the National Clearinghouse for Educational Facilities (www.edfacilities.org) provide information about designing and commissioning high-performance schools. The Healthy School Environments Assessment Tool (HealthySEAT v2) (www.epa.gov/schools/healthyseat), developed by the US Environmental Protection Agency (EPA), is a free downloadable program that can be used to systematically track and manage information about school environmental conditions as well as school compliance with government regulations and voluntary school program requirements.

Utilization of Space

Understanding the school environment requires an assessment of how space in schools is used. Schools are primarily established to provide children with an education, and they may also serve other community functions. They often serve as sites for before- and after-school child care and enrichment programs, recreation, adult education, artistic performances, and public meetings. Health clinics and social service providers may colocate in schools. During disasters and other emergencies, schools often serve as shelters or command posts. These uses raise concerns about safety and security as well as the possibility that utilizing makeshift and converted spaces exposes users to existing environmental hazards. Information about the benefits and challenges of schools serving as focal points for academic, health, social service, community development, and community engagement efforts is available (www.communityschools.org).

Crowding

Objectively, crowding occurs when people inhabit a space beyond its capacity or when people in a space have very little room per person. Subjectively, crowding occurs when an individual feels that his or her ability to control interaction with other people is impaired or that other people interfere with their activities. Crowding is linked to increased transmission of infectious diseases. Crowding is stressful. It can cause overstimulation, interfere with concentration, create social friction, and increase aggression. This, in turn, can interfere with learning and precipitate problematic behavior—especially for children with autism spectrum disorders (ASDs), attention-deficit/hyperactivity disorder (ADHD) or other attention disorders, sensory integration dysfunction, or learning disorders. Teachers are likely to feel stressed in crowded environments, where they often spend more time on discipline and classroom management.

Acoustics and Noise

Poor classroom acoustics can interfere with children's ability to learn and communicate.[3] Noise—unwanted sound—can interfere with student concentration, motivation, and memory. It can be stressful, especially if loud or persistent, and can result in elevated blood pressure.[4] Students with sensory impairment, auditory processing disorders, ADHD, and ASDs may be particularly sensitive to noise.[5,6] In many cases, improved acoustics and noise reduction can be achieved by simple interventions such as furniture reconfiguration, designation of "quiet" areas, replacement of noisy lighting fixtures and equipment, and changes in scheduling (eg, staggering lunchtimes to reduce hallway traffic during instructional periods). In other cases, soundproofing and other building modifications may be necessary. Information on classroom acoustics and noise reduction is available from the Acoustical Society of America (http://asa.aip.org/classroom.html) and Quiet Classrooms (www.quietclassrooms.org).

Learning Environments and Activities

Certain learning activities may pose health risks because of the nature of the learning space or the materials and equipment used.

- Industrial arts projects often involve potentially toxic chemicals. Students should be taught about the toxicity and how to avoid exposure. Workshops typically contain tools and equipment that may cause cuts, abrasions, burns, lifting injuries, or more serious injuries, such as amputations. Students may be exposed to noise, flying objects, chemical fumes, intense heat, and sharp edges; protective gear (eg, goggles, ear plugs, gloves, masks) must be used in potentially hazardous situations. In wood shops, dust and shavings in the air can trigger asthma exacerbations and use of a protective mask should be considered.
- Certain materials used for art and craft projects are potentially toxic (see Chapter 42). Nontoxic materials certified by the Art & Creative Materials Institute (www.acminet.org) should be used whenever possible. Kilns can emit chemicals that may cause respiratory problems. Adequate ventilation is crucial.
- Chemistry and biology classrooms and labs may contain potentially toxic materials that require proper storage and handling. The EPA's School Chemical Cleanout Campaign (http://www.epa.gov/epawaste/partnerships/sc3) provides information and tools for managing these risks. Other potential injuries include burns and cuts. Handling live animals may lead to bites, scratches, allergic reactions, or zoonotic diseases.[7] Animals should only be maintained as necessary for curricula and should be carefully confined in suitable, sanitary, self-contained enclosures appropriate for their size.[8]
- Traumatic injuries are especially likely in gym classes and with recreational activities involving movement. Risks can be reduced by ensuring adequate

supervision and space. Floors and equipment should be in good repair and cleaned regularly. Indoor pools should be properly maintained and well ventilated.

Bathrooms and Locker Rooms

Bathrooms and locker rooms are just some of the locations where students may be exposed to microorganisms, such as molds, especially when plumbing leaks or toilets overflow. Students may come in contact with infectious agents by interacting with other students and through fomites. Waste containers, soap, and paper towels should be readily available. Students should be encouraged to wash their hands or use hand sanitizer throughout the day, especially after toileting, outdoor play, and before eating. Bathroom areas should be well ventilated, because sewer gasses, cigarette smoke, air fresheners, hair sprays, and perfumes may contribute to poor air quality. Good lighting and antislip measures should be used to reduce the risk of injuries in showers and areas where water tends to be tracked. The water temperature should be set low enough to prevent scalding.

Food Preparation, Storage, and Service Areas

Pest management is particularly important in food-related areas. Food service staff and students involved in food preparation or service should be trained in proper food storage and handling techniques to reduce the risk of spread of infectious disease, food contamination, and spoilage. Equipment should be cleaned and maintained properly to reduce the risk of biological contaminants or nonfood objects affecting food. It is also important to clean equipment properly to avoid cross-contamination that can trigger food allergy. The National Coalition for Food-Safe Schools (www.foodsafeschools.org) and the EPA (http://www.epa.gov/pesticides/ipm/) are excellent sources of information on this topic.

Lighting

Lighting quality affects students' ability to see and process visual information. Students may have difficulty attending and learning if available light is insufficient, unbalanced (contrasting bright spots and shadows), or gloomy. Glare may cause fatigue, eye strain, and headaches. Modern school designs tend to better integrate natural light into lighting design, because students tend to perform better when natural light contributes to classroom lighting and may experience a subtle, positive effect on their mood and behavior.[9]

Children with visual impairment, learning disabilities, sensory processing/integration disorder, ADHD, and ASDs are often very sensitive to lighting environments. They may disengage from the learning process or engage in problematic behavior if distracted, annoyed, or stressed by glare or malfunctioning (flickering, humming) light fixtures. Interventions include repairing or replacing lighting fixtures, strategic use of window coverings, repositioning of classroom furniture, and assigning students to optimally lighted classroom areas.

Ergonomics

Ergonomics is the science of taking human characteristics into account when designing and using objects or equipment. Providing child-friendly seating, workstations, equipment, and furniture can be especially challenging given the wide variation in children's sizes, body proportions, and growth rates. Children who use adaptive equipment or who have specific areas of difficulty or disability may present additional challenges. Information about ergonomic aspects of backpacks, computers, and other items associated with school is available through Healthy Computing (www.healthycomputing.com/kids), the Cornell University Ergonomics Web (http://ergo.human.cornell.edu/MBergo/school-guide.html), and Ergonomics 4 Schools (http://ergonomics4schools.com). Information on inspecting and retrofitting bleachers to reduce the risk injury is available from the US Consumer Product Safety Commission (http://www.cpsc.gov/CPSCPUB/PUBS/330.pdf).

Thermal Conditions

Temperature, relative humidity, and air velocity are important parts of the physical environment (see Chapter 26). Thermal conditions influence mold growth and the release of chemical and microbiological agents into the air. Relatively small changes in thermal conditions can influence student comfort. Students are less able to learn if they are uncomfortable. Factors such as student clothing and activity level; radiant heat transfer from very hot equipment (eg, computers); season; air flow; heating, ventilating, and air conditioning (HVAC) unit performance; sunlight penetration; and building construction should be considered when managing the thermal environment.

The national consensus standard for outside air ventilation is ASHRAE (American Society of Heating, Refrigerating and Air-Conditioning Engineers) Standard 62.1-200, Ventilation for Acceptable Indoor Air Quality (available online via www.ashrae.org) and its published Addenda. This standard is often incorporated into state and local building codes and specifies the amounts of outside air that must be provided by natural or mechanical ventilation systems to various areas of the school, including classrooms, gymnasiums, kitchens, and other special-use areas. Airflow in schools should be between 15 and 20 cubic feet/minute per person and result in more than 4 air changes per hour.[10,11] Carbon dioxide levels, which are useful in determining the adequacy of ventilation, should be less than 1000 parts per million (ppm) when a room has been occupied for 4 to 6 hours.[12] The optimal temperature for most classrooms is 69.8°F to 73.4°F (21°C–23°C).[13] The relative humidity should be between 30%

and 50%. High temperature, especially in combination with low relative humidity, can increase eye, skin, and mucosal irritation and may also result in fatigue, lethargy, poor concentration, and headache. High relative humidity, often manifested as surfaces that feel damp, is problematic, because it stimulates dust mite multiplication as well as growth of bacteria and mold. This is a particular problem in portable classroom structures. Mold can be a potent trigger for asthma. High humidity may be caused by flooding, wet carpet, inadequate bathroom ventilation, and kitchen-generated moisture. Other sources of moisture include humidifiers, dehumidifiers, air conditioners, and drip pans under refrigerator cooling coils. Means of reducing moisture include proper maintenance of HVAC systems, use of exhaust fans in high-moisture environments (eg, kitchens, pool areas), repairing leaks, and prompt drying or removal of wet carpeting. Regular walk-throughs and inspections can help to identify these hazards before they cause harm.

Air Quality

Poor air quality in schools places children at risk of short- and long-term health problems and can have a negative effect on learning and performance. An analysis of school-level data from the 2006 School Health Policies and Programs Study shows that 51.4% of schools had a formal indoor air quality management program and that those schools were significantly more likely than were schools without a program to have policies and use strategies to promote indoor air quality.[14]

Outdoor Air Pollution

Air quality around schools depends on factors such as traffic patterns, nearby industrial activities, proximity to waste sites, local herbicide and pesticide use, atmospheric conditions, and geography. Outdoor air pollution is linked to respiratory problems in children, including decreased lung function, coughing, wheezing, more frequent respiratory illness, and asthma exacerbation (see Chapter 21). Children are primarily exposed to outdoor air pollutants while traveling to or from school and when playing outside. Pollutants may also enter through doors, windows, vents, and drains. Carbon monoxide (see Chapter 25), nitrogen dioxide, and particles found in vehicle exhaust may be present at high levels in schools located close to busy roadways or where busses, delivery trucks, or passenger vehicles idle nearby for long periods of time. School officials can reduce traffic-related emissions by discouraging vehicle idling and improving school-related traffic flow and by using the free toolkit available from the EPA's Clean School Bus USA program (www.epa.gov/otaq/schoolbus). They should also consider outdoor air quality when scheduling recess, sports, and other outdoor activities. Information about ozone levels and smog alerts is available through local media and the EPA's Air Now Web site (http://airnow.gov).

Indoor Air Quality

Many factors contribute to indoor air quality (see Chapter 20). The concentration of indoor air pollutants can vary from room to room and even within a single classroom. Levels may also vary according to the activity occurring in the space (eg, higher levels during craft activities) and variations in airflow (eg, caused by opening windows).

Pollen, soot, fiberglass fibers, chalk dust, lead, and other airborne particulates can cause respiratory and other health problems. Smoking should not be allowed within the school or any part of the school property, including sporting fields and bleachers. Secondhand smoke exposure (see Chapter 40) can occur if schools restrict smoking to designated areas.

Toxic gasses can affect air quality. Although some can be detected by odor, others are odorless and require specific equipment for detection. An estimated 19.3% of US schools have at least 1 room with radon levels at or above 4 picocuries per liter (pCi/L).[15] Formaldehyde may cause irritation of the mouth, throat, nose, and eyes; worsen asthma symptoms; and cause headache and nausea. Exposure may be especially likely in portable classrooms containing composite wood products (eg, plywood, particleboard).[16] Paints, adhesives, carpets, cleaning products, and building materials may contain volatile organic compounds (VOCs), which are associated with respiratory and other health problems. Unhealthy concentrations of volatile organic compounds may be especially common in portable classrooms, where thermal conditions tend to facilitate off-gassing, especially in the first few years of use.[16]

Poor indoor air quality may give rise to a building-related illness or sick building syndrome. Building-related illnesses are disorders that can be directly attributed to chemical or physical agents in a particular building.[17] Sick building syndrome is a phenomenon whereby several occupants in the same building experience similar acute or lingering symptoms with no obvious etiology. Symptoms appear to be linked to a particular building or area within a building. Sick building syndrome has been linked to biological and chemical contaminants, poorly designed and maintained HVAC systems, overly warm temperatures, and high relative humidity.[18,19] Very low levels of specific pollutants and other physical factors may act synergistically or in combination to cause sick building syndrome.[20] Often, symptoms of sick building syndrome and building-related illnesses disappear when the people are not in the building. Some of the symptoms of sick building syndrome may overlap with symptoms of multiple chemical sensitivities (see Chapter 55).[21,22]

Free materials related to indoor air quality in schools are available on the EPA's Tools for Schools Web site (www.epa.gov/iaq/schools).

Biological air pollutants are found to some degree in every school. They may generate toxic or allergic reactions, particularly with excessive exposure.

Sources include outdoor air, animals, human occupants, insects, and water reservoirs (eg, humidifiers).

- Molds characteristically thrive in warm, moist climates and release spores into the air that are associated with allergic reactions in susceptible individuals, asthma exacerbations, coughing, wheezing, and upper respiratory symptoms in otherwise healthy people with an allergic predisposition. Mold toxins are associated with headache and fatigue.[23]

- Hair and dander of cats, dogs, and other animals may be shed by classroom pets, laboratory animals, service animals, visiting pets, and vermin. They may be carried to school on children's clothes. Classroom allergen levels may become high enough to cause sensitization or induce asthma in children who do not have pets at home or come into direct contact with animals. Other than service dogs, animals should be avoided or limited in schools and in child care settings.[8]

- Dust mite allergens may become airborne and cause asthma, rhinitis, or atopic dermatitis in predisposed individuals. Reservoirs in schools include upholstered furniture, pillows, carpets, and books.

- Cockroach allergens can be a significant factor in the development and exacerbation of asthma in children.[24]

Among children with clinical complaints related to the environment, appropriate allergic and psychological consultation should be considered. Viral respiratory tract infections peak in prevalence at the onset of school, and children with asthma have increased respiratory symptoms from those viral respiratory tract infections. Mold spores and animal dander in the school can cause inhalant allergy symptoms in susceptible allergic children; these problems can be identified by appropriate clinical assessment and often are readily treatable. For the individual child in whom treatment is not successful, special arrangements may be needed.

Although it is important to eliminate undesirable insects, routine spraying of pesticides inside and outside the building can adversely affect indoor air quality and can leave toxic residue that can be ingested or absorbed through the skin (see Chapter 37). To control pests in a more environmentally sensitive and cost-effective way, many schools adopt integrated pest management (IPM) programs. Integrated pest management involves the judicial use of pesticides in conjunction with other strategies informed by knowledge about specific pests and their interactions with the environment. When chemicals are used, the treatments are timed according to the pest's life cycle (eg, breeding, egg laying) to maximize effect. Materials related to integrated pest management in schools are available from the EPA (www.epa.gov/pesticides/ipm), the National School IPM Information Source (http://schoolipm.ifas.ufl.edu), and the National Pest Management Association (www.pestworld.org).

Cleaning Materials and Practices

Children's health and well-being may be enhanced or compromised by the products and practices used to clean and maintain schools.[25] Cleaning, sanitizing, and disinfecting are useful methods for protecting people against viruses and bacteria. Cleaning refers to using soaps or detergents and water to physically remove visible dirt and contamination from surfaces or objects. Sanitizing is the process used after visible dirt is removed from a surface. Sanitizing greatly reduces the number of pathogens to levels that are unlikely to cause disease. Disinfecting, a process that is more rigorous than sanitizing, involves applying cumulative heat or a chemical to result in the elimination of almost all microorganisms from inanimate surfaces.

Routine procedures differ from place to place and may include use of disinfectants on frequently touched surfaces and objects. More information on cleaning, sanitizing, and disinfecting can be found in Chapter 10.

Many chemicals used to clean floors, desks, and tables are potentially toxic. String mops used to clean bathroom floors may promote the spread of infectious agents to uncontaminated areas. Although cleaning is important to remove particulate matter from floors, carpets, and other surfaces, many cleaning activities, such as rag dusting and use of a vacuum cleaner with a cloth bag, simply resuspend particulate matter rather than remove it. School staff should vacuum regularly using well-constructed cleaners with high-efficiency particulate air (HEPA) filters or near-HEPA filters. Dusters should be made of materials that trap, rather than simply push, dust particles.

Many schools have adopted "green" cleaning programs that minimize the effects of cleaning materials on health and also protect the environment. Such programs emphasize the thoughtful use and proper storage of cleaning materials. They incorporate healthy, environmentally conscious policies, procedures, and training. Information can be obtained from the Healthy Schools Campaign (www.healthyschools.org), the National Clearinghouse for Educational Facilities (www.edfacilities.org), and The Cleaning for Healthy Schools Toolkit (www.cleaningforhealthyschools.org).

Water Quality

Lead contamination (see Chapter 31) may be a significant water-related concern in schools. One study found that more than 57% of Philadelphia's public schools had water lead levels exceeding the EPA action level at the time of 20 parts per billion (ppb).[26] More than 28% had water with mean lead levels in excess of 50 parts per billion. Lead most frequently enters drinking water by leaching from plumbing materials and fixtures as water moves through plumbing.[27] High concentrations of lead can accumulate in water overnight, on weekends, and over school holidays because of the increased time that the water remains in the water distribution system. Schools should meet or exceed federal and state laws for lead and other water quality measures. Those with private wells should have water tested periodically for bacterial and chemical contamination. Information about water quality is available from the EPA Safewater program (www.epa.gov/safewater).

Outdoor Environments

Playgrounds, athletic fields, and green areas provide spaces for play, physical activity, socializing, and relaxation (see Chapter 9). They allow contact with the natural world and can facilitate learning about local wildlife. With these benefits come potential risks related to air pollution, ultraviolet (UV) radiation, contaminated soil, contaminated groundwater, play surfaces, and equipment, as well as contact with birds, animals, and human members of the larger community.

Excessive exposure to UV radiation places children at higher risk of skin cancers and other serious health problems ater in their lives[28] (see Chapter 41). Schools can schedule children's outdoor activities before and after the hours when UV rays are strongest (ie, avoiding outdoor activities from 10 AM–4 PM). They can implement policies that encourage students to wear protective clothing, hats, and sunglasses and to apply sunscreen during outdoor activities. They can also implement educational programs, such as the EPA's SunWise Program (www.epa.gov/sunwise), to encourage and reinforce preventative behaviors. Information on increasing outdoor shading using strategies is suggested by Shade Planning for America's Schools (www.cdc.gov/cancer/skin/pdf/shade_planning.pdf).

Toxicants may be present the soil and groundwater near schools, especially those built in areas of high air pollution or on land contaminated by industrial waste. Lead (see Chapter 31) may be found in high concentrations near school walls, where paint has flaked off and accumulated, or throughout the grounds if the school is located near a point source, such as a smelter or battery manufacturing plant. High levels of polychlorinated biphenyls (PCBs) may be found near buildings with PCB-containing caulk.[29] Sufficient exposure to herbicides and pesticides used on school grounds can cause skin and eye irritation as well as abdominal pain and vomiting.

Hazards around school driveways, parking lots, and other paths of travel increase the risk of injury. These areas should be clearly marked, well-lighted, and well-maintained, especially when weather conditions cause them to be slippery or difficult to traverse. Areas where students are picked up and dropped off should offer adequate protection from the elements as well as from traffic and vehicle exhaust. During peak traffic times, additional safety measures, such as crossing guards and alterations in traffic light timing, can help reduce the risk of accidents. The Pedestrian and Bicycle Information Center (www.pedbikeinfo.org)

provides information to enhance biking and walking safety. The Centers for Disease Control and Prevention (CDC)'s KidsWalk-to-School program (www.cdc.gov/nccdphp/dnpa/kidswalk) and the National Center for Safe Routes to School (http://www.saferoutesinfo.org) provide information to encourage children to walk and bicycle to and from school.

Children who walk, bicycle, or take public transportation may be vulnerable to street crime. Students may be more inclined to engage in truant, delinquent, or risky behavior if nearby parks, stores, abandoned buildings, or wooded areas prove to be tempting hangouts. It is prudent for school officials to investigate any potential dangers in nearby areas such as construction sites, industrial sites, and water bodies.

Playgrounds and Outdoor Athletic Spaces

Play areas should be designed and maintained to meet the needs of all students, including students with disabilities. An informative reference on this topic, *Accessible Play Areas: A Summary of Accessibility Guidelines for Play Areas*, is available at http://www.access-board.gov/play/guide/guide.pdf. Additional materials are available at www.beyondaccess.org.

Playgrounds are common sites of serious injury at school. Between 1996 and 2005, playground equipment injuries accounted for more than 2.1 million emergency department visits in the United States.[30] The most common injuries were fractures (35%), contusions or abrasions (20%), and lacerations (20%). Such injuries can often be reduced by modifying playground equipment and layout, as well as installing shock-absorbing safety surfaces. Information is available from the National Program for Playground Safety (www.playgroundsafety.org) and in the Public Playground Safety Handbook developed by the Consumer Product Safety Commission (CPSC) (www.cpsc.gov/cpscpub).

The risk of athletic injuries increases if students have insufficient space, are exposed to physical hazards (eg, rocks, holes, sharp objects, animal droppings) on playing fields, or engage in sports on hard, loose, or uneven terrain. Artificial turf may contain toxicants and increase the risk of certain types of injuries and infections.[31] Playing spaces should be clearly marked. Where appropriate, nets and other barriers should be used to protect spectators from stray balls or other play-related hazards.

THE SCHOOL NUTRITIONAL ENVIRONMENT

Most children eat meals or snacks each day at school. Although some food and beverages are brought from home or purchased off-site, much is obtained from the cafeteria or purchased from on-site vending machines. Schools may play an important role in influencing children's food intake, eating habits, and knowledge of nutrition. Food often plays a significant part in school events (eg, fund-raising, class parties). Food should not be used as a reward for good performance. Information about food and nutrition is often incorporated into health, science, home economics, and vocational curricula. Status among peers may be affected by a child's eating habits, such as whether a child eats a school lunch or brings lunch from home, contents of lunches and lunch containers brought from home or provided by a family member during the lunch period, whether one shares food, where and with whom (if anyone) one sits at lunch, and whether the environment provides opportunity for activities that might make a child rush or skip lunch.[32] Students, especially girls, may feel pressured to engage in unhealthy eating practices or use potentially dangerous diet supplements. Other students may be inclined to overeat if they find the school environment stressful or are on restrictive diets at home.

Although significant effort has been undertaken to improve the nutritional value of the foods offered and eaten at school, some foods consumed at school can be high in calories and have limited nutritional value, thereby increasing the risk of obesity and diabetes. This risk may be especially relevant for children from low-income families, whose diets may be especially lacking in nutrients. Ideally, food and drinks available at schools should conform to the federal nutrition guidelines established for schools participating in the National School Lunch and Breakfast programs. Foods served at schools have been occasionally linked to widespread illness among children.[33]

Meal planning can be challenging given budgetary constraints, bulk food purchasing policies, concerns about food allergies, and children's food preferences. The US Department of Agriculture's Food and Nutrition Services Web site (www.fns.usda.gov/fns) and the School Nutrition Association (www.school-nutrition.org) offer information on school nutrition assistance programs, school meal planning, and nutrition. Information on improving the school nutritional environment and encouraging physical activity is available from the Action for Healthy Kids (www.actionforhealthykids.org) and the Healthy Schools campaign (www.healthyschoolscampaign.org).

PSYCHOSOCIAL DIMENSIONS OF THE SCHOOL ENVIRONMENT

Historically, environmental health research and practice has focused on toxicants and physical hazards. A more holistic perspective recognizes the significant influence of psychosocial factors. School affords children the opportunity to develop social skills, form friendships, learn teamwork, achieve a sense of belonging, and develop a positive self-image. School can also be a site where animosities foment and children feel physically or emotionally vulnerable to other students, teachers, cliques, or gangs.

School Violence and Intimidation

Violent crime on school grounds represents a real threat to student health and well-being. Some 628 000 violent crimes on school property—including sexual offenses and 14 homicides—were reported during the 2005–2006 school year alone.[34] Many students' school experiences are colored by concerns about violence.[35] The 2005 School Crime Supplement to the National Crime Victimization Survey found that more than 12% of respondents 12 to 18 years of age did not feel safe at school. Those attending schools with minority enrollment greater than 49% were particularly likely to feel unsafe. Approximately 1 in 3 students attending urban schools reported the presence of gangs in their school. Those attending suburban or rural schools reported lower but still concerning rates (21% and 16%, respectively). Among students in grades 9 through 12, 10% of males and 6% of females reported having been threatened or injured with a weapon on school property in the past year. Some 6% reported having skipped classes or extracurricular activities, avoided certain places on school grounds, or stayed home from school in the previous 6 months because of fear of attack or harm. Six percent reported having carried a weapon on school property during the previous 30 days.

The National Crime Victimization Survey also found that 11% of students 12 to 18 years of age reported that someone at school had used hate-related words against them, having to do with their race, ethnicity, religion, disability, gender, or sexual orientation. Thirty-eight percent reported seeing hate-related graffiti at school. Twenty-eight percent of students had been bullied at school during the previous 6 months.[35] Of these, 53% said that the bullying had happened once or twice during that period; another 25% reported experiencing it once or twice a month; the remainder reported the frequency as once or twice a week (11%) or almost daily (8%). The bullying involved pushing, shoving, tripping, or spitting approximately 9% of the time. When this occurred, about 1 in 4 students reported having been injured. Resources are available from the Stop Bullying Now campaign at http://www.stopbullyingnow.hrsa.gov/adults/default.aspx. The prevalence of "cyberbullying" (through e-mail, text messages, or Web sites) is not known.

Substance Use

Substance use and abuse occurs on school property. Four percent of students 12 to 18 years of age reported having consumed at least 1 alcoholic drink on school property during the previous 30 days. One in 4 (25.7%) students smoked cigarettes, cigars, cigarillos, or little cigars or used chewing tobacco, snuff, or dip (a form of smokeless tobacco) at least 1 day during the past 30 days.[36] Information about youth tobacco use is available from the CDC Youth Risk Behavior Surveillance System (YRBSS) (http://www.cdc.gov/HealthyYouth/yrbs/)

and the Youth Tobacco Survey (YTS) (http://www.cdc.gov/tobacco/data_statistics/surveys/yts/index.htm). One in 4 National Crime Victimization Survey respondents reported that someone had offered, sold, or given them an illegal drug on school property in the past 12 months.[35]

One in 4 students who reported using marijuana anywhere during the past 30 days (20% of the total respondents) reported having used marijuana on school property during that period. The use of inhalants ("huffing") at school is a concern, because students may be able to access glues, markers, paints, solvents, and other substances with mind-altering effects. Information about youth substance abuse is available from the National Institute on Drug Abuse (www.drugabuse.gov) and the National Inhalant Prevention Coalition (www.inhalants.com).

Positive Influences and Effects

School is a place where children are taught facts and develop academic skills. It is also a place where children can learn how to ask questions, problem-solve, relate, communicate, act responsibly, and lead. For many children, school is a place where their learning disabilities, emotional and behavioral problems, social difficulties, or maltreatment are first noticed and addressed. School may serve as a temporary haven for those with chaotic home lives.

Many children encounter teachers and other positive role models who inspire, encourage, and support them. They are afforded opportunities to feed their curiosity and expand their interests, as well as develop and be recognized for their artistic, athletic, and intellectual talents. School is often a place where good memories are formed and important friendships take root. These positive aspects can enhance mental health, bolster resiliency, and pave the way for healthy adult relationships and personal success.

STUDENTS AS ACTIVE PARTICIPANTS IN SCHOOL ENVIRONMENTAL HEALTH EFFORTS

Students can play an active role in promoting a healthy school environment. For example, they can participate in school walk-throughs to identify potential health hazards; initiate and promote recycling programs, help cultivate schoolyard wildlife habitats (see the Georgia Wildlife Federation's downloadable guide at http://www.gwf.org), help implement antibullying campaigns. Student interest in school environmental health can be sparked through materials and lessons such as those offered by the Environmental Health Perspectives Science Education Program (www.ehponline. org/science-ed-new), the National Environmental Education Foundation (http://www.neefusa.org), National Institute of Environmental Health Sciences (http://www.niehs.nih.gov/health/scied), and the EPA Teaching Center (http://www.epa.gov/teachers/teachresources.htm).

THE PEDIATRICIAN'S ROLE IN SCHOOL ENVIRONMENTAL HEALTH

Taking a School Environmental Health History

Taking a school environmental health history can be important when a child presents with respiratory problems; unexplained illness and nonspecific symptoms suggestive of toxicant exposure; or behavioral and social problems associated with sensory integration difficulties, ADHD, or autism spectrum disorders. It can be valuable when addressing chronic conditions with implications across multiple domains, such as obesity, asthma, diabetes, hypertension, and mood disorders. The history-taking process provides opportunities to educate children, families, and educators about how school environmental factors can enhance or compromise children's health and well-being.

It can be helpful to ask the student to recount their activities and interactions over the course of a typical week. Younger children may have difficulty providing detailed information, but their input is nonetheless valuable, because it may yield information about the physical environment and provide insight into their experience of school. Older students are likely to have more complicated schedules that vary from one day or marking period to the next.

In addition to focusing on the health of individual children, pediatricians are uniquely poised to promote the health, development, and wellness of children in the community. Pediatricians' expertise, interests, and concerns afford the opportunity to contribute to or lead efforts to improve the school environment by participating in on-site inspections of school buildings, grounds, and play equipment; encouraging schools to promote good nutrition; supporting efforts to increase physical activity; educating parents, students, and school personnel about using protective clothing and equipment; encouraging exploration of and integrating concern for nature and the environment into curricula (see Appendix B) and into students' daily experiences; serving on school committees addressing health, wellness, and emergency preparedness; and supporting school nurse efforts to make the school a positive focus for child health in the community.

Frequently Asked Questions

Q *Asbestos was recently discovered in ceilings at my child's school. What should the school do? Should my child have a chest x-ray? Will she develop cancer?*

A Asbestos was extensively used as insulation in school construction until the 1970s. Because asbestos release is typically episodic (eg, when materials are fractured during renovation) and usually missed by air sampling, visual inspection is required to establish the nature of the asbestos risk. All schools must maintain an asbestos management plan and undergo systematic inspection every 3 years. Normally, asbestos removal is not necessary unless children are likely to come into direct contact with it or building renovation is about to occur. More often, the fibers are simply contained by installing drywall, drop ceilings, or other enclosures. Under federal law, you have the right to request a copy of your school's asbestos management plan, which provides information about building inspections, as well as asbestos removal and containment activities. The risk of lung cancer or mesothelioma from a brief exposure is very low. A chest x-ray will not be helpful, because asbestos does not produce acute changes in the lungs.

Q *How do I know if there is a problem with lead in our school?*

A Schools built before the 1970s are likely to contain leaded materials on walls, woodwork, stairwells, and window casings and sills. Other sources include deteriorating paint, lead pipes, lead-lined water coolers, water fixtures, and lead-containing art supplies. You can contact school officials to ask for copies of any inspections or test results. You can also contact health department officials to learn about regulations related to lead hazards.

Q *Where else can I find information about school health issues?*

A School health information on a variety of topics is available from the American Academy of Pediatrics (AAP) school health Web site maintained by the AAP Council on School Health (http://www.aap.org/sections/school-health), the American School Health Association, (www.ashaweb.org), the CDC Division of Adolescent and School Health (DASH) (http://www.cdc.gov/HealthyYouth/index.htm), Center for Health and Health Care in Schools (www.healthinschools.org), and the National Association of School Nurses (www.nasn.org).

Resources

Healthy Schools Network, Inc.

Advocates for the protection of children's environmental health in schools. Web site: www.healthyschools.org

References

1. Silva E. *On the Clock: Rethinking the Way Schools Use Time.* Washington, DC: Education Sector; 2007

2. National Center for Education Statistics. *How Old Are America's Public Schools?* Washington, DC: National Center for Education Statistics; 1999

3. Shield BM, Dockrell JE. The effects of noise on children at school: a review. *Building Acoustics.* 2003;10(2):97-106

4. Evans GW, Lercher P, Meis M, Ising H, Kofler WW. Community noise exposure and stress in children. *J Acoust Soc Am.* 2001;109(3):1023–1027

5. Alcántara, JI, Weisblatt EJ, Moore BC, Bolton PF. Speech-in-noise perception in high-functioning individuals with autism or Asperger's syndrome. *J Child Psychol Psychiatry.* 2004;45(6):1107-1114

6. Dobbins M, Sunder T, Soltys S. Nonverbal learning disabilities and sensory processing disorders. *Psychiatric Times*. August 1, 2007:24(9). Available at: http://www.psychiatrictimes.com/display/article/10168/54261#. Accessed September 23, 2010

7. Pickering LK; Marano N; Bocchini JA; Angulo FJ; American Academy of Pediatrics, Committee on Infectious Diseases. Exposure to nontraditional pets at home and to animals in public settings: risks to children. *Pediatrics*. 2008;122(4):876–886

8. American Academy of Pediatrics, Committee on School Health; National Association of School Nurses. *Health, Mental Health and Safety Guidelines for Schools*. Taras H, Duncan P, Luckenbill D, et al, eds. Elk Grove Village, IL: American Academy of Pediatrics; 2004

9. Heschong Mahone Group. *Daylighting in Schools: An Investigation into the Relationship Between Daylighting and Human Performance*. HMG Project No. 9803. San Francisco, CA: Pacific Gas and Electric Company; 1999

10. Etzel RA. Indoor air pollutants in homes and schools. *Pediatr Clin North Am*. 2001;48(5): 1153–1165

11. US Environmental Protection Agency. Heating, Ventilation, and Air-Conditioning (HVAC) Systems. Codes and Standards. Available at: http://www.epa.gov/iaq/schooldesign/hvac. html#Codes and Standards. Accessed September 23, 2010

12. American Society of Heating, Refrigerating and Air-Conditioning Engineers Inc. Standard 62-2007, Ventilation for Acceptable Indoor Air Quality. Atlanta, GA: American Society of Heating, Refrigerating and Air-Conditioning Engineers Inc; 2007

13. Jaakkola JJK. Temperature and humidity. In: Frumkin H, Geller R, IL Rubin, Nodvin J, eds. *Safe and Healthy School Environments*. New York, NY: Oxford University Press; 2006:46-57

14. Everett Jones S, Smith AM, Wheeler LS, McManus T. School policies and practices that improve indoor air quality. *J Sch Health*. 2010;80(6):280-286

15. US Environmental Protection Agency. Radon Measurement in Schools (Rev Ed). EPA Publication 402-R-92-014. Washington, DC: US Environmental Protection Agency; 1993. Available at: http://www.epa.gov/radon/pdfs/radon_measurement_in_schools.pdf. Accessed September 23, 2010

16. Jenkins PL, Phillips TJ, Waldman J. *California Portable Classrooms Study Project: Executive Summary. Final Report, Vol. III*. Sacramento, CA: California Department of Health Services; 2004. Available at: http://www.arb.ca.gov/research/indoor/pcs/leg_rpt/pcs_r2l.pdf. Accessed September 23, 2010

17. Menzies D, Bourbeau J. Building-related illnesses. *N Engl J Med*. 1997;337(21):1524–1531

18. Gammage RB, Kaye SV. *Indoor Air and Human Health*. Chelsea, MI: Lewis Publishers; 1985

19. Reinikainen LM, Jaakkola JJK. Effect of temperature and humidification in the office environment. *Arch Environ Health*. 2001;56(4):365–368

20. US Environmental Protection Agency. *Indoor Air Facts No. 4: Sick Building Syndrome (Rev)*. Washington, DC: US Environmental Protection Agency; 1991. Available at: http://www.epa. gov/iaq/pdfs/sick_building_factsheet.pdf. Accessed September 23, 2010

21. Salvaggio JE. Psychological aspects of "environmental illness," "multiple chemical sensitivity," and building-related illness. *J Allergy Clin Immunol*. 1994;94(2 Pt 2):366-370

22. Ryan CM, Morrow LA. Dysfunctional buildings or dysfunctional people: an examination of the sick building syndrome and allied disorders. *J Consult Clin Psychol*. 1992;60(2):220-224

23. Institute of Medicine. *Damp Indoor Spaces and Health*. Washington, DC: National Academy of Sciences; 2004

24. Gruchalla RS, Pongracic J. Plaut M, et al. Inner City Asthma Study: relationships among sensitivity, allergen exposure, and asthma morbidity. *J Allergy Clin Immunol*. 2005;115(3): 478-485

25. American Academy of Pediatrics. Red Book: 2009 Report of the Committee on Infectious Diseases. Pickering LK, Baker CJ, Long SS, McMillan JA, eds. 28th ed. Elk Grove Village, IL: American Academy of Pediatrics; 2009

26. Bryant D. Lead-contaminated drinking waters in the public schools of Philadelphia. *J Toxicol Clin Toxicol.* 2004;42(3):287-294

27. US Environmental Protection Agency. *3 Ts for Reducing Lead in Drinking Water in Schools: Revised Technical Guidance.* Washington, DC: US Environmental Protection Agency; 2006. Available at: http://www.epa.gov/safewater/schools/pdfs/lead/toolkit_leadschools_guide_3ts_ leadschools.pdf. Accessed September 23, 2010

28. Balk SJ; American Academy of Pediatrics, Council on Environmental Health and Section on Dermatology. Technical Report—ultraviolet radiation: a hazard to children and adolescents. *Pediatrics.* 2011;127(3):e791–e817

29. Herrick RF, Lefkowitz DJ, Weymouth GA. Soil contamination from PCB-containing buildings. *Environ Health Perspect.* 2007;115(2):173–175

30. Vollman D, Witsaman R Comstock RD, Smith GA. Epidemiology of playground equipment-related injuries to children in the United States, 1996–2005. *Clin Pediatr (Phila).* 2009;48(1): 66-71

31. Claudio L. Synthetic turf: health debate takes root. *Environ Health Perspect.* 2008;116(3): A116–A122

32. Thorne B. Unpacking school lunch: structure, practice, and the negotiation of differences. In: Cooper CR, ed. *Developmental Pathways Through Middle Childhood: Rethinking Contexts and Diversity as Resources.* Philadelphia, PA: Lawrence Erlbaum; 2005:63-87

33. Centers for Disease Control and Prevention. Outbreaks of gastrointestinal illness of unknown etiology associated with eating burritos—United States, October 1997-October 1998. *MMWR Morb Mortal Wkly Rep.* 1999;48(10):210-213

34. Dinkes R, Cataldi EF, Lin-Kelly W. *Indicators of school crime and safety: 2007.* Washington, DC: National Center for Education Statistics; 2007. NCES Publication 2008-021/NCJ 219553

35. DeVoe JF, Peter K, Noonan M, Snyder TD, Baum K. *Indicators of School Crime and Safety: 2005.* Washington, DC: US Departments of Education and Justice; 2005. NCES Publication 2006–001/NCJ 210697

36. Centers for Disease Control and Prevention. Youth Risk Behavior Surveillance—United States, 2007. *MMWR Surveill Summ.* 2008;57(SS-4):1-131

Chapter 12

Waste Sites

■ ■ ■ ■ ■ ■

According to the US Environmental Protection Agency (EPA), "hazardous waste is waste that is dangerous or potentially harmful to our health or the environment."[1] An uncontrolled hazardous waste site is an area where an accumulation of hazardous substances creates a threat to the health and safety of individuals or the environment or both (http://www.lni.wa.gov/WISHA/Rules/HazardousWaste/PDFs/296-843-300.pdf). Uncontrolled hazardous waste sites are prevalent throughout the world. Locations or sites containing hazardous waste may be a source of concern to families and health professionals. The Agency for Toxic Substances and Disease Registry (ATSDR), a component of the US Department of Health and Human Services, estimates that 3 to 4 million American children live within 1 mile of a hazardous waste site.[2] In addition, on the basis of data from 1255 waste sites, ATSDR estimates that 1 127 563 children younger than 6 years live within 1 mile of one of these sites.[3]

On the basis of a hazard ranking system, 1245 waste sites were listed on the National Priorities List (NPL). The NPL is a list of hazardous waste sites with high levels of contamination requiring long-term remediation and funding under the Superfund program (the federal program that locates, investigates, and cleans up the worst uncontrolled and abandoned toxic waste sites).[4] The EPA determines which sites are eligible for placement on this list through a formal assessment process. With the exception of North Dakota (which has none), all states have at least one NPL site; 5 states (California, Michigan, New Jersey, New York, and Pennsylvania) contain 36% of all the sites and 29% of the children and youth (from birth through 17 years of age) in the United States.[5,6] Most (65%–70%) uncontrolled hazardous waste sites in the United States are waste storage/treatment facilities (including landfills) or former industrial properties.[7]

Many of these properties have been abandoned, and most have more than one chemical contaminant that poses serious risk to human health. Less common are waste recycling facilities and mining sites, which may be active, inactive, or abandoned.

Some of the substances found in uncontrolled hazardous waste sites are heavy metals, such as lead, chromium, and arsenic; and organic solvents, such as trichloroethylene and benzene.[7] Arsenic has been found in more than 1000 current and former NPL sites and ranks No. 1 on the ATSDR/EPA priority list of hazardous chemicals.[8] Children living in urban areas may have greater risks of exposure to hazardous waste because of nearby "brownfield" sites. A brownfield is a tract of land that has been developed for industrial purposes, polluted, abandoned, and later designated by municipalities for commercial and/or residential redevelopment. An additional group of hazardous waste sites is associated with federal government facilities, in particular military facilities and nuclear energy complexes. See Table 12.1 for federal legislation covering waste sites and unintentional releases. The National Research Council has cited 17 482 contaminated sites at 1855 military installations and 3700 sites at 500 nuclear facilities.[9] Some of these sites cover large geographic areas and are contaminated with complex mixtures of wastes.

Certain types of waste sites and chemical contaminants are in preponderance in distinct regions of the country. For example, the New England states have

Table 12.1: US Legislation Covering Waste Sites and Unintentional Releases	
1980	The Comprehensive Environmental Response, Compensation, and Liability Act (CERCLA) of 1980 established ATSDR as an agency of the Public Health Service with mandates to (1) establish a National Exposure and Disease Registry; (2) create an inventory of health information on hazardous substances; (3) create a list of closed and restricted-access sites; (4) provide medical assistance during hazardous substance emergencies; and (5) determine the relationship between hazardous substance exposures and illness.
1984	The Resource Conservation and Recovery Act (RCRA), as amended in 1984, mandated that ATSDR work with the EPA to (1) identify new hazardous waste sites to be regulated; (2) conduct health assessments at RCRA sites at EPA's request; and (3) consider petitions for health assessments by the public or states.
1986	The Superfund Amendments and Reauthorization Act (SARA) of 1986 broadened ATSDR's responsibilities in the areas of public health assessments, establishment and maintenance of toxicologic databases, information dissemination, and medical education.

National Priorities List

When the EPA places a site on the National Priorities List, the Superfund Act (passed in 1980* and amended in 1986†) provides monies for remediation (cleanup) of the site and an array of public health actions in nearby communities. The Superfund Act also holds the potentially responsible party for the contamination legally liable. The ATSDR conducts public health assessments to evaluate the potential health hazards faced by communities in proximity to every proposed, listed, or former NPL site and in response to petitions from individuals. In many cases, this work is conducted by state health departments under ATSDR sponsorship and review. A site is assigned a hazard category according to the human health hazard it poses on the basis of professional judgment and weight-of-evidence criteria.[7] In the 3-year period from 1993 to 1995, this process indicated a health hazard at 49% of sites and an urgent hazard at 4% of sites.[7] A site-specific epidemiologic investigation or other type of investigation is needed to establish the actual hazard to health. Of the public health assessments conducted at 1371 sites, 60% to 70% have included recommendations that address the need for intervention to interrupt ongoing exposure pathways.[10] These interventions have included provision of alternate drinking water, issuance of fish consumption advisories, posting of warning notices, restriction of site access, and (rarely) relocation of community residents.

*The Comprehensive Environmental Response, Compensation, and Liability Act of 1980.
†The Superfund Amendment and Reauthorization Act of 1986.

many sites related to old economy industries, such as mills, radium clock factories, and metal plating and tanning facilities; the common contaminants are lead, arsenic, chromium, radium, and mercury. In contrast, several southwestern states have waste sites related to oil refining and petrochemicals, wood treatment, and mining and smelting; the common contaminants are volatile organic compounds (VOCs), pentachlorophenol, lead, arsenic, and creosote.[10]

ROUTES AND SOURCES OF EXPOSURE

Routes of exposure are ingestion, inhalation, and dermal absorption. Children may be exposed through contaminated groundwater, surface water, drinking water, air, surface soil, sediment, dust, or consumable plants or animals.

Children often find waste sites interesting. They may ignore or fail to notice warning signs, find or create openings in fences, or otherwise gain access to restricted places on or near a site.[11] Often, there is considerable variation in exposure depending on climate, season, and time of day.

Recognizing that proximity to a waste site may be an important risk factor for children, ATSDR initiated a process of routinely collecting standardized information on populations and demographics at NPL sites. This process uses geographic information systems to determine the number of people living within 1 mile of the boundaries of a hazardous waste site. The process ascertains the number of children living within the 1-mile polygon and alerts site investigators to the children's presence.

CLINICAL EFFECTS

The effect that exposure to a hazardous substance(s) has on an infant's or child's health is related to the nature of the pollutant, the total and peak dose received, the toxicity of the substance, and the individual's susceptibility.

The overall impact of hazardous waste sites on national health is difficult to assess because of conflicting information from epidemiologic studies and limitations of the methodologies used.[12] Many studies have been interpreted as "negative," meaning that no statistically significant increase in adverse health effects was found. These observations may reflect the true absence of adverse effects or the inability to detect such effects because of inadequacies in study design or sample size. For example, many studies that found little, if any, excess risks of adverse effects defined their target populations crudely, based on linear distance from a site, instead of documented environmental pathways and routes of exposure. Likewise, studies interpreted as "positive" may reflect a true effect or other types of study design flaws, such as misclassification of exposure or inappropriate choice of comparison groups. Improved study methods, such as those that generate real-time exposure models via computerized geographic information systems mapping tools, hold greater promise for associating exposure to site contaminants with adverse health effects.

Adverse health effects have been reported in some, but not all, investigations of communities around hazardous waste sites.[12,13] These effects have ranged from nonspecific symptoms (eg, headache, fatigue, and skin rashes)[14] to congenital heart defects[15] and neurobehavioral deficits.[16] Most investigations have included some children in the study population, but only a few have focused primarily on health effects among infants and children. In these studies, it is difficult to know whether proximity to the waste site or some other factor(s) is responsible for the health outcome. Some of the studies that support concerns were conducted by governmental agencies and findings of those studies have not been reported in peer-reviewed literature, making access to such documents difficult. The following are examples of findings considered "positive":

- Children living near waste sites with persistent organic pollutants (POPs) had higher rates of hospitalization for asthma and infectious respiratory disease.[17]

- Among Washington State women, residing within 1 mile of waste sites containing pesticides was associated with increased risk of fetal death.[18]
- Maternal residence during pregnancy of 1 mile or less from urban waste sites in Washington State was associated with a wide variety of infant malformations.[19]
- In New York State, women living within a zip code close to a waste site contaminated with polychrominated biphenyls (PCBs) had increased risk of giving birth to a male infant of low birth weight.[20]
- Children exposed to trichloroethylene in drinking water supplies at 15 different sites in 5 states had increased reporting of speech and hearing impairments.[21]
- In California, neural tube defects in newborn infants of minority races were associated with maternal residence in a census tract that had a Superfund site, with the biggest association found between birth defects and toxic substance class in the following order: cytochrome oxidase inhibitors, nitrates or nitrites, inorganic compounds not otherwise classified, pesticides, and volatile organic compounds.[22]
- Preterm birth was associated with exposure to iodine-131 (^{131}I) at the Hanford nuclear site in Washington state.[23]
- Gestational exposure to drinking water contaminated with perchlorate was associated with measures of decreased thyroid function in neonates.[24]
- Children exposed to lead from a smelter showed lower than normal neurobehavioral and peripheral nerve function when tested as young adults 15 to 20 years after exposure.[25]
- Children living near a municipal waste incinerator had a threefold increase in risk of lower respiratory tract illnesses.[26]

An array of information resources is available on the health hazards of 275 individual toxic substances. This information is provided in a variety of formats intended for different audiences. The ATSDR Toxicological Profiles, in particular, systematically review the toxicology, pharmacokinetics, epidemiology, exposure, environmental fate, and transport of the substances. Additional information specific to children's health and developmental issues is provided in profiles covering most commonly encountered substances. Individual profiles are available on CD-ROM and at http://www.atsdr.cdc.gov/toxprofiles/index.asp.

Disruption of community cultures and daily life has been observed following toxic releases. For example, persistently high indoor air levels of mercury vapor forced authorities to relocate residents from their own condominium building.[27] The source of the mercury was residual pools of condensed liquid metal from a factory that had been housed in the same building decades before its renovation. The awareness of environmental risks and hazards in communities with waste sites has often led to increased concern and stress within these communities.

DIAGNOSTIC METHODS

An exposed infant or child can remain asymptomatic, develop nonspecific symptoms, or develop signs and symptoms frequently associated with common medical conditions. Because of this range of outcomes, a history of exposure should be obtained when evaluating the etiology of unexplained symptoms. Standardized approaches to taking an exposure history are available.[28,29]

Individual Evaluation

As in other aspects of medicine, the history guides laboratory testing. Blood or urine tests may be indicated when a child is symptomatic and there is a recent history of a specific exposure (eg, when a child has climbed over a fence and played in a site known to be contaminated with a specific toxicant). Generally, laboratory tests to document exposure are not recommended in the absence of signs or symptoms. However, a diagnostic blood test of children potentially exposed to lead may be indicated, and other diagnostic tests may be indicated for specific children on the basis of known effects of the particular contaminant.

Community Studies

In formal epidemiologic studies, laboratory biological tests may be useful to determine whether there is an association between exposure and any adverse health effects.

A biomarker of exposure provides a reasonable measure of the internal body level of a substance over a period that depends on the pharmacokinetics of that substance. Testing may be performed on blood (for lead), urine (for metallic mercury, arsenic), or tissue specimens. Analytical methods and human reference ranges are available for many of the substances found most commonly at hazardous waste sites. In some cases, age-specific reference ranges are available to facilitate interpretation of levels found in infants and children. It may be difficult to interpret the results, however, when reference ranges for children are not available.

Highly sensitive standardized medical test batteries are available for use in epidemiologic studies to evaluate subclinical and clinical organ damage or dysfunction related to noncancer health conditions, such as immune function disorders,[30] kidney dysfunction,[31] lung and respiratory diseases,[32] and neurotoxic disorders.[16] Because of their low specificity, these test batteries are not useful to assess effects of community exposures outside the context of a formal research study.

TREATMENT

Treatment of acute exposure to one or more substances from a hazardous waste site depends on the substance; the route, dose, and duration of exposure;

and the presence of any symptoms or ill effects.[33] Treatment should generally be undertaken in consultation with a toxicologist or expert in pediatric environmental health.

A 2-part video titled "ATSDR's Community Challenge" gives emergency medical services personnel and hospital emergency departments the necessary guidance to plan for incidents involving human exposure to hazardous materials. "Community Challenge" is available in CD-ROM format, which includes:

- **Volume I:** Hazardous Materials Response and the Emergency Medical System
- **Volume II:** Hazardous Materials Response and the Hospital Emergency Department

CONSULTATION

Consultation is available on potentially toxic exposures and possible ill effects from such exposures. A North American network of Pediatric Environmental Health Specialty Units has been formed to provide information, receive referrals, and offer training in the diagnosis and treatment of illnesses associated with exposure to toxic substances and other environmental health risks (see Resources).

PREVENTION OF EXPOSURE

In the United States, the EPA is responsible for cleaning up waste sites under the Superfund Act. Experience at hundreds of communities near waste sites has demonstrated the value and importance of early and extensive community involvement. This is usually not a simple process. However, government agencies have made considerable progress in these areas by forming community assistance panels; awarding assistance grants; and developing valid methods of needs assessment, health risk communication, and community outreach. These methods have enhanced the agencies' abilities to recognize the value of community input, address community needs, and focus attention on those needed areas.[10] Table 12.2 lists ways to prevent or limit exposure to waste site contaminants.

Frequently Asked Questions

Q *I am confused by the conflicting information I hear about the risks to my children from waste sites. Can you clarify this?*

A The risks depend on the amount, type, and duration of exposure and the types of chemicals involved. However, it is difficult to know the exact details of a child's exposure, so it is difficult to know the risk precisely. In addition, for many chemicals, the effects of exposure in childhood are not well known and only can be estimated from the toxic effects found in experiments with animals.

Table 12.2: Preventing or Limiting Exposure

Personal Preventive Actions

Comply with advisories (eg, warnings about eating fish or swimming in certain waters).

Connect to a safer water supply.

Establish play areas through fencing and landscape methods to reduce potential for exposures to contaminated soil.

Engineering Controls

Destroy contaminants by incineration or by chemical or biological reactions.

Remove the contaminants to a safer location.

Disrupt the exposure pathway (eg, an alternate water supply or perimeter fence).

Use dust control and other measures to protect workers and neighbors during the cleanup process.

Develop engineering solutions to eliminate relatively small, acute problems (removal actions).

Develop "remedial actions," engineering solutions that involve complex planning to permanently solve a complicated waste site problem.

Administrative Controls

Temporarily or permanently relocate residents.

Restrict deeds (eg, to prevent future use of the land for residential or child care purposes).

Enact ordinances to control future land use.

Communicate health advisories.

Q *Did exposure from a waste site cause my child's illness? or One of my children has an illness that is linked to the waste site. Will my other children become ill also?*

A It is difficult to prove that one child's illness was caused by exposure to one particular waste site. Most of the illnesses that can be caused by exposure to toxic chemicals have more than one possible cause. Also, not every child who is so exposed becomes ill. A linkage is more likely if several children (or adults) become ill at about the same time, the same place, or following the same exposure.

Q *Will my child get cancer from exposure to a waste site?*

A Although a number of chemicals found at waste sites are carcinogens (known or predicted to cause cancer), the chance of getting cancer from exposure to a waste site is thought to be small. If the child was exposed to one or more carcinogens, the risk to the child depends on the amount and duration of the exposure and type of carcinogen, among other considerations. Most experts believe that development of cancer is unlikely unless there has been exposure for many years (see Chapter 45).

Q   *Is my child's learning disability (or attention-deficit/hyperactivity disorder) caused by exposure to a waste site?*

A   A number of chemicals found at waste sites may affect the nervous system, including a child's developing nervous system. These chemicals include heavy metals (eg, lead and mercury), organic solvents (eg, toluene), and certain types of pesticides (eg, carbamates and organophosphates). The risk to the child depends on how long the child was exposed, the child's age at exposure, the degree of exposure, and the child's genetic susceptibility.

Q   *How can I protect my child from future exposure to hazardous waste sites?*

A   It is best to avoid areas where soil is contaminated by hazardous waste. Explain to children the meaning and importance of posted warning signs, and strongly advise children to stay out of restricted areas. Do not let children swim in streams or other bodies of water that are known to be contaminated. Such conditions usually are posted, but if there is doubt, contact the local health department. Know the source of your household drinking water, and if uncertain about contaminants, have it tested. Children, pregnant women, and others should not eat certain fish caught from contaminated waters. Fishing license brochures available locally list advisories about which fish are safe to eat. If a parent or other caregiver works at a hazardous waste site, soiled work clothes should not be brought into the home. Dust can be a source of exposure for children. Stay engaged and vigilant during the development of remediation plans and the actual remediation process to ensure proper dust control and other safety procedures are in place and followed.

Q   *My home is near a landfill. Is my child at risk?*

A   The risk depends on the types of chemicals at the site and the quantity, kind, and duration of exposure. Because it is extremely difficult to determine the precise nature of any exposure, it is not easy to measure the real risk for your child. In addition, more scientific information is needed about the ways that many chemicals, such as those found in landfills, affect children's health. It is best to keep your child away from the site, monitor activities that could cause exposure to chemicals, and regularly test drinking water from nearby wells. Investigate whether your local community holds household hazardous waste collection days, which help prevent toxic chemicals from entering municipal waste streams and landfills. Substitute less toxic alternatives in your home, minimize your family's use of hazardous chemicals and advocate for these healthier practices within your local community.

For more information, see Chapters 17 and 45.

Resources

Agency for Toxic Substances and Disease Registry (ATSDR)

Educational materials, medical management guidelines for acute toxicity, toxicity information for individual chemicals, Toxicological Profiles, publications, and information: www.atsdr.cdc.gov

Phone: 888-42-ATSDR (888-422-8737) or 404-498-0110;

Chemical emergencies and accidental releases: 770-488-7100
(information available 24 hours a day).

The ATSDR provides 24-hour technical and scientific support (emergency response hotline: 770-488-7100) for chemical emergencies (including terrorist threats) such as spills, explosions, and transportation accidents throughout the United States. The ATSDR also provides health consultations for people exposed to individual substances or mixtures. The 3-volume reference text, *Managing Hazardous Materials Incidents: Medical Management Guidelines for Acute Chemical Exposures,* contains the following information:

- **Volume I:** Emergency Medical Services: A Planning Guide for the Management of Contaminated Patients
- **Volume II:** Hospital Emergency Departments: A Planning Guide for the Management of Contaminated Patients
- **Volume III:** Medical Management Guidelines for Acute Chemical Exposures

In particular, ATSDR has addressed issues related to children with respect to the prehospital (Volume I) and hospital (Volume II) management of children who may be chemically contaminated. Appropriate revisions, including pediatric updates, also are included in Volume III, which addresses medical management of patients who have been exposed to specific chemicals.

Other resources provided by ATSDR include:

— Cases Studies in Environmental Medicine
(information for clinicians on specific exposures)
www.atsdr.cdc.gov/csem/csem.html

— Chemical Mixtures Program
(information about the human health effects of chemical mixtures)
www.atsdr.cdc.gov/mixtures.html

— ToxFAQs
(Frequently Asked Questions about Contaminants Found at Hazardous Waste Sites)
www.atsdr.cdc.gov/toxfaqs/index.asp

— Public Health Statements
(a series of summaries about hazardous substances)
www.atsdr.cdc.gov/PHS/Index.asp

Association of Occupational and Environmental Clinics
  Web site: www.aoec.org
  Phone: 202-347-4976; Toll free: 1-888-347-2632

Center for Children's Environmental Health and Disease Prevention Research at the Harvard School of Public Health
  Web site: www.hsph.harvard.edu/children

Chemical poisoning emergencies
  Web site: www.disastercenter.com/poison.htm

Dartmouth Toxic Metals Research Program
  Web site: www.dartmouth.edu/~toxmetal

EPA Superfund Program (general description)
  Web site: www.epa.gov/superfund

EPA Search Engine (for finding toxic waste sites in your community)
  Web site: http://cfpub.epa.gov/supercpad/cursites/srchsites.cfm

Harvard NIEHS Center for Environmental Health — Metals Core
  Web site: www.hsph.harvard.edu/research/niehs/research-cores
  metals-research-core/

National Library of Medicine TOXNET
  (a collection of toxicology and environmental health databases)
  Web site: http://toxnet.nlm.nih.gov/cgi-bin/sis/htmlgen?TOXLINE.

National Center for Environmental Health (NCEH)
  Government agency that addresses diverse environmental health issues
  Web site: www.cdc.gov/nceh

Pediatric Environmental Health Specialty Units
  Web site: www.aoec.org/PEHSU.htm

Poison Control Centers
  Web site: www.aapcc.org/dnn/About/FindLocalPoisonCenters/tabid/130/
  Default.aspx
  National toll-free phone: 1-800-222-1222

Additional Information
Superfund Record of Decision System
  Web site: www.epa.gov/superfund/sites/rods/index.htm

US Environmental Protection Agency–Oil Spills and Chemical Spills
Phone: 800-372-9473

Web site: www.epa.gov/epaoswer/non-hw/reduce/wstewise/index.htm

Chemical spills, oil spills, threats
Phone: 800-424-8802

Web site: www.epa.gov/oilspill/oilhow.htm

References

1. US Environmental Protection Agency. *Wastes – Hazardous Waste.* Available at: http://www.epa.gov/osw/hazard/index.htm. Accessed August 2, 2010
2. Amler RW, Smith L, eds. *Achievements in Children's Environmental Health.* Atlanta, GA: US Department of Health and Human Services, Agency for Toxic Substances and Disease Registry; 2001
3. Agency for Toxic Substances and Disease Registry. Case Studies in Environmental Medicine. Pediatric Environmental Health. 2002. ATSDR Publication number ATSDR-HE-CS-2002-0002. Page 10. Available at: http://www.atsdr.cdc.gov/csem/pediatric/docs/pediatric.pdf
4. US Environmental Protection Agency. Final National Priorities List (NPL) Sites – by State. Available at: http://www.epa.gov/superfund/sites/query/queryhtm/nplfin.htm. Accessed August 2, 2010
5. US Environmental Protection Agency. *National Priorities List (NPL).* Available at: http://www.epa.gov/superfund/sites/npl/index.htm. Accessed August 2, 2010
6. US Census Bureau. *State Population Estimates as of July 2006.* Available at: http://www.census.gov/popest/states/asrh/. Accessed August 2, 2010
7. Agency for Toxic Substances and Disease Registry. *Report to Congress,* 1993, 1994, 1995. Atlanta, GA: US Department of Health and Human Services, Public Health Service, Agency for Toxic Substances and Disease Registry; 1999
8. Chou CH, De Rosa CT. 2003. Case studies—arsenic. *Int J Hyg Envir Health.* 2003;206 (4-5):381-386
9. National Research Council. *Ranking Hazardous-Waste Sites for Remedial Action.* Washington, DC: National Academies Press; 1994;29, 37
10. Amler RW, Falk H. Opportunities and challenges in community environmental health evaluations. *Environ Epidemiol Toxicol.* 2000;2:51–55
11. Agency for Toxic Substances and Disease Registry. *Healthy Children–Toxic Environments: Acting on the Unique Vulnerability of Children Who Dwell Near Hazardous Waste Sites. Report of the Child Health Workgroup, Board of Scientific Counselors.* Atlanta, GA: US Department of Health and Human Services, Public Health Service, Agency for Toxic Substances and Disease Registry; 1997
12. Elliott P, Briggs D, Morris S, et al. Risk of adverse birth outcomes in populations living near landfill sites. *BMJ.* 2001;323(7309):363–368
13. Johnson BL. *Impact of Hazardous Waste on Human Health.* Boca Raton FL: Lewis Publishers; 1999
14. Brender JD, Pichette JL, Suarez L, Hendricks KA, Holt M. 2003. Health risks of residential exposure to polycyclic aromatic hydrocarbons. *Arch Environ Health.* 2003;58(2):111-118
15. Savitz DA, Bornschein RL, Amler RW, et al. Assessment of reproductive disorders and birth defects in communities near hazardous chemical sites. I. Birth defects and developmental disorders. *Reprod Toxicol.* 1997;11(2-3):223–230

16. Amler RW, Gibertinin M, eds. *Pediatric Environmental Neurobehavioral Test Battery.* Atlanta, GA: US Department of Health and Human Services, Public Health Service, Agency for Toxic Substances and Disease Registry; 1996

17. Ma J, Kouznetsova M, Lessner L, Carpenter DO. Asthma and infectious respiratory disease in children—correlation to residence near hazardous waste sites. *Paediatr Respir Rev.* 2007;8(4):292-298

18. Mueller BA, Kuehn CM, Shapiro-Mendoza CK, Tomashek KM. 2007. Fetal deaths and proximity to hazardous waste sites in Washington State. *Environ Health Perspect.* 2007;115(5):776-780

19. Kuehn CM, Mueller BA, Checkoway H, Williams M. Risk of malformations associated with residential proximity to hazardous waste sites in Washington State. *Environ Res.* 2007;103(3):405-412

20. Baibergenova A, Kudyakov R, Zdeb M, Carpenter DO. Low birth weight and residential proximity to PCB-contaminated waste sites. *Environ Health Perspect.* 2003;111(10):1352-1357

21. Agency for Toxic Substances and Disease Registry. *National Exposure Registry Trichloroethylene (TCE) Subregistry Baseline Technical Report (Revised).* Atlanta, GA: US Department of Health and Human Services, Public Health Service, Agency for Toxic Substances and Disease Registry; 1994

22. Orr M, Bove F, Kaye W, Stone M. Elevated birth defects in racial or ethnic minority children of women living near hazardous waste sites. *Int J Hyg Environ Health.* 2002;205(1-2):19–27

23. US Department of Energy Office of Health Studies. *Agenda of HHS Public Health Activities (For Fiscal Years 2005-2010) at US Department of Energy Sites.* Washington, DC: US Department of Energy Office of Health Studies and US Department of Health and Human Services; 2005

24. Brechner RJ, Parkhurst GD, Humble WO, Brown MB, Herman WH. Ammonium perchlorate contamination of Colorado River drinking water is associated with abnormal thyroid function in newborns in Arizona. *J Occup Environ Med.* 2000;42(8):777–782

25. Agency for Toxic Substances and Disease Registry. *A Cohort Study of Current and Previous Residents of the Silver Valley: Assessment of Lead Exposure and Health Outcomes.* Atlanta, GA: US Department of Health and Human Services, Public Health Service, Agency for Toxic Substances and Disease Registry; 1997

26. Agency for Toxic Substances and Disease Registry. *Study of Effect of Residential Proximity to Waste Incinerators on Lower Respiratory Illness in Children.* Atlanta, GA: US Department of Health and Human Services, Public Health Service, Agency for Toxic Substances and Disease Registry; 1995

27. Centers for Disease Control and Prevention. Mercury exposure among residents of a building formerly used for industrial purposes—New Jersey, 1995. *MMWR Morb Mortal Wkly Rep.* 1996;45(20):422–424

28. Agency for Toxic Substances and Disease Registry. *Case Studies in Environmental Medicine: Taking an Exposure History.* Atlanta, GA: US Department of Health and Human Services, Public Health Service, Agency for Toxic Substances and Disease Registry; 2000. ATSDR Publication ATSDR-HE-CS-2001-0002. Available at: http://www.atsdr.cdc.gov/csem/exphistory/ehcover_page.html. Accessed August 3, 2010

29. Agency for Toxic Substances and Disease Registry. *Case Studies in Environmental Medicine: Pediatric Environmental Medicine. Principles of Environmental Medical Evaluation.* Atlanta, GA: US Department of Health and Human Services, Agency for Toxic Substances and Disease Registry; 2003:24

30. Straight JM, Kipen HM, Vogt RF, Amler RW. *Immune Function Test Batteries for Use in Environmental Health Field Studies.* Atlanta, GA: US Department of Health and Human Services, Public Health Service, Agency for Toxic Substances and Disease Registry; 1994

31. Amler RW, Mueller PW, Schultz MG. *Biomarkers of Kidney Function for Environmental Health Field Studies.* Atlanta, GA: US Department of Health and Human Services, Public Health Service, Agency for Toxic Substances and Disease Registry; 1998

32. Metcalf SW, Samet J, Hanrahan J, Schwartz D, Hunninghake G. *A Standardized Test Battery for Lungs and Respiratory Diseases for Use in Environmental Health Field Studies.* Atlanta, GA: US Department of Health and Human Services, Public Health Service, Agency for Toxic Substances and Disease Registry; 1994

33. Agency for Toxic Substances and Disease Registry. *Managing Hazardous Materials Incidents: Medical Management Guidelines for Acute Chemical Exposures.* Atlanta, GA: US Department of Health and Human Services, Public Health Service, Agency for Toxic Substances and Disease Registry; 2001

Chapter 13

Workplaces

■ ■ ■ ■ ■ ■

Although most people consider that an adolescent's main occupation is "student," 3 of 4 high school seniors visiting a pediatrician's office also work. Although work potentially has positive effects on adolescent development, every year thousands of workers younger than 18 years are injured, and more than a classroom-full die on the job.[1] Although adolescent risk-taking behaviors often are blamed for work-related injuries, a 2007 Canadian review confirmed that work conditions, expectations, and exposures were consistently more important than the adolescent's individual behavior in causing injury. The presence of more hazards in the workplace, pressure to work faster, and minority status were associated with injuries. Workers in their first jobs may be at increased risk.[2] Adolescent exposures to dangerous machinery and hazardous chemicals are seldom addressed by health care providers. Adult occupational medicine professionals rarely see teenagers, and pediatricians do not usually become involved in occupational health and safety issues of their adolescent patients. Given that so many teenagers are injured and some are killed, there is a need for pediatricians to better advocate and educate about improved workplace health and safety for their individual patients, in their communities, and when policy is being developed. Issues of acute toxicity and safety need to be addressed most urgently, but chronic or delayed health effects also must be considered.

This chapter discusses youth employment with a focus on hazardous exposures, especially to chemicals. Other occupational hazards include those stemming from using dangerous equipment in large-scale industries, such as agriculture, construction, forestry, and some service industries, as well as hazards found in small industries, such as fishing and canning, retailing, and food service. Workplace violence, although extremely important, is not addressed in this chapter.

ADOLESCENT WORKERS

One quarter of 8th graders and 75% of high school seniors report that they work at a formal paid job during the year through a combination of after-school, weekend, and summer hours. In 2007, 2.6 million adolescents 15 to 17 years of age worked. Food services employed 37%; retail employed 24%.[1] Younger adolescents also work, especially in agricultural settings and family businesses, but official employment statistics are not available for these teenagers. Many teenagers also work as babysitters, doing small cleaning jobs, or lawnmowing. Official counts are also not available for the estimated 20% of youth who work "off the books" in violation of some wage, hour, or safety regulations.[3]

The number of working teenagers in the United States varies from year to year without any obvious trend. It is not entirely clear how the recent recession (2009-2010) altered youth employment statistics. Although there have been fewer government-supported summer jobs, and the number of work hours of 16- and 17-year-olds declined from 2000-2004, there was an increase in the number of self-employed teenagers during this time, and occupational fatality reports suggest that students continue to have jobs.[4]

Efforts to improve school-to-work transitions for typical and special needs students are resulting in more teenagers entering the workplace. School-based vocational and technical education that simulates employment conditions may involve hazardous conditions, including chemical exposures. There are concerns that high school students with disabilities may be placed in menial jobs at school for which they have minimal or no training and that increase their risk of injury or expose them to chemical and biological hazards. National priorities for volunteer community involvement that support increased participation of adolescents in nonpaid activities (such as rehabilitation of old housing) may carry the same risks of exposures as doing similar work for pay.[5]

Regulation of Hours and Hazards in Adolescent Employment

The Fair Labor Standards Act (FLSA) of 1938 remains the major federal law that regulates work for individuals younger than 18 years.[6] The law has 2 parts— protecting education through regulating permitted hours of work in a day and in a week, and protecting health and safety through prohibiting work on dangerous machinery or with hazardous chemicals via Hazard Orders (a list of tasks designated as dangerous). Under the Fair Labor Standards Act, adolescents younger than 18 years are prohibited from working with hazardous chemicals in nonagricultural jobs.[7] Prohibitions regarding chemical work in agriculture extend only to age 16 years, and work by children and adolescents on their own family farms is unregulated.[8] A list of permitted hours and prohibited occupations can be found on the National Institute for Occupational Safety and Health (NIOSH) Web site (see Resources).

Many states also have laws regulating child labor, and if state law is more stringent than the federal law, state law supersedes. Many businesses, particularly small ones, may not be covered by federal or state law; discerning exactly who, if anyone, has jurisdiction for child labor in small business or agriculture often is complex. Labor trends toward increased use of contract workers (workers who are not company employees but are hired for a specific task), especially for newspaper delivery and janitorial services, are problematic, because they leave unclear who is responsible for education, supervision, health, and safety.

Another area of legal exemption is vocational/technical training. Because such training is assumed to occur with supervision in a safe environment, restrictions based on safety concerns may be waived for students in these settings. No systematic surveillance of exposure resulting in illness or injury has been conducted in school-based learning sites or on job sites, but studies of shop-related injuries and of work-related poison control center calls suggest that there is reason for concern.[9,10] From 1992 to 1996, 1008 Utah children in grades 7 through 12 were reported to be injured in shop class. Of the 7 (all high school students) who were injured badly enough to require hospital admission, 6 were injured using a table saw, and 1 was injured using automotive cleaning fluid. That student sustained second-degree burns of the face and upper extremity.[9]

The Fair Labor Standards Act has remained essentially unchanged since 1938 except for one update in 2005. In 2010 the US Department of Labor Wage and Hour Division published a Final Rule, the purpose of which was to better protect working children from hazards not previously addressed. At the same time, the Final Rule recognized the value of safe work to children and their families by removing restrictions considered to be outdated.[11] Major changes for 14- and 15-year-olds in nonagricultural employment pertain primarily to issues of injury, but there are 3 potential effects on adolescent exposures. First, the Final Rule incorporates provisions enacted in 2004 allowing 14- and 15-year-olds to be employed in businesses that process wood products (brought about in response to the Amish shift from farming to woodworking). This change created a new group of young workers at risk of respiratory problems resulting from inhaling wood dust. Second, the Final Rule permits 15-year-olds to work as lifeguards at swimming pools and water parks; previously, the permitted age was 16. Because maintaining pools is often associated with water testing and treatment, this change increases the number of teenagers potentially exposed to pool chemicals, such as chlorine. Third, the Final Rule bans peddling and door-to-door sales by individuals younger than 16 years, potentially protecting more youth from motor vehicle and interpersonal violence risks seen in this employment sector and from the potential risk of sexual abuse and resulting exposure to sexually transmitted infections. Most changes in nonagricultural employment for 16- and 17-year-olds also pertain to injury prevention and expanded prohibitions in forest fire fighting protect against potential exposure to smoke and extreme heat.

Work Permits

In approximately half of states, adolescents must obtain a work permit issued by their school before seeking or starting a job. Some states require the signature of a physician certifying that the teenager is physically fit for employment. This offers an opportunity to provide anticipatory guidance about safety at work.

Enforcement of Child Labor Laws

Child labor laws are enforced by federal and state labor departments. Labor inspectors are responsible for enforcing wage, hour, and safety laws for all workers. Most child labor is investigated only when a complaint is made, usually by a parent or occasionally by business personnel. The number of inspectors available to enforce child labor laws is small, and the fines for violations historically have been small. Hours violation problems include keeping teenagers at work too late on school nights and having them clock out at an appropriate time but continue to work without pay.

The most critical aspect of child labor law violation relates to safety because of the repeated association between safety violations and fatalities. If an employer does not abide by wage and hour laws, it is reasonable to assume that he or she may not follow laws to protect the teenager's health and safety.[12,13] Exposures of legally employed youth to potentially hazardous materials may occur in job activities that violate the law, jobs not covered by the law because of business size or production, or activities (especially cleaning) outside the major job title. Family businesses, especially agriculture, are disproportionately represented among child work injury fatalities, including in children younger than 14 years,[14] suggesting that exposures also are important in these businesses. Current economic pressures may render employed teenagers even more at risk: refusing to perform a hazardous or prohibited task may be more difficult if doing so jeopardizes employment, especially if the teenager is aware that family hardships necessitate work.

Occupational Death, Injury, Hazardous Exposures, and Illness

During the 1990s, despite laws intended to protect teen workers, every year at least 70 children younger than 18 years died in work-related deaths.[15,16] From 1998-2007, the fatality rate for "younger workers" (15 to 24 years of age) decreased by an estimated 14%.[17] However, when occupational fatality counts for 1992-1997 were compared with counts for 1998-2002, fatalities among 14- and 15-year-olds increased 34%.[5] In 2007, 38 individuals younger than 18 years died; almost half of those occupational fatalities were among children younger than 16 years. In

2008, 37 teenagers younger than 18 years died from work-related injuries. Among workers 15 to 17 years of age, males accounted for 90% of fatalities; 65% of those who died were white, 5% were black, and 27% were Hispanic. Rates of occupational fatality among Hispanic teenagers exceeded those of others. Transportation incidents accounted for almost half of the occupational fatalities among all young workers, including those 14 to 15 years of age, who are generally prohibited from working on or around a vehicle. Exposure to harmful substances or environments (including electrocutions) accounted for 40 (11%) of the fatalities.[17]

Although there are no large-scale studies that describe illness or death resulting from exposures in the workplace among teenagers, large studies do document occupational injuries among working adolescents. Each study contains information about small numbers of exposures to hazardous substances. Concern about occupational exposures is reinforced by knowledge about exposure-related fatalities.[18-24] Approximately 3% of the more than 70 yearly youth occupational deaths may be attributable to poisonings rather than injuries. The percentage varies, ranging from 4% of North Carolina medical examiner reports of youth occupational fatalities[25] to 7% of deaths among New York State adolescent workers' compensation fatality cases.[19] Consultations requested of the Massachusetts Poison Control Center from 1991 to 1996 included 124 cases of working teenagers 14 to 17 years of age with occupational exposures. Moderate to severe injuries were sustained by 18 of these youth, with almost half being related to caustics or cleaning compounds.[26]

Each year during the 1990s, approximately 65 000 to 70 000 children and adolescents were injured on the job severely enough to seek care in emergency departments.[20] In 2007, an estimated 48 600 work-related injuries and illnesses among youth 15 to 17 years of age were treated in hospital emergency departments. Because only approximately one third of people with work-related injuries are seen in emergency departments, it is likely that approximately 146 000 youth sustain work-related injuries and illnesses each year.[17] These numbers likely still underestimate the extent of the problem, because many people assume a child or adolescent's occupation is "student" and never inquire or record further information about employment. Some workers may not want the occupational connection to be known. The current trend of including 18- and 19-year-olds when reporting some "young worker" injury and fatality statistics results in more difficulty in separating out the true situation for workers younger than 18 years, most of whom are still in school and not full-time employees.

CLINICAL EFFECTS

There is no surveillance system in the United States for monitoring children's occupational exposures. With the exception of noise, for which there are studies of clinical effects and preventive interventions,[27] information on clinical effects is gathered piecemeal. Five major sources of data are (1) the Census of Fatal Occupational Injuries (CFOI), which includes death from occupational exposure; (2) the National Electronic Injury Surveillance System occupational supplement (NEISS-Work); (3) case reports of exposures and acute poisonings from the literature and from within adolescent occupational injury studies; (4) adult occupational medicine literature about exposures that may be extrapolated to adolescents in similar jobs; and (5) concerns about the safety of exposures based on knowledge of chemical toxicology and of adolescent growth, development, physiology, and anatomy.

ROUTES OF EXPOSURE

An adolescent worker may incur multiple types of exposures simultaneously or may be exposed to a single chemical by multiple routes simultaneously (as with inhalation of a pesticide and ingestion from hands). It is useful to separately examine each route.

Dermal

Some chemicals are absorbed through the skin or through breaks in the skin. Examples include pesticides absorbed during lawn care and agriculture,[28] nicotine absorbed while harvesting tobacco,[29] and solvents used in screen printing shops,[30] leather shops, and auto body shops. Cloth gloves and sneakers do not provide adequate protection. If soaked with a chemical, clothing may worsen exposure if not promptly removed.

Although generally considered with injury rather than exposures, radiation and sun exposure are important because of the increased risks that these exposures confer for causing cancers later in life.

Electrocutions, usually considered with injury rather than exposure, represent exposure to the dermal hazard of electrical current. More than 50% of electrocutions involved contact with power lines and were the third-leading cause of occupational death among 16- and 17-year-olds from 1980 to 1989.[31] From 1998-2002, electrocutions accounted for 5% of young farmworker fatalities in the 14- to 18-year age range, a doubling from 5 years before. This is in contrast to the simultaneous decrease in occupational fatalities from suffocation in oxygen-deficient environments and fire/explosion fatalities.[5]

Inhalation

Inhalational injuries may result from breathing chemical fumes, particles or molds. Health effects may involve immediate symptoms or be inapparent for years.

- Adolescents involved in new home construction as part of school programs may be exposed to spray foam around windows.[32] They may also be exposed to lead fumes and isocyanates found in auto body paint and some types of shellac that are pulmonary sensitizers.

- Secondhand tobacco smoke (SHS) is a hazard for workers in restaurants in which smoking is allowed.[33]
- Farm environments may be associated with several asthma precipitants, such as animal dander, mold, and grain dust.
- When a Tennessee high school with leaky roofs developed mold contamination in air conditioners and students developed allergies and respiratory illness, the school administration turned to students in an air conditioning maintenance class to help with cleaning. Students wore "masks and protective clothing and that sort of thing." The school reported feeling that the students were safe. Local professionals, however, said that their standard for remediating a mold problem included full respirators, protective suits, areas sealed with plastic, and negative air pressure to prevent contamination with toxins from molds.[34]
- In May 2010, executives of a now-defunct California nonprofit organization that provided job training were charged with knowingly placing dozens of teenagers in jobs that exposed them to asbestos from 2005-2006.[35] All exposed students face an increased risk of lung cancer and mesothelioma later in life (see Chapter 23). Similar issues have been seen among farm youth with pesticide exposure.[36]
- Moving to a farm during adolescence (ages 11-20) rather than in adulthood was associated with a higher risk of developing primary intracranial gliomas.[37]
- Inhalation of solvents, which may lead to neurotoxic and hepatotoxic effects, may occur during cleanup activities in workplaces, ranging from fast food establishments to shop classes.[26]
- Inhalation of heated solvent cleaning mixtures can result in fatal cardiac arrhythmias.
- Inhaling adhesives and general cleaning substances has been shown to increase the incidence of asthma among nurses.[38]
- Bronchiolitis obliterans, an illness seen in adult occupational medicine, is awaiting regulation by the US Occupational Safety and Health Administration (OSHA). Bronchiolitis obliterans ("popcorn lung") is caused by workers' exposure to diacetyl in food flavorings (butter flavoring) used in the manufacture of popcorn.[39-41] Given that teenagers are employed in movie theaters at snack counters, it is possible that this serious illness may result after teenagers prepare enormous quantities of popcorn.

Ingestion

Lead and other heavy metals may be ingested. Lead hazards have been found in auto body shops.[42] Children whose functional age is younger than their chronologic age often exhibit more oral behaviors than is normal for age, potentially placing them at higher risk of ingestion of toxicants. Such children are commonly preferentially channeled into vocational education in the United States; these risks must be considered in planning for placement.

EXAMPLES OF ACUTE POISONINGS AND OTHER ACUTE EXPOSURES

Data from a study of more than 17 000 Washington state workers' compensation awards to adolescents (11–17 years of age) from 1988 to 1991 included almost 900 (4.9%) awards for toxic exposures.[6] Eighteen cases from Massachusetts and Kentucky have suggested that acute occupational exposures are occurring in adolescents; the most common agents are cleaning solutions, and the most common work site is food service.[10,43] A typical example would be a teenager working in a fast-food restaurant who is hired to work at the counter but becomes part of the cleanup crew at the end of a shift. Cleaning involves various chemicals, sometimes informally mixed. The adolescent usually has had no training in safe handling or use of those chemicals, with potentially life-threatening results. Cases of illness are significantly undercounted, because many teenagers do not die or become sick enough to be reported to a poison control center or workers' compensation system.

Teenagers employed on farms or with lawn care companies also may be at risk of hazardous exposures. A 1989 survey of 50 migrant farmworkers younger than 18 years in New York State found that 11% had mixed or applied pesticides despite child labor laws that prohibit work with hazardous chemicals.[36] No protective equipment was used other than gloves, and it was unclear whether the gloves were impermeable. More than 15% of the youth surveyed reported having had symptoms consistent with organophosphate poisoning, but few sought medical care. More than 40% had worked in fields wet with pesticides, violating field reentry times suggested by chemical manufacturers, and 40% had been directly sprayed with pesticides by crop-dusting planes, or indirectly by drifting chemicals from planes or tractors. Similar observations were made among 323 North Carolina 4-H students, 69% of whom were working on a relative's farm. Use of pesticides or other farm chemicals was reported by 29% of girls and 59% of boys. Sickness related to pesticide or other chemical exposures was reported by 3% of girls and 11% of boys.[44]

EXAMPLES OF EXPOSURES WITH CHRONIC EFFECTS

Noise

Wisconsin high school students with active involvement in farm work had more than twice the risk of early noise-induced hearing loss than their peers who did not work on farms.[27,45] There was a relationship between amount of noise exposure and degree of hearing loss. Among farming students with greater noise exposure, 74% had evidence of some hearing loss in at least one ear. Only 9% of farming students reported using any hearing protection devices.

Repetitive Motion

Although there are few data about adolescents, a study including slightly older female supermarket cashiers was notable for the prevalence of self-reported carpal tunnel symptoms (62.5%) related to use of laser scanners, years worked as a cashier, and number of hours worked per week.[46] This is a concern because of the large number of female teenagers employed as supermarket cashiers and because teenagers often have additional school or leisure computer time, adding to the potential for repetitive motion problems.[35]

DIAGNOSTIC METHODS

When a teenager presents with a symptom without an obvious cause, a thorough history (including an occupational history) and physical examination are most important. Patients should be screened for exposure to heavy metals or other substances if appropriate (for example, for lead when renovating old houses). When the substance itself cannot be measured, end-organ effects of exposure may be measured (eg, hepatocellular enzymes following solvent exposure). In acute events, the substance and its original container(s) should be saved for analysis if needed.

TREATMENT OF CLINICAL SYMPTOMS

Treatment ranges from determining and eliminating the source of low-level chronic exposure to advanced cardiac life support in some acute poisonings. It is critical to have knowledge of proper rescue measures to ensure the safety of the rescuer, especially if the first victim is in an oxygen-deficient or chemically toxic environment, such as 2 teens killed in a Michigan silo in 2010.[47,48] Specific information about medical treatment may be provided by pediatric toxicologists or personnel in a poison control center.

PREVENTION OF EXPOSURE

Community-Based Strategies

Prevention involves a combination of training and engineering controls. Knowledge of substances used and potential routes of exposure is needed. Proper ergonomics are important in preventing repetitive motion disorders. Back problems may be better prevented if the size of the teenager and the size of the load are carefully matched.

Evidence-based prevention programs are in their infancy. A program in Wisconsin illustrates how a culture of safety may influence teenagers' workplace behaviors and may help to form protective job-safety habits for life. A 4-year program to prevent noise-induced hearing loss was effective in having Wisconsin farm tractor-driving adolescents wear hearing protection devices. Students' reports of their planned future use of hearing protection devices increased from 23% to 81% among the 375 study students, whereas it increased from 24% to only 43% in a comparison group.[27]

Table 13.1: Examples of Job-Related Exposures

- Asbestos in auto brake repair, renovation/demolition of old buildings
- Asthma-exacerbating wood dusts in shop and furniture making
- Benzene when pumping gas
- Bloodborne pathogens in nursing homes/hospitals
- Cleaning agents in restaurants, nursing homes, and schools
- Cold in areas with cold weather and outdoor jobs, potentially exacerbated by wet conditions contributing to faster heat loss (in gas station work, construction work, ski area work, and whitewater guiding)
- Cosmetology chemicals and dyes
- Heat in dishwashing and outdoor work in the summer or in hot climates
- Isocyanates (pulmonary sensitizers) during auto body repair or roofing with newer forms of roofing materials
- Lead from radiators in auto body repair and from paint and plaster in home renovation
- Nicotine in harvest of tobacco (green tobacco sickness)
- Noise-induced hearing loss in farming and factory work
- Pesticides in lawn care work, farm work, and when buildings are sprayed
- Secondhand smoke in waitstaff jobs
- Solvents in t-shirt screening
- Sun exposure in lifeguard work, farm work, and other outdoor work
- Tetanus and other biological/infectious hazards in farming (hypersensitivity pneumonitis), veterinary clinics
- Welding fumes resulting in eye exposures

Office-Based Strategies

As part of well visits and other visits, such as sports physicals and visits for working papers, pediatricians are encouraged to find out which patients work, job duties, types of chemicals, and/or types of equipment used and whether teenagers have received training about working safely with chemicals or equipment. Because more than 75% of teenagers work at some point in the year, every teenager needs an occupational history, with a focus on potential hazards (Table 13.1). Such a history includes asking about unpaid work (such as helping at a family farm or nonfarm business), vocational training at school in shop and other classes, and school-related work-study or other on-the-job site placements. Pediatricians should ask whether adolescents are volunteers on projects such as summer housing rehabilitation work, which may result in exposures. An occupational history is recommended for teenagers with learning disabilities, developmental delays, or intellectual disabilities. Asking about the presence of an adult supervisor on-site is important, as is asking about the presence of someone who knows first aid. Although some workplaces are exempt from the Fair Labor Standards Act, all workers legally have the right to know about the chemicals with which they work. Discussing these issues may start with a patient-reported checklist. Although the discussion may be brief, it provides an opportunity for pediatricians to educate teenagers about occupational safety and health.

Pediatricians should become familiar with state child labor laws. Each state Department of Labor provides a 1-page poster summarizing work hours, wages, and occupations permitted for adolescents of different ages. This poster must be posted prominently in every workplace, and could be posted in the adolescent area of a practice or clinic. In some states, the office of the US Department of Labor also can provide information. Pediatricians should have some familiarity with state workers' compensation laws, because adolescents may be eligible for compensation for medical expenses, lost wages, and lost time because of illnesses from occupational exposures.

Pediatricians are not expected to be experts in harmful work exposures. Rather, in a model similar to that of child passenger safety, pediatricians should be aware of basic information and know where to turn for expert advice. Pediatric Environmental Health Specialty Units are staffed by pediatricians and occupational medicine specialists. Information about exposures can also be obtained from industrial hygienists, union or corporate health and safety employees, and local Committee on Occupational Safety and Health groups. State-based Occupational Safety and Health Administration training sections may be helpful. Employers are legally responsible for educating workers about chemical exposures and use.

An adolescent's employment should be considered when diagnosing an illness. For example, chronic fatigue in an adolescent who makes silk screens can be caused by chronic solvent intoxication if the teenager works or sleeps in an area with inadequate ventilation. The adolescent's employment should be considered in the management of known illnesses (for example, asthma previously under control may flare when the teenager works in a restaurant with a smoking section).

Pediatricians can provide guidance about the choice of occupations for adolescents with chronic conditions. Employment opportunities, which may be fewer than those for their peers, are important for development and future adult employment.

Pediatricians are urged to advocate for age-appropriate rehabilitation and follow-up for those injured on the job. Although agriculturally related injuries often are not covered, workers' compensation should pay for many cases of rehabilitation resulting from occupational injury or exposure.

HELPING PARENTS TO MAKE INFORMED DECISIONS ABOUT ADOLESCENT WORK SAFETY

Pediatricians should talk with parents and guardians about the potential risks and benefits of their teenager's employment situation. Many adults are unaware of the risks of injury or chemical exposures and the need for adolescents to receive training about safety. Guidance may help reduce risks. Parents should be educated about normal patterns of adolescent growth and development and appropriate expectations for the teenager's developmental stage. Teenagers who are small for age, especially those do farm work, may be unable to fit into adult-size protective equipment, potentially resulting in exposures. Teenagers who are large for age may be cognitively or emotionally immature and should not be expected to perform physical tasks needing the judgment of an experienced adult. Realizing that responsibilities for teenagers should increase within safe limits, parents need support in their decisions about safety. Faced with pressure from children or children's friends, parents may doubt the wisdom of their decisions. Support for safety is important as families weigh the appropriate limits of independence for their teenagers.

Parents also should be encouraged to be role models for safety. Parents who are farmers or farmworkers, for example, can demonstrate and discuss safe use, handling, storage, and disposal of chemicals with their adolescent. Parents should be encouraged to discuss exposures to noise and dust and to share information on protective measures and minimizing exposures.

TAKE-HOME EXPOSURES

A "take-home" exposure refers to exposure of a child (or other household member) to chemicals, fibers, metals, or dusts brought home from a work site by a parent. Exposures may result in poisoning. Lead is one of the best known examples: a parent employed in a job such as bridge repair, auto battery repair, painting, or work at a firing range may inadvertently bring home sufficient lead dust on clothing to give a child lead poisoning (see Chapter 31).[49-53] Mercury, pesticides, fiberglass, and asbestos are among other known take-home exposures. In evaluating a child with known heavy metal poisoning, parental occupations should be considered.

IN-HOME EXPOSURES

Work conducted by parents or others in a home setting may put children at risk. Kitchen-table assembly of radar detectors, which involves dipping wires in lead, may create a poisoning hazard. Backyard work on car batteries has caused lead poisoning in children living in that home or neighbors' homes.[49]

A new and widespread hazard involves the clandestine home manufacture of methamphetamine ("meth" [see Chapter 49]).[54] Children at home during methamphetamine production are at risk of death or injury from explosions, fire, and burns. They are also at risk of death from ingestion of severely corrosive materials. Chemicals involved with methamphetamine production are so toxic that law enforcement personnel treat such sites as hazardous for their own protection.[54]

Frequently Asked Questions

Q *My teenager has asthma, for which she takes daily medication. She wants to get a part-time job. Can I help direct her to work that won't cause her asthma to flare up?*

A Teenagers need to ask potential employers about the tasks they will be doing and whether they may be exposed to any chemicals. A restaurant with a smoking section is not a wise choice for a teenager with asthma. A customer service or cashier job should provide a better respiratory environment, or the teenager with asthma may seek work in an ice cream store without smoking, as long as he or she is not also required to use cleaning materials that are respiratory irritants. In any job, parents should be concerned about adult supervision, job training, and safety instruction. It is important for parents to visit the workplace. A job that requires personal protective equipment suggests a possible risk that should be explored. Potential chemical exposures in vocational education, shop class, work-study, and volunteer work should be considered.

Q *Are teenagers less vulnerable to workplace exposures because they're young and healthy? When we were young, we worked without all these protections.*

A Risks of exposures can be small or life-threatening, depending on the chemical. Teenagers and children are just as vulnerable to enclosed space exposures. Like adults, they will die in an oxygen-deprived environment, such as in a tank they are cleaning that was previously full of chemicals. Theoretically, if a chemical becomes less toxic when metabolized, and teenagers metabolize better or faster than adults, then its effects could be less toxic for a young worker. If the metabolite itself is poisonous, teenagers could be at increased risk. Because one is unlikely to know in advance which situation pertains for any given chemical, testing the situation may involve risking illness or death. Thus, protection from exposure is always the best approach.

Q *Are teenagers more vulnerable to work exposure than adults because their systems (especially immune systems) aren't yet fully developed?*

A Adolescents may be more vulnerable from some respects but not because of their immune systems. Although there are no definitive data to answer this question at present, by adolescence, the immune system is essentially fully developed, so it is not likely to be more vulnerable. When advocating for adolescent occupational health and safety, it is important not to exaggerate the risks that exist; this may lessen our credibility about the real risks.

If we know, however, that an exposure is hazardous for adults, we should assume that it is likely to be at least as hazardous for adolescents and protect them from that exposure. Exposure to potentially cancer-causing (carcinogenic) substances and to substances that may produce birth defects (teratogens) may create increased risk for adolescents. There may be higher risks of early life exposure to substances (especially carcinogenic ones) associated with diseases that occur only after long latency periods. If a substance accumulates in the body over time, and the effects are dose-related, teen workers may be at risk, because their exposure started earlier in life. It is possible that exposure to a potential carcinogen during the rapid growth period of adolescence may increase cancer risk. Given that adolescence is a time of endocrine changes, there may be increased vulnerability to chemicals (including certain pesticides) that are endocrine disrupters. Because adolescents are of childbearing age, acute and latent reproductive effects of chemicals are potentially of concern.

Q   Is it safe for a teenager who is still growing to do manual labor with heavy equipment?

A   Our knowledge about occupational back injury and about overuse injuries among young gymnasts and baseball players suggests that periods of rapid growth may put an individual at increased risk of severe and chronic musculoskeletal injuries, especially if there are too many repetitions of a movement.[55] This has implications for farm work, cashier work, and any work with repetitive motion.

Resources

National Institute for Occupational Safety and Health (NIOSH)
Phone: 800-356-4674
Web site: www.cdc.gov/niosh/homepage.html
The Web site of this federal agency contains information on hours and safety regulations, hazards, and how to protect against them, including a sheet for teenagers. The Division of Safety Research in the Morgantown, WV, NIOSH office (phone: 304-285-5894) has expertise in the scientific, research, and educational aspects. The NIOSH office in Cincinnati, OH, works on exposures in vocational/technical education settings. In May 1995, NIOSH published *Alert-Request for Assistance in Preventing Deaths and Injuries of Adolescent Workers*. This booklet (Department of Health and Human Services Publication No. 95-125, available from NIOSH) has background information and a tear-out page to post in the office or to copy for adolescent patients and their parents or for community work. NIOSH funds educational resource centers and academic departments of occupational medicine.

Labor Departments

Each state Department of Labor has information on child labor laws; wages; hours of work; safety regulations, including Hazard Orders that prohibit specific types of hazardous exposures; and problems with any of those areas. A poster summarizing child labor law often is available. In some states, a caller will be told to call the local office of the US Department of Labor.

Youthwork E-mail List

Web site: www.youthwork.com/ywnetlists.html
This mailing list for professionals and volunteers working with youth addresses programs and issues relating to work. Questions are posted, as are information and opinions from the federal, state, university, and front-line sources on issues pertaining to health and safety.

Occupational Safety and Health Administration (OSHA)

Phone: 800-321-OSHA (6742)
Web site: www.osha.gov
This federal agency deals with regulatory and enforcement issues. If a teenager has a question about a specific hazard, the teenager or parent (with permission) can call OSHA for assistance. This can be done anonymously, but sometimes an employee may be identifiable. Pediatricians should consider this agency especially when there is concern about imminent danger to other adolescents in that workplace. OSHA offices can be found in local phone directories.

Committees on Occupational Safety and Health (COSH)

Most community-based COSH groups maintain staff capable of answering questions about occupational exposures. The New York Committee for Occupational Safety and Health publishes an update every few days of current worker health and safety issues including those relevant to employed adolescents.

Poison Control Centers

Information on toxicity of specific chemicals and clinical guidance is available. Poison control centers provide expertise and treatment advice by phone. All poison control centers can be reached by calling the same telephone number: 1-800-222-1222.

North American Guidelines for Children's Agricultural Tasks

Web site: www.nagcat.org/nagcat
The North American Guidelines for Children's Agricultural Tasks (NAGCAT), published by the Marshfield Clinic Research Foundation, were developed to assist parents in assigning farm jobs to their children

7 to 16 years of age, living or working on farms. The NAGCAT can help answer questions from parents and professionals about the role of their child in agricultural work.

Child Labor Coalition

Web site: www.stopchildlabor.org/index.html

This is a coalition of diverse organizations and individuals (including the American Academy of Pediatrics, consumer groups, medical professionals, universities, unions, and religious organizations) interested in international and US child labor. They organize conferences, meet monthly, and maintain one of the most up-to-date watches in the nation on federal and state child labor law changes.

National Child Labor Committee

Phone: 212-840-1801

Web site: www.kapow.org/nclc.htm

The committee, founded in 1904, has historical and legal information and continues to advocate for the safe employment of adolescents.

References

1. National Institute for Occupational Safety and Health, Centers for Disease Control and Prevention. *Young Worker Safety and Health.* Available at: http://www.cdc.gov/niosh/topics/youth/. Accessed March 1, 2011

2. Breslin FC, Day D, Tompa E, et al. Non-agricultural work injuries among youth—a systematic review. *Am J Prev Med.* 2007;32(2):151-162

3. American Academy of Pediatrics Committee on Environmental Health. The hazards of child labor. *Pediatrics.* 1995;95(2):311–313

4. Windau J, Meyer S. Occupational injuries among young workers. *Monthly Labor Review.* October 2005:11-23

5. Institute of Medicine, Committee on Health and Safety Implications of Child Labor. *Protecting Youth at Work: Health, Safety and Development of Working Children and Adolescents in the United States.* Washington, DC: National Academies Press; 1998

6. Fair Labor Standards Act, 29 USC 201, CFR 570–580 (1938)

7. US Department of Labor. *Child Labor Requirements in Nonagricultural Occupations Under the Fair Labor Standards Act.* Child Labor Bulletin 101. Washington, DC: Employment Standards Administration, Wage and Hour Division; 1985

8. US Department of Labor. *Child Labor Requirements in Agriculture Under the Fair Labor Standards Act.* Child Labor Bulletin 102. Washington, DC: Employment Standards Administration, Wage and Hour Division; 1984

9. Knight S, Junkins EP Jr, Lightfood AC, Cazier CF, Olson LM. Injuries sustained by students in shop class. *Pediatrics.* 2000;106(1 Pt 1):10–13

10. Woolf AD, Flynn E. Workplace toxic exposures involving adolescents aged 14 to 19 years: one poison center's experience. *Arch Pediatr Adolesc Med.* 2000;154(3):234–239

11. US Department of Labor, Wage and Hour Division. Youth Rules. Available at: http://www.youthrules.dol.gov/index.htm. Accessed March 1, 2011

12. Suruda A, Halperin W. Work-related deaths in children. *Am J Ind Med.* 1991;19(6):739–745

13. Dunn KA, Runyan CW. Deaths at work among children and adolescents. *Am J Dis Child.* 1993;147(10):1044–1047

14. Derstine B. Youth workers at risk of fatal injuries. Presented at: 122nd Annual Meeting of the American Public Health Association; November 1, 1994; Washington, DC

15. Castillo DN, Malit BD. Occupational injury deaths of 16 and 17 year olds in the US: trends and comparisons with older workers. *Inj Prev.* 1997;3(4):277–281

16. Centers for Disease Control and Prevention. Work-related injuries and illnesses associated with child labor—United States, 1993. *MMWR Morb Mortal Wkly Rep.* 1996;45(22):464–468

17. Centers for Disease Control and Prevention. occupational injuries and deaths among younger workers—United States, 1998-2007. *MMWR Morb Mortal Wkly Rep.* 2010;59(15):449-455

18. Miller M. *Occupational Injuries Among Adolescents in Washington State, 1988–91: A Review of Workers' Compensation Data.* Olympia, WA: Safety and Health Assessment and Research for Prevention, Washington State Department of Labor and Industries; 1995. Technical Report No. 35-1-1995

19. Bellville R, Pollack SH, Godbold JH, Landrigan PJ. Occupational injuries among working adolescents in New York State. *JAMA.* 1993;269(21):2754–2759

20. Brooks DR, Davis LK, Gallagher SS. Work-related injuries among Massachusetts children: a study based on emergency department data. *Am J Ind Med.* 1993;24(3):313–324

21. Bush D, Baker R. *Young Workers at Risk: Health and Safety Education and the Schools.* Berkeley, CA: Labor Occupational Health Program; 1994

22. Cooper SP, Rothstein MA. Health hazards among working children in Texas. *South Med J.* 1995;88(5):550–554

23. Banco L, Lapidus G, Braddock M. Work-related injury among Connecticut minors. *Pediatrics.* 1992;89(5 Pt 1):957–960

24. Parker DL, Carl WR, French LR, Martin FB. Characteristics of adolescent work injuries reported to the Minnesota Department of Labor and Industry. *Am J Public Health.* 1994;84(4):606–611

25. Loomis DP, Richardson DB, Wolf SH, Runyan CW, Butts JD. Fatal occupational injuries in a southern state. *Am J Epidemiol.* 1997;145(12):1089–1099

26. Woolf AD. Health hazards for children at work. *J Toxicol Clin Toxicol.* 2002;40(4):477–482

27. Knobloch MJ, Broste SK. A hearing conversation program for Wisconsin youth working in agriculture. *J Sch Health.* 1998;68(8):313–318

28. Curwin B, Sanderson W, Reynolds S, Hein M, Alavanja M. Pesticide use and practices in an Iowa farm family pesticide exposure study. *J Agric Saf Health.* 2002;8(4):423–433

29. Gelbach SH, Williams WA, Perry LD, Woodall JS. Green-tobacco sickness. An illness of tobacco harvesters. *JAMA.* 1974;229(14):1880–1883

30. Horstman SW, Browning SR, Szeluga R, Burzycki J, Stebbins A. Solvent exposures in screen printing shops. *J Environ Sci Health Part A Tox Hazard Subst Environ Eng.* 2001;36(10): 1957–1973

31. National Institute of Occupational Safety and Health. *Alert-Request for Assistance in Preventing Deaths and Injuries of Adolescent Workers.* Washington, DC: US Department of Health and Human Services; 1995. DHHS (NIOSH) publication No. 95-125

32. Hosein HR, Farkas S. Risk associated with the spray application of polyurethane foam. *Am Ind Hyg Assoc J.* 1981;42(9):663–665

33. Husgafvel-Pursiainen K, Sorsa M, Engstrom K, Einisto P. Passive smoking at work: biochemical and biological measures of exposure to environmental tobacco smoke. *Int Arch Occup Environ Health.* 1987;59(4):337–345

34. WVLT-TV. Students Used to Help Fix Mold Problem. Knoxville, TN: WVLT-TV, reported on September 14, 2004

35. Nonprofit execs indicted on health risks to teens. *Associated Press*. November 11, 2010. Available at: http://www.signonsandiego.com/news/2010/nov/11/nonprofit-execs-indicted-on-health-risks-to-teens/. Accessed March 1, 2011

36. Pollack S, McConnell R, Gallelli M, Schmidt J, Obregon R, Landrigan P. Pesticide exposure and working conditions among migrant farmworker children in western New York State [abstr 317]. In: Proceedings of the 118th Annual Meeting of the American Public Health Association; September 30-October 4, 1990; New York, NY

37. Ruder AM, Waters MA, Carreon T, et al. The Upper Midwest Health Study: a case-control study of primary intracranial gliomas in farm and rural residents. Brain Cancer Collaborative Study Group. *J Agric Saf Health*. 2006;12(4):255-274

38. Arif AA, Delclos GL, Serra C. Occupational exposures and asthma among nursing professionals. *Occup Environ Med*. 2009;66(4):274-278

39. Egilman D, Mailloux C, Valentin C. Popcorn-worker lung caused by corporate and regulatory negligence: an avoidable tragedy. *Int J Occup Environ Health*. 2007;13(1):85-98

40. van Rooy FGBGJ, Smit LAM, Houba R, Zaat VAC, Rooyackers JM, Heederik DJJ. A cross-sectional study of lung function and respiratory symptoms among chemical workers producing diacetyl for food flavourings. *Occup Environ Med*. 2009;66:105-110

41. US Department of Labor, Occupational Safety and Health Administration. OSHA National News Release: US Secretary of Labor Hilda L. Solis announces convening of rulemaking panel on worker exposure to food flavorings containing diacetyl. Washington, DC: US Department of Labor; April 28, 2009. National News Release: 09-431-NAT

42. Enander RT, Gute DM, Cohen HJ, Brown LC, Desmaris AM, Missaghian R. Chemical characterization of sanding dust and methylene chloride usage in auto refinishing: implications for occupational and environmental health. *AIHA J (Farifax, VA)*. 2002;63(6):741–749

43. Pollack SH, Scheurich-Payne SL, Bryant S. The nature of occupational injury among Kentucky adolescents. Presented at: Occupational Injury Symposium; February 24-27, 1996; Sydney, Australia

44. Cohen LR, Runyan CW, Dunn KA, Schulman MD. Work patterns and occupational hazard exposures of North Carolina adolescents in 4-H clubs. *Inj Prev*. 1996;2(4):274–277

45. Broste SK, Hansen DA, Strand RL, Stueland DT. Hearing loss among high school farm students. *Am J Public Health*. 1989;79(5):619–622

46. Margolis W, Krause JF. The prevalence of carpal tunnel syndrome symptoms in female supermarket checkers. *J Occup Med*. 1987;29(12):953–956

47. Newschannel 3, Barry County, Michigan. Families remember two teens who died in silo accident. Aired July 13, 2010. Available at: http://www.wwmt.com/articles/silo-1378978-jose-victor.html. Accessed March 1, 2011

48. Lynch Ryan. Two farmworking teens killed in silo; media is mystified, blog on Workers' Comp Insider. July 13, 2010. Available at: http://www.workerscompinsider.com/2010/07/two-farmworking.html. Accessed March 1, 2011

49. Gittleman JL, Engelgau MM, Shaw J, Wille KK, Seligman PJ. Lead poisoning among battery reclamation workers in Alabama. *J Occup Med*. 1994;36(5):526–532

50. Piacitelli GM, Whelan EA, Ewers LM, Sieber WK. Lead contamination in automobiles of lead-exposed bridgeworkers. *Appl Occup Environ Hyg*. 1995;10:849–855

51. Gerson M, Van den Eeden SK, Gahagan P. Take-home lead poisoning in a child from his father's occupational exposure. *Am J Ind Med*. 1996;29(5):507–508

52. Piacitelli GM, Whelan EA, Sieber WK, Gerwel B. Elevated lead contamination in homes of construction workers. *Am Ind Hyg Assoc J*. 1997;58(6):447–454

53. Whelan EA, Piacitelli GM, Gerwel B, et al. Elevated blood lead levels in children of construction workers. *Am J Public Health.* 1997;87(8):1352–1355
54. Willers-Russo LJ. Three fatalities involving phosphine gas, produced as a result of methamphetamine manufacturing. *J Forensic Sci.* 1999;44(3):647–652
55. Hutchinson MR, Ireland ML. Overuse and throwing injuries in the skeletally immature athlete. *Instr Course Lect.* 2003;52:25–36

Chapter 14

Environmental Health Considerations for Children in Developing Nations

■ ■ ■ ■ ■ ■

A majority of the world's children live in developing nations, including nations with environmental conditions that are detrimental to health. Awareness of the environmental health conditions in other parts of the world provides a perspective on the importance of the United States and other governments, nonprofit institutions, and international organizations in improving global child health.

In addition, pediatricians in the United States, particularly in urban areas and areas with large immigrant populations, may examine and care for patients who were not born in this country. Every year, approximately 17 000 children are adopted internationally (http://adoption.state.gov/news/total_chart.html). Currently, most children arrive from Guatemala, China, Russia, Ethiopia, and South Korea. Each year, thousands of persons who face persecution in their country of nationality seek asylum or refugee status in the United States. In recent years, according to the Department of Homeland Security, the majority of refugees come from Burma, Somalia, Iran, Burundi, and Cuba (www.dhs.gov/ximgtn/statistics). When a child comes from a developing country, it is important to be aware of the lifestyle, cultural, and environmental differences that greatly influence health status.

This chapter is intended to 1) provide an overview of global pediatric environmental health issues; and 2) discuss the key exposures to consider in the care of international adoptees, refugees, and immigrants from developing nations.

GLOBAL PEDIATRIC ENVIRONMENTAL HEALTH: DEFINING THE POPULATION, KEY PROBLEMS, AND ORGANIZATIONS

Although there is no single accepted definition of developing countries, the *Cambridge International Dictionary of English* defines them as: "the poorer countries of the world, which include many of the countries of Africa, Latin America and Asia, which have less advanced industries."[1] The World Trade Organization (WTO) does not define "developed" and "developing" countries; members announce for themselves whether they are "developed" or "developing" countries.[2]

Ninety-one percent of the world's 1.8 billion children 0 to 14 years of age live in developing countries.[3] The total global population is projected to increase from the current 6.7 billion to 9.2 billion by the year 2050, with essentially all growth in developing countries, concentrated among the poorest populations in urban areas.[4]

The World Health Organization (WHO) estimates that approximately one third of the disease burden in developing countries is attributable to environmental factors, 2 to 3 times higher than that in the most developed countries.[5] Fig 14.1 summarizes the disparate burden of disease for children in developing countries attributable to air, water, soil, and food contamination, compared with children in the more developed nations. This unequal disease burden on the poorer nations may be further aggravated by differences in access to health care.

Urbanization, unregulated industrialization, population growth and displacement, and increased pressure on limited natural resources underlie the environmental hazards in poorer nations. Mitigation measures are often unaddressed in the quest for economic development. Obstacles to protecting pediatric environmental health in developing countries include inadequate medical and public health infrastructure and financial resources, shortage of laboratory equipment and trained technical personnel, and distrust between the public and governmental agencies.

The United Nations (UN) has core agencies that monitor trends, identify priorities, and promote programs and activities designed to improve pediatric environmental health in developing countries. The WHO, the UN's public health arm, supports a pediatric environmental health program that provides national profiles and tracks health indicators in the developing regions of the world. In addition, capacity-building activities and resource development relevant to developing countries are ongoing. The International Pediatric Association, an organization of national pediatric societies, has a program focusing on environmental health. The International Network for Children's Health, Environment and Safety and the International Society of Doctors for the Environment also focus on this topic (see Resources).

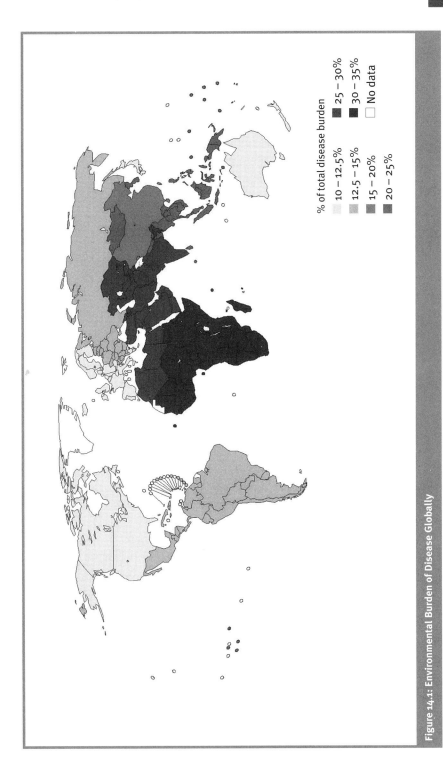

Figure 14.1: Environmental Burden of Disease Globally

Reprinted with permission from World Health Organization © 2005. http:-//www.who.int/heli/risks/en/ebdtotal.pdf. Accessed August 3, 2011

The following primary areas of concern in global child health and environment are well recognized and briefly described in this chapter. In many cases, their etiologies and solutions are intertwined:

- Unsafe water, poor sanitation, and hygiene
- Vectorborne diseases
- Indoor air pollution
- Tobacco and secondhand tobacco smoke
- Traffic-related pollution and traffic injury
- Industrialization and hazardous materials
- Pesticides
- Climate change

Unsafe Water, Poor Sanitation, and Hygiene

Nearly 1.1 billion people in the world are still without access to safe drinking water.[6] Forty-two percent of these people are in East Asia and the Pacific, 25% are in Sub-Saharan Africa, and 19% are in South Asia.[7] Access to safe drinking water is particularly low in the poor, rural areas of developing countries. Nearly 2.4 billion people, including half of all Asians, lack access to sanitary means of excreta disposal.[6]

With proper sanitation, proper hygiene, and safe drinking water, diarrhea can be decreased by 22%, and deaths resulting from diarrhea can be decreased by 65%.[8] However, rapid growth of cities in developing countries represents a serious challenge to efforts to provide proper housing, drinking water, and sanitation. Given that diarrhea accounts for 12% of the deaths of children younger than 5 years, improvements in water and sanitation are critical to child health. Additionally, improved sanitation and safe drinking water will help to eradicate guinea worm disease, hookworm, schistosomiasis, and other waterborne diseases that greatly influence the health and development of children in developing countries, especially in Sub-Saharan Africa.

High levels of chemical contaminants, such as nitrates, arsenic, and fluoride, are common in the drinking water supply in many rural areas. High levels of naturally occurring arsenic have been found in 10 developing countries, including Taiwan, China, India, Bangladesh, Mexico, Argentina, Chile, and Romania, exposing approximately 45 million individuals.[9] In Bangladesh, 57.5% of 1630 exposed adults had skin lesions caused by arsenic poisoning.[9] Fluorosis is a potentially crippling disease caused by the ingestion of too much fluoride in drinking water.[10] High concentrations of fluoride occur naturally in groundwater and coal in many of these countries.[11] Fluorosis is endemic in at least 25 countries, including India, Mexico, China, and Bangladesh. Pesticide and herbicide contamination from agricultural uses is also common, because approximately 80% of rural people in developing countries are engaged in agricultural work.[8] Persistent organic pollutants have been documented in water supplies throughout developing countries.[12]

Vectorborne Diseases

Environmental degradation can lead to increased vectorborne disease. In addition to the waterborne diseases described above, poorly designed irrigation and water systems and poor waste disposal and water storage can contribute to malaria, dengue fever, and leishmaniasis. Malaria kills more than 1.2 million people annually, mostly African children younger than 5 years.[13] Dengue fever, with associated dengue hemorrhagic fever, is the world's fastest growing vector-borne disease.[13]

The United Nations Environment Programme has identified a number of links between increased malaria and worsening environmental conditions.[14] The expansion of mining and other extractive industries has been associated with an increase in the incidence of malaria. For example, in Sri Lankan gem-mining areas, shallow pits left behind by gem miners become ideal mosquito breeding areas. Studies from Brazil suggest that mercury used in small-scale gold mining may increase peoples' susceptibility to malaria by depressing their immune systems. Deforestation and road building disrupt forest and river systems that may increase the habitats for malaria-carrying mosquitoes. Migration of workers into previously inaccessible areas increases the population at risk. In addition, the WHO recently estimated that some 6% of malaria cases in parts of the world during the last 25 years are the result of climate change.

Indoor Air Pollution

In developing countries, indoor air pollution is an important risk factor that contributes to disease and death overall.[15] This is because 90% of rural households in low-income countries and two thirds of households in developing countries rely on unprocessed biomass (plant materials and animal waste) fuels for cooking and/or heating.[16] These fuels include wood, dung, and crop residues, which are burned indoors on open fires or in poorly ventilated stoves. This creates levels of gas and particulate pollutant mixtures that are many times greater than permitted under typical regulatory limits.[17] As part of the WHO's Comparative Quantification of Health Risks study, it was estimated that 3.6% of the global burden of disease can be attributed to indoor air pollution from the use of solid fuels.[18]

Women of childbearing age are traditionally responsible for cooking, and consequently, the exposures are highest for them and for their infants and young children, who are often carried on the backs of their mothers. Child exposures occur not only at home but also at school, where biomass fuel is commonly used. Indoor air pollution is estimated to cause 1 million deaths in infants and young children by causing acute lower respiratory infections.[19]

In some countries, kerosene is used as a substitute because it seems to burn "cleaner." As with biomass fuel, indoor kerosene burning leads to the accumulation of volatile organic compounds and polyaromatic hydrocarbons. Intervention studies using improved stoves are ongoing in poor, rural communities where access to alternative fuels is very limited. These studies demonstrate that pollution levels can be lowered significantly.[20]

Tobacco and Secondhand Tobacco Smoke

Tobacco use is currently the world's leading killer, causing 1 in 10 (or 5.4 million) deaths annually among adults worldwide. Unless urgent action is taken, there will be more than 8 million tobacco deaths annually by 2030, with more than 80% of these deaths occurring in developing countries. Smokers are not the only ones sickened and killed by tobacco. Secondhand smoke (SHS) also has serious and potentially fatal health consequences[21] (http://www.who.int/tobacco/mpower/mpower_report_full_2008.pdf).

Secondhand smoke is composed of sidestream smoke (the smoke released from the burning end of a cigarette) and exhaled mainstream smoke (the smoke exhaled by the smoker). The 2006 Report of the United States Surgeon General states that there is no risk-free level of exposure to secondhand smoke: even small amounts of secondhand smoke exposure can be harmful to people's health. According to the report, almost 60% of children 3 through 11 years of age are exposed to secondhand smoke in the United States. These children are at increased risk of multiple serious health effects including asthma, respiratory infections, decreased lung growth and exercise tolerance, and sudden infant death syndrome. Smoking by parents or primary caregivers in the home is the primary source of exposure for preschoolers. This exposure is most dangerous for the youngest children, because they have immature lungs and spend more time in close proximity to parents. The most effective method for reducing exposure is to establish and maintain smoke-free environments[22] (http://www.surgeongeneral.gov/library/secondhandsmoke).

Nearly two thirds of the world's smokers live in 10 countries, with tobacco use growing fastest in low-income countries as populations grow, and as tobacco companies turn their attention away from the increasingly regulated US and European markets. With approximately 350 million smokers, China has the biggest smoking population in the world. Smokers in China consume an estimated 1.7 trillion cigarettes per year and roughly 540 million Chinese people are exposed to secondhand smoke. Of Chinese smokers, 61% are men, and smoking fathers account for 60% of children's exposure to secondhand smoke; 98% of smokers smoke at home,[23] and an estimated 43% of Chinese people are exposed to secondhand smoke outside the home.

India is the third-largest tobacco producing country in the world after China and Brazil, and a large part of that production is consumed within the country.

With a population of 1.15 billion people, India represents 17% of the Earth's population. There is a high prevalence of tobacco use in the Indian population, with 57% of males and 3% of females using tobacco; 26.6% of Indian children are exposed to secondhand smoke indoors and more than 40% are exposed outside their homes.[23]

Although there are strong cultural differences in smoking behaviors in different countries and regions, the WHO Framework Convention on Tobacco Control, a multilateral treaty that has been ratified by 173 parties, developed a blueprint for countries to halt the tobacco epidemic and move toward a tobacco-free world. Although the United States signed the Framework Convention on Tobacco Control, it has never been ratified by the Senate; thus, the United States is not among the parties to the treaty. To help countries fulfill the promise of the Convention, the WHO established the MPOWER package, which includes the 6 most important and effective tobacco-control policies that are proven to reduce tobacco use and secondhand smoke exposure: raising taxes and prices; banning advertising and promotion of tobacco products and sponsorship of sporting events by tobacco companies; protecting people from secondhand smoke; warning people about the dangers of tobacco; offering help to people who want to quit; and carefully monitoring the epidemic and prevention policies.[21]

Traffic-Derived Pollution and Traffic Injury

Urban air pollution is largely and increasingly derived from vehicular combustion and power generation (see Chapter 21). In the rapidly growing megacities of Asia, Africa, and Latin America, concentrations of pollutants rival and exceed those experienced in the industrialized countries in the early 20th century.[24] Outdoor air pollution is made worse in many developing countries because of the types of vehicles driven. In Southeast Asia and several other developing countries, most vehicles are 2- and 3-wheelers, including mopeds, motorcycles, scooters, and auto rickshaws. These types of vehicles use the more polluting 2-stroke engine technology, which contributes greatly to air pollution in urban areas.

Because leaded gasoline is still used in a few developing countries, many vehicles in developing countries do not have catalytic converters, which help to reduce carbon monoxide and hydrocarbon emissions. Lead contamination from leaded gasoline has been a significant problem in rapidly industrializing countries. Currently, all but 9 countries have phased out the use of lead in gasoline.[25]

A WHO review of published childhood blood lead surveillance data found that 40% of children worldwide had blood lead concentrations >5 µg/dL, and 20% had blood lead concentrations >10 µg/dL.[26] Ninety percent of these high blood lead concentrations were observed in children who lived in developing countries. Fewer than 10% of the children had blood lead concentrations >20 µg/dL, but 99% of those children lived in developing regions.

An epidemic of road traffic injuries in developing countries is also linked to urbanization and was summarized in a 2003 WHO report.[27] The WHO notes that more than 90% of road traffic deaths occur in low-income and middle-income countries. Fatality rates are twice as high as in high-income countries and are rapidly accelerating in the developing world, especially in Asia. By 2020, road traffic deaths are expected to increase by 92% in China and 147% in India, with an average increase of 80% in many other developing countries. Unlike the situation in high-income countries, where traffic injuries predominantly affect drivers, a far higher proportion of road deaths in developing countries occur among pedestrians, bicyclists, other nonmotorized traffic, motorcyclists and moped riders, and passengers of buses and trucks.

Industrialization and Hazardous Materials

Coal-burning fuel plants, steel factories, and mining operations without regulatory oversight or environmental impact reduction procedures have created severe air, water, and soil contamination in much of Central and Eastern Europe and other parts of the world. Sixty percent of the world's smelters are located in developing nations.[28] Pollutants from these operations include mercury vapor, sulfur dioxide, nitrogen oxides, particulate matter, lead, chromium, arsenic, cadmium, zinc, copper, and heavy metals in mine tailings.

Metal contamination with mercury from gold mining and other heavy metals from uranium mines is a serious problem, because these waste products are often disposed of in open dumps. Scavenging in these open dumps, particularly by children, has become a cottage industry and a means of support for many young people. Small-scale industries such as mining and battery recycling are present in many developing countries.[29] Children living in Trinidad and Tobago, whose blood lead concentrations averaged 72.1 µg/dL, resided in a locality contaminated by wastes from battery recycling.[30] Mercury contamination associated with small-scale gold mining and processing presents a major hazard in at least 25 countries in Latin America, Asia, and Africa.[31]

Pesticides

Pesticides, including some that have been banned in more developed countries, are widely used in less-developed countries. Lack of regulatory oversight, protective measures, and education increases the risk of significant exposure. Children experience exposure through a take-home pathway from household members who work with pesticides, drift from nearby spraying, residue on crops and foliage, contaminated water, or their own occupational or residential use of pesticides.

Although the sale of pesticides is higher in developed countries, pesticide-related poisoning is more frequent in less-developed countries.[32] Approximately 30% of pesticides marketed in developing countries do not meet internationally accepted quality standards and frequently contain hazardous substances and impurities that have been banned or severely restricted elsewhere.[33] In Latin America, 12% to 13% of workers have been acutely poisoned with pesticides at least once.[32] Data on worldwide prevalence of poisoning is difficult to obtain, given the limited efforts at surveillance even in developed countries. Few worldwide data specific to children's exposures and poisonings are available. Most regional estimates are derived from hospitalizations and represent the most severe cases. A WHO task group estimated that (for all age groups) there may be 1 million serious unintentional poisonings each year with 2 million additional hospitalizations for suicide attempts with pesticides. It is estimated that 99% of the deaths related to pesticide poisonings occur in developing regions.[32] On the basis of a survey of self-reported minor poisoning in the Asia region, 25 million agricultural workers in the developing world experience pesticide poisoning each year.[34]

Climate Change

The primary public health impacts of climate change include increased heat stress, worsened air quality, changes in vectorborne disease, and extreme weather events (see Chapter 54). Developing countries are the most vulnerable to these effects by virtue of having fewer resources to adapt socially, technologically, and financially. The rapid economic development and the concurrent urbanization of poorer countries mean that cities in developing countries may also become increasing contributors to the problem, although at present, their contribution is lowest in terms of greenhouse gas emissions. In the most comprehensive, peer-reviewed analysis of climate change effects on health available, the WHO estimates that changes that have already occurred since the mid-1970s are causing more than 150 000 deaths and approximately 5 million disability-adjusted life years (DALYs) lost per year. These effects are the result of increases in diarrheal diseases (temperature effects only), malaria, and malnutrition that occur mainly in developing countries.[35] Regions at highest risk of the adverse health effects of climate change include coastlines along the Pacific and Indian oceans and Sub-Saharan Africa. Large sprawling cities, with their urban "heat island" effect, are also prone to temperature-related health problems. The African region is gravely at risk of warming-related effects on infectious disease incidence and consequences.[36]

IMPLICATIONS OF ENVIRONMENTAL HEALTH CONDITIONS IN DEVELOPING COUNTRIES FOR IMMIGRANT CHILDREN, INCLUDING FOREIGN ADOPTEES

An infant or child's previous environmental setting or cultural identity and practices will guide the pediatrician's specific environmental health evaluation beyond the routine screening and preventive health guidelines for adoptees and

Table 14.1: Identified Sources of Toxic Environmental Exposures Among Immigrant Populations

POTENTIAL TOXICANT	POSSIBLE EXPOSURE
Lead	Imported spices Herbal, traditional, or imported medicinals Imported, traditional cosmetics Work in lead battery recycling Lead glaze in dishware or crystal
Mercury	Contaminated fish Proximity to or work in gold mining operations Rituals (eg, Santeria)
Arsenic	Imported spices Herbal, traditional, or imported medicinals Groundwater contamination
Alcohol	Prenatal exposure
Radioactivity	Residential proximity to waste sites, spills
Hazardous waste materials	Residential proximity to waste sites, spills
Tobacco, secondhand tobacco smoke	Prenatal or postnatal exposure Work in tobacco fields

immigrant children.[37] Table 14.1 summarizes the key environmental exposures to consider for immigrant children. An environmental history can reveal potential hazardous exposures, such as residence in proximity to waste dumps, gold-mining operations, home-based cottage industries involving lead exposure, consumption of potentially contaminated fish, or family use of ethnic remedies that may present heavy metal exposure. If a pediatrician identifies a potential hazardous exposure but is not acquainted with appropriate assessment of the exposure or its toxicity, consultation with a pediatric environmental health specialist is advised.

Because elevated blood lead concentrations have been commonly observed among immigrant, refugee, and foreign adoptees from developing countries, screening with a blood lead test is appropriate for these high-risk groups. The Centers for Disease Control and Prevention has issued specific guidance for screening of all immigrant and refugee children (http://www.cdc.gov/nceh/lead/Publications/RefugeeToolKit/Refugee_Tool_Kit.htm).

Alcohol consumption patterns vary widely among countries. Data on fetal alcohol exposure and related morbidity by country are limited, although Eastern

Europe and Russia are often cited as countries with a high prevalence of fetal alcohol syndrome and effects.[37] Established protocols for assessment of fetal alcohol syndrome and effects should be used if there is suspicion based on phenotype or other features noted on physical examination or exposure assessment.

Biological assessment of mercury exposure may be considered for children who have lived in settings with presumed environmental contamination (eg, gold-mining operations) or where consumption of contaminated fish, medicinals, or spices is suspected.

People from a number of ethnic groups may use remedies that could contain toxic substances. Such remedies may include azarcon, a lead-containing orange powder, and greta, a lead-containing yellow powder used by Mexican and Mexican-American people; pay-loo-ah, a lead- and arsenic-containing orange powder used by Hmong people; and ghasard, bala goli, and kandu, lead-containing brown, black, or red powders used by some American Indian people. Some Ayurvedic (pertaining to a traditional system of medicine native to India) medicines contain arsenic and can cause typical skin changes. Use in rituals results in potential exposure to environmental contaminants. For example, some Hispanic people who practice Santeria may sprinkle elemental mercury in the house, possibly resulting in elevated levels of mercury in the indoor air.

With increasing attention and monitoring, the known population affected by arsenic contamination of groundwater is expanding. A careful physical examination can identify any stigmata of arsenic exposure (eg, hyperkeratotic lesions of the palms and/or soles), although skin changes are unlikely until years after chronic exposure and generally occur only in settings of very high exposure. Biomarker assessment of arsenic exposure is limited by its rapid excretion. Urinary arsenic concentrations are useful for exposure assessment only if conducted within days of exposure, so measurement will not be useful in most situations. In most cases of suspected exposure, consultation with a pediatric environmental health specialist may be required to best assess risk and improve communication with families (see Chapter 22).

FUTURE DIRECTIONS AND NEEDS IN GLOBAL CHILDREN'S ENVIRONMENTAL HEALTH

There are sparse data sources on specific contaminants, disease incidence, and biological monitoring in many low- and middle-income countries. Efforts to measure children's environmental health risks, develop policies and programs to mitigate such exposures worldwide, and strengthen efforts to address the problem are needed. This includes further educating pediatricians and others who care for children to recognize, treat, and promote prevention of pediatric environmental health hazards.

Resources

World Health Organization (WHO) Children's Environmental Health
Web site: www.who.int/ceh/en
Links to publications and resources regarding national profiles, fact sheets, workshops, and statistics.

International Network for Children's Health, Environment and Safety
Web site: www.inchesnetwork.net

International Pediatric Association
Web site: www.ipa-world.org

International Society of Doctors for the Environment
Web site: www.isde.org
The site provides links to environmental topics and international programs within each topic area.

Foreign adoption medicine resources
www.aap.org/sections/adoption/default.cfm
Many universities and hospitals have specialty international adoption medicine clinics that can provide specialty expertise for caring for foreign adoptees. The American Academy of Pediatrics Section on Adoption and Foster Care can help locate the closest resource.

References

1. *Cambridge International Dictionary of English.* Cambridge, United Kingdom: Cambridge University Press; 2001
2. World Trade Organization. *Who are the developing countries in the WTO?* Available at: http://www.wto.org/english/tratop_e/devel_e/d1who_e.htm. Accessed September 27, 2010
3. Baris E, Yurekli AA. World Bank Data 2000. Available at: http://www1.worldbank.org/tobacco/presentations/ETSFinlandEditedFinalVersionSept03.ppt#14. Accessed September 27, 2010
4. United Nations Population Fund. *Population Trends: Rapid Growth in Less Developed Regions.* Available at: http://www.unfpa.org/pds/trends.htm. Accessed September 27, 2010
5. World Health Organization. *Health and Environment Linkages Initiative. Priority Environmental and Health Risk.* Available at: http://www.who.int/heli/risks/en/. Accessed September 27, 2010
6. World Health Organization. *Global Water Supply and Sanitation Assessment 2000 Report.* Geneva, Switzerland: World Health Organization; 2000. Available at: http://www.who.int/docstore/water_sanitation_health/Globassessment/GlobalTOC.htm. Accessed September 27, 2010
7. UNICEF. *Progress Since the World Summit for Children: A Statistical Review. New York, NY: UNICEF; 2001.* Available at: http://www.unicef.org/specialsession/about/sgreport-pdf/sgreport_adapted_stats_eng.pdf. Accessed September 27, 2010
8. UNICEF. *We the Children: Meeting the Promises of the World Summit for Children. New York, NY: UNICEF; 2001.* Available at: http://www.unicef.org/specialsession/about/sgreport-pdf/sgreport_adapted_eng.pdf. Accessed September 27, 2010

9. Yanez L, Ortiz D, Calderon J, et al. Overview of human health and chemical mixtures: problems facing developing countries. *Environ Health Perspect.* 2002;110(Suppl 6):901-909

10. UNICEF. *State of the Art Report on Fluoride and Resulting Endemicity for Fluorosis in India.* New York, NY: UNICEF; 1999

11. UNICEF. Water, Sanitation, and Hygiene. New York, NY: UNICEF; 2002. Available at: http://www.unicef.org/wash/index_water_quality.html

12. European Environment Agency. *Children's Health and Environment: A Review of Evidence. A Joint Report from the European Environment Agency and the WHO Regional Office for Europe.* Environmental Issue Report No. 29. Copenhagen, Denmark: European Environment Agency; 2002. Available at: http://www.eea.europa.eu/publications/environmental_issue_report_2002_29. Accessed September 27, 2010

13. World Health Organization. Health and Environmental Linkages Initiative: Vector-Borne Disease. Available at: http://www.who.int/heli/risks/vectors/vector/en/index.html. Accessed September 27, 2010

14. United Nations Environment Programme. *Geo YearBook 2004/5: An Overview of Our Changing Environment.* Nairobi, Kenya: United Nations Environment Programme; 2005. Available at: http://www.unep.org/GEO/pdfs/yearbook04/EmergingChallenges.pdf. Accessed September 27, 2010

15. World Health Organization. *World Health Report 2002. Reducing Risks, Promoting Healthy Life.* Available at: http://www.who.int/whr/2002/en/whr02_en.pdf. Accessed September 27, 2010

16. Chapter 10. Rural Energy in Developing Countries. Goldemberg J, ed. Available at: http://www.undp.org/energy/activities/wea/pdfs/chapter10.pdf. Accessed September 27, 2010

17. Samet J, Tielsch J. Commentary: Could biomass fuel smoke cause anaemia and stunting in early. *Int J Epidemiol.* 2007;36(1):130-131. doi:10.1093/ije/dyl278

18. Smith KR, Mehta S, Maeusezahl-Feuz M. Indoor air pollution from household use of solid fuels. In: Ezzati M, Lopez AD, Rodgers A, Murray CJL, eds. *Comparative Quantification of Health Risks: Global and Regional Burden of Disease Attributable to Selected Major Risk Factors.* Geneva: World Health Organization; 2004:1435–1493

19. Rinne ST, Rodas EJ, Rinne ML, Simpson JM, Glickman LT. Use of biomass fuel is associated with infant mortality and child health in trend analysis. *Trop Med Hyg.* 2007;76(3):585–591. Available at: http://www.ajtmh.org/cgi/reprint/76/3/585.pdf. Accessed September 27, 2010

20. Bruce N, McCracken J, Albalak R, et al. Impact of improved stoves, house construction and child location on levels of indoor air pollution exposure in young Guatemalan children. *J Expo Anal Environ Epidemiol.* 2004;14(Suppl):S26-S33

21. World Health Organization. WHO Report on the Global Tobacco Epidemic, 2008. The MPOWER Package. Geneva, Switzerland: World Health Organization; 2008. Available at: http://www.who.int/tobacco/mpower/mpower_report_full_2008.pdf. Accessed September 27, 2010

22. Centers for Disease Control and Prevention. *The Health Consequences of Involuntary Exposure to Tobacco Smoke: A Report of the Surgeon General.* Atlanta, GA: US Department of Health and Human Services, Centers for Disease Control and Prevention, Coordinating Center for Health Promotion, National Center for Chronic Disease Prevention and Health Promotion, Office on Smoking and Health; 2006

23. Wipfli H, Avila-Tang E, Navas-Acien A, et al; FAMRI Homes Study Investigators. Secondhand smoke exposure among women and children: evidence from 31 countries. *Am J Public Health.* 2008;98(4):672-679

24. Krzyzanowski M, Schwela D. Patterns of air pollution in developing countries. In: Holgate ST, Koren HS, Samet JM, Maynard RL, eds. *Air Pollution and Health.* San Diego, CA: Academic Press; 1999:105-113

25. World Health Organization. *Childhood Lead Poisoning.* Geneva, Switzerland, 2010, page 37, available at: http://www.who.int/ceh/publications/leadguidance.pdf. Accessed September 27, 2010

26. World Health Organization. *Quantifying Environmental Health Impacts. Annex 4. Estimating the Global Disease Burden of Environmental Lead Exposure.* Available at: http://www.who.int/quantifying_ehimpacts/publications/en/9241546107ann4-5.pdf. Accessed September 27, 2010

27. World Health Organization. Chapter 6: Neglected Global Epidemics: three growing threats. Road Traffic Hazards: Hidden Epidemics. In: *The World Health Report 2003. Shaping the Future.* Geneva, Switzerland: World Health Organization; 2003. Available at: http://www.who.int/whr/2003/chapter6/en/index3.html. Accessed September 27, 2010

28. International Lead and Zinc Study Group. Lead and Zinc New Mine and Smelter Projects, 2011. Available at: http://www.ilzsg.org/generic/pages/list.aspx?table=document&ff_aa_document_type=B&from=1. Accessed September 27, 2010

29. Heath RGM. Small scale mines, their cumulative environmental impacts and developing coutnries best practice guidelines for water management. *J Water Environ Technol.* 2005;3(2):175-182. Available at: http://www.jstage.jst.go.jp/article/jwet/3/2/175/_pdf. Accessed September 27, 2010

30. Romieu I, Lacasana M, McConnell R. Lead exposure in Latin America and the Caribbean. *Environ Health Perspect.* 1997;105(4):398-405

31. United Nations Environment Programme. *Global Mercury Assessment. Draft.* Geneva, Switzerland: United Nations Environment Programme; 2002

32. McConnell R, Henao S, Nieto O, Rosenstock L, Trape AZ, Wesseling C. Plaguicidas. In: *Epidemiologia Ambiental: Un Proyecto para America Latina y el Caribe.* Mexico City, Mexico: PAHO; 1994:153-210

33. World Health Organization. FAO/WHO amount of poor quality pesticide in developing countries alarmingly high [press release]. Geneva, Switzerland: World Health Organization; February 1, 2001

34. Jayaratnam J. Acute pesticide poisoning: a major global health problem. *World Health Stat Q.* 1990;43:139-144

35. McMichael AJ, Campbell-Lendrum D, Kovats S, et al. Global climate change. In: Ezzati M, Lopez AD, Rodgers A, Murray CJL, eds. *Comparative Quantification of Health Risks: Global and Regional Burden of Disease Attributable to Selected Major Risk Factors.* Geneva, Switzerland: World Health Organization; 2004:1543–1649

36. Patz, JA, Campbell-Lendrum D, Holloway T, Foley JA. Impact of regional climate change on human health. *Nature.* 2005;438(7066):310-317

37. Jenista JA. The immigrant, refugee, or internationally adopted child. *Pediatr Rev.* 2001;22(12): 419-43

Chapter 15

Human Milk

■ ■ ■ ■ ■ ■

Breastfeeding is good for infants. The World Health Organization,[1,2] the US Surgeon General,[3] and the American Academy of Pediatrics (AAP), both in previous editions of this book and in a policy statement,[4] have considered the problem of environmental contaminants in human milk and continue to recommend breastfeeding. Extensive research has documented the broad and compelling advantages for infants, mothers, families, and society related to breastfeeding. Some of the many benefits include immunologic advantages, lower obesity rates, and greater cognitive development for the infant as well as a variety of health advantages for the lactating mother. Even though a number of environmental pollutants readily pass to the infant through human milk, the advantages of breastfeeding continue to greatly outweigh the potential risks in nearly every circumstance. So far, despite literature that is more than 50 years old, there are very few instances in which morbidity has been described in a nursling from a pollutant chemical in milk. There is good evidence that little, if any, morbidity is occurring from the more common and well-studied chemical agents. This chapter will discuss chemicals that are known to appear in human milk.

In 1951, Laug and colleagues[5] reported the presence of the persistent pesticide dichlorodiphenyltrichloroethane (DDT) in human milk. DDT or one of its derivatives, usually the very stable metabolite dichlorodiphenyldichloroethylene (DDE), has since been found in the lipid of essentially all human milk tested worldwide. Hexachlorobenzene; the cyclodiene pesticides, such as dieldrin, heptachlor, and chlordane (all organochlorines); and industrial chemicals, such as polychlorinated biphenyls (PCBs) and similar compounds, have been, and in some cases continue to be, common contaminants. These residues are present

Table 15.1: Pollutants That May Be Found in Human Milk

CHEMICAL AGENT

DDT (dichlorodiphenyltrichloroethane), DDE (dichlorodiphenyldichloroethylene)	Perchlorate
PCBs (polychlorinated biphenyls), PCDFs (polychlorinated dibenzofurans), polychlorinated dibenzodioxins	PBDEs (polybrominated diphenyl ethers)
	PFOS, (perfluorooctane sulfonate), PFOA (perfluorooctanoic acid)
Chlordane	Phthalates
Heptachlor	Volatile organic compounds
Hexachlorobenzene	Metals
Nicotine and other components of tobacco smoke	Sunscreens (ultraviolet [UV] filters)

in the milk of women without occupational or other special exposure (see Table 15.1).[6] Following regulations aimed at reducing exposure to these compounds, levels of PCBs and persistent pesticides have declined. Levels of the flame retardants polybrominated diphenyl ethers, however, have increased.[7] Infant formula is free of these residues, because the lipid comes from coconuts or other sources low on the food chain. Dairy cows do not have much exposure; in addition, a cow makes tons of milk during her lifetime production, keeping the concentrations of pollutants low in any given volume of cow milk.

Human milk is the major dietary source of these stable pollutants for young children. The quantities transferred can leave breastfed children with detectably higher body burdens of pollutants for years.[8] The relatively high concentration of fat in human milk means that fat-soluble substances will, in effect, concentrate there. Because hind milk is reported to have higher fat concentrations (approximately 4% or more), compared with foremilk (approximately 2.5%), it is likely that contaminants that are fat-soluble would have higher concentrations in hind milk. The persistent fat-soluble agents that are discussed here are the most studied human milk contaminants, but volatile organic hydrocarbons, phthalates, metals, and organometals can contaminate human milk, although almost always at levels that are of much less toxicologic concern than the persistent fat-soluble agents. Asbestos fibers or fine particulate air pollutants are not found in human milk. Much of this material was reviewed in a "mini-monograph" of the journal *Environmental Health Perspectives* in June 2002 (http://www.ehponline.org/docs/2002/110-6/toc.html). There are also Internet sources—the Natural Resources Defense Council, for example, maintains a Web site with updated links at http://www.nrdc.org/breastmilk.

SPECIFIC AGENTS

DDT and DDE

DDT, an organochlorine pesticide once used widely in the United States, was banned from manufacture in 1972 after 4 decades of extensive global use. This decision was based on, among other things, its widespread appearance in human tissue and its effects on wildlife, especially reproduction in pelagic birds (those living in open oceans or seas rather than in waters near land). The metabolites *o,p'*-DDT and DDE are weak estrogens. An estrogen-like effect of DDE (ie, shortened duration of lactation) was seen in 2 studies, one in North Carolina and the other in Mexico.[9] Although a similar-sized effect was seen among Michigan women,[10] studies in upstate New York[11] and another Mexican study[12] saw no association between DDE and weaning. The possibility that DDE might interfere with lactation performance or have other toxicity (an association with preterm birth has been reported)[13] became topical with the resurgence of interest in DDT for malaria control.[14] Control of malaria vectors with affordable, effective methods in developing countries will present public health dilemmas if DDT is deemed the most suitable agent and yet has the potential to increase mortality by producing preterm birth and early weaning.[15] Results from a Catalonian[16] birth cohort showed that prenatal exposure to *p,p'*-DDE was associated with a delay in mental and psychomotor development at 13 months of age; a study in mostly migrant women in California showed similar developmental delays, but in association with DDT, the parent compound.[17] Long-term breastfeeding was found to be beneficial to neurodevelopment in both studies, despite exposure to these chemicals through human milk.

PCBs, Polychlorinated Dibenzofurans, and Polychlorinated Dibenzodioxins

Exposure to commonly encountered levels of PCBs is associated with lower developmental/IQ test scores, including lower psychomotor scores from the newborn period through 2 years of age, defects in short-term memory in 7-month-olds and 4-year-olds, lowered IQs in 42-month-olds and 11-year-olds, and other effects. Prenatal exposure to PCBs from the mother's body burden, rather than exposure through human milk, seems to account for most of the findings.[18]

Polychlorinated dibenzofurans are partially oxidized PCBs that appear in PCB mixtures subjected to high heat or explosions. They were responsible for some of the toxicity seen in workers cleaning up office building transformer fires[19] and also in 2 Asian outbreaks of PCB poisoning from contaminated cooking oil[20] (see Chapter 35). In the Asian poisonings, infants seem to have been affected by exposure through human milk.[21,22] Background exposure to polychlorinated dibenzofurans probably comes mostly from diet, especially contaminated fish.[23]

Polychlorinated dibenzodioxins are similar to PCBs and polychlorinated dibenzofurans in that they have 2 linked phenyl rings with varying numbers of chlorines. The dioxins have 2 oxygen molecules between the phenyl rings. These compounds were formed during the manufacture of hexachlorophene, pentachlorophenol, and the phenoxy acid herbicides 2,4,5 trichlorophenoxyacetic acid (a component of Agent Orange, used as a defoliant during the Vietnam War) and silvex, under what would now be considered poorly controlled conditions. They also are formed, albeit at very low yield, during paper bleaching and waste incineration. One dioxin congener, 2,3,7,8-tetrachlorodibenzo-*p*-dioxin, may be the most toxic synthetic chemical known.[24]

Chlordane

In 1970, inadvertent injection of chlordane, an organochlorine insecticide, into the heating ducts of a military home resulted in air contamination when the heat was turned on. The US Air Force performed studies in almost 500 dwellings and found that although most homes had very little chlordane in the air, occasionally values were as high as 260 µg/m³. The symptoms abated and the air cleared when appropriate repairs were made.[25] Among women who lived in homes treated with chlordane, human milk levels of chlordane increased during the following 5 years.[26] There are no reports of morbidity attributable to this exposure.

Heptachlor

The agricultural use of heptachlor, an organochlorine cyclodiene pesticide, resulted in 2 major mishaps, one in Hawaii and the other in Arkansas. In January 1982, routine analysis of cow milk by the Hawaii State Health Department turned up an unexpected amount of heptachlor epoxide, the stable metabolite. The contamination was traced to the practice of feeding dairy cows "green chop," which is the leafy portion of the pineapple plant. In this case, the pineapple plants had been treated with heptachlor to control aphids and were harvested too soon. Retrospective testing of green chop samples showed that heptachlor was present as far back as June 1981. Human milk in Hawaii had previously been quite low in heptachlor epoxide; during this episode, the levels increased threefold but into the range of values of those reported from the US mainland.[27] In 1986, cow milk in Arkansas was found to be contaminated. This time, the cows had been fed mash left over from the fermentation of grain to produce ethanol for addition to gasoline. Nine hundred forty-two samples collected contemporaneously with the exposure were analyzed, and human milk concentrations of heptachlor epoxide did not seem to be higher in Arkansas than in the adjoining southeastern states.[28] There has, thus far, been no morbidity attributable to these exposures, but research continues in Hawaii.[29]

Hexachlorobenzene

The fungicide hexachlorobenzene in human milk has caused disease in nurslings. After an epidemic of hexachlorobenzene poisoning in Turkey (1957–1959), breastfed children did not get porphyria as seen in adults but rather *pembe yara* (pink sore), characterized by weakness, convulsions, and an annular papular rash. The case-fatality rate was approximately 95%, and cohorts of children died in some of the villages. The chemical was present in human milk but not quantitated at the time; 20 years later, 20 samples that were analyzed had an average of 0.23 ppm of hexachlorobenzene.[30] If it is assumed that analysis was per g of milk fat, then levels were still approximately 15 times background levels 20 years after the original poisoning.

Nicotine and Other Components of Tobacco Smoke

Nicotine, cotinine,[31] thiocyanate (a compound present in tobacco smoke derived from hydrogen cyanide),[32] and other components of cigarette smoke[33] appear in the milk of smokers. Smokers tend to wean their infants early, but whether this is caused by smoking is not known.[34] There is no evidence of a smoking effect on the child from components of smoke in human milk—indeed, there is some evidence that the increase in lower respiratory tract infections seen in the offspring of smoking mothers is prevented by 6 months of breastfeeding. Chapter 40 contains more information about tobacco.

Perchlorate

Perchlorate is a common contaminant of human milk, because it is commonly in water and food. It competes with iodide for uptake into the thyroid, thus interfering with thyroid hormone production.[35] One study found that 9 out of 13 breastfeeding infants were ingesting perchlorate at a level exceeding the reference dose (an estimate of a daily oral exposure that is likely to be without an appreciable risk of adverse health effects over a lifetime) suggested by the National Academy of Sciences, and 12 of 13 infants did not have an adequate intake of iodine as defined by the Institute of Medicine.[32] To get sufficient iodine, lactating women should be encouraged to use iodized salt.

Polybrominated Diphenyl Ethers and Persistent Perfluorinated Chemicals

Polybrominated diphenyl ethers (see Chapter 35) are flame-retardant compounds used in a wide variety of consumer products throughout the world. They have been detected in human milk for the last 2 decades, and concentrations in North America are among the highest. Some of these compounds have neurologic or developmental toxicity in the laboratory, but there is dispute about whether sufficient exposure is occurring to produce detectable toxicity.[36]

Persistent perfluorinated chemicals, such as perfluorooctane sulfonate (PFOS) and perfluorooctanoic acid (PFOA), can be found in human milk.

These manmade organic chemicals have developmental toxicity in laboratory animals. Their effects on human infants have yet to be determined.[37,38]

Phthalates

Phthalates are plasticizers found in flooring, personal care products, medical devices, and some food packaging. Some of the phthalates have been demonstrated to be antiandrogens in laboratory studies; a Danish study of boys with cryptorchidism measured phthalates in human milk and endogenous sex hormones in the boys at 3 months of age. Although they found no difference in phthalate exposure between the boys with cryptorchidism and controls, boys whose mothers had higher levels of certain phthalates in their milk had lower concentrations of serum testosterone and higher concentrations of luteinizing hormone.[39] The clinical significance of this finding is unknown, and it has not yet been replicated. Phthalates are discussed further in Chapter 38, and endocrine disrupters are discussed in Chapter 28.

Volatile Organic Compounds

Because halothane has been detected in the milk of a lactating anesthesiologist,[40] it may be presumed to be present in lactating women who undergo anesthesia using halothane. Volatile agents similar to anesthetic gases may be excreted through expired air, and their concentration in human milk should decline rapidly once exposure ceases. Many other commonly encountered volatile organic compounds, such as benzene, Freon, and methylene chloride, have been found in human milk but are of no known clinical significance.[41]

Metals

Lead concentrations in human milk are low, and there are no modern reports of lead toxicity in a child who was breastfed by an asymptomatic mother. Lead was known historically to be toxic to the nurslings of women who worked with it. Decades ago, there was much more lead in canned formula and evaporated milk than in human milk because of the soldered seams in the cans. The levels in formula are now quite low; formula must be prepared with lead-free water to remain that way (see Chapters 16 and 17). Lead in human milk might be a problem among women with unusually high exposures, such as among foreign-born women, women with occupational exposures, and women with pica. The Centers for Disease Control and Prevention's Advisory Committee on Childhood Lead Poisoning Prevention has published guidance on this topic.[42] Levels of cadmium, arsenic, and metallic mercury are low in human milk. Methyl mercury, although relatively nonpolar, associates with protein and appears in human milk at concentrations lower than those in serum. In Iraq in 1972, methyl mercury-treated seed wheat inadvertently used to make bread produced mercury concentrations in human milk of approximately 200 ppb, which is 50 to 100 times the background exposure. There were thousands of cases of illness (see Chapter 32), including some that may have resulted from exposure to human milk alone.[43] The upper end of background exposure to methyl mercury has been studied among children in the Seychelles Islands[44] and Faroe Islands,[45] who have relatively high dietary exposure from ocean fish or mammals; these studies show inconsistent results, with some effects seen from transplacental exposure in the Faroe Islands but not in the Seychelles. In neither case were effects seen that could be attributed to human milk exposure.

Sunscreens (UV filters)

Researchers in Europe asked nursing mothers about their use of sunscreens and cosmetics that contained the sunscreen ingredients benzophenone 2, benzo-phenone 3, 3-benzylidene camphor, 4-methyl-benzylidene camphor (4-MBC), octyl methoxycinnamate (OMC), homosalate, octocrylene, and octyl-dimethyl para amino benzoic acid (PABA). Responding to questionnaires, 78.8% of the women reported using products that contained sunscreens; 76.5% of human milk samples contained these chemicals. A high correlation was reported between mothers' use of these chemicals and their concentrations in human milk. Except for lipsticks (the ingestion of which is probably important), the authors stated that their results agree with studies in animals and humans showing dermal sunscreen absorption. Given that some of these chemicals have endocrine activity in animals, the authors suggested that exposure could be lessened if mothers abstained from using these products during their children's sensitive life stages.[46]

DIAGNOSTIC METHODS

Many laboratories have equipment to measure some or all of the contaminant residues in human milk. However, any such analysis must be regarded as research, because there are no standard quality assurance methods, no established normal values, and some evidence that, at least for PCBs, the variability of test results between laboratories is too great to allow a single sample to be interpretable. Analysis of human milk for these chemicals is not clinically useful.

REGULATIONS

There are no regulations for chemical contaminants in human milk. Although it is tempting to apply the numbers used for infant formula, the risk-benefit situation is not comparable. There likely is no such thing as uncontaminated human milk. The most difficult situation is encountered with the persistent fat-soluble agents, such as PCBs, because their levels in human milk have been at or near the upper regulatory allowances for formula or infant foods. For the other environmental contaminants, amounts in human milk are relatively low.

The most important action is to eliminate exposure to persistent bioaccumulating toxic chemicals. The manufacture and use of DDT, all the cyclodienes, and most PCBs have been stopped in the United States, but not in many other parts of the world. Because 25% of the US food supply is imported, global action is necessary.

Frequently Asked Questions

Q *Should I get my breast milk tested for chemical pollutants?*

A No. Residue levels of many chemicals can be found in milk; quantitating them is difficult, and there are no programs to promote quality assurance. Even if a very good laboratory generates results, there are no accepted normal or safe values against which to evaluate them.

Q *Could my child's illness be caused by a contaminant in my breast milk?*

A Nursing infants have been poisoned by contaminant chemicals in human milk, although in most cases, the mother herself also was ill. The phenomenon is extraordinarily rare. Investigating such a case would be regarded as research.

Q *If I diet while I am breastfeeding, will that increase the levels of contaminants in my body because the same amount of contaminants will be dissolved in a smaller amount of fat? If I lose weight, will that lead to the contaminants coming out of fat and allow them to increase in my breast milk?*

A No one has measured the levels of these chemicals in human milk during weight loss. The greatest reported average weight loss among women who breastfeed long-term is 4.4 kg[47] at 1 year, compared with a 2.4-kg loss in nonbreastfeeding women. Other studies find little or no weight loss among breastfeeding women.[48] Overweight breastfeeding women who exercise and restrict calories can achieve that weight loss faster and lose it mostly as fat.[49] Theoretically, because the same amount of chemical would be stored in 4.4 kg less tissue, mostly fat, weight loss might increase the concentration of the fat-soluble contaminants by up to 25%.

Breastfeeding does decrease the amount of these contaminants in a mother's body. The concentration per unit of milk would be higher if the mother had lost body fat, but there should be no "mobilization" beyond that. There is little evidence that background exposure to contaminated human milk produces any ill consequences in children. On the other hand, there is reasonable evidence that obesity in the mother does have consequences. Therefore, it is reasonable for a woman to follow a sensible diet and to exercise while she is breastfeeding her baby.

Q *If I smoke, should I breastfeed?*

A Human milk is the best food for infants, regardless of whether a mother smokes. However, for the same reasons it is recommended that pregnant women do not smoke, breastfeeding mothers should not smoke because nicotine, thiocyanate, and other toxicants are transferred through the human milk to the infant. Another reason not to smoke and breastfeed is that infants of women who smoke are weaned at an earlier age. If a mother does continue to smoke, she should never breastfeed while smoking, because a high concentration of smoke will be in close proximity to the infant. It is also advised not to smoke immediately before breastfeeding.[34]

Q   *What advice can be given to women affected by a radiation disaster, such as a reactor meltdown?*

A   Radioiodine and KI are secreted into human milk. For lactating women and their infants, expert consultants have firmly recommended that infants of exposed mothers should not breastfeed because of the risk to exposed infants of additional exposure to radioiodine from human milk. Exposed women should temporarily cease breastfeeding unless there are no alternatives.

References

1. Consultation on assessment of the health risks of dioxins; re-evaluation of the tolerable daily intake (TDI): executive summary. *Food Addit Contam.* 2000;17(4):223-240
2. Pronczuk J, Moy G, Vallenas C. Breast milk: an optimal food. *Environ Health Perspect.* 2004; 112(13): A722-A723
3. US Department of Health and Human Services, Office on Women's Health. *HHS Blueprint for Action on Breastfeeding.* Washington, DC: US Department of Health and Human Services; 2000. Available at: http://www.womenshealth.gov/pub/hhs.cfm. Accessed September 29, 2010
4. American Academy of Pediatrics, Committee on Environmental Health. PCBs in breast milk. *Pediatrics.* 1994;94(1):122-123
5. Laug EP, Kunze FM, Prickett CS. Occurrence of DDT in human fat and milk. *Arch Ind Hyg Occup Med.* 1951;3(3):245-246
6. Solomon GM, Weiss PM. Chemical contaminants in breast milk: time trends and regional variability. *Environ Health Perspect.* 2002;110(6):A339-A347
7. Noren K, Meironyte D. Certain organochlorine and organobromine contaminants in Swedish human milk in perspective of past 20-30 years. *Chemosphere.* 2000;40(9-11):1111-1123
8. Longnecker MP, Rogan WJ. Commentary: persistent organic pollutants in children. *Pediatr Res.* 2001;50(3):322-323
9. Gladen BC, Rogan WJ. DDE and shortened duration of lactation in a Northern Mexican town. *Am J Public Health.* 1995;85(4):504-508
10. Karmaus W, Davis S, Fussman C, Brooks K. Maternal concentration of dichlordiphenyl dichloroethylene (DDE) and initiation and duration of breast feeding. *Paediatr Perinat Epidemiol.* 2005;19(5):388-398
11. McGuiness B, Vena JE, Buck GM, et al. The effects of DDE on the duration of lactation among women in the New York State Angler Cohort. *Epidemiology.* 1999;10(4):359
12. Cupul-Uicab LA, Gladen BC, Hernandez-Avila M, Weber JP, Longnecker MP. DDE, a degradation product of DDT, and duration of lactation in a highly exposed area of Mexico. *Environ Health Perspect.* 2008;116(2):179-183
13. Longnecker MP, Klebanoff M, Zhou H, Brock J. Association between maternal serum concentration of the DDT metabolite DDE and preterm and small-for-gestational-age babies at birth. *Lancet.* 2001;358(9276):110-114

14. Roberts DR, Manguin S, Mouchet J. DDT house spraying and re-emerging malaria. *Lancet.* 2001;356(9226):330-332

15. Longnecker MP. Invited commentary: why DDT matters now. *Am J Epidemiol.* 2005;162(8): 726-728

16. Ribas-Fito N, Julvez J, Torrent M, Grimalt JO, Sunyer J. Beneficial effects of breastfeeding on cognition regardless of DDT concentrations at birth. *Am J Epidemiol.* 2007;166(10):1198-1202

17. Eskenazi B, Marks AR, Bradman A, et al. In utero exposure to dichlorodiphenyltrichloroethane (DDT) and dichlorodiphenyldichloroethylene (DDE) and neurodevelopment among young Mexican American children. *Pediatrics.* 2006;118(1):233-241

18. Schantz SL, Widholm JJ, Rice DC. Effects of PCB exposure on neuropsychological function in children. *Environ Health Perspect.* 2003;111(3):357-376

19. Schecter A, Tiernan T. Occupational exposure to polychlorinated dioxins, polychlorinated furans, polychlorinated biphenyls, and biphenylenes after an electrical panel and transformer accident in an office building in Binghamton, NY. *Environ Health Perspect.* 1985;60:305-313

20. Rogan WJ, Gladen BC, Hung KL, Koong SL, Shih LY, Taylor JS, et al. Congenital poisoning by polychlorinated biphenyls and their contaminants in Taiwan. *Science.* 1988;241(4863): 334-336

21. Harada M. Intrauterine poisoning: Clinical and epidemiological studies and significance of the problem. *Bull Inst Constit Med.* 1976;25(Suppl):1-66

22. Yu ML, Hsu CC, Gladen BC, Rogan WJ. In utero PCB/PCDF exposure: relation of developmental delay to dysmorphology and dose. *Neurotoxicol Teratol.* 1991;13(2):195-202

23. Wang RY, Needham LL. Environmental chemicals: from the environment to food, to breast milk, to the infant. *J Toxicol Environ Health Part B Crit Rev.* 2007;10(8):597-609

24. Baarschers W. *Eco-Facts and Eco-Fiction: Understanding the Environmental Debate.* New York, NY: Routledge; 1996:221

25. Lillie TH. *Chlordane in Air Force Family Housing: A Study of Houses Treated After Construction.* Brooks Air Force Base, TX: USAF Occupational and Environmental Health Laboratory, Brooks Air Force Base; 1981. Report No: OEHL 81-45

26. Taguchi S, Yakushiji T. Influence of termite treatment in the home on the chlordane concentration in human milk. *Arch Environ Contam Toxicol.* 1988;17(1):65-71

27. Pesticide HAP. *Hepatochlor Epoxide in Mother's Milk, Oahu, August 1981-November 1982.* Manoa, HI: University of Hawaii at Manoa; 1983

28. Mattison DR, Wohleb J, To T, et al. Pesticide concentrations in Arkansas breast milk. *J Ark Med Soc.* 1992;88(11):553-557

29. Maskarinec G. The difficulties in detecting effects of population-based exposures: the heptachlor contamination episode in Hawaii as an example. *Epidemiology.* 2006;17(6):S313

30. Cripps DI, Peters HA, Gocmen A, et al. Porphyria turcica due to hexachlorobenzene— a 20 to 30 year follow-up-study on 204 patients. *Br J Dermatol.* 1984;111(4):413-422

31. Dahlstrom A, Ebersjo C, Lundell B. Nicotine exposure in breastfed infants. *Acta Paediatrica.* 2004;93(6):810-816

32. Dasgupta PK, Kirk AB, Dyke JV, Ohira S. Intake of iodine and perchlorate and excretion in human milk. *Environ Sci Technol.* 2008;42(21):8115-8121

33. Zanieri L, Galvan P, Checchini L, et al. Polycyclic aromatic hydrocarbons (PAHs) in human milk from Italian women: influence of cigarette smoking and residential area. *Chemosphere.* 2007;67(7):1265-1274

34. Counsilman JJ, MacKay E. Cigarette smoking by pregnant women with particular reference to their past and subsequent breast feeding behavior. *Aust N Z J Obstet Gynaecol.* 1985;25(2) 101-107

35. Ginsberg GL, Hattis DB, Zoeller RT, Rice DC. Evaluation of the U.S. EPA/OSWER preliminary remediation goal for perchlorate in groundwater: focus on exposure to nursing infants. *Environ Health Perspect.* 2007;115(3):361-9

36. Costa LG, Giordano G. Developmental neurotoxicity of polybrominated diphenyl ether (PBDE) flame retardants. *Neurotoxicology.* 2007;28(6):1047-67

37. von Ehrenstein OS, Fenton SE, Kato K, Kuklenyik Z, Calafat AM, Hines EP. Polyfluoroalkyl chemicals in the serum and milk of breastfeeding women. *Reprod Toxicol.* 2009;27(3-4): 239-245

38. Kärrman A, Ericson I, van Bavel B, et al. Exposure of perfluorinated chemicals through lactation: levels of matched human milk and serum and a temporal trend, 1996-2004, in Sweden. *Environ Health Perspect.* 2007;115(2):226-230

39. Main KM, Mortensen GK, Kaleva MM, et al. Human breast milk contamination with phthalates and alterations of endogenous reproductive hormones in infants three months of age. *Environ Health Perspect.* 2006;114(2):270-276

40. Cote CJ, Kenepp NB, Reed SB, Strobel GE. Trace concentrations of halothane in human breast milk. *Br J Anaesth.* 1976;48(6):541-543

41. Pellizari ED, Hartwell TD, Harris BS, Waddell RD, Whitaker DA, Erickson MD. Purgeable organic compounds in mothers' milk. *Bull Environ Contam Toxicol.* 1982;28(3):322-328

42. Centers for Disease Control and Prevention. *Guidelines on the Identification and Management of Lead Exposure in Pregnant and Lactating Women.* Atlanta, Georgia: 2010. Available at: http://www.cdc.gov/nceh/lead/publications/LeadandPregnancy2010.pdf

43. Bakir F, Damluji SF, Amin-Zaki L, et al. Methylmercury poisoning in Iraq. *Science.* 1973; 181(96):230-241

44. Clarkson TW, Magos L, Myers GJ. The toxicology of mercury—current exposures and clinical manifestations. *N Engl J Med.* 2003;349(18):1731-1737

45. Grandjean P, Weihe P, White RF, et al. Cognitive deficit in 7-year-old children with prenatal exposure to methylmercury. *Neurotoxicol Teratol.* 1997;19(6):417-428

46. Schlumpf M, Kypkec K, Vöktd CC, et al. Endocrine active UV filters: developmental toxicity and exposure through breast milk. *Chimia (Aarau).* 2008;62:345–351).

47. Dewey KG, Heinig MJ, Nommsen LA. Maternal weight-loss patterns during prolonged lactation. *Am J Clin Nutr.* 1993;58(2):162-166

48. Schauberger CW, Rooney BL, Brimer LM. Factors that influence weight loss in the puerperium. *Obstet Gynecol.* 1992;79(3):424-429

49. Lovelady CA, Garner KE, Moreno KL, Williams JP. The effect of weight loss in overweight, lactating women on the growth of their infants. *N Engl J Med.* 2000;342(7):449-453

Chapter 16

Phytoestrogens and Contaminants in Infant Formula

■ ■ ■ ■ ■ ■

INTRODUCTION

Although breastfeeding is recommended by the American Academy of Pediatrics (AAP), formula is widely used for infant feeding. In the United States in 2003, approximately 30% of newborn infants and 60% of 6–month-olds were fed formula. Although other formulas are available for special purposes, nearly all formula sold in the United States is based on protein from cow milk or soybeans; soy formula achieves approximately 25% of the market in the United States.[1] Soy formula contains no lactose and, thus, is indicated for infants with galactosemia, primary lactase deficiency (an extremely rare condition), and some infants with secondary lactase deficiency.[1] Its proteins are dissimilar enough from cow milk protein that it can be given to many children with cow milk protein allergy.

Soy formula contains isoflavones, a class of phytoestrogens. Phytoestrogens are plant-based compounds found in many foods, including tofu and soy milk,[2] that are able to produce some or all of the effects of estrogen. It is the presence of these compounds that has led to the promotion of soy products for the alleviation of menopausal and other symptoms in adults. Genistein and daidzein, the isoflavones at highest concentration in soy formula, have structures similar to 17-β estradiol and can bind to estrogen receptors and have weak estrogenic effects.[3] A soy formula-fed infant's daily exposure to total isoflavones may be 6 to 11 times higher on a body weight basis than the dose that may affect menstrual cycle function in women ingesting soy proteins.[3] The United

Kingdom, Australia, New Zealand, and Israel have issued position statements suggesting restricted use of soy infant formula.[4] The concern is based largely on studies in laboratory animals and *in vitro* experiments. The policy statement from the AAP Committee on Nutrition regarding soy formula provides relatively limited indications for US infants.[1] Soy infant formula also contains phytates that bind iron and zinc, but current soy protein-based formula is fortified with iron and zinc. Soybean protease inhibitor has been mostly removed by heating soybean protein isolate. Even though animal studies demonstrated adverse reproductive and developmental toxicity of soy exposure,[5] soy formula use for infant feeding in the past 50 years has been relatively uneventful. Few studies in humans have identified clinical or subclinical effects from soy formula use.[2,3] Currently, there are insufficient human data to determine whether there are any adverse effects of soy infant formula on reproduction, development, thyroid hormones, or immune function.[1,2]

This chapter focuses mainly on isoflavones in soy infant formula and briefly mentions other contaminants in or from the use of soy formula or cow milk-based formula (ie, aluminum and manganese, bacteria, melamine, and plasticizers in baby bottles). Some of these contaminants are described in Chapters 18 and 38.

ROUTES OF EXPOSURE

The route of exposure to isoflavones in soy formula is ingestion. Infants ingesting human milk or cow milk-based formula consume less than 1/200th as much isoflavones daily as do infants ingesting soy formula. Infants and adults who consume soy products can absorb isoflavones.

SYSTEMS AFFECTED AND CLINICAL EFFECTS

Epidemiologic Studies on Effects of Soy Infant Formula

Studies have documented normal growth in full-term babies fed soy infant formula.[1] Soy formula is not recommended for preterm babies, because studies of mostly very low birth weight (<1500 g) infants who ingested soy formula showed decreased growth rates, albumin concentrations, and bone mineralization in the first several months of life.[1,5] Evidence from human studies on adverse effects of soy formula is scarce and insufficient to draw firm conclusions. Studies have examined precocious thelarche (early breast development), persistence of breast buds, menstruation, thyroid function, and allergy and immune function, but these results are inconclusive because of limitations in study design and sample size. These studies are summarized in Table 16.1. The short- and long-term effects of soy formula use remain to be determined by well-designed, large-scale epidemiologic studies.

Table 16.1: Human Studies of Soy Infant Formula Use

OUTCOME	AUTHOR, YEAR OF PUBLICATION	METHODS AND SUBJECTS	FINDINGS
Premature thelarche	Freni-Titulaer et al, 1986[6]	Case-control study of 120 girls with premature thelarche and 120 matched controls	Soy formula use increased risk
Reproductive development	Giampietro et al, 2004[8]	48 soy formula-fed children and 18 controls	No signs of precocious puberty in girls or of gynecomastia in boys
Breast bud persistence	Zung et al, 2008[9]	Cross-sectional study of 92 soy formula-fed and 602 human milk- or cow milk formula-fed female infants	Soy group had higher prevalence of breast buds (≥1.5cm) than milk group in the second year of life but not in the first year
Adult reproduction	Strom et al, 2001[11]	Controlled but not randomized feeding study in infancy, follow-up at early adulthood, 120 males and 128 females fed soy formula, 295 males and 268 females fed cow milk formula	Soy formula use increased duration of menstrual bleeding and discomfort with menstrual periods but did not affect puberty or menstrual cycle length or regularity
Autoimmune thyroid disease	Fort et al, 1990[13]	Case-control study of 59 children with auto-immune thyroid disease, 76 healthy siblings, and 54 healthy unrelated control children	Patients with autoimmune thyroid disease had higher percentages of soy formula feeding (31%) than did healthy siblings (12%) or healthy controls (13%)
Immune function	Ostrom et al, 2002[15] Cordle et al, 2002[16]	Randomized feeding study of 94 infants fed soy formula with added nucleotides and 92 infants fed soy formula without added nucleotides, plus nonrandomized groups of 81 infants fed human milk or cow milk formula	Total IgG concentrations similar. Soy-fed infants had higher H influenzae type b antibody and lower polio neutralizing antibody concentrations. Soy-fed infants had more physician-reported diarrhea. Immune cell (B, T, natural killer cells) status similar; soy-fed infants had lower CD57⁺ natural killer T-cells

Reproductive Effects

A report in Puerto Rico found that soy formula use was associated with precocious thelarche in girls before 2 years of age.[6] Other factors, however, including maternal history of ovarian cysts and consumption of fresh chicken, have also been suggested.[6] This study has not been replicated elsewhere; thus, the association between soy formula use and precocious thelarche remains speculative. Phthalate exposure was also considered by other investigators.[7] Another study attempted to compare children who were fed soy formula with those who were fed other formula for signs of precocious puberty, but the sample was very small.[8] An Israeli study found that girls fed soy formula had higher prevalence of palpable breast buds in the second year of life, suggesting prolonged presence of infantile breast tissue.[9] In a very small pilot study, 6-month-old girls fed soy formula had a tendency toward a more "estrogenized" profile of their vaginal epithelial cells (shed cells collected with a cotton-tipped swab of the introitus); the authors emphasized the potential utility of this method for assessing estrogen exposure rather than any effect of formula.[10]

The only epidemiologic study among adults who were fed soy formula during infancy indicated longer duration of menstrual bleeding and more discomfort with menstrual periods in women but did not find associations with age at menarche or with menstrual cycle length or regularity.[11] This study was not large enough to demonstrate the safety of soy formula use on reproduction, and there has been no similar study with a larger sample size on adult fertility and pregnancy outcome.

Thyroid Function

Before 1959, goiter after soy formula consumption was reported,[12] but its incidence was eliminated after adding iodine to soy infant formula. There were case reports of insensitivity to thyroxine treatment in infants with congenital hypothyroidism at the time of soy formula use, and switching to cow milk-based formula improved the treatment effect. It may be that phytates in soy protein isolate interfere with iodine metabolism and thyroid hormone.[5] A case-control study of autoimmune thyroid diseases (Hashimoto thyroiditis or Graves' disease) indicated a higher percentage of soy formula use in cases than in healthy siblings or unrelated control children.[13] It is not clear whether this can be explained by a greater likelihood of soy formula consumption in atopic infants who have such antibodies. Currently, there is a lack of studies of soy infant formula use and thyroid-stimulating hormone (TSH) and thyroid hormone.

Immune Function

There is good evidence that soy infant formula does not prevent allergic diseases.[14] Although some older soy formulations may have interfered with immune response,[2] more recent studies have found that soy formula-fed babies have normal immune response to vaccinations.[15,16] In these newer studies, soy formula-fed infants had total immunoglobulin (Ig)G, IgA, anti-diphtheria IgG, and anti-tetanus IgG concentrations similar to infants fed human milk or cow milk formula. However, soy formula-fed babies had higher levels of antibody to *Haemophilus influenza* type b at 7 and 12 months compared with the group fed cow milk formula or human milk, and their polio viral neutralization antibody at 12 months was lower (but still within normal range).[15] Soy formula-fed babies had immune cell counts similar to those fed cow milk formula or human milk, except that the percentage of CD57+ natural killer T-cells was lower at 12 months of age in infants fed soy formula.[16]

Other Effects

One study compared cholesterol fractional synthesis rate (FSR), an indicator of endogenous cholesterol synthesis, in infants fed human milk, cow milk-based formula, and soy formula at 4 months of age.[17] Soy formula-fed babies had the highest fractional synthesis rate, probably because of the absence of cholesterol contents in soy formula. Human milk-fed infants had the lowest fractional synthesis rate, and supplementing soy formula with cholesterol only slightly lowered fractional synthesis rate, compared with no supplementation. Other studies examined the effect of soy infant formula on type 1 diabetes and cognitive function in children, but these studies were relatively small or designed for other purposes.[18,19]

Experimental Studies on Effects of Soy Infant Formula

There have been few studies of the effects of soy infant formula on reproduction and development in experimental animals; thus, direct observation of soy formula's adverse effect has been limited. More often, ingestion or injection of genistein is used in these animal studies. Although the effects of genistein ingestion or injection may not be directly extrapolated to human infants fed soy formula, the endpoints in animal studies were relevant in pinpointing possible effects of soy formula in humans, given the scarcity of human studies. In experimental animal models or in vitro studies, adverse effects included lower neonatal testosterone concentration, multi-oocyte follicles, uterine adenocarcinoma, mammary gland adenoma or adenocarcinoma, and decreased thyroid peroxidase concentration.

Reproductive Effects

A feeding study that strived to mimic human infant soy formula use in twin male marmoset monkeys found that soy formula feeding suppressed the increase in neonatal testosterone concentration.[20] The early postneonatal period activation of the hypothalamic-pituitary-testicular axis is characteristic of male primates, including humans. It may be related to pubertal maturation, sexual and social behavior, and fertility. Subsequent follow-up into adolescence and adulthood, however, did not find continuous differences in serum testosterone concentrations between marmosets fed soy formula and cow milk formula.[21] Puberty onset, progression, and adulthood fertility was not affected in the soy formula-fed marmosets. Soy formula-fed marmosets, however, had higher testis weight and more Sertoli and Leydig cells, which may indicate some degree of "compensated Leydig cell failure."[21] The effects of soy formula use on male reproductive hormone levels, fertility, and testicular function remain to be determined by additional studies.

In contrast to male reproduction, the effects of genistein exposure on female reproductive function have received more attention. Studies in rodents given subcutaneous injections of genistein revealed increased numbers of multi-oocyte follicles in the ovary.[22] The response was in a dose-dependent pattern from 0.5 to 50 mg/kg genistein. Other endogenous and synthetic estrogens (ie, 17-β estradiol, diethylstilbestrol [DES], bisphenol A [BPA]) can also cause multi-oocyte follicles. Although the reproductive consequences related to multi-oocyte follicles were not clearly defined, this may signal permanently altered ovarian differentiation and decreased fertility later in life. Genistein may also affect hypothalamic-pituitary-gonadal function, disrupt estrous cyclicity, and reduce fertility. Neonatal exposure to genistein induced uterine adenocarcinoma. An equal estrogenic dose of DES at 0.001 mg/kg and of genistein at 50 mg/kg caused similar incidence of uterine adenocarcinoma (~30%) in these experimental animal models.[23] New studies from the National Toxicology Program (NTP) also suggested higher risk of mammary gland adenoma or adenocarcinoma and pituitary gland adenoma or carcinoma in female rats fed genistein for up to 2 years.[24] Other reproductive effects of genistein exposure included accelerated vaginal opening, decreased anogenital distance, and alterations in uterine and ovarian histopathology.[25]

Thyroid Function

An experimental study found that genistein inhibited thyroid peroxidase in rats but had no effect on serum triiodothyronine, thyroxine, and TSH concentrations.[26] There is no similar study in humans.

Immune Function

Results of animal studies on genistein's immunotoxicity are not consistent.[25] Early studies in rodents found decreased thymic weight and reduced number of thymocytes. The feeding study in twin marmosets did not find a difference in thymic weight between soy formula-fed and cow milk-fed monkeys.[21] Genistein was found to inhibit both humoral and cell-mediated immune responses in some studies, but other studies did not find such effects.[27] The effect of isoflavones on immune function may vary by age, sex, species, and dosing regimens.

Controversies Regarding Effects of Isoflavones in Soy Infant Formula

There has been debate about whether soy infant formula poses potential health risks to infants. Soy infant formula has been used for about 50 years, and relatively few studies are available to describe the potential health risks in human infants or children. Many effects of environmental exposure, however, can only be revealed by well-designed epidemiologic studies, such as in the cases of secondhand smoke and lead exposure. High levels of isoflavone intake and strong evidence in animals of genistein's toxicity leads to legitimate concern, but clear advice on soy formula use in infants will need relevant studies in humans. Studies in laboratory animals found that high doses of genistein can disrupt reproduction and development. There are documented differences, however, in physiology between humans and laboratory animals, exposures (soy formula vs genistein), route of exposure (ingestion vs injection), and dosage (ad lib feeding vs repeated high dose). Integration of human studies with the results of laboratory experiments is not yet possible. A better estimate of the estrogenicity of isoflavones is still needed, because this is relevant to the strength of an estrogenic effect in humans. Genistein has higher affinity for estrogen receptor β than for estrogen receptor α. The 2 estrogen receptors are not equally distributed in tissues; thus, the estrogenic effects vary by tissue. In vitro and in vivo studies showed variable estrogenicity potency estimates, ranging from 10^{-5} to 10^{-1} relative to estradiol. How this uncertainty of estrogenicity translates into human effects is unknown. The lack of large-scale epidemiologic and clinical observations in children who were fed soy formula as infants complicates the situation. Recognizing the controversy, several advisory committees in Australia, New Zealand, and Europe have suggested limiting soy formula use in infants if other alternatives are available.[4] In 2006, the National Toxicology Program Center for Evaluation of Risk to Human Reproduction evaluated reproductive and developmental toxicity of genistein and soy formula. The expert panel found that purified genistein can produce reproductive and developmental toxicity in rodents[25] but that the effects of soy infant formula in both humans and experimental animals could not be determined because of insufficient data.[2] In 2008, the AAP Committee on Nutrition reviewed the existing studies on isoflavones in soy formula and child health but found no conclusive evidence that dietary soy isoflavones may adversely affect human development, reproduction, or endocrine function.[1] In 2009, the National Toxicology Program Center for Evaluation of Risk to Human Reproduction convened an expert panel to reevaluate reproductive and developmental toxicity of soy formula. The expert panel had minimal concern for adverse developmental effects in infants fed soy infant formula.[28]

DIAGNOSTIC METHODS

Soy formula use can be identified through infant feeding history. Isoflavone concentrations in plasma samples have been quantified.[29] Urine samples in diaper and saliva can be used to analyze isoflavone excretion in infants.[30,31] These assays, however, are only available in research settings.

TREATMENT OF CLINICAL SYMPTOMS

Currently, data are insufficient to define clinical symptoms from isoflavones in soy infant formula. However, if isoflavones cause any symptoms, switching to cow milk-based formula may alleviate the symptoms.

PREVENTION OF EXPOSURE

Consumption of soy infant formula is voluntary (ie, at the discretion of the parents of infants). To prevent isoflavone intake, parents can simply decide to use human milk or cow milk-based formula. Human milk may contain other environmental chemicals, such as dichlorodiphenyltrichloroethane (DDT) and its metabolite dichlorodiphenyldichloroethylene (DDE), polychlorinated biphenyls (PCBs), lead, and methylmercury. However, current evidence suggests these contaminants in human milk pose little risk to infants as compared with documented benefits of breastfeeding.[32] Infants who have cow milk protein-induced enteropathy or enterocolitis can be provided formula with hydrolyzed protein or synthetic amino acid.[1]

Infant formula is regulated as food by the Food and Drug Administration (FDA). The FDA has requirements for nutrients in infant formulas; however, it does not regulate isoflavone levels in soy infant formula. Isoflavone levels in soybeans can vary by geographic location, climate, and other environmental conditions. Depending on isoflavone levels in soy infant formula and daily formula consumption, infants consuming soy formula have an estimated intake of total isoflavones (in unconjugated isoflavone equivalents) of 2 to 12 mg/kg of body weight per day.[2] Efforts can probably to be made to reduce isoflavone concentrations in soy protein isolates in the future (ie, using ion exchange technology) if isoflavones in soy formula are a continuing source of concern.

OTHER CONTAMINANTS RELATED TO INFANT FORMULA USE

Aluminum and Manganese

The AAP Committee on Nutrition noted relatively high amounts of aluminum in soy infant formulas in 1996. Soy formula had aluminum concentrations of 600 to 1300 ng/mL, much higher than human milk (4-65 ng/mL).[5] Mineral salts used in formula production were considered to be the source of contamination. The effects from aluminum exposure in soy infant formula do not seem to be substantial in term infants. Infants fed soy infant formula also consume greater amounts of manganese than do breastfed infants, but the effects of manganese on neurodevelopment have not been clearly defined.[33]

Bacteria

Infant formula consumption has been associated with reported cases of *Enterobacter sakazakii* infection, which can kill 40% to 80% of infected infants.[34] *E sakazakii* was found in 2.4% of powdered infant formula samples in 2003, but a recent review found invasive *E sakazakii* disease was rare (only 46 cases reported from 1958-2005).[34] Other bacteria have also been found in powdered infant formula. Formula also may be contaminated during preparation if it is mixed with contaminated water or dirty bottles or utensils are used.

Bisphenol A

Infants who are formula fed use baby bottles that often contain bisphenol A (BPA), a weak estrogenic compound. Bisphenol A can migrate from the bottle to the liquid it contains, especially when the liquid is hot. Increased migration of bisphenol A from the bottle occurs after repeated dishwashing, boiling, and brushing.[35] A report from the National Toxicology Program has estimated that formula-fed infants have a range of exposure to BPA of 1 to 11 µg/kg per day.[36] Low-dose exposure to bisphenol A is linked to reproductive and neurodevelopmental alterations in rodents. The National Toxicology Program considers current exposure levels to cause some concern for possible adverse effects on the brain, behavior, and prostate gland in infants and children.[36] See Chapter 38 for more detailed information.

Melamine

In September 2008, an outbreak of kidney stones and renal failure in infants consuming melamine-contaminated powered milk formula occurred in China, resulting in at least 3 deaths and 13 000 hospitalizations.[37] Melamine, an industrial material that is not permitted for use as food additive, and its derivative cyanuric acid, were associated with renal failure in US pets in 2007.[38] Melamine was deliberately added to raw milk in China to increase protein readings, but its renal toxicity in human infants led to the large-scale international market withdrawal of contaminated formulas and other dairy products. No such infant formulas, however, were imported to the US market. In experimental studies, melamine and cyanuric acid produced significant renal damage and crystals in nephrons.[38] Reports of adverse effects among human infants consuming melamine-contaminated formulas have been published.[39-42]

Frequently Asked Questions

Q *Can my daughter switch to soy formula because she has lactose intolerance? Will isoflavones in soy formula cause harmful effects in her?*

A When thinking about what formula to give to an infant, it is important to remember that it is very unusual for an infant to be born with lactose intolerance. Lactose intolerance, if it develops, usually comes on later in childhood. Nevertheless, many infants are given soy infant formula because soy protein-based formula is lactose free. Lactose-free and reduced-lactose cow milk-based formulas are also available. Soy formula contains much higher levels of isoflavones than does human milk or cow milk-based formula. Experimental studies in animals have found that high level genistein (one compound in the isoflavone category) can cause adverse effects in reproduction and development. However, studies using soy infant formula in experimental animals were not conclusive. Currently, there are some data in human infants on the effects of isoflavone exposure in soy formula. More research is needed in this area.[43]

Q *Are the phytoestrogens in soy formula related to precocious puberty?*

A Soy infant formula contains phytoestrogens that are weak estrogenic compounds. However, isoflavones in soy formula have estrogenic effects that are probably orders of magnitude lower than estradiol, the natural human estrogen. There is one report of soy infant formula use and precocious breast development in girls younger than 2 years, but that study was small and inconclusive.[6] Precocious puberty in girls younger than 8 years or boys younger than 9 years may be caused by exogenous hormone exposure, but the role of soy infant formula has not been clearly demonstrated.

Q *Is it possible to reduce isoflavone levels in soy infant formula?*

A Isoflavone levels vary in soybeans depending on geographic location and meteorologic conditions. This variation can probably be exploited to produce soy protein isolates with lower concentrations of isoflavones. In the future, manufacturers may be able to consider processes that modify isoflavone levels from soy protein isolates. Isoflavone levels are not currently labeled on soy infant formula packages.

Q *Is BPA in the baby bottle harmful to my formula-fed baby?*

A Experimental studies in animals have found adverse effects of bisphenol A (BPA) on reproduction and development from relatively low level exposures that may be experienced by infants. Research is needed to clarify whether similar adverse effects occur in formula-fed infants. Many baby bottles contain BPA, which may be a concern for parents.

Q *Can melamine contamination happen again, and does internationally produced formula come into the United States?*

A In the Chinese incident of adulterated infant formula, melamine was added to falsely increase apparent protein content, because melamine contains nitrogen. This practice has been banned in China. Melamine is not approved in the United States for addition to foods. When the FDA tested milk (Yili Pure Milk and Yili Sour Milk produced by Nationwide HUA XIA Food Trade, USA, Flushing, NY), they found melamine contamination.[44] Currently, there are no Chinese-made infant formulas for sale in the United States.

Q *What is the recommended way to prepare infant formula?*

A Water used for mixing infant formula must be from a safe water source as defined by the state or local health department. If you are concerned or uncertain about the safety of tap water, you may use bottled water or bring cold tap water to a rolling boil for 1 minute (no longer), then cool the water to room temperature for no more than 30 minutes before it is used. Warmed water should be tested in advance to make sure it is not too hot for the infant. The easiest way to test the temperature is to shake a few drops on the inside of your wrist. Otherwise, a bottle can be prepared by adding powdered formula and room temperature water from the tap just before feeding. Bottles made in this way from powdered formula can be ready for feeding as no additional refrigeration or warming would be required. Prepared formula must be discarded within 1 hour after serving to an infant. Prepared formula that has not been given to an infant may be stored in the refrigerator for 24 hours to prevent bacterial contamination. An open container of ready-to-feed, concentrated formula, or formula prepared from concentrated formula should be covered, refrigerated, and discarded after 48 hours if not used.

Resources

National Institute of Environmental Health Sciences

Web site: www.niehs.nih.gov

Available publications include Final CERHR Expert Panel Report on Soy Infant Formula (http://cerhr.niehs.nih.gov/evals/genistein-soy/SoyFormulaUpdt/FinalEPReport_508.pdf) and NTP-CERHR Expert Panel Report on the Reproductive and Developmental Toxicity of Genistein (http://www.ncbi.nlm.nih.gov/pmc/articles/PMC2020434)

US Food and Drug Administration

Web site: www.fda.gov

Frequently Asked Questions about FDA's Regulation of Infant Formula:
http://www.fda.gov/Food/GuidanceComplianceRegulatoryInformation/
GuidanceDocuments/InfantFormula/ucm056524.htm

References

1. Bhatia J; Greer F; American Academy of Pediatrics, Committee on Nutrition. Use of soy protein-based formulas in infant feeding. *Pediatrics*. 2008;121(5):1062-1068
2. Rozman KK, Bhatia J, Calafat AM, et al. NTP-CERHR expert panel report on the reproductive and developmental toxicity of soy formula. *Birth Defects Res B Dev Reprod Toxicol*. 2006;77(4):280-397
3. Chen A, Rogan WJ. Isoflavones in soy infant formula: a review of evidence for endocrine and other activity in infants. *Annu Rev Nutr*. 2004;24:33-54
4. Agostoni C, Axelsson I, Goulet O, et al. Soy protein infant formulae and follow-on formulae: a commentary by the ESPGHAN Committee on Nutrition. *J Pediatr Gastroenterol Nutr*. 2006;42(4):352-361
5. Simmen, R. C., et al. Inhibition of NMU-induced mammary tumorigenesis by dietary soy. *Cancer Lett* 2005;224, 45-52.
6. Freni-Titulaer LW, Cordero JF, Haddock L, Lebron G, Martinez R, Mills JL. Premature thelarche in Puerto Rico. A search for environmental factors. *Am J Dis Child*. 1986;140(12):1263-1267
7. Colon I, Caro D, Bourdony CJ, Rosario O. Identification of phthalate esters in the serum of young Puerto Rican girls with premature breast development. *Environ Health Perspect*. 2000;108(9):895-900
8. Giampietro PG, Bruno G, Furcolo G, et al. Soy protein formulas in children: no hormonal effects in long-term feeding. *J Pediatr Endocrinol Metab*. 2004;17(2):191-196
9. Zung A, Glaser T, Kerem Z, Zadik Z. Breast development in the first 2 years of life: an association with soy-based infant formulas. *J Pediatr Gastroenterol Nutr*. 2008;46(2):191-195
10. Bernbaum JC, Umbach DM, Ragan NB, et al. Pilot studies of estrogen-related physical findings in infants. *Environ Health Perspect*. 2008;116(3):416-420
11. Strom BL, Schinnar R, Ziegler EE, et al. Exposure to soy-based formula in infancy and endocrinological and reproductive outcomes in young adulthood. *JAMA*. 2001;286(7):807-814
12. Shepard TH, Pyne GE, Kirschvink JF, Mclean M. Soy bean goiter: report of three cases. *N Engl J Med*. 1960;262:1099-1103
13. Fort P, Moses N, Fasano M, Goldberg T, Lifshitz F. Breast and soy-formula feedings in early infancy and the prevalence of autoimmune thyroid disease in children. *J Am Coll Nutr*. 1990;9(2):164-167
14. Osborn DA, Sinn J. Soy formula for prevention of allergy and food intolerance in infants. *Cochrane Database Syst Rev*. 2006;(4):CD003741
15. Ostrom KM, Cordle CT, Schaller JP, et al. Immune status of infants fed soy-based formulas with or without added nucleotides for 1 year: part 1: vaccine responses, and morbidity. *J Pediatr Gastroenterol Nutr*. 2002;34(2):137-144
16. Cordle CT, Winship TR, Schaller JP, et al. Immune status of infants fed soy-based formulas with or without added nucleotides for 1 year: part 2: immune cell populations. *J Pediatr Gastroenterol Nutr*. 2002;34(2):145-153
17. Cruz ML, Wong WW, Mimouni F, et al. Effects of infant nutrition on cholesterol synthesis rates. *Pediatr Res*. 1994;35(2):135-140

18. Fort P, Lanes R, Dahlem S, et al. Breast feeding and insulin-dependent diabetes mellitus in children. *J Am Coll Nutr*. 1986;5(5):439-441

19. Malloy MH, Berendes H. Does breast-feeding influence intelligence quotients at 9 and 10 years of age? *Early Hum Dev*. 1998;50(2):209-217

20. Sharpe RM, Martin B, Morris K, et al. Infant feeding with soy formula milk: effects on the testis and on blood testosterone levels in marmoset monkeys during the period of neonatal testicular activity. *Hum Reprod*. 2002;17(7):1692-1703

21. Tan KA, Walker M, Morris K, Greig I, Mason JI, Sharpe RM. Infant feeding with soy formula milk: effects on puberty progression, reproductive function and testicular cell numbers in marmoset monkeys in adulthood. *Hum Reprod*. 2006;21(4):896-904

22. Jefferson WN, Couse JF, Padilla-Banks E, Korach KS, Newbold RR. Neonatal exposure to genistein induces estrogen receptor (ER)alpha expression and multioocyte follicles in the maturing mouse ovary: evidence for ER-beta-mediated and nonestrogenic actions. *Biol Reprod*. 2002;67(4):1285-1296

23. Newbold RR, Banks EP, Bullock B, Jefferson WN. Uterine adenocarcinoma in mice treated neonatally with genistein. *Cancer Res*. 2001;61(11):4325-4328

24. National Toxicology Program. NTP Toxicology and Carcinogenesis Studies of Genistein (CAS No. 446-72-0) in Sprague-Dawley Rats (Feed Study). *Natl Toxicol Program Tech Rep Ser*. 2008;(545):1-240

25. Rozman KK, Bhatia J, Calafat AM, et al. NTP-CERHR expert panel report on the reproductive and developmental toxicity of genistein. *Birth Defects Res B Dev Reprod Toxicol*. 2006;77(6): 485-638

26. Chang HC, Doerge DR. Dietary genistein inactivates rat thyroid peroxidase in vivo without an apparent hypothyroid effect. *Toxicol Appl Pharmacol*. 2000;168(3):244-252

27. Cooke PS, Selvaraj V, Yellayi S. Genistein, estrogen receptors, and the acquired immune response. *J Nutr*. 2006;136(3):704-708

28. National Toxicology Program, Center for Evaluation of Risks to Human Reproduction. Final CERHR Expert Panel Report on Soy Infant Formula. Research Triangle Park, NC: 2010. Available at: http://cerhr.niehs.nih.gov/evals/genistein-soy/SoyFormulaUpdt/ FinalEPReport_508.pdf

29. Setchell KD, Zimmer-Nechemias L, Cai J, Heubi JE. Exposure of infants to phyto-oestrogens from soy-based infant formula. *Lancet*. 1997;350(9070):23-27

30. Irvine CH, Shand N, Fitzpatrick MG, Alexander SL. Daily intake and urinary excretion of genistein and daidzein by infants fed soy- or dairy-based infant formulas. *Am J Clin Nutr*. 1998;68(6 Suppl):1462S-1465S

31. Cao YA, Calafat AM, Doerge DR, et al. Isoflavones in urine, saliva, and blood of infants: data from a pilot study on the estrogenic activity of soy formula. *J Expo Sci Environ Epidemiol*. 2009;19(2):223-234

32. Berlin CM Jr, LaKind JS, Sonawane BR, et al. Conclusions, research needs, and recommendations of the expert panel: technical workshop on human milk surveillance and research for environmental chemicals in the United States. *J Toxicol Environ Health A*. 2002;65(22):1929-1935

33. Golub MS, Hogrefe CE, Germann SL, et al. Neurobehavioral evaluation of rhesus monkey infants fed cow's milk formula, soy formula, or soy formula with added manganese. *Neurotoxicol Teratol*. 2005;27(4):615-627

34. Bowen AB, Braden CR. Invasive *Enterobacter sakazakii* disease in infants. *Emerg Infect Dis*. 2006;12(8):1185-1189

35. Brede C, Fjeldal P, Skjevrak I, Herikstad H. Increased migration levels of bisphenol A from polycarbonate baby bottles after dishwashing, boiling and brushing. *Food Addit Contam.* 2003;20(7):684-689

36. Center for the Evaluation of Risks to Human Reproduction, National Toxicology Program. *NTP-CERHR Monograph on the Potential Human Reproductive and Developmental Effects of Bisphenol A.* Research Triangle Park, NC: National Toxicology Program, US Department of Health and Human Services; 2008. NIH Publication No. 08-5994

37. World Health Organization. Outbreak news. Melamine contamination, China. *Wkly Epidemiol Rec.* 2008;83(40):358

38. Dobson RL, Motlagh S, Quijano M, et al. Identification and characterization of toxicity of contaminants in pet food leading to an outbreak of renal toxicity in cats and dogs. *Toxicol Sci.* 2008;106(1):251-262

39. Guan N, Fan Q, Ding J, et al. Melamine-contaminated powdered formula and urolithiasis in young children. *N Engl J Med.* 2009;360(11):1067-1074

40. Ho SS, Chu WC, Wong KT, et al. Ultrasonographic evaluation of melamine-exposed children in Hong Kong. *N Engl J Med.* 2009;360(11):1156-1157

41. Wang IJ, Chen PC, Hwang KC. Melamine and nephrolithiasis in children in Taiwan. *N Engl J Med.* 2009;360(11):1157-1158

42. Langman CB. Melamine, powdered milk, and nephrolithiasis in Chinese infants. *N Engl J Med.* 2009;360(11):1139-1141

43. Nielsen IL, Williamson G. Review of the factors affecting bioavailability of soy isoflavones in humans. *Nutr Cancer.* 2007;57(1):1-10

44. Ingelfinger JR. Melamine and the global implications of food contamination. *N Engl J Med.* 2008;359(26):2745-2748

Chapter 17

Water

■ ■ ■ ■ ■ ■

Water safety is of primary importance to child health. Water is used for drinking, cooking, and preparing infant formulas for children who are not breastfed. The food supply may become contaminated when crops are irrigated with polluted water or when fish and shellfish from polluted waters are consumed. Water is important for bathing and swimming; contaminated water can result in exposures to children who may swallow or have skin contact with pollutants. In developing countries, access to safe water is a major determinant of child health (see Chapter 14). Drowning is the second-leading cause of unintentional injury death among children 1 to 14 years of age in the United States[1] and is the cause of very high morbidity and mortality worldwide, mostly in the same settings in which access to safe drinking water is a problem.

Although 70% of the earth is covered by water, only 3% of the earth's water is fresh. Of that 3%, two thirds is frozen in glaciers and ice caps, leaving only 1% available for human use. Freshwater is classified as either groundwater, such as underground aquifers (0.7%), or surface water, such as lakes and rivers (0.3%), but less than half of the liquid freshwater in the world is readily accessible.[2] In the United States, approximately half of drinking water comes from groundwater, with the other half coming from either surface water or mixed surface water and groundwater sources. Preserving an adequate supply of quality freshwater is essential to public health and ecologic integrity but is threatened by increasing population pressure and industrial and agricultural production, which can result in pollution.

Water pollution results from sources of contamination termed either point or nonpoint. Point sources of pollution include municipal wastewater treatment plant discharges and industrial wastewater discharges into surface waters.

Nonpoint sources are more difficult to identify and control and include agricultural runoff, urban runoff, soil contamination, and atmospheric deposition. Pollutants contaminate surface waters or soils directly and also seep into underground aquifers to contaminate groundwater.

Contaminated drinking water has long been identified as a potential threat to public health, going back to prehistory with the construction in ancient Rome of systems to purify and purvey drinking water to urban communities. Water pollutants can be categorized as biological agents, chemicals, or radionuclides (see Table 17.1). Hundreds of biological agents and thousands of chemical agents may be found in water. For many water pollutants, little is known of their long-term health effects. In the United States, federal water regulations were not required until passage of the Safe Drinking Water Act of 1974; regulations exist for only a small percentage of the contaminants that have been identified in water. Federal standards apply to community water supplies serving 25 or more customers. Some states have standards for smaller suppliers, but private wells are not regulated. Internationally, similar systems are in place in many countries. Moreover, the World Health Organization (WHO) has established guidelines for drinking water quality.[3] Modern water treatment facilities have made drinking water safe in most of the world, eliminating most waterborne infectious illnesses as well as contamination by lead and other harmful substances. However, in many parts of the United States, the drinking water supplies are threatened by contaminants. The true effects of drinking water contamination are difficult to determine, but it is estimated that in the United States, millions of illnesses each year are caused by microbial contaminants. Even where water treatment facilities are regulated, drinking water outbreaks can be caused by breaches in municipal water treatment and distribution processes, source water contamination, treatment plant inadequacies, and minor intrusions in the distribution system caused by water main breaks.[4]

The discussion in this chapter will be limited to a few representative examples of each of the categories of water pollutants. Although biological contamination of drinking water represents the largest threat to human health worldwide, it will not be extensively discussed in this chapter. See the American Academy of Pediatrics (AAP) *Red Book* for information about infectious diarrheal diseases.[5] Details about specific pollutants can be found in other chapters in this book.

ROUTES AND SOURCES OF EXPOSURE

Children drink more water per kg of body weight than do adults. For example, 6- to 12-month-old infants consume 4 times the amount of water per unit of body weight compared with adults. Drinking water is consumed in a number of forms: as water; as an addition to infant formula powder or concentrate, juice, and other drinks; and in cooking. To the extent that children consume human milk or drinks from outside the home (eg, fresh milk and juice, premixed formulas, and sodas), they have less consumption of household tap water.

Household water supplies can result in inhalation exposures. If volatile substances (eg, organic solvents) or gases (eg, radon gas) are present, these will enter the home during showering, bathing, and other activities. It has been estimated that 50% of the total exposure to volatile organic compounds in drinking water is via this inhalation route.

Water can cause exposure via other pathways. When contaminated water is used for the irrigation of foods, the foods may become contaminated (see Chapter 18). Fish and shellfish harvested from polluted fresh and marine waters also are important sources of exposure to water pollutants; in many cases, pollutants are concentrated by shellfish and fish. Contaminated bathing water can result in exposures via ingestion or dermal contact. Young children particularly are at risk, because they swallow more water when bathing than do older children and adults. Flood water may adversely affect human health by bringing children in contact with metals, such as lead and cadmium in flood-plain soils.[6]

The fetus also may be exposed to pollutants when a pregnant woman ingests foods in the aquatic food chain in which water pollutants have bioaccumulated. Methylmercury and polychlorinated biphenyls (PCBs) in fish are particularly important in this regard, because they accumulate in the body and are not readily excreted. These toxicants may be found in the body years after exposure.

CONTAMINANTS IN WATER

Biological Agents

Microorganisms

Drinking and bathing water may contain numerous pathogens, which have the ability to survive in the water for variable periods. Some of these agents are listed in Table 17.1. Some (eg, certain parasites) form small cysts, which pass through standard filters and are quite resistant to water disinfectants. Waterborne illness usually results in mild gastroenteritis with diarrhea but can also result in nongastrointestinal tract disease. Even when water systems are in compliance with federal and local regulations, sporadic and epidemic illnesses occur.[4] This is of particular concern for infants and immunocompromised persons exposed to pathogens such as *Cryptosporidium* species despite state-of-the-art water treatment. In the United States, it is rare to have serious dysentery or enteric fever attributable to *Vibrio cholerae* and *Salmonella typhi*, even in areas where water quality is compromised. Viral upper respiratory and gastrointestinal tract infections can be transmitted by contaminated bathing water. Syndromes associated with illnesses from various pathogens are described in the *Red Book*.[5]

Table 17.1: Examples of Some Water Pollutants, Common Sources, and Systems Affected

POLLUTANT CATEGORY (SPECIFIC EXAMPLES)	COMMON SOURCES	SYSTEMS AFFECTED/ HEALTH EFFECTS
BIOLOGICAL AGENTS		
Bacteria		
Campylobacter species	Feces: human, animal	Gastrointestinal tract
Escherichia coli	Feces: human, animal	Gastrointestinal tract
Salmonella species	Feces: human, animal	Gastrointestinal tract
Shigella species	Feces: human	Gastrointestinal tract
Vibrio species	Feces: human, animal	Gastrointestinal tract
Viruses		
Calicivirus	Feces: human	Gastrointestinal tract
Enterovirus	Feces: human	Gastrointestinal tract, neurologic
Hepatitis A virus	Feces: human	Gastrointestinal tract (liver)
Rotavirus	Feces: human	Gastrointestinal tract
Parasites		
Balantidium coli	Feces: human, animal	Gastrointestinal tract
Cryptosporidium parvum	Feces: human, animal	Gastrointestinal tract
Entamoeba histolytica	Feces: human	Gastrointestinal tract
Giardia intestinalis	Feces: human, animal	Gastrointestinal tract
Natural Toxins		
Microcystins	Cyanobacteria	Gastrointestinal tract, neurologic
Pfiesteria toxins	*Pfiesteria piscicida*	Neurologic, dermatologic
Phytoplankton (Dinoflagellate) toxins	*Alexandria catarella* *Pseudonitzchia pungens*	Neurologic
CHEMICALS		
Inorganic		
Arsenic	Ores, smelting, pesticides	Lung, kidney, and skin cancer; cardiovascular; neurodevelopmental
Chromium	Ores, steel and pulp mills	Cancer (chromium VI)
Lead	Pipes, solder, soil	Neurologic, cardiovascular
Mercury (inorganic)	Waste incineration, burning coal, mercury use, volcanoes	Kidney damage, neurologic

Table 17.1: Examples of Some Water Pollutants, Common Sources, and Systems Affected, *continued*

POLLUTANT CATEGORY (SPECIFIC EXAMPLES)	COMMON SOURCES	SYSTEMS AFFECTED/ HEALTH EFFECTS
CHEMICALS		
Inorganic		
Nitrates	Nitrogen fertilizer, leaching from septic tanks, sewage; erosion of natural deposits	Methemoglobinemia in infants
Organic		
Benzene, other organic chemicals	Leaking gasoline storage tanks	Leukemia, aplastic anemia
Pesticides	Agricultural use, urban runoff	Multiple
Polychlorinated biphenyls	Transformers, industry	Multiple
Trichloroethylene	Degreasing, dry cleaning	Cancer
DISINFECTANTS AND DISINFECTION BY-PRODUCTS		
Chloramines	Water chlorination	Eye irritation, upper and lower airway irritation; stomach discomfort, anemia
Chlorine	Water chlorination	Eye/nose irritation; stomach discomfort
Chlorine dioxide	Water chlorination	Anemia; nervous system effects
Haloacetic acid	Byproduct of drinking water disinfection	Increased risk of cancer
Trihalomethanes	Byproduct of drinking water disinfection	Increased risk of cancer
RADIONUCLIDES		
Radon	Natural uranium	Lung cancer

Natural Toxins

Natural toxins may produce acute or chronic illnesses and a variety of clinical syndromes. Water from ponds and lakes as well as municipal and recreational waters, under certain conditions, may contain toxin-producing cyanobacteria (blue-green algae [eg, *Microcystis aeruginosa*]) or phytoplankton, which may result in toxic shellfish poisoning. Cyanotoxins, such as microcystins, are hepatotoxic and neurotoxic compounds.[7] Microcystins produced by cyanobacteria have been linked to liver failure and death in patients who underwent hemodialysis at a dialysis center in Brazil supplied by untreated water from a lake with massive growth of blue-green algae; many water treatment systems do not effectively remove cyanotoxins.[8] Water from the rivers flowing into the Chesapeake Bay on the eastern shore of the United States or mussel-growing areas in the Pacific Northwest periodically may be contaminated with dinoflagellates (*Pfiesteria piscicida, pseudonitzchia pungens*) that can produce neurotoxins.[9] The rate of contamination by toxin-producing organisms is not well characterized but thought to be infrequent.

Chemical Contaminants

Water and sediments in water are the ultimate sinks for many chemicals produced and used by humans. Each year in the United States, more than 15 000 chemicals are produced at more than 10 000 pounds each, and thousands of new chemicals are introduced into use each year. Few of these chemicals have been evaluated with regard to their effects on human health. Even among the 2800 chemicals used at more than a million pounds per year, more than half have not been tested for toxic effects on humans.[10] Thousands of synthetic organic chemicals are used in agricultural and industrial processes. For example, drinking water supplies near natural gas production sites can be contaminated from hydraulic fracturing ("hydrofracking" or "fracking"), a process to extract natural gas from shale. This practice uses million of gallons of water containing sand and some very toxic chemicals. The water is pumped deep into the ground under extreme pressure. Most of the water is never recovered; the water that is recovered needs to be disposed of in some "safe" way. The process is repeated over and over again.

According to the US Geological Survey, many industrial chemicals, antibiotics and other pharmaceuticals (including estrogens), and pesticides frequently are found in the waters of the United States, particularly downstream from factories and cities.[11]

Inorganic Chemicals

Arsenic

Arsenic, a ubiquitous metal, can be found in the environment in organic and inorganic forms and in valence states of 0, 3, and 5. Drinking water and food are the major sources of arsenic for humans. Clinical effects of arsenic are discussed in Chapter 22 and include skin and lung cancer, peripheral neuropathy (in adults), hyperkeratotic skin lesions, and chronic lung disease (in adults). Arsenic is a known human carcinogen; its natural occurrence in drinking water and the expense of removal, however, have led the US Environmental Protection Agency (EPA) to allow a drinking water standard that is less protective than is usual for carcinogens.[12] Increasingly, associations are being made between high levels of arsenic in drinking water and neurodevelopmental effects, including loss of IQ points.[13,14]

Chromium

Chromium in drinking water is regulated to protect against exposure to one of the valence states of chromium—chromium VI (hexavalent chromium)— a carcinogen (see Chapter 24).

Fluoride

In 2011, the US Department of Health and Human Services and the US EPA set the recommended level of fluoride in drinking water at 0.7 mg/L, which is the lower limit of the prior standard (0.7-1.2 mg/L). This new standard is expected to reduce the incidence of fluorosis.[15]

Lead

Drinking water represents a potential source of exposure to lead. In the past 2 decades, expanded regulations and monitoring have made most large municipal water supplies safe from exposure to lead. Nevertheless, water in some homes and schools in the United States contains lead above acceptable levels. Chicago, Boston, and other cities historically used 100% lead piping to connect water mains to homes. Millions of these lead connectors still exist. In addition, lead solder, used to connect copper pipes, was widely used until the late 1980s. Drinking water, particularly water that is "soft" (ie, low in calcium or magnesium), or below a neutral pH, causes lead to leach from connector pipes, soldered joints, or lead-containing fixtures. Clinical effects of lead exposure are discussed in Chapter 31. Lead in drinking water is controlled by limiting the corrosiveness of the water (ie, the ability of the water to leach lead from these materials) and eliminated by removing lead pipes or pipes with lead solder. In recent years, increased levels of lead in drinking water were found in some older systems with lead service lines after the disinfectant chlorine was replaced with less explosive chloramines.[16]

Methylmercury

Mercury in fish originates from natural sources (such as volcanoes) and from combustion sources that release mercury into the air, such as coal-fired power plants used for generating electrical energy and municipal waste incinerators that burn garbage.[17] Atmospheric mercury is ultimately deposited into lakes and rivers by dustfall, rain, and snow. In the aquatic environment, mercury is converted by sediment bacteria into methylmercury, which becomes concentrated in the muscle tissues of fish by direct absorption from the water and by biomagnification up through the aquatic food chain. Clinical effects of mercury exposure are discussed in Chapter 32. Although mercury is regulated as a drinking water contaminant, the most important source of methylmercury exposure for most children is through consumption of contaminated fish (typically long-lived species such as swordfish and shark).

Organic Chemicals

Gasoline and its Additives

Gasoline stored in underground tanks may develop leaks over the years, causing toxic chemicals to rapidly move into groundwater and eventually into drinking water. Probably the most toxic component of gasoline is benzene. Along with other gasoline constituents (some of which also are very toxic), it enters the water when gasoline is spilled or when gasoline tanks leak into the ground and from other industrial sources. Benzene is known to cause leukemia in humans and aplastic anemia at high doses. Thousands of other compounds in gasoline are of unknown toxicity. One toxic compound in gasoline that has been found in drinking water sources is methyl tertiary butyl ether (MTBE).[18] The EPA has issued a drinking water advisory for methyl tertiary butyl ether, including recommendations for preventing unpleasant odor and taste (occurring at levels between 20 and 40 parts per billion [ppb]). California regulates methyl tertiary butyl ether both on the basis of taste and odor (5 parts per billion) and as a carcinogen (13 parts per billion [see Chapter 29]).

Nitrates

Nitrates enter the water supply from urban and agricultural runoff of nitrogen fertilizers and also may be produced by bacterial action on animal waste runoff. Nitrates themselves are not toxic to humans but can be converted by gut bacteria to more reactive and toxic nitrites. Nitrates in drinking water above the EPA level of 10 mg/L may cause fatal methemoglobinemia in infants (see Chapter 33).

Pesticides

Pesticides may not be removed by conventional drinking water treatment (see Chapter 37). As detection technologies have improved, increasingly low concentrations of common insecticides, herbicides, and fungicides have been documented in drinking water sources.[11] Some older pesticides (such as dichlorodiphenyltrichloroethane [DDT]) were designed to persist in the environment for years and can be found distributed worldwide in water and soil. Newer pesticides degrade more quickly but still contaminate water and may persist for long durations in groundwater. Concentrations in water often correlate with growing seasons in agricultural areas and rainy seasons in more urban settings. Private drinking water wells are particularly susceptible to contamination by agricultural chemicals, especially in higher-risk agricultural areas with sandy soils and high water tables. The EPA is now required to consider contributions of exposures from drinking water when establishing standards for pesticides in foods.

Polychlorinated Biphenyls and Dioxins

Polychlorinated biphenyls and dioxins have very low solubility in water and are not found in drinking water. They are a problem because they readily bioaccumulate in the fat of wildlife, are very resistant to biological degradation, and remain in the environment for decades. The sediments of many lakes and rivers are contaminated with PCBs and/or dioxins. Contaminated sediments, a nonpoint source, are still the major source of PCBs and dioxins found in fish and wildlife. Certain dioxins and PCBs are associated with risks of cancer and developmental toxicity[19,20] (see Chapter 35).

Trichloroethylene

In 1986, an association was found between childhood leukemia and drinking water supplied from 2 municipal wells in Woburn, MA.[21] Childhood leukemia rates in Woburn reported between 1964 and 1983 were twice the national rates. Some chemical disposal pits, used for several decades, were suspected as the source of trichloroethylene, a chlorinated product, and other chlorinated chemicals. Although the 2 affected wells were shut down immediately on discovery of the contamination, exposure to these carcinogens is believed to have occurred for many years. At this time, trichloroethylene is classified as "reasonably anticipated" to be a human carcinogen based on strong evidence in animals and much weaker human epidemiologic evidence.[19]

Disinfectants and Disinfection Byproducts

In the 1970s, chlorination of waters with high natural organic content (eg, humic and tannic acids) was found to cause the formation of chloroform and other chlorinated compounds called trihalomethanes. Some residual levels of the disinfectants chlorine and chlorine dioxide are found in tap water. Epidemiologic studies show a correlation between drinking water containing trihalomethanes and increased rates of rectal and bladder cancer.[22] As a result of extensive testing of the water supplies in the United States, cancer risk analysis of the chemicals found, and suggestive epidemiologic studies in 1981, the EPA issued a maximum contaminant level for trihalomethanes in water. Studies have found associations between trihalomethanes and spontaneous abortion and birth defects; it appears, however, that the evidence for this association is not strong at currently allowable levels in the United States.[23,24] A consistent conclusion has been that disinfecting drinking water reduces waterborne diseases, a benefit that far outweighs the risks resulting from traces of disinfection byproducts in drinking water. Chlorination of swimming pool water is also a common practice. Although some studies have indicated a possible relationship between chloramines found in pool water and childhood asthma among swimmers, a recent meta-analysis was unable to conclude that a causal relationship exists.[25]

Radionuclides

Radon

Radon gas, a product of the radioactive decay of uranium, enters the water supply naturally and becomes aerosolized during use of tap water. Radon further breaks down into radon "daughters" or "progeny." Radon in water is important, because radon may be inhaled during showering. Lung cancer in adults has been linked to inhalation of radon progeny.[26] For a more extensive discussion of radon hazards, see Chapter 39.

PREVENTION OF EXPOSURE

The public health successes of the 20th century in eliminating epidemic cholera and typhoid fever are dramatic evidence of the importance of prevention in managing drinking and recreational water supplies. Historically, water and waste management were local responsibilities. During the environmental movement in the 1970s, Congress enacted laws that unified standards, resulting in the development of high-quality drinking and recreational waters.

Public Water Supplies

The EPA and state agencies require that municipal or commercial water suppliers serving more than 25 people meet all standards developed under the Safe Drinking Water Act of 1974 and its amendments (see Table 17.2). The Water Pollution Control Act (1972) and the Resource Conservation and Recovery Act (1976) require industrial, commercial, and municipal facilities to meet requirements to prevent contamination of surface and groundwaters. The EPA and state environmental agencies also require municipal water supplies to meet specific standards for pesticides that have been found in groundwater and surface water. Restrictions have been placed on the use of certain pesticides that have a propensity to leach into waters.

Table 17.2: Selected National Primary Drinking Water Regulations
(http://www.epa.gov/safewater/contaminants/index.html)[a]

CONTAMINANT	TYPE OF STANDARD[b]	STANDARD
Microbiologic Contaminants		
Cryptosporidium species	TT	99% removal[c]
Giardia lamblia	TT	99.9% removal/inactivation
Heterotrophic plate count (HPC)[d]	TT	≤500 bacterial colonies/mL
Legionella species	TT	No limit, but EPA believes that if *Giardia* and viruses are removed/inactivated, *Legionella* will also be controlled.
Total coliforms (including fecal coliforms and *Escherichia coli*)	MCL	≤5.0% of samples/month allowed to contain fecal coliforms and *Escherichia coli*
Turbidity[e]	TT	Can never exceed 1 turbidity unit; <0.3 unit in 95% of daily samples (per month)
Viruses (enteric)	TT	99.99% removal/inactivation
Inorganic Chemicals		**Standard (mg/L = parts per million)**
Antimony	MCL	0.006
Arsenic	TT	0.010
Asbestos (fiber >10 μm)	MCL	7 million fibers/L
Barium	MCL	2
Beryllium	MCL	0.004
Cadmium	MCL	0.005
Chromium (total)	MCL	0.1
Copper	TT	1.3
Cyanide	MCL	0.2
Fluoride	MCL	4.0
Lead	TT	Action level = 0.015
Mercury (inorganic)	MCL	0.002
Nitrate (measured as nitrogen)	MCL	10
Nitrite (measured as nitrogen)	MCL	1

continued on page 236

continued from page 235

Table 17.2: Selected National Primary Drinking Water Regulations
(http://www.epa.gov/safewater/contaminants/index.html)[a] *continued*

CONTAMINANT	TYPE OF STANDARD[b]	STANDARD
Inorganic Chemicals		**Standard (mg/L = parts per million)**
Selenium	MCL	0.05
Thallium	TT	0.002
Organic Chemicals		
Acrylamide	TT	If used, 0.05% dosed at 1 mg/L (or equivalent)
Alachlor	MCL	0.002
Atrazine	MCL	0.003
Benzene	MCL	0.005
Benzo(a)pyrene	MCL	0.0002
Carbofuran	MCL	0.04
Carbon tetrachloride	MCL	0.005
Chlordane	MCL	0.002
Chlorobenzene	MCL	0.1
2,4-D	MCL	0.07
Dalopon	MCL	0.2
1,2-Dibromo-3-chloropropane (DBCP)	MCL	0.0002
o-Dichlorobenzene	MCL	0.6
p-Dichlorobenzene	MCL	0.075
1,2-Dichloroethane	MCL	0.005
1,1-Dichloroethylene	MCL	0.007
Cis-1,2-Dichloroethylene	MCL	0.07
Trans-1,2-Dichloroethylene	MCL	0.1
Dichloromethane	MCL	0.005
1,2-Dichloropropane	MCL	0.005
Di(2-ethylhexyl) adipate	MCL	0.4

Table 17.2: Selected National Primary Drinking Water Regulations
(http://www.epa.gov/safewater/contaminants/index.html)[a] *continued*

CONTAMINANT	TYPE OF STANDARD[b]	STANDARD
Organic Chemicals		
Di (2-ethylhexyl) phthalate	MCL	0.006
Dinoseb	MCL	0.007
Dioxin (2,3,7,8-TCDD)	MCL	0.00000003
Diquat	MCL	0.02
Endothall	MCL	0.1
Endrin	MCL	0.002
Epichlorohydrin	TT	If used, 0.01% dosed at 20 mg/L (or equivalent)
Ethylbenzene	MCL	0.7
Ethelyne dibromide	MCL	0.00005
Glyphosate	MCL	0.7
Heptachlor	MCL	0.0004
Heptachlor epoxide	MCL	0.0002
Hexachlorobenzene	MCL	0.001
Hexachlorocyclopentadiene	MCL	0.05
Lindane	MCL	0.0002
Methoxychlor	MCL	0.04
Oxamyl	MCL	0.2
Polychlorinated biphenyls	MCL	0.0005
Pentachlorophenol	MCL	0.001
Picloram	MCL	0.5
Simazine	MCL	0.004
Styrene	MCL	0.1
Tetrachloroethylene	MCL	0.005
Toluene	MCL	1
Toxaphene	MCL	0.003

continued on page 238

continued from page 237

Table 17.2: Selected National Primary Drinking Water Regulations
(http://www.epa.gov/safewater/contaminants/index.html)[a] *continued*

CONTAMINANT	TYPE OF STANDARD[b]	STANDARD
Organic Chemicals		
2,4,5-T, Silvex	MCL	0.05
1,2,4-Trichlorobenzene	MCL	0.07
1,1,1-Trichloroethane	MCL	0.2
1,1,2-Trichloroethane	MCL	0.005
Trichloroethylene	MCL	0.005
Vinyl chloride	MCL	0.002
Xylenes (total)	MCL	10
Disinfectants/Disinfectant Byproducts		
Bromate	MCL	0.01
Chloramines (as Cl_2)	MRDL	4.0
Chlorine (as Cl_2)	MRDL	4.0
Chlorine dioxide (as ClO_2)	MRDL	0.8
Chlorite	MCL	1.0
Haloacetic acid	MCL	0.06
Total trihalomethanes	MCL	0.08
Radionuclides		
Alpha particles	MCL	15 pCi/L
Beta particles and photon emitters	MCL	4 mrem/y
Radium-226 & radium-228 (combined)	MCL	5 pCi/L
Uranium	MCL	30 µg/L

[a] From US Environmental Protection Agency.[33]

[b] MCL indicates maximum contaminant level; TT, treatment technique; MRDL, maximum residual disinfectant level; pCi, picocurie; mrem, millirem.

[c] http://www.epa.gov/envirofw/html/icr/gloss_path.html

[d] Heterotrophic plate count (HPC): HPC has no health effects but is an analytic method used to measure the variety of bacteria common in water. The lower the concentration of bacteria in water, the better maintained is the water system.

[e] Turbidity: a measure of water cloudiness used to determine water quality and filtration effectiveness. Higher turbidity levels are often associated with higher levels of disease-producing organisms.

Private Wells

Private wells are not federally regulated. The EPA estimates that 15% to 20% of the US population obtains drinking water from private wells. Infants and children may drink well water at home and also if they are on vacation, are traveling, or are in child care or other locations. Contamination of well water can occur if the well is shallow, in porous soil, old, poorly maintained, near a leaky septic tank, or downhill from agricultural fields or intensive livestock operations. Flooding associated with extreme weather events can carry pollutants into private wells. Each state has different testing procedures, sometimes requiring testing only at transfer of land ownership. Testing of private wells is the responsibility of individual homeowners but in some states may be performed at no cost by the health department if testing is recommended by a health care provider. In rural areas, physicians can ask patients if their wells have been tested for coliforms and nitrates by local or county health departments within the last year. Guidance for testing and water treatment for owners of private wells is available from the State of Wisconsin[27] and the American Academy of Pediatrics.[28] The EPA includes guidance on its Web site, including what to do after a flood (http://www.epa.gov/privatewells/publications.html).

In agricultural areas, higher-than-normal levels of nitrates or coliform bacteria may indicate the presence of pesticides. If so, parents can contact state health and environmental agencies to determine whether their well water should be tested for specific pesticides. State agencies may conduct the testing without cost or may recommend private laboratories. Extensive pesticide testing should not be encouraged because of the cost and the rarity of pesticide contamination.

Home Water-Treatment Systems

Home water-filtration and treatment systems that remove lead, chlorine byproducts, traces of organic compounds, and bacteria are increasingly popular. These systems, which may attach to the end of a water faucet, generally provide limited health benefits. Most drinking water sources keep contaminants below EPA standards and state criteria. In addition, small, end-of-the-faucet filtration systems or water pitcher-based filters are not always highly effective in removing trace substances.[29] If not properly maintained, filters using activated carbon can provide media for the growth of bacteria. Unless the carbon filter is frequently replaced, the first morning draw of tap water can have unacceptable levels of bacteria. Despite potential drawbacks, some home water-filtration systems can be effective in removing lead and other toxic substances. These systems, however, do not remove fluoride.

Home drinking treatment systems or filters are not encouraged unless a chemical problem has been identified. Even then, it is more effective, on a community-wide basis, to have the municipal or commercial water source

To reduce hazards from fish consumption, inform parents to:

- Eat pan fish rather than predator fish (shark, swordfish, tuna).

- Eat small game fish rather than large fish.

- Eat fewer fatty fish (mackerel, carp, catfish, lake trout), which accumulate higher levels of chemical toxicants.

- Trim skin and fatty areas where contaminants such as PCBs and dichlorodiphenyltrichloroethane accumulate (Note: Trimming fatty areas will have no effect on removing methylmercury, which accumulates in fish muscle).

- Follow fish advisories for women of childbearing age, pregnant women, nursing mothers, and young children.

- Be aware of federal and state fish advisories issued by state health, environmental, and conservation departments.

personnel correct the problem as required by law than to have homeowners assume the responsibility. However, if families prefer to treat water, it is important to ensure that the treatment system removes the pollutants of concern and that the system is maintained so that it functions well and does not become contaminated.

The environmental history should include questions about the source of the child's drinking water (private well or municipal water supply) and use of home water-filtration systems.

Contaminants in Fish

Physicians living in active fishing areas with advisories related to PCBs or mercury should ask patients if their consumption of fish is in accordance with federal- and state-issued fish advisories. Freshwater fish generally have higher levels of contaminants than do saltwater fish. Saltwater fish, generally low in contaminants, are the main fish purchased in the marketplace. However, a few saltwater fish may have higher levels of contaminants than freshwater fish. They include swordfish, shark, king mackerel, tuna, and tilefish, which are long-lived, predatory fish capable of bioaccumulating methylmercury. See Chapter 32 for more detailed information regarding methylmercury content in fish.

Frequently Asked Questions

Q *Does my pitcher-based water filter remove lead?*

A Water-filtration pitchers are commonly used because of their affordability. Most water pitchers use granular-activated carbon and resins to bond with and trap contaminants. These filters are effective at improving the taste of water, and many will also reduce levels of lead and other contaminants. Specific contaminants removed vary by model. Carbon filters have a specified shelf life and should be replaced regularly according to the manufacturer's instructions (http://water.epa.gov/aboutow/ogwdw/upload/2005_11_17_faq_fs_healthseries_filtration.pdf).

Q *Are the chemicals in swimming pools a health concern?*

A Concern is emerging about the health effects of chemicals accumulating above a swimming pool, "off-gassed" from the water into the air breathed by swimmers or pool workers. Chemicals used in pools are irritating to eyes, skin, and upper and lower airways. Exposures may also be associated with development of asthma in predisposed atopic children.[30] Children who swim or work frequently in poorly ventilated indoor pools may be at higher risk.[31,32] Swimming is a popular and healthy form of exercise for children. Showering before swimming to remove organic matter (eg, sweat, dirt, and lotions) which can react with pool chemicals to form chloramines helps to prevent their formation. Proper disinfection practices and ventilation will reduce exposure.

Q *Should I buy bottled water?*

A Unless there are known contamination problems of drinking water, families should not be encouraged to buy bottled water. Bottled water is not required to meet any higher standards than tap water and can cost 500 to 1000 times as much. Bottled water is regulated by the US Food and Drug Administration (FDA); for more information, see http://www.fda.gov/Food/ResourcesForYou/Consumers/ucm046894.htm.

Q *Should I boil my baby's water or use a home water-treatment system?*

A If a family uses a public water supply that meets standards, parents should not boil their infant's drinking water or use a home water treatment system unless the drinking water is contaminated. Drinking water should be boiled only when the water supplier or health or environmental agency issues such instructions. The Centers for Disease Control and Prevention and the EPA state that people with special health needs (eg, those who are immunocompromised) may wish to boil or treat their drinking water. Boiling tap water for 1 minute inactivates or destroys biological agents, but boiling water longer than 1 minute may concentrate contaminants. Point-of-use filters also may be considered but only if they are clearly labeled to remove particles

1 μm or less in diameter. Unless they are well maintained on schedule, home water-treatment systems often are ineffective and may even contribute to exposure to waterborne bacteria.

Q *Is it true that federal and state regulations ensure the safety of drinking water?*

A Federal and state regulations have oversight for water distributions systems that serve at least 25 homes. In most cases, regulations result in very safe water. Nonetheless, almost 10% of the population drinks water that does not meet regulations. Violations are higher where water supply systems serve fewer than 1000 people. Some standards (eg, for *Cryptosporidium* species) only apply to systems that serve more than 10 000 people. Information on drinking water quality and violations can be obtained from the water supplier or state health and environmental agencies. Even water in compliance with all standards may contain harmful contamination. Consumers are given annual written statements of any violations by their public water supply in consumer confidence reports. Many public water suppliers maintain Web sites with current surveillance information. Private wells are not regulated, so determining safety of water from those sources requires the attention of well owners.

Q *Should I get my water tested?*

A Under most circumstances, it is not necessary to have drinking water tested. If the local water supply fails to meet a standard, pressure should be exerted on politicians to correct the problem, rather than having people test their own water. As a precaution, people who use private wells less than 50 ft (15 m) deep and who have septic systems should have wells tested yearly for coliforms (see Table 17.2). In the case of private wells, quarterly testing for 1 year is recommended, followed by yearly nitrate testing if results of quarterly tests are normal.

Q *Is it okay to flush unused prescription drugs down the toilet?*

A Residues of birth control pills, antidepressants, painkillers, shampoos, and many other pharmaceuticals and personal care products have been found in water, in trace amounts. These chemicals are flushed into rivers from sewage treatment plants or leach into groundwater from septic systems. The discovery of these substances in water probably reflects better sensing technology. The health effects, if any, from exposure to these substances in water is not yet known.

In many cases, these chemicals enter water when people excrete them or wash them away in the shower. Some chemicals, however, are flushed or washed down the drain when people discard outdated or unused drugs. Recent federal guidelines state that prescription or over-the-counter medications should not be flushed down the toilet or poured down a sink unless

patient information material specifically states that it is safe to do so (http://lists.dep.state.fl.us/pipermail/pharmwaste/2007-February/000894.html). Follow these guidelines to dispose of these products properly:
— First, check with your police department to see if they have a drug collection program.
— Second, check to see if your community household hazardous waste program collects medications (they must have law enforcement officials present).
— Lastly, if no collection options exist, follow these steps:
  ☐ Remove all personal identification from prescription bottles;
  ☐ Mix all unused drugs with coffee grounds, kitty litter, or another undesirable substance; and
  ☐ Place this mixture in a sealed container before disposing in the trash.

Resources

Agency for Toxic Substances and Disease Registry, Information Center
Web site: www.atsdr.cdc.gov

US Environmental Protection Agency
Web site: www.epa.gov/ost/fish
EPA Safe Drinking Water Hotline: 800/426-4791. Regional offices are listed in the local telephone book.

US Environmental Protection Agency: Private Drinking Water Wells
Web site: www.epa.gov/privatewells/publications.html

US Fish and Wildlife Service, Department of the Interior
Web site: www.fws.gov

US Food and Drug Administration
FDA Regulates the Safety of Bottled Water Beverages Including Flavored Water and Nutrient-Added Water Beverages
Web site: www.fda.gov/Food/ResourcesForYou/Consumers/ucm046894.htm

Wisconsin Department of Natural Resources
Information for Homeowners with Private Wells
Web site: www.dnr.state.wi.us/org/water/dwg/prih2o.htm

References

1. Borse NN, Gilchrist J, Dellinger AM, Rudd RA, Ballesteros MF, Sleet DA. *CDC Childhood Injury Report: Patterns of Unintentional Injuries among 0-19 Year Olds in the United States, 2000-2006.* Atlanta, GA: Centers for Disease Control and Prevention, National Center for Injury Prevention and Control; 2008. Available at: http://www.cdc.gov/safechild/images/CDC-ChildhoodInjury.pdf. Accessed March 2, 2011

2. Okum D. Water quality management. In: Last JM, Wallace RB, eds. *Maxcy-Rosenau-Last Public Health and Preventive Medicine*. 13th ed. East Norwalk, CT: Appleton & Lange; 1992;619-648

3. World Health Organization. *Guidelines for Drinking-Water Quality. Incorporating First Addendum. Vol 1, Recommendations*. 3rd ed. Geneva, Switzerland: World Health Organization; 2006

4. Reynolds KA, Mena KD, Gerba CP. Risk of waterborne illness via drinking water in the United States. *Rev Environ Contam Toxicol*. 2008;192:117-158

5. American Academy of Pediatrics. *Red Book: 2009 Report of the Committee on Infectious Diseases*. Pickering LK, Baker CJ, Kimberlin DW, Long SS, eds. 28th ed. Elk Grove Village, IL: American Academy of Pediatrics; 2009

6. Albering HJ, van Leusen SM, Moonen EJC, et al. Human health risk assessment: a case study involving heavy metal soil contamination after the flooding of the river Meuse during the winter of 1993-1994. *Environ Health Perspect*. 1999;107(1):37-43

7. Codd GA, Morrison LF, Metcalf JS. Cyanobacterial toxins: risk management for health protection. *Toxicol Appl Pharmacol*. 2005;203(3):264-272

8. Pouria S, de Andrade A, Barbosa J, et al. Fatal microcystin intoxication in haemodialysis unit in Caruaru, Brazil. *Lancet*. 1998;352(9121):21-26

9. Friedman MA, Levin BE. Neurobehavioral effects of harmful algal bloom (HAB) toxins: a critical review. *J Int Neuropsychol Soc*. 2005;11(3):331-338

10. Goldman LR, Koduru S. Chemicals in the environment and developmental toxicity to children: a public health and policy perspective. *Environ Health Perspect*. 2000;108(Suppl 3):443-448

11. Focazio MJ, Kolpin DW, Barnes KK, et al. A national reconnaissance for pharmaceuticals and other organic wastewater contaminants in the United States—II. Untreated drinking water sources. *Sci Total Environ*. 2008402(2-3):201-216

12. National Research Council, Committee on Toxicology. *Arsenic in Drinking Water: 2001 Update*. Washington, DC: National Research Council.

13. Calderon RL, Abernathy CO, Thomas DJ. Consequences of acute and chronic exposure to arsenic in children. *Pediatr Ann*. 2004;33(7):461-466

14. Wang SX, Wang ZH, Cheng XT, et al. Arsenic and fluoride exposure in drinking water: children's IQ and growth in Shanyin county, Shanxi province, China. *Environ Health Perspect*. 2007;115(4):643-647

15. Centers for Disease Control and Prevention. Community Water Fluoridation: Questions and Answers. Available at: http://www.cdc.gov/fluoridation/fact_sheets/cwf_qa.htm. Accessed March 2, 2011

16. Miranda ML, Kim D, Hull AP, Paul CJ, Galeano MA. Changes in blood lead levels associated with use of chloramines in water treatment systems. *Environ Health Perspect*. 2007;115(2): 221-225

17. Goldman LR, Shannon MW. Technical report: mercury in the environment: implications for pediatricians. *Pediatrics*. 2001;108(1):197-205

18. Moran MJ, Zogorski JS, Squillace PJ. MTBE and gasoline hydrocarbons in ground water of the United States. *Ground Water*. 2005;43(4):615-627

19. US Department of Health and Human Services, National Toxicology Program. *Report on Carcinogens, 11th ed*. Research Triangle Park, NC: US Department of Health and Human Services, Public Health Service; 2005

20. Jacobson JL, Jacobson SW. Prenatal exposure to polychlorinated biphenyls and attention at school age. *J Pediatr*. 2003;143(6):780-788

21. National Research Council. *Environmental Epidemiology: Public Health and Hazardous Wastes*. Washington, DC: National Academies Press; 1991

22. Villanueva CM, Fernandez F, Malats N, Grimalt JO, Kogevinas M. Meta-analysis of studies on individual consumption of chlorinated drinking water and bladder cancer. *J Epidemiol Community Health*. 2003;57(3):166-173

23. Savitz DA, Singer PC, Herring AH, Hartmann KE, Weinberg HS, Makarushka C. Exposure to drinking water disinfection by-products and pregnancy loss. *Am J Epidemiol*. 2006;164(11):1043-1051

24. Nieuwenhuijsen MJ, Toledano MB, Eaton NE, Fawell J, Elliott P. Chlorination disinfection byproducts in water and their association with adverse reproductive outcomes: a review. *Occup Environ Med*. 2000;57(2):73-85

25. Goodman M, Hays S. Asthma and swimming: a meta-analysis. *J Asthma*. 2008;45(8):639-647

26. Bean JA, Isacson P, Hahne RM, Kohler J. Drinking water and cancer incidence in Iowa. II. Radioactivity in drinking water. *Am J Epidemiol*. 1982;116(6):924-932

27. Wisconsin Department of Natural Resources. Information for Homeowners with Private Wells. Available at: http://www.dnr.state.wi.us/org/water/dwg/prih2o.htm. Accessed March 2, 2011

28. American Academy of Pediatrics, Committee on Environmental Health and Committee on Infectious Diseases. Policy statement—drinking water from private wells and risks to children. *Pediatrics*. 2009;123(6):1599–1605

29. NSF International. *Home Water Treatment Devices*. Available at: http://www.nsf.org/consumer/drinking_water/dw_treatment.asp?program=WaterTre. Accessed March 2, 2011

30. Bernard A, Carbonnelle S, de Burbure C, Michel O, Nickmilder M. Chlorinated pool attendance, atopy, and the risk of asthma during childhood. *Environ Health Perspect*. 2006;114(10):1567–1573

31. Centers for Disease Control and Prevention. Ocular and respiratory illness associated with an indoor swimming pool—Nebraska, 2006. *MMWR Morb Mortal Wkly Rep*. 2007;56(36):929-932

32. Jacobs JH, Spaan S, van Rooy GB, et al. Exposure to trichloramine and respiratory symptoms in indoor swimming pool workers. *Eur Respir J*. 2007;29(4):690–698

33. US Environmental Protection Agency, Office of Ground Water and Drinking Water. *List of Drinking Water Contaminants and MCLs*. Washington, DC: US Environmental Protection Agency; updated January 2011. http://www.epa.gov/safewater/contaminants/index.html. Accessed April 12, 2011

Chapter 18

Food Safety

This chapter focuses on a variety of contaminants in foods, including microbes, prions, pesticides, certain food additives, and mycotoxins. The chapter also discusses food irradiation and organic foods. Contamination of food by lead and mercury is described in Chapters 31 and 32, respectively.

PATHOGENIC HAZARDS

Although the US food supply is among the safest in the world, there are 76 million foodborne illnesses every year in the United States and an estimated 325 000 hospitalizations and 5000 deaths per year, mostly among the elderly and the very young.[1] The American Academy of Pediatrics (AAP) *Red Book* describes the diagnosis and treatment of illnesses caused by foodborne pathogens.[2] Contaminants in foods include:

- Viruses such as hepatitis A, norovirus, and rotavirus
- Bacteria such as *Salmonella* species, *Shigella* species, *Campylobacter* species, *Escherichia coli*, *Vibrio cholerae*, *Vibrio vulnificus*, *Yersinia enterocolitica*, *Brucella* species, and *Listeria* species
- Toxins from bacteria including *Staphylococcus aureus*, *Bacillus cereus*, *Clostridium perfringens*, *Clostridium botulinum*, and *E coli* O157:H7
- Toxins such as aflatoxins and vomitoxin produced by molds
- Parasites such as *Toxoplasma gondii*, *Cryptosporidium parvum*, *Cyclospora* species, *Giardia lamblia*, *Taenia* species, and *Trichinella spiralis*
- Products accumulated in the food chain of fish and shellfish, such as scombroid, saxitoxin, ciguatera toxin, tetrodotoxin, and domoic acid
- Prions, the agents of mad cow disease and other transmissible spongiform encephalopathies

The American Medical Association, Centers for Disease Control and Prevention (CDC), Food Safety and Inspection Service (FSIS), and US Food and Drug Administration (FDA) have produced a primer for physicians that describes the diagnosis and management of these foodborne illnesses.[3]

Infectious organisms are ubiquitous in the environment and can enter the food supply in a multitude of ways. Chickens infected with *Salmonella* species can excrete these organisms into their eggs before the shells are formed or excrete the organisms in feces that can contaminate egg shells. Shellfish and other seafood can become contaminated by pathogens, such as the hepatitis A virus in manure runoff and sewage overflows and *Anisakis simplex* (herring worm, a roundworm) in sushi. Animal feces can contaminate foods via polluted irrigation water, unsafe handling of manure, and unsanitary production and processing activities. Food can become contaminated in retail facilities, institutional settings, and homes because of inappropriate food handling. The major nonhuman use of antibiotics is in food animal production, and millions of pounds are used annually at nontherapeutic doses in healthy animals, contributing to increased antibiotic resistance in humans (see Chapter 56).

The food production system is becoming more centralized and global, adding to the complexity of foodborne pathogen exposures. For example, in the United States, there have been large outbreaks of infection attributable to *Cyclospora* species associated with raspberry consumption.[4,5] Extensive investigation identified the source as *Cyclospora*-contaminated irrigation water in Guatemalan raspberry fields. Severe outbreaks of hemolytic-uremic syndrome (HUS) and death attributable to *E coli* O157:H7-contaminated hamburger meat have involved the transport and blending of meats from various parts of the country, often with distribution to regions quite remote from the source of the contamination.[6,7] More recently, widespread outbreaks of salmonellosis have occurred, traceable to contaminated ground peanut products (*Salmonella typhimurium*) and contaminated imported jalapeño peppers (*Salmonella Saintpaul*).[8]

Since 1996, the CDC has used the FoodNet system to track incidence and trends of foodborne infections. From 2003-2008, no change was observed in the incidence of infections caused by *Campylobacter* species, *Cryptosporidium* species, *Cyclospora* species, *Listeria* species, Shiga toxin-producing *E coli* O157, *Salmonella* species, *Shigella* species, *Vibrio* species, and *Yersinia* species. Generally incidence of these infections was highest among children aged <4 years.[8] Many pathogens are particularly virulent for children. *Salmonella, Listeria, Cyclospora, Cryptosporidium, E coli* O157:H7, *Shigella*, and *Campylobacter* are among many foodborne pathogens that pose risks to young children.[1] In 2007 in the 10 FoodNet surveillance states, there were 77 cases of postdiarrheal hemolytic-uremic syndrome in children <18 years (0.73 cases/100 000 children). Most of these (68%) were in children younger than 5 years (1.75 cases/100 000 children).[8] Standards for pathogens are established for meat, poultry, and egg products by the Food Safety and Inspection Service and for all other foods by the FDA. State public health agencies, along with local public health officers, monitor the incidence of foodborne illness, and the US Environmental Protection Agency (EPA) regulates the discharge of pollutants into waters that may later contaminate food.

Powdered infant formula is not a sterile product and may be contaminated with bacteria. During 2001, powdered formula contaminated with *Enterobacter sakazakii* caused an epidemic of illnesses, including a fatal case of neonatal meningitis in Tennessee.[9]

The prion, the agent responsible for transmissible spongiform encephalopathies, is neither a virus nor a bacterium but an abnormal form of a normal glycoprotein. Prion diseases include bovine spongiform encephalopathy (mad cow disease), scrapie in sheep, chronic wasting disease in deer and elk, and Creutzfeldt-Jakob disease and variant Creutzfeldt-Jakob disease in humans.[10] In the United Kingdom, an epidemic of variant Creutzfeldt-Jakob disease has followed the epidemic of bovine spongiform encephalopathy.[11] Although one case of variant Creutzfeldt-Jakob disease has been identified in the United States, the patient was born in the United Kingdom in 1979 and moved to the United States in 1992.[12] This case is to be differentiated from the cases of Creutzfeld-Jakob disease in the United States secondary to injection of pituitary growth hormone extracted from pituitaries of infected individuals. Those cases resulted in removal of pituitary-derived growth hormone from the market, so now only recombinant growth hormone is available.

TOXIC HAZARDS

Toxic chemicals in food can be grouped into the following broad categories:

- Residues of pesticides deliberately applied to food crops or to stored or processed foods
- Colorings, flavorings, and other chemicals deliberately added to food during processing (direct food additives) and substances used in food-contact materials including adhesives, dyes, coatings, paper, paperboard, and polymers (plastics) that may come into contact with food as part of packaging or processing equipment but are not intended to be added directly to food (indirect food additives)
- Contaminants that inadvertently or purposely enter the food supply, such as aflatoxins, nitrites, polychlorinated biphenyls (PCBs), dioxins, metals including mercury, persistent pesticide residues such as dichlorodiphenyltrichloroethane (DDT), and vomitoxin

Pesticides

The diet is a major route of exposure of children to pesticides; exposure by other routes is described in Chapter 37.

Pesticides are applied extensively to food crops around the world. More than 400 different pesticidal active ingredients are formulated into thousands of products. Pesticides are used at all stages of food production to protect against pests in the field and in shipping and storage. In 2007, over 1.1 billion pounds of pesticides were used in the United States.[13] The EPA sets standards for allowable levels of pesticides on food, called "tolerances." In the United Status, pesticides must be registered with the EPA and the state before distribution. The FDA and the Food Safety and Inspection Service monitor the food supply for pesticide residues.

The Food Quality Protection Act of 1996 required that when the toxic risks for children are uncertain, the EPA will provide an additional margin of safety, referred to as an uncertainty factor, to ensure that children are adequately protected from excessive pesticide exposure. Significant features of the Food Quality Protection Act are shown in Table 18.1 (see also the Food Quality Protection Act text box in Chapter 37.)

Pesticide residues on individual commodities may be extremely variable. In the past, the EPA established residue levels to ensure that average levels were safe. However, in 1992, the EPA discovered that it is possible for individual food items (eg, potatoes and bananas) to have high enough levels to make a child acutely ill, even when the average level for the crop is within EPA standards. Such illnesses would be expected to be sporadic and, thus, not detectable by disease surveillance efforts.[14] Since enactment of the Food Quality Protection Act, the EPA has completed reassessing the 9721 food pesticide standards that existed in 1996; this involved a number of intensive studies of the pesticides on food commonly eaten by children.

Food Additives

Some food additives may cause adverse reactions in children. Tartrazine (also known as FD&C—food dye and coloring—yellow No. 5) is a dye used in some foods and beverages. Cake mixes, candies, canned vegetables, cheese, chewing gum, hot dogs, ice cream, orange drinks, salad dressings, seasoning salts, soft drinks, and catsup may contain tartrazine. An estimated 0.12% of the general population is intolerant to tartrazine. In those who are sensitive to it, tartrazine may cause urticaria and asthma exacerbations.

Monosodium glutamate (MSG) is associated with the so-called "Chinese restaurant syndrome" of headache, nausea, diarrhea, sweating, chest tightness, and a burning sensation along the back of the neck. It seems to be linked to the consumption of large amounts of MSG, not only in Chinese food but also in any other food in which a large concentration of MSG is used as a flavor enhancer.

Table 18.1: Food Quality Protection Act of 1996

Health-based standard
A new standard of a "reasonable certainty of no harm," with special consideration of children's special sensitivity and exposure to pesticide chemicals.

Additional margin of safety for children
Requires that the US EPA use an additional 10-fold margin of safety when setting standards for pesticides on food to account for prenatal and postnatal exposures when there are limited data on infants and children. Less than a 10-fold margin of safety may be used when there are adequate data to assess prenatal and postnatal risks.

Account for children's diets
Requires the use of age-appropriate estimates of dietary consumption in establishing allowable levels of pesticides on food to account for children's unique dietary patterns.

Account for all exposures
In establishing acceptable levels of a pesticide on food, the EPA must account for exposures that may occur via other routes, such as drinking water and residential application of the pesticide.

Cumulative effects
The EPA must consider the cumulative effects of all pesticides that share a common mechanism of action.

Tolerance reassessments
All existing pesticide food standards must be reassessed over a 10-year period to ensure that they meet the new health-based standard.

Endocrine disrupter testing
Incorporates provisions for endocrine testing by the EPA and also provides new authority to require that chemical manufacturers provide data on their products, including data on potential endocrine effects.

Registration renewal
Requires EPA to periodically review pesticide registrations, with a goal of establishing a 15-year cycle, to ensure that all pesticides meet updated safety standards.

Sulfites are used to preserve foods and sanitize containers for fermented beverages. They may be found in soup mixes, frozen and dehydrated potatoes, dried fruits, fruit juices, canned and dehydrated vegetables, processed seafood products, jams and jellies, relishes, and some bakery products. Some beverages, such as hard cider, wine, and beer, also contain sulfites. Because sulfites can cause asthma exacerbations in sulfite-sensitive patients, the FDA has ruled that packaged foods be labeled if they contain more than 10 parts per million (ppm) of sulfites.

Food Contact Substances

Indirect food additives are substances that enter the food supply through contact with food in manufacturing, packing, packaging, transporting, or holding, even though that substance is not intended to have any technical effects on the food. More than 3000 such substances are recognized by the FDA. One category is called "food contact substances"; these include packaging materials (adhesives and compounds of coatings, paper and paperboard products, polymers, adjuvants [agents added to increase the effect of the product], and production aids) and a wide array of other materials.

Recently, certain plastic substances have come under increased scrutiny as food contact items. One is bisphenol A (BPA, 2,2-bis[4-hydroxyphenyl] propane), which is made by combining acetone and phenol and is one of the highest-volume chemicals produced worldwide. Bisphenol A acts as a weak estrogen. It is used mainly as a material for the production of epoxy resins that are used to line metal cans and in hard plastics. Bisphenol A has been found in hard plastic baby bottles, water bottles, and many other food containers. The FDA has approved these uses; however, new scientific data on bisphenol A are accumulating. In a 2003-2004 US national sample, the median intake of bisphenol A was approximately three orders of magnitude below health-based guidance values of 50 µg/kg/day, with higher levels for children and teenagers than for older individuals.[15]

Phthalates are another class of plasticizers that may come into contact with food. Phthalates are used in soft plastics.[16] Phthalates are weak estrogens and antiandrogenic (androgen blocking) chemicals. Phthalates have numerous industrial uses (in industrial plastics, inks, and dyes and adhesives in food packaging), consumer uses (eg, in cosmetics and vinyl clothing), and medical uses (as a softener in polyvinyl chloride intravenous tubing, blood bags, and dialysis equipment). Over the years, phthalate compounds were used in pacifiers, baby bottle nipples, and teething toys and then removed from these uses by the US Consumer Product Safety Commission (CPSC).

As of February 2009, the Consumer Product Safety Improvement Act mandated that it is unlawful for any person to manufacture for sale, offer for sale, distribute in commerce, or import into the United States any children's toy or child care article that contains concentrations of more than 0.1% of the most commonly used phthalates (di[2-ethylhexyl] phthalate [DEHP], dibutyl phthalate [DBP], or benzyl-butyl phthalate [BBP]) and that it is unlawful for any person to manufacture for sale, offer for sale, distribute in commerce, or import into the United States any children's toy that can be placed in a child's mouth or child care article that contains concentrations of more than 0.1% of di-isononyl phthalate (DINP), di-isodecyl phthalate (DIDP), or di-n-octyl phthalate (DnOP).

The FDA allows the use of phthalates in food contact items and in the past has found that exposures are very low. The CDC tracks trends of phthalates in the human population. Bisphenol A and phthalates are further discussed in Chapter 38.

Mycotoxins

Mycotoxins, toxins produced by certain molds, are present in many agricultural products, such as peanuts, corn, and wheat.[17] The best known mycotoxin, aflatoxin, is produced by the *Aspergillus* fungus. Others include patulin, citrinin, zearalenone, vomitoxin, and the trichothecenes.

The principal human exposure to aflatoxins is from food. The International Agency for Research on Cancer (IARC) has concluded that aflatoxin is a carcinogen[18] on the basis of studies conducted in areas with a high incidence of hepatocellular carcinoma, such as Asia, where the incidence of chronic hepatitis B viral infections also is high. Aflatoxin B_1 is an important risk factor for the development of hepatocellular carcinoma in humans.[19-21]

Vomitoxin, a frequent contaminant of corn and wheat products, can lead to epidemics of vomiting within hours of consuming contaminated food. The disease usually is self-limiting.[22]

Dioxins and PCBs

Dioxins and furans are produced inadvertently during the manufacture of certain chemicals and by incineration. PCBs were manufactured for use as fire retardants and in electrical transformers and capacitors. Dioxins and PCBs are persistent and bioaccumulative chemicals and are found at highest levels in fish in contaminated areas. They can also enter the food supply via animal feed. In the United States in 1998 and in Belgium in 1999, there were episodes in which a large proportion of the food supply (chickens, eggs, and catfish in the United States and chicken and eggs in Belgium) became contaminated by dioxins as a result of adulteration of animal feeds.[23,24] In 2001, the European Commission established a tolerable weekly intake of dioxins and dioxin-like PCBs in the diet.[25] There is no regulatory standard for these compounds in food in the United States (see Chapter 35).

Melamine

Melamine is a monomeric chemical that, when polymerized, makes a hard material that can be molded into dishes or containers or used as a laminate. The polymer also is called melamine. Each molecule of melamine contains 4 nitrogen atoms. Melamine was recently identified as an illegal additive found in certain foods from China including infant formula, various milk and milk-derived products, and dog and cat food. The melamine problem was first identified in China in 2007 when a number of cats and small dogs developed mysterious illnesses involving urinary stones, renal failure, and death. Illnesses were traced to the presence of melamine in a wide variety of pet foods, eventually traced to a single source of protein powder.[26] It had been a standard practice to test the protein content of foods through chemical assessment of total nitrogen atoms. Melamine was used as a food additive for the purpose of defrauding purchasers by artificially inflating protein content of foods, thereby making them appear suitable for consumption by pets or infants, when they were not. In urine, melamine and its breakdown products precipitate and form calculi. In 2007 and 2008, thousands of infants across China were reported to have urinary tract symptoms involving calculi; there were an unknown number of deaths linked to melamine-contaminated infant formula.[27,28] One specific brand of infant formula was identified; it is not marketed in the United States. However, melamine has now been identified in other foods in the United States, at much lower levels. At this time, the FDA is not concerned about these lower levels of melamine. Melamine dishware has not been implicated as a source of melamine contamination of food.

FOOD IRRADIATION

Food irradiation is a process by which food is exposed to a controlled source of ionizing radiation to prolong shelf life and reduce food losses, improve microbiological safety, and/or reduce the use of chemical fumigants and additives. It can be used to reduce insect infestation of grain, dried spices, and dried or fresh fruits and vegetables; inhibit sprouting in tubers and bulbs; retard postharvest ripening of fruits; inactivate parasites in meats and fish; eliminate spoilage microbes from fresh fruits and vegetables; extend shelf life in poultry, meats, fish, and shellfish; decontaminate poultry and beef; and sterilize foods and feeds.[29]

The dose of ionizing radiation determines the effects of the process on foods. Food generally is irradiated at levels from 50 Gray (Gy) to 10 kiloGray (kGy) (1 kGy = 1000 Gy), depending on the goals of the process. Low-dose irradiation (up to 1 kGy) primarily is used to delay ripening of produce or kill or render sterile insects and other higher organisms that may infest fresh food. Medium-dose irradiation (1–10 kGy) reduces the number of pathogens and other microbes on food and prolongs shelf life. High-dose irradiation (>10 kGy) sterilizes food.[30]

Food irradiation is considered a "process" by many nations. The US Congress explicitly included sources of irradiation as "food additives" under the 1958 Food Additives Amendment to the Federal Food, Drug, and Cosmetic Act of 1938.[31] Thus, irradiated food is defined as adulterated and illegal to market unless irradiation conforms to specified federal rules. The technical effect on the food, dosimetry, and environmental controls must be defined and in compliance with the Federal Food, Drug, and Cosmetic Act. Facilities also must pass an environmental impact study to comply with the National Environmental Policy Act of 1969. Nutritional adequacy as well as radiologic, toxicologic, and microbiological safety must be ensured under FDA regulations.

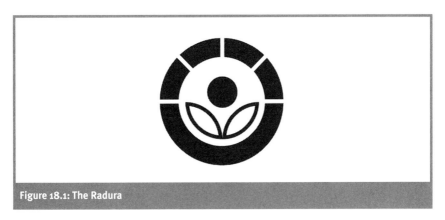

Figure 18.1: The Radura

All irradiated food sold in the United States must be labeled with the international sign of irradiation, the radura (Fig 18.1). Current labeling rules do not require that the dose of the irradiation or the purpose of the irradiation be specified.[32] Thus, it is not possible for consumers to know whether food has been treated to reduce pathogen loads or merely to prolong shelf life. Furthermore, current rules do not require food services to identify irradiated foods they serve.

In considering the safety of irradiated food, radiologic, toxicologic, micro-biologic, nutritional and, palatability factors are considered. In terms of radio-logic safety, neither the food nor the packaging materials become radioactive as a result of irradiation.[33] The sources of radiation approved for use in food irradiation are limited to those producing energy too low to induce formation of radioactive compounds or radioactive atomic species. Although in theory, radiation could cause undesired reactions of food chemicals and creation of toxic compounds, hundreds of studies have failed to identify any unique toxic compounds created during irradiation (versus canning, freezing, drying, etc) in amounts large enough to cause harm. Feeding studies and analytical chemical modeling studies have failed to identify any unusual toxicity associated with irradiation.[34] Further, heat-processed foods can contain 50 to 500 times the number of changed molecules than do irradiated foods.[35] Microbial safety of irradiated foods mainly has to do with pathogens that are relatively resistant to radiation. Microbes in food include those added intentionally to produce fermentation, those that cause spoilage, rendering it unpalatable, and patho-gens including invasive and toxigenic bacteria, toxigenic molds, viruses, and parasites.[30] Irradiation kills microbes primarily by fragmenting DNA. Viruses, spores, cysts, toxins, and prions are quite resistant to the effects of irradiation, because they contain little or no DNA and/or are in highly stable resting states. Generally, irradiated food would most likely spoil long before becoming pathogenic.[36] However, sporulating toxin-producing bacteria are approximately 10 times more resistant to radiation than are nonspore formers. For example,

Clostridium botulinum type E, found in fish and seafood, can survive nonsterilizing doses of irradiation intended to extend shelf life. When refrigerated long enough at 10°C or higher, toxin formation can occur. Thus, it may be possible for food to become toxic with botulinum toxin before it is obviously spoiled.[37] Conditions that allow for toxin formation before spoilage, such as inadequate refrigeration, are well understood, and regulations can be designed to mitigate against such occurrences. This concern also applies to other nonsterilizing food processing technologies, such as heat, to which spore-forming bacteria also are relatively resistant. Similar concerns exist about mycotoxins. Experimental data are conflicting, but some studies show an increase in mycotoxin formation after irradiation.[38]

Irradiation can have a negative effect on some nutrients, similar to those resulting from cooking, canning, and other heat processing of foods. Slight loss of essential polyunsaturated fatty acids does occur with irradiation, but fats and oils that are major dietary sources of these nutrients tend to become rancid when irradiated and are not good candidates for this treatment.[39] Vitamin loss is the largest nutritional concern when foods are irradiated. Whole foods exert a protective effect on vitamins, because most of the radiation dose is absorbed by macromolecules (proteins, carbohydrates, and fats). Losses can be minimized by irradiating at low temperatures, at low doses, and by excluding oxygen and light.[30] When studied in pure solution, the water-soluble vitamins most sensitive to irradiation are thiamine (B_1), pyridoxine (B_6), and riboflavin (B_2). Of the fat-soluble vitamins, E and A are sensitive.[35] More than 50% of thiamine (found in meats, milk, whole grains, and legumes) can be lost after irradiation.[35] If all sources of thiamine come from irradiated products, a deficiency condition could develop, but this is unlikely in the United States. Likewise, vitamin E loss can be significant after irradiation, especially in conjunction with cooking.[35] Many of the sources of vitamin E—cereal grains, seed oils, peanuts, soybeans, milk fat, and turnip greens—are unlikely to be treated with radiation and should provide for adequate alternative sources in a balanced and varied diet. In general, irradiated food is quite nutritious. As long as a diet is balanced and food choices are varied, deficiency states are unlikely to develop.

Palatability—taste, texture, color, and smell—can be affected by food irradiation, particularly in foods with high fat content. Modified conditions, such as excluding oxygen from the atmosphere, lowering the temperature, excluding light, reducing water content, or lowering the radiation dose, can minimize or eliminate these changes. These same modifications also can minimize vitamin loss.

Irradiated food is safe and nutritious and produces no unusual toxicity as long as best management practices are followed. However, irradiation of food does not substitute for careful food handling from farm to fork.[38] Widespread use of food irradiation would require construction of irradiation facilities in the United

States and other countries. The benefits of expanding this technology and the risks involved must be thoroughly debated. Pediatricians should participate in the dialogue. As with any technology, unforeseen consequences are possible. Therefore, careful monitoring and continuous evaluation of this and all food processing techniques are prudent precautions.

ORGANIC FOODS

Organic farming uses an approach to growing crops and raising livestock that avoids synthetic chemicals, hormones, antibiotics, genetic engineering, and irradiation. In response to the Organic Foods Production Act (http://www.ams. usda.gov/AMSv1.0/getfile?dDocName=STELPRDC5060370&acct=nopgen info), the US Department of Agriculture (USDA) implemented the National Organic Program (http://www.ams.usda.gov/AMSv1.0/nop). Labeling standards set by the National Organic Program have been in effect since October 2002. The National Organic Program organic food production standards include many specific requirements for crops and livestock. To qualify as organic, crops must be produced on farms that meet requirements that include avoiding the use of most synthetic pesticides, herbicides, and fertilizer for 3 years before harvest, and having a sufficient buffer zone to decrease contamination from adjacent lands. Organic livestock must be reared without the routine use of antibiotics or growth hormones, be provided with access to the outdoors, and meet other requirements. The USDA certifies organic products according to these guidelines. Organic farmers must apply for certification, pass a test, and pay a fee. The National Organic Program requires annual inspections to ensure ongoing compliance with these standards.

Although some consumers believe that organic produce is more nutritious, the research has not substantiated this belief. A large systematic review published in 2009 found that less than 20% of 292 articles with potentially relevant titles met criteria for quality, leaving only 55 studies to assess. Because of the large number of nutrients reported in the various articles, the authors grouped the nutrients into large categories. They found no significant differences in most nutrients with the exception of higher nitrogen in conventional produce and higher titratable acidity and phosphorus in organic produce.[40]

The primary form of exposure to pesticides in children is via dietary intake.[41] Organic produce consistently has lower levels of pesticide residues than conventionally grown produce.[42] Several studies also clearly demonstrate that an organic diet protects against exposure to pesticides commonly used in conventional agricultural production. A small longitudinal cohort of children who regularly consumed conventional produce demonstrated that urinary pesticide residues were reduced to almost nondetectable levels (from approximately 1.5 µg/L to 0.3 µg/L for malathion dicarboxylic acid, for example) when they were changed to an organic produce diet for 5 days.[43] It remains unclear whether such a reduction in exposure is clinically relevant.

One major concern with organic food is its higher price to consumers. Organic products typically cost 10% to 40% more than similar conventionally produced products. A number of factors contribute to these higher costs, including higher-priced organic animal feed, lower productivity, and higher labor costs because of the increased reliance on hand weeding. Of potential concern is that the higher price of organically produced fruits and vegetables might lead consumers to eat less of these foods, decreasing the well-established health benefits of eating fruits and vegetables.

SEX STEROIDS AND BOVINE GROWTH HORMONE

Cattle may be treated with sex steroids to increase their lean muscle mass, thus promoting meat yield. It has been postulated that estrogen ingested from food may play a role in earlier development of puberty and an increased risk of breast cancer. A 7-year longitudinal study of more than 39 000 women assessing their history of foods eaten while they were in high school revealed an increased risk (relative risk of 1.34) of developing premenopausal breast cancer in those who recalled eating more red meat. However, study findings were limited by reliance on the subjects' long-term memory of the amount of food eaten while in high school and lacked direct measurement of hormonal exposure.[44]

Examinations of the nutrient content of milk must account for the breed of cows and food supplements provided to the cows. In general, milk from both organic and conventionally reared cows has the same protein, vitamin, trace mineral content and lipids. Another consideration is the potential effect of using bovine growth hormone (ie, recombinant bovine somatotropin), which is applied to cows by injection to increase milk yield. There is no evidence that the gross composition of milk is altered by treatment with bovine growth hormone, nor is there any evidence that the vitamin and mineral contents of milk are changed by growth hormone treatment. Approximately 90% of bovine growth hormone in milk is destroyed during pasteurization. There is no evidence that conventional milk contains significantly increased amounts of bovine growth hormone as compared with organic milk. Growth hormone is destroyed in the gastrointestinal tract when given orally and must be injected to retain biologic activity. Furthermore, bovine growth hormone is very species specific and is biologically inactive in humans. Because of this, any bovine growth hormone present in food products has no physiological effect on humans.[45]

PREVENTION OF FOOD CONTAMINATION

Care must be taken during food production and preparation to prevent the introduction of pathogens and other contaminants into the food supply. When used in the manufacturing process, these methods are referred to as Hazard

Analysis and Critical Control Point systems. These systems require that food manufacturers identify points at which contamination is likely to occur and implement control processes to prevent it. Also important are efforts to prevent antibiotic resistance; control use of pesticides and food additives; prevent environmental contamination of food; provide consumer education about proper preparation and storage of foods, pasteurization, irradiation of food, protection of animal health, and prevention of discharge of pathogens and nitrogen into water bodies; and other efforts.

Food contamination is best prevented by application of appropriate agricultural and manufacturing practices. Integrated pest management, which uses information about pest biology to control pests, is a means to reduce the risks and use of pesticides (see Chapter 37).

Enforcement of food safety laws is important in prevention at all levels. Regulation and enforcement involve a complex network of federal, state, and local laws and regulations. Some enforcement efforts involve routine monitoring and surveillance of the food supply; other efforts are in response to reports of problems and incidents. Pediatricians have an important role in reporting foodborne illnesses to local and state public health agencies. For example, physician reports of outbreaks of hemolytic-uremic syndrome caused by *E coli* O157:H7 led to stronger enforcement efforts to ensure that foods such as hamburger meat and apple juice are safe to consume. Table 18.2 lists steps to reduce the likelihood of foodborne illness resulting from pathogens.

FOODS DEVELOPED USING BIOTECHNOLOGY

Food engineered through biotechnology is now common. Through genetic engineering, unique traits can be inserted into the genes of plants and animals, thereby causing the organism to predictably express the new trait. This technology has been very controversial. Many argue that newly expressed traits are harmless and that selecting desirable traits has gone on for centuries. Others argue that there are too many uncertainties in the new technology and that the scientific information used to develop regulation is inconclusive.

Although the debate continues, genetically engineered food likely will be maintained in the United States as new products are developed and approved. Genetically modified foods now include corn, soybeans, rice, potatoes, milk, and a dozen or so other products. Before genetically modified food products are commercialized, the FDA, EPA, and USDA conduct scientific reviews to help ensure the safety of these products. Specifically, the FDA conducts a premarket notification and safety review of bioengineered foods to ensure they meet the safety standards in the Federal Food, Drug, and Cosmetic Act. If products have been genetically modified to express a pesticide for insect or disease control, the EPA is responsible for conducting a rigorous scientific review process to ensure the product will not cause unreasonable adverse effects on people or the

Table 18.2: Steps to Reduce the Likelihood of Foodborne Illness Resulting From Pathogens in Food
■ Thoroughly wash fruits and vegetables with water to remove some pathogens and many pesticide residues. Wash before you peel. Don't peel anything you wouldn't normally peel. It is unnecessary to use soap or chemicals when washing food.
■ Raw eggs, fish, and meat should not be eaten, and unpasteurized milk products should not be consumed.
■ Thoroughly cook meat, poultry, and eggs to ensure that pathogens are killed. For hamburgers, a thermometer inserted into the center should read 160°F.
■ After poultry is prepared, hands, cutting boards, and implements used on raw poultry should be washed with soap and hot water. Cook stuffings for poultry separately rather than inside the birds.
■ Store food appropriately. Refrigeration of prepared food prevents growth of many microorganisms responsible for food poisoning.
■ Use soap and water to wash hands and surfaces in order to prevent transmission of pathogens from food. At this time, incorporation of chemical agents into high-chair trays and cutting boards, and similar practices do not have a role in preventing foodborne infections. It also is unnecessary to use chemical disinfectants for washing hands in the home; soap and water are quite effective.

environment. To ensure that the new technology does not jeopardize existing plants or animals, the USDA conducts premarket reviews.

It may be difficult to determine whether a food has been genetically modified. Although there are simple and inexpensive testing procedures available to identify genetically modified corn, there are not simple tests available for many other food products produced using biotechnology. Because the genetic modifications vary according to trait, the testing regimen can require identification of exact gene sequences and sophisticated equipment. To expand the testing capacity, there are a variety of products under development (eg, strip tests) that will detect the presence of genetically modified material.

As the government regulatory process and the science underlying biotechnology are evolving and improving, questions still remain on the safety of these products. It is important that the government and scientific and medical communities remain vigilant to monitor possible adverse effects from and ensure the safety of foods produced using biotechnology.

Frequently Asked Questions

Q *Are there pesticides on fresh vegetables found in the store?*

A Pesticides commonly are found on fruits and vegetables in the store. Because no labeling is required, parents and other consumers cannot tell which fruits and vegetables contain pesticides. Even organically grown fruits and vegetables are not necessarily pesticide free. Parents should be advised to scrub all fruits and vegetables under running water to remove superficial particle residues. Fruits and vegetables are good for children, because they provide vitamins, minerals, and roughage. Because of these health benefits, children should continue to consume a wide variety of fruits and vegetables, particularly those grown in season.

Q   *Are there pesticides in store-bought baby food?*

A   Processed foods generally contain lower residues of pesticides than fresh fruits and vegetables, in part because federal standards are stricter for processed foods. Some makers of baby foods voluntarily make their products free of all pesticide residues, although they do not advertise this action.

Q   *Could cancer develop in my child because of exposure to pesticides?*

A   Many factors contribute to cancer, including genetics, contact with viruses, and diet. More research is needed to determine how and why cancers develop during childhood. No causal relationship between exposure to pesticides in food and childhood cancer has been established. A number of pesticides can cause tumors in laboratory animals and are associated with cancer in some farm workers exposed to very high doses.

Q   *Are organic foods safer than other foods?*

A   It is not known whether organic foods are safer than other foods. However, under standards set by the National Organic Program, organic foods must meet additional requirements. They must be grown without pesticides or chemical fertilizers and they must not use biotechnology-bred plants. There should be lower levels of pesticide residues on foods marketed as organic. (This was true even before the standard was in place.)

Q   *What is the concern about peanut butter?*

A   There have been several concerns. The first concern is that many children are allergic to peanuts. Peanuts are among the most potent of food allergens; for some individuals, even a minute amount of peanut can cause serious or even fatal allergic responses. Therefore, it is important that children who have allergies to peanuts strictly avoid peanut butter; this avoidance sometimes means that other children in close contact with such a child should not have peanut butter (or other foods containing peanuts), because children often share foods. Children who have had an anaphylactic reaction to peanuts should have an auto-injector epinephrine device available. The second concern is that peanuts can contain higher levels of carcinogenic aflatoxins. In the United States, there are standards for aflatoxins; however, peanut butter is not frequently monitored. The third is the possibility of microbial contamination of peanut butter and other peanut products, as evidenced by the discovery of *Salmonella*-contaminated peanut products in the United States in 2009. Fourth, there have been past concerns with arsenical pesticides used for other crops drifting into peanut fields and, thus, into peanut butter. In the United States today, stricter enforcement of pesticide laws has addressed this situation. Finally, another significant concern with peanut butter is the potential for choking. Similar to latex balloons, peanut butter can conform to the airway and form a tenacious seal difficult to dislodge or extract.

Q *Are pesticides in foods 10 times more hazardous for children than adults?*

A Many scientists recognize that children may be more susceptible to the effects of pesticides and other chemicals. To account for this difference, which often has not been quantified, standards for pesticides in foods generally include a 10-fold margin of safety.

Q *I heard that hot dogs can cause brain cancer in children. Should my children avoid hot dogs?*

A Sodium nitrite prevents the growth of *Clostridium botulinum* in meat products. In the early 1990s, consumption of nitrite-cured hot dogs was reported to be associated with brain cancer in a group of children in California. Although more research needs to be performed to confirm this association, manufacturers have been working to reduce the amount of nitrite in their cured meat products. Children should eat a balanced diet, and an occasional hot dog may be a part of that diet. Young children, however, should not be given hot dogs, because of the danger of choking.

Q *What can I do to prevent my children from eating products contaminated with prions (the agents of mad cow disease)?*

A Avoid consumption of brains or any food containing nerve tissue. Although there have been no cases of bovine spongiform encephalopathy (mad cow disease) reported in the United States, there have been confirmed cases of chronic wasting disease, a spongiform encephalopathy of deer and elk, in the western and midwestern states. Avoid feeding children products made with deer or elk from areas known to have chronic wasting disease.

Q *Are bioengineered food products required to be labeled?*

A No. The FDA does not require labeling to indicate whether a food or food ingredient is a bioengineered product. Currently, the FDA has guidance available for companies that wish to voluntarily label their bioengineered food products.

Q *I'm worried that the nonnutritive or artificial sweeteners will cause cancer, but I'm also worried about my child's weight, so what should I do?*

A There are 5 nonnutritive sweeteners that have FDA approval in the United States. These substances are hundreds of times sweeter than sugar, so only minute amounts are needed to sweeten foods. No studies have found a link between use of nonnutritive sweeteners and cancer in humans. A study in rats performed in the 1970s found an association between bladder cancer and use of saccharine; however, the mechanism for cancer development in rats from saccharine exposure may not apply to humans. There is a wide range of nutritive and nonnutritive sweeteners available in the food supply that can be blended to keep intakes of nonnutritive sweeteners in children well below acceptable daily intakes and reduce excessive calories or other negative effects of nutritive sweeteners. Drinking water is a good alternative to artificially sweetened drinks.

Q *Can I safely feed my children rare hamburger if it has been irradiated?*
A No. Do not feed children rare hamburger. The label is not required to specify the dose of irradiation used or the purpose for use, so irradiated food can be legally labeled as such when it has received very low-dose irradiation designed only to prolong shelf life but not to reduce pathogen loads. Irradiation can never replace careful food handling and adequate cooking. Children (and others) should not consume undercooked hamburger.

Q *Doesn't irradiation create toxic chemicals in food that are dangerous to children?*
A During early reviews of the safety of irradiated foods, the FDA coined the term "unique radiolytic products" to describe the theoretical possibility that molecules unique to the process of food irradiation could be generated.[46] This term has been abandoned, because any product produced through food irradiation has eventually been found in foods processed in more conventional ways.

Q *Can irradiation be used to hide the fact that food has spoiled and allow bad food to be sold to the public?*
A Spoiled food has undergone irreversible changes in texture, flavor, smell, and color. Irradiation cannot mask these.

Q *When food is irradiated in the package, do chemicals from the packaging get into the food? Is that dangerous for children?*
A One great advantage of irradiation is that it can be accomplished after foods are packaged, preventing recontamination during subsequent handling. Breakdown products of packaging do migrate into food as a result of irradiation. Components that migrate into food from packaging are classified by the FDA as indirect food additives. Toxicologic testing of indirect food additives is required if anticipated exposure levels exceed a regulatory limit.[47] These exposure levels are calculated for adults and may not be safe for infants and children. Additionally, indirect food additives after irradiation were evaluated based on packaging materials available 10 to 30 years ago. Studies of the effects of irradiation on foods packaged in modern materials are ongoing.

Q *Can increased use of food irradiation create resistant or mutant bacteria and viruses that could cause human disease?*

A Induction of radiation-resistant microbial populations occurs when cultures are experimentally exposed to repeated cycles of radiation.[48,49] Mutations in bacteria and other organisms develop with any form of food processing; ionizing radiation does not produce mutations by unique mechanisms. Mutations from any cause can result in greater, less, or similar levels of virulence or pathogenicity from parent organisms. Although it remains a theoretical risk, several major international reviews cite no reports of the induction of novel pathogens attributable to food irradiation.[50]

Q *Are the benefits of food irradiation worth the risks of the technology?*

A This is the central issue that is debated by proponents and detractors of the technology.[51,52] In the United States, there are sufficient alternatives to food production, handling, storage, and preparation to make irradiation unnecessary for most foods and for most people in the population. Individuals who are opposed to nuclear technologies can easily and safely avoid consumption of irradiated foods.

Q *Will irradiation eliminate foodborne illness?*

A No. Most foodborne illness (approximately 67%) is caused by viruses, which are not killed by food irradiation. Among all illnesses attributable to foodborne transmission, only about 30% are caused by bacteria, and about 3% are caused by parasites. Thus, an estimated 33% of foodborne illness (those attributable to bacteria and parasites) may potentially be prevented by food irradiation.[53]

Q *Will irradiation kill prions?*

A No. Irradiation does not kill prions, the agents of bovine spongiform encephalopathy.

Resources

Gateway to Government Food Safety Information: Food Irradiation
Web site: www.foodsafety.gov/~fsg/irradiat.html

International Atomic Energy Agency
Web site: www.iaea.org/programmes/nafa/d5/index.html
Facts about food irradiation: www.iaea.org/icgfi/documents/foodirradiation.pdf

Iowa State University
Web site: www.extension.iastate.edu/foodsafety/rad/irradhome.html

US Department of Agriculture
Meat and Poultry Hotline: 800-535-4555
Web site: www.usda.gov

References

1. Mead PS, Slutsker L, Dietz V, et al. Food-related illness and death in the United States. *Emerg Infect Dis.* 1999;5(5):607-625
2. American Academy of Pediatrics. *Red Book: 2009 Report of the Committee on Infectious Diseases.* Pickering LK, Baker CJ, Kimberlin DW, Long SS, ed. 28th ed. ed. Elk Grove Village, IL: American Academy of Pediatrics; 2009
3. American Medical Association, Centers for Disease Control and Prevention, Food and Drug Administration, Food Safety and Inspection Service. *Diagnosis and Management of Foodborne Illnesses: A Primer for Physicians.* Chicago, IL: American Medical Association; 2004
4. Herwaldt BL, Beach MJ. The return of *Cyclospora* in 1997: another outbreak of cyclosporiasis in North America associated with imported raspberries. *Cyclospora* Working Group. *Ann Intern Med.* 1999;130(3):210-220
5. Ho AY, Lopez AS, Eberhart MG, et al. Outbreak of cyclosporiasis associated with imported raspberries, Philadelphia, Pennsylvania, 2000. *Emerg Infect Dis.* 2002;8(8):783-788
6. Slutsker L, Ries AA, Maloney K, Wells JG, Greene KD, Griffin PM. A nationwide case-control study of *Escherichia coli* O157:H7 infection in the United States. *J Infect Dis.* 1998;177(4):962-966
7. Tuttle J, Gomez T, Doyle MP, et al. Lessons from a large outbreak of *Escherichia coli* O157:H7 infections: insights into the infectious dose and method of widespread contamination of hamburger patties. *Epidemiol Infect.* 1999;122(2):185-192
8. Centers for Disease Control and Prevention. Preliminary FoodNet Data on the incidence of infection with pathogens transmitted commonly through food—10 states, 2008. *MMWR Morb Mortal Wkly Rep.* 2009;58(13):333-337
9. Centers for Disease Control and Prevention. *Enterobacter sakazakii* infections associated with the use of powdered infant formula—Tennessee, 2001. *MMWR Morb Mortal Wkly Rep.* 2002;51(14):297-300
10. American Academy of Pediatrics, Committee on Infectious Diseases. Technical report: transmissible spongiform encephalopathies: a review for pediatricians. *Pediatrics.* 2000;106(5):1160-1165
11. Spencer MD, Knight RS, Will RG. First hundred cases of variant Creutzfeldt-Jakob disease: retrospective case note review of early psychiatric and neurological features. *BMJ.* 2002;324(7352):1479-1482
12. Centers for Disease Control and Prevention. Probable variant Creutzfeldt-Jakob disease in a U.S. resident—Florida, 2002. *MMWR Morb Mortal Wkly Rep.* 2002;51(41):927-929
13. Aspelin AL, Grube AH. *Pesticide Industry Sales and Usage: 2006 and 2007 Market Estimates.* Washington, DC: US Environmental Protection Agency, Office of Chemical Safety and Pollution Prevention; February 2011. Report No. EPA 733-R-11-001.
14. Goldman LR. Children—unique and vulnerable. Environmental risks facing children and recommendations for response. *Environ Health Perspect.* 1995;103(Suppl 6):13-18
15. Lakind JS, Naimanb DQ. Bisphenol A (BPA) daily intakes in the United States: estimates from the 2003–2004 NHANES urinary BPA data. *J Expo Sci Environ Epidemiol.* 2008;18(6):608–615
16. Shea KM; American Academy of Pediatrics, Committee on Environmental Health. Pediatric exposure and potential toxicity of phthalate plasticizers. *Pediatrics.* 2003;111(6 Pt 1):1467-1474

17. Morgan MR, Fenwick GR. Natural foodborne toxicants. *Lancet.* 1990;336(8729):1492-1495
18. International Agency for Research on Cancer. Aflatoxins: naturally occurring aflatoxins (group 1). Aflatoxin M₁ (group 2B). *IARC Monogr.* 2002;82:171
19. Alpert ME, Hutt MS, Wogan GN, Davidson CS. Association between aflatoxin content of food and hepatoma frequency in Uganda. *Cancer.* 1971;28(1):253-260
20. Yeh FS, Yu MC, Mo CC, Luo S, Tong MJ, Henderson BE. Hepatitis B virus, aflatoxins, and hepatocellular carcinoma in southern Guangxi, China. *Cancer Res.* 1989;49(9):2506-2509
21. Yeh F. Aflatoxin consumption and primary liver cancer: a case control study in the USA. *J Cancer.* 1989;42:325–328
22. Etzel RA. Mycotoxins. *JAMA.* 2002;287(4):425-427
23. Bernard A, Hermans C, Broeckaert F, De Poorter G, De Cock A, Houins G. Food contamination by PCBs and dioxins. *Nature.* 1999;401(6750):231-232
24. Hayward D, Nortrup D, Gardiner A, Clower M. Elevated TCDD in chicken eggs and farm-raised catfish fed a diet containing ball clay from a Southern United States mine. *Environ Res.* 1999;81(3):248-256
25. European Commission. Commission Press Release: Dioxin in food. Byrne welcomes adoption by Council of dioxin limits in food [press release]. Brussels, Belgium: European Commission; November 29, 2001. Report No. IP/01/1698
26. Melamine adulterates component of pellet feeds. *J Am Vet Med Assoc.* 2007;231(1):17
27. Zhang L, Wu LL, Wang YP, Liu AM, Zou CC, Zhao ZY. Melamine-contaminated milk products induced urinary tract calculi in children. *World J Pediatr.* 2009;5(1):31-35
28. Chen JS. A worldwide food safety concern in 2008—melamine-contaminated infant formula in China caused urinary tract stone in 290,000 children in China. *Chin Med J (Engl).* 2009;122(3):243-244
29. American Academy of Pediatrics, Committee on Environmental Health. Technical report: irradiation of food. *Pediatrics.* 2000;106(6):1505-1510
30. Murano E. *Food Irradiation: A Source Book.* Ames, Iowa: Iowa State University Press; 1995
31. Derr D. International regulatory status and harmonization of food irradiation. *J Food Prot.* 1993;56:882-886, 892
32. US Food and Drug Administration. Irradiation in the production, processing, and handling of food. *Fed Regist.* 1999;64:7834–7837
33. Urbain W. *Food Irradiation.* Orlando, FL: Academic Press Inc; 1986
34. World Health Organization. *High-Dose Irradiation: Wholesomeness of Food Irradiated With Doses Above 10 kGy.* Report of a Joint FAO/IAEA/WHO Study Group. Geneva, Switzerland: World Health Organization; 1999. Report No. WHO Technical Report Series 890
35. Diehl J. *Safety of Irradiated Food.* 3rd ed. New York: Marcel Dekker; 1999
36. US Food and Drug Administration. Irradiation in the production, processing, and handling of food. *Fed Regist.* 1997;62:64107-64121
37. Farkas J. Microbiological safety of irradiated foods. *Int J Food Microbiol.* 1989;9(1):1-15
38. Thayer D. Food irradiation: benefits and concerns. *J Food Qual.* 1990;13:147-169
39. World Health Organization. *Safety and Nutritional Adequacy of Irradiated Food.* Geneva, Switzerland: World Health Organization; 1994
40. Dangour AD, Dodhia SK, Hayter A, Allen E, Lock K, Uauy R. Nutritional quality of organic foods: a systematic review. *Am J Clin Nutr.* 2009;90(3):680-685
41. National Research Council. *Pesticides in the Diets of Infants and Children.* Washington, DC: National Academies Press; 1993
42. Baker B, Benbrook C, Groth III E, Benbrook K. Pesticide residues in conventional, IPM grown and organic foods: Insights from three U.S. data sets. *Food Addit Contam.* 2002;19(5):427-446

43. Lu C, Barr DB, Pearson MA, Waller LA. Dietary intake and its contribution to longitudinal organophosphorus pesticide exposure in urban/suburban children. *Environ Health Perspect.* 2008;116(4):537-542

44. Linos E, Willett WC, Cho E, Colditz G, Frazier LA. Red meat consumption during adolescence among premenopausal women and risk of breast cancer. *Cancer Epidemiol Biomarkers Prev.* 2008;17(8):2146–2151

45. Food and Drug Administration. *Report on the Food and Drug Administration's Review of the Safety of Recombinant Bovine Somatotropin.* Available at: http://www.fda.gov/AnimalVeterinary/SafetyHealth/ProductSafetyInformation/ucm130321.htm. Accessed March 3, 2011

46. Lagunas-Solar M. Radiation processing of foods: an overview of scientific principles and current status. *J Food Prot.* 1995;58:186-192

47. Food and Drug Administration, Center for Food Safety and Applied Nutrition, Office of Premarket Approval. *Guidance for Submitting Requests Under Threshold of Regulation for Substances Used in Food-Contact Articles.* Washington, DC: US Department of Health and Human Services; 2005. Report No. 21 CFR 170.39

48. Corry JE, Roberts TA. A note on the development of resistance to heat and gamma radiation in *Salmonella. J Appl Bacteriol.* 1970;33(4):733-737

49. Davies R, Sinskey AJ. Radiation-resistant mutants of *Salmonella typhimurium* LT2: development and characterization. *J Bacteriol.* 1973;113(1):133-144

50. World Health Organization. *Wholesomeness of Irradiated Food. Report of a Joint FAO/IAEA/WHO Study Group.* Geneva, Switzerland: World Health Organization; 1981. Report No. WHO Technical Report Series 659

51. Tauxe RV. Food safety and irradiation: protecting the public from foodborne infections. *Emerg Infect Dis.* 2001;7(3 Suppl):516-521

52. Louria DB. Counterpoint on food irradiation. *Int J Infect Dis.* 2000;4(2):67-69

53. Etzel R. Epidemiology of foodborne illness—role of food irradiation. In: Loaharanu P, Thomas P, eds. *Irradiation for Food Safety and Quality.* Lancaster PA: Technomic Publishing Co; 2001:50-54

Chapter 19

Herbs, Dietary Supplements, and Other Remedies

■ ■ ■ ■ ■ ■

A dietary supplement can be defined as a product (other than tobacco) that contains one or more of the following ingredients: a vitamin, a mineral, an herb or other botanical, or an amino acid; a dietary substance that supplements the normal diet; or a concentrate, metabolite, constituent, extract, or combination of the above ingredients (see Table 19.1).[1] This chapter will not address caffeine or botanicals, such as marijuana or *Salvia divinorum*, which are used to alter the sensorium.

PREVALENCE AND TRENDS

The use of herbs and dietary supplements by Americans is growing. In 1997, a telephone survey of adults found that an estimated 15 million US adults (1 in 5 adults who responded that they were taking prescription medicine) took prescription medications concurrently with herbal remedies and/or high-dose vitamins.[2] US sales of herbs and dietary supplements have continued to increase at an accelerated rate—by 2003, total sales exceeded $18.8 billion, an increase of more than 100% in less than 10 years.[3] Such products are now being marketed to parents for the treatment of their children. In one survey, 11% of 1911 families using the clinics of the University of Montreal sought alternative therapies for their children's medical conditions.[4] A study of 348 Washington, DC, families interviewed in pediatricians' offices revealed that 21% of parents used alternative therapies for their children's health problems. Of these, 25% used nutritional supplements or diets, and 40% used herbal therapies for their children.[5] The rate of complementary and alternative medicine use by children in a Detroit, MI,

Table 19.1: Categories of Dietary Supplements*

The term "dietary supplement" means

1. A product (other than tobacco) intended to supplement the diet that bears or contains one or more of the following dietary ingredients:
   - Vitamin
   - Mineral
   - Herb or other botanical
   - Amino acid
   - Dietary substance that supplements the normal diet
   - Concentrate, metabolite, constituent, extract, or combination of any ingredients described in the previous entries

2. A product that is
   - Intended for ingestion
   - Not represented for use as a conventional food or as a sole item of a meal in the diet

*Food and Drug Administration, Center for Food Safety and Applied Nutrition.[1]

survey of 1013 families was 12%.[6] Of these, the most frequent therapies used included herbs (43%), high-dose vitamins and other nutritional supplements (34.5%), and folk/home remedies (28%). Most families did not report the use of complementary and alternative medicine to their primary care physician, and parental use of complementary and alternative medicine was the strongest predictor of use of complementary and alternative medicine by the children.[6]

Use of herbal products increases in adolescence. A national, population-weighted online survey of 1280 adolescents found that 46.2% had used dietary supplements in their lifetime—29.1% in the previous month.[7] Another study of youth in Monroe County, NY, found that more than 25% of high school students reported that they use herbs.[8] In that study, herbal use by adolescents was associated with substance abuse.

Families whose children have chronic conditions, such as autism or cystic fibrosis, may be particularly likely to use dietary supplements as part of their treatment regimen. The American Academy of Pediatrics has published guidelines for discussing such issues with parents.[9]

A "natural" product is advertised as such to imply that it is not synthetic in origin; "organic" implies growing methods that eschew the use of hormones, pesticides, and other chemicals. However, consumers frequently confuse terms such as "natural" or "organic" with "safe." "Natural" strychnine, extracted from the nut of the plant *Strychnos nux vomica,* still has the same potentially life-threatening toxicity. The definitions are ambiguous, because the terms are used in different contexts by food and dietary supplement manufacturers, consumers, scientists, and policy makers. Chemical structures do not change, regardless of their origin. Synthesized ascorbic acid has the same structure as ascorbic acid found in orange juice or rose hips. Marketing of herbs in the form of pills or capsules, using terms such as "safe" or "natural" may be misleading to consumers. A survey of dietary supplements advertised in popular health and bodybuilding magazines showed that no human toxicology data were available in the peer-reviewed scientific literature for approximately 60% of ingredients in the products advertised.[10] Herbals containing caffeine also are marketed as "safe" dietary aids and as a source of energy or for improved alertness. Student athletes may be influenced by the performance-enhancing claims of the purveyors of herbs and dietary supplements that contain ingredients such as caffeine, amino acids, proteins, or creatine. Adolescents and young adults are particularly easy targets for such promotional tactics.

DEFINITIONS

Herbs used for medicinal purposes come in a variety of forms. Active parts of a plant may include leaves, flowers, stems, roots, seeds and/or berries, and essential oils.[11] They may be taken internally as liquids, capsules, tablets, or powders; dissolved into tinctures or syrups; or brewed in teas, infusions, and decoctions. Although few products are available as rectal suppositories, a wide variety of substances, in particular herbal products, are used in solutions for "therapeutic enemas." Table 19.2 lists some terms used in the context of herbal therapy.

THERAPEUTIC EFFICACY

To give better advice to patients and their families, pediatricians should understand the pharmacologic activity of the active ingredients in the product and whether animal or human studies demonstrate effectiveness.[12] In clinical studies, some herbs have shown promising results. For example, *Artemisia* species compared favorably with chloroquine in the treatment of some types of malaria,[13] *Astragalus membranaceus* extracts enhanced the antibody response in immunosuppressed mice,[14] and herbal teas containing chamomile seemed to have a salubrious effect on infantile colic.[15] Table 19.3 describes studies of some herbs commonly used in pediatrics.[16]

ETHNIC REMEDIES

Pediatricians should be culturally competent in their approach to the diagnosis and treatment of children in families from diverse ethnic backgrounds, whose health beliefs and practices may differ from those of Western medicine. For example, "*empacho,*" described as an illness in which food, saliva, or other matter becomes "stuck" to the intestines, is accepted among some Hispanic people as the etiology of gastrointestinal tract symptoms and treated with a variety of

Table 19.2: Definitions and Types of Preparations

PREPARATION	DEFINITION
Abortifacient	Agent that induces an abortion.
Aromatherapy	Inhalation of volatile oils in the treatment of certain health conditions.
Carminative	Agent that aids in expelling gas from the gastrointestinal tract.
Carrier oil	A fixed oil (nonvolatile, long-chain fatty acid, such as safflower oil) into which a few drops of the potent, essential oils are added to dilute them for topical uses.
Decoction	A dilute aqueous extract prepared by boiling an herb in water and straining and filtering the liquid, similar to an infusion.
Discipline of signatures	Historical term suggesting that the appearance of a plant gives a clue as to its medical value (eg, the extract of St John's wort is red, thus it is believed to be restorative for conditions involving the blood).
Elixir	A clear sweetening hydroalcoholic solution for oral use.
Emmenagogue	Agent that influences menstruation.
Essential oil	Class of volatile oils composed of complex hydrocarbons (often terpenes, alkaloids, and other large molecular weight compounds) extracted from a plant.
Excipient	Another ingredient, such as a binder or filler, used to make a supplement product.
Extract	A concentrated form of a natural substance, which can be a powder, liquid, or tincture. The concentration varies from 1:1 in a fluid extract to 1:0.1 in a tincture.
"Natural" product	The term "natural" defies accurate definition because, strictly speaking, everything is derived from nature. In common usage it is intended to imply a substance that is not synthetic or is not grown using pesticides or other chemicals.
Poultice	Salve used in a preparation that is applied to skin, scalp, or mucous membrane.
Resin	Solid or semisolid organic substance found in plant secretions and applied topically in a cream or ointment.
Rubefacient	Agent that warms and reddens the skin by local cutaneous vasodilation.

Table 19.3: Herbs Commonly Used in Pediatrics

DIETARY SUPPLEMENT	SCIENTIFIC STUDIES	POTENTIAL SIDE EFFECTS AND CONTRAINDICATIONS
Echinacea	One trial of *Echinacea purpurea* in children who had upper respiratory tract infection found no significant difference in duration or symptoms.[17]	Allergic reactions.
German chamomile *(Matricaria recutita)*	Chamomile/pectin combinations have had positive effects on diarrhea.[18,19] Chamomile in combination with other herbs was found effective for treating infantile colic.[15,20]	Individuals allergic to the *Compositae* family (ragweed, chrysanthemum) may be allergic to chamomile.[21] Chamomile can cause atopic and contact dermatitis and rare cases of anaphylaxis.[22]
Ginger *(Zingiber officinale)*	Clinical trials showed good results for ginger as a treatment for postoperative nausea and vomiting.[23] Ginger has proven helpful in treating hyperemesis gravidarum.[24]	Heartburn. Contraindications: patients who have gallstones (ginger's cholagogue effect).
Lemon balm *(Melissa officinalis)*	Clinical trials of lemon balm/valerian combinations have shown modest enhanced sleep quality.[25-27]	Allergic reactions.
Valerian *(Valeriana officinalis)*	See 'lemon balm' category above.	Allergic reactions, headaches, insomnia.

Table modified from Gardner and Riley.[16]

home-based remedies (such as greta or azarcon) as well as visits to a traditional healer.[28] More than half of patients of Southeast Asian descent using one Seattle, WA, primary care clinic used one or more traditional practices, such as moxibustion, cupping, coining, aromatic oils, or massage.[29] The formation of a therapeutic alliance among physician, parent, and child requires a sensitivity to the family's background and interests, with the goals of optimizing communications and facilitating a team approach in the clinical care of the child. For example, ethnomedical remedies practiced by the Puerto Rican community may hold some medical risks but also considerable benefits in decreasing the symptoms of asthma.[30] *Cao gio,* or coin rubbing of the skin to alleviate symptoms of illness, is an innocuous traditional Vietnamese practice that has unfortunately been

Table 19.4: Examples of Toxicity of Some Ethnic Remedies and Dietary Supplements

PRODUCT/REMEDY	TOXIC AGENT	ADVERSE EFFECTS	REFERENCE
Ayurvedic remedies	Lead, arsenic	Plumbism, arsenic poisoning (weight loss, myalgias, neuropathy, shock, death)	33
Azarcon	Lead	Plumbism	34
Ghasard, bala goli, kandu	Lead	Plumbism	35
Glycerite asafoetida	Terpenes, undifferentiated	Methemoglobinemia	36
Greta	Lead	Plumbism	34
Pay-loo-ah	Lead, arsenic	Plumbism, arsenic poisoning	37
Santeria, palo, voodoo, espiritismo	Mercury	Rash, neuropathy, seizures	38
Tongue powders	Lead, metals	Plumbism	39

confused by some Western physicians as traumatic abuse, leading to instances of distrust and avoidance of health care by people who practice it.[31] Certain Afro-Caribbean and Hispanic practices, such as the exposure to vapors of elemental mercury, may have risks of toxicity.[32] Some treatments for *empacho*, such as greta or azarcon, are contaminated by significant amounts of lead. Table 19.4 lists some of the common folk remedies that can produce toxic effects. Authorities recommend an approach of education and community outreach to effect changes in potentially harmful practices. The pediatrician can be helpful in assessing the traditional practices families may be using to treat their children by listening carefully to their rationales, beliefs, and concerns. In the course of building a therapeutic alliance, the pediatrician can then counsel them knowledgeably about possible benefits and/or adverse or harmful effects of such ethnic remedies, including interactions with other currently prescribed medications.

ADVERSE EFFECTS

Products that are natural are frequently promoted to consumers as having no adverse effects; however, many potent drugs are derived from natural products (eg, ergot alkaloids, opiates, digitalis, estrogen), and other natural substances and plants are poisonous (eg, aconite, certain types of molds and mushrooms, snake venom, hemlock). On occasion, foragers who seek herbal remedies will mistakenly collect one plant, confusing it with another. This can be a lethal error if, for example, water hemlock is mistakenly harvested and eaten after being identified as wild ginseng.[40] Table 19.5 provides other examples of some of the potent chemicals present in certain herbs and ethnic remedies and their potential uses, toxic effects, and/or drug-herb interactions.

The concentration of active ingredients as well as other chemicals in plants varies by the part of the plant harvested and sold as a remedy, the maturity of the plant at the time of harvest, and the time of year at harvest. Geography and soil conditions where the plant is grown; soil composition and its contaminants; and year-to-year variations in soil acidity, water, and weather conditions and other growth factors also can affect the concentration of the herb's active ingredients. Because of this variability in herbal product ingredients, the actual dose of active ingredients being consumed often is variable, unpredictable, or simply unknown. Children are particularly susceptible to such dosage considerations by virtue of their smaller size and different capacity for detoxifying chemicals compared with adults. For some herbs, such as those containing pyrrolizidine alkaloids (eg, coltsfoot, comfrey, red tassel flower, golden ragwort), there may be no safe dose for children. The duration of use is another consideration, with longer courses of herbal therapy exposing the patient to a higher risk of acute and cumulative or chronic adverse effects.

Adverse effects resulting from consumption of dietary supplements may involve one or more organ systems. In some cases, a single ingredient can have multiple adverse effects. More than one dietary supplement product may be consumed concurrently, and many products may contain more than one physi-ologically active ingredient. Plants have complex mixtures of terpenes, sugars, alkaloids, saponins, and other chemicals. For example, more than 100 different chemicals have been identified in tea tree oil.[75] Certain herbs and dietary supple-ments can cause unexpected reactions when used with medications. Effects on a drug's pharmacokinetics may be pronounced and lead either to toxicity or thera-peutic ineffectiveness. For example, St John's wort induces hepatic cytochromes and may decrease blood levels of medications such as indinavir,[76] digoxin,[77] and cyclosporin,[78] causing loss of their effectiveness. Pediatric patients who take oral anticoagulants, cardiovascular medications, psychiatric drugs, diabetes medications, immunosuppressive agents, or antiretroviral agents for HIV may experience a serious reduction in the efficacy of their medications with the concomitant use of certain herbs or dietary supplements.[79]

Contaminants and adulterants of herbal products can be pharmacologically active and responsible for unexpected toxicity. For example, infants have suffered significant lead poisoning from spices brought into the United States from other countries.[80] Herbal plants may be harvested from contaminated soils or cleaned improperly such that they contain illness-producing microorganisms or

Table 19.5: Examples of Known Herbal Ingredients and Their Associated Toxic Effects

HERBAL PRODUCT	TOXIC CHEMICALS	EFFECT OR TARGET ORGAN	REFERENCES
Chamomile *Matricaria chamomilla* *Anthemis nobilis*	Allergens: *Compositae* species	Anaphylaxis, contact dermatitis	41
Chaparral *Larrea divericata* *Larrea tridentate*	Nordihydroguaiaretic acid	Nausea, vomiting, lethargy Hepatitis	42,43
Cinnamon oil *Cinnamomum spp*	Cinnamaldehyde	Dermatitis, stomatitis, abuse syndrome	44,45
Coltsfoot *Tussilago farfara*	Pyrrolizidines	Hepatic veno-occlusive disease	46-50
Comfrey *(Symphytum officinale)*	Pyrrolizidines	Hepatic veno-occlusive disease	46-50
Crotalaria spp	Pyrrolizidines	Hepatic veno-occlusive disease	46-50
Echinacea *Echinacea augustifolia* *(Compositae* spp)	Polysaccharides	Asthma, atopy, anaphylaxis, urticaria, angioedema	51
Eucalyptus *Eucalyptus globules*	1,8 cineole	Drowsiness, ataxia, seizures, coma Nausea, vomiting, respiratory failure	52,53
Garlic *Allium sativum*	Allicin	Dermatitis, chemical burns	54
Germander *Teucrium chamaedrys*		Hepatotoxicity	55
Ginseng *Panax ginseng*	Ginsenoside	Ginseng abuse syndrome: diarrhea, insomnia, anxiety, hypertension	56
Glycerated asafetida	Oxidants	Methemoglobinemia	36
Groundsel *Senecio longilobus*	Pyrrolizidines	Hepatic veno-occlusive disease	46-50
Heliotrope, turnsole *Heliotropium* species *Crotalaria fulva* *Cynoglossum officinale*	Pyrrolizidines	Hepatic veno-occlusive disease	46-50

Table 19.5: Examples of Known Herbal Ingredients and Their Associated Toxic Effects, *continued*

HERBAL PRODUCT	TOXIC CHEMICALS	EFFECT OR TARGET ORGAN	REFERENCES
Jin bu huan *Stephania* species *Corydalis* species	L-Tetrahydro palmitin	Hepatitis, lethargy, coma	57,58
Kava kava *Piper methysticum*	Kawain, methysticine	Hepatic failure, "kawaism," neurotoxicity	59,60
Laetrile	Cyanide	Coma, seizures, death	61
Licorice *Glycyrrhiza glabra*	Glycyrrhetic acid	Hypertension, hypokalemia, cardiac arrhythmias	62
Ma huang *Ephedra sinica*	Ephedrine	Cardiac arrhythmias, hypertension, seizures, stroke	63,64
Monkshood *Aconitum napellus* *Aconitum columbianum*	Aconite	Cardiac arrhythmias, shock, seizures, weakness, coma, paresthesias, vomiting	65,66
Nutmeg *Myristica fragrans*	Myristicin, eugenol	Hallucinations, emesis, headache	67,68
Strychnine *Nux vomica*	Strychnine	Seizures, abdominal pain, respiratory arrest	69
Pennyroyal *Mentha pulegium* or *Hedeoma* species	Pulegone	Centrilobular liver necrosis, shock Fetotoxicity, seizures, abortion	70-72
Ragwort (golden) *Senecio jacobaea* *(Senecio aureus* or *Echium)*	Pyrrolizidines	Hepatic veno-occlusive disease	46-50
Wormwood	Thujone	Seizures, dementia, tremors, headache	73,74

soil contaminants. Contaminated Ayurvedic medications have been known to cause lead poisoning in children. (Ayurvedic medicine, or "ayurveda," is a system of health that has been practiced in India for more than 5000 years.) Saper and his colleagues tested a "market basket" of Ayurvedic remedies purchased in the United States and found that 20% were contaminated with metals such as lead, cadmium, arsenic, or mercury.[81] Asian patent remedies contain drugs such as phenylbutazone, barbiturates, benzodiazepines, or warfarin-like chemicals as well as contaminants, such as lead, cadmium, or arsenic. An analysis by the California Department of Health of 260 imported traditional Chinese medicines found high levels of contaminants in almost half of them.[82]

Parents may be tempted to give herbs to children on the basis of product advertising, information from a magazine or Web site, or advice from friends or relatives, without any guidance from a knowledgeable source. Such experimentation can be expensive and risks exposure of the child to adverse effects. Herbal products are misused in excessive doses or in combinations without any known rationale. Some products are sold as mixtures of 10 or more different plants, vitamins, minerals, etc. The "stacking" of many different herbs increases the risk of toxicity from any of them or from their interactions.

The allergic potential of plants is well known. Infants and young children may be particularly sensitive to their first introduction to chemicals in herbs and dietary supplements. Manifestations may include dermatitis, wheezing, rhinitis, conjunctivitis, itchy throat, and other allergic manifestations. In infants, allergies also may cause nonspecific effects, such as irritability, colic, poor appetite, or gastrointestinal tract disturbances. Angelica and rue, which contain psoralen-type furocoumarins, and hypericin, the active ingredient in St John's wort, are capable of causing photosensitization.[83]

Children differ from adults in their absorption and detoxification of some substances. However, they also have developing nervous and immune systems that may make them more sensitive to the adverse effects of herbs. For example, some herbs, such as buckthorn, senna, and aloe, are known cathartics, and some herbal teas and juniper oil contain powerful diuretic compounds.[83,84] Their actions may cause clinically significant dehydration and electrolyte disturbances quickly in an infant or young child.

Although the chemicals in herbs may have carcinogenic effects, this concern has not been adequately investigated. Some chemicals found in plants are known carcinogens, for example, pyrrolizidines (comfrey, coltsfoot, *Senecio*), safrole (*Sassafras*), aristolochic acids (wild ginger), and catechin tannins (betel nuts).[84] Whether such chemicals pose a threat for children, who are particularly vulnerable, because their developing organ systems and their longer life spans allow a long latency to tumor induction, is unknown.

Toxic effects of herbs on the male or female reproductive systems are of concern but have not been adequately investigated. Some essential oils, for example, have cytotoxic properties or cause cellular transformation in cell culture studies performed in vitro.[85] In many cases, the effects of herbs on the embryo and fetus are not known. It is possible that herbal chemicals may be transported through the placenta to cause toxic effects on the sensitive growing fetus. For example, Roulet and associates[49] reported the case of a newborn infant whose mother drank senecionine-containing herbal tea daily for the duration of her pregnancy

---

Dietary Supplement Health and Education Act of 1994

■ Premarketing testing or oversight protections of the FDA licensing process for an herbal remedy or dietary supplement are not required.

■ The use of child-resistant containers or safe packaging for herbs or dietary supplements is not mandated.

■ Nutritional support claims made in the labeling or marketing of an herb or dietary supplement do not require FDA approval.

■ Pharmacologically active substances can be marketed as dietary substances, provided no unsubstantiated claims concerning the cure of specific illnesses or conditions are made for them.

■ The Secretary of the US Department of Health and Human Services is empowered to act to remove a dietary supplement only when it "poses an imminent hazard to public health or safety."

■ There is no regulatory provision for mandatory reporting of adverse health effects associated with the use of herbs or dietary supplements.

(senecionine is one of the pyrrolizidine alkaloids associated with hepatic venous injury). The infant was born with hepatic veno-occlusive disease and died. Animal studies have confirmed the teratogenicity of some herbs (eg, the popular Eastern European herb *Plectranthus fruticosus*).[86] The excretion of chemicals from herbs and dietary supplements into human milk is a concern to pediatricians, because some have lipophilic ingredients that might be expected to concentrate in human milk, although there are little data to confirm or refute this.

REGULATION AND ADVERSE EFFECT REPORTING

Clinicians can play an important role in identifying, reporting, and preventing adverse effects from dietary supplements. Unfortunately, herbal products and dietary supplements are virtually unregulated. Congress passed legislation, the Dietary Supplement Health and Education Act of 1994, which does not include all of the consumer protections that are applied to medications and generally responds only when the outcome is death.[1] Pharmacologically active substances, such as melatonin, yohimbine, and dehydroepiandrosterone, can be marketed as dietary supplements, provided no therapeutic claims are made for them.

There are no international conventions in naming plants, and many confusing synonyms exist. The common names of plants and herbal remedies can be archaic and variable depending on the geographic region. For example, *cohosh* can refer to several different species of plants depending on where a person lives. There is little regulation of the manufacture, quality, purity, concentration, or labeling claims of herbal remedies and dietary supplements. Errors in labeling may be inadvertent; however, intentional mislabeling also has been problematic. For example, one study revealed that products sold as ginseng actually contained such substitutes as scopolamine and reserpine.[87]

Clinicians may play a critical role in recognizing toxicity associated with herbal products and dietary supplements. A special segment of the MedWatch program, administered by the US Food and Drug Administration (FDA), has been targeted to adverse events involving such products. To report adverse reactions to the FDA, the MedWatch telephone number is 800-FDA-1088; the fax number is 800-FDA-0178. Consumers can report adverse events to the FDA Consumer Hotline at 888-INFO-FDA. Local or regional poison control centers also are a valuable resource for information on the adverse effects of dietary supplements and can be reached at 800-222-1222.

ADVICE TO PARENTS

The assessment of children whose parents may be seeking complementary and alternative medicine options requires strategies that promote the therapeutic interaction among physician, parent, and child. Physicians and other health professionals should ask questions about use of dietary supplements, minerals, vitamins, or herbs as well as the reasons or health conditions for which these products are used.[88] Guidelines have been suggested for practitioners in the assessment of a patient whose parents may be seeking medical solutions involving complementary and alternative medicine.[89] These suggestions are modified here to make them more specific to the needs of pediatricians.

- Carry out a thorough medical evaluation.
- Explore conventional therapeutic options—establish a dialogue with the parents about what, in your opinion, is the best treatment for the condition as well as what may be established or untested alternatives. Keep an open mind and research what beliefs the parents may bring to the assessment.
- Ask the unasked question—find out about the current beliefs of the parents and any current alternative therapies, herbs, or other remedies in use by the family and given to children. In one study, up to 50% of families using complementary and alternative medicine did not reveal this to their primary care physician.[4]
- Obtain consultations as needed—for example, if the child has frequent unresolved ear infections, suggest that the parents follow up on your referral of the child to an otolaryngologist before trying herbs.
- Document requests for complementary and alternative medicine or therapeutic refusals in the medical record.
- If you disagree with the plan, discuss why and document your disagreement in the record.

The best interests of the child are always paramount. When the pediatrician disagrees with the family's intended actions, such disagreement should be voiced along with the reasons behind it. In other circumstances, the pediatrician can and should support the parents' decision to pursue herbal remedies or dietary supplements when the risk of harm is low, the possibility of benefit is backed by scientific evidence, and the parents can be engaged in an integrative approach to the child's care. All of this presumes that the pediatrician has adequately educated himself or herself about the health aspects of the herbs and dietary supplements in question, using reliable sources of information.

Frequently Asked Questions

Q *Conventional medications have many side effects. Shouldn't I worry more about the known side effects?*

A Conventional pharmaceutical products have been through extensive testing for safety and efficacy by manufacturers and through FDA review processes, and through this process, side effects and prevalence have been identified and are listed in package inserts or available sources. Less is known about side effects associated with children's use of certain herbs and dietary supplements, since they do not need to undergo this level of premarketing scrutiny.

Q *Does my child need extra vitamins/food supplements? Won't they help my child grow, eat, and study better?*

A A diet that provides enough calories and is balanced in all the major food groups generally provides adequate nutrition for an otherwise healthy growing child. Infants and young children may gain dental benefits from fluoride supplements if they drink only unfluorinated bottled or well water or live in communities that do not fluoridate public water sources. Additional vitamin or dietary supplements may be necessary for children to reach recommended amounts of vitamin D. AAP guidelines recommend that breastfed infants, formula-fed infants, children, and teenagers who are consuming less than 1 quart per day of vitamin D-fortified formula or milk should receive a vitamin D supplement of 400 IU per day.[90] New guidelines from the Institute of Medicine recommend that children 1 year and older have a total of 600 IU of vitamin D daily from food and supplemental sources.[91] Guidelines for supplementation with iron, zinc, and other essential nutrients should be followed.[92]

Q *Doesn't the FDA approve herbs and dietary supplements?*

A No. Legislation enacted in 1994 made dietary ingredients exempt from FDA premarket approval that apply to drugs and food additives. Manufacturers no longer must prove that an ingredient is safe. The FDA needs to prove the ingredient is hazardous if it believes there is a risk.

Q Is it OK to give my child chamomile or spearmint tea?

A Weak teas made from the leaves and flowers of chamomile or spearmint probably pose a negligible threat of an adverse effect, although there is little evidence of clear therapeutic benefits on children's health from such teas. Parents should keep in mind that children as well as adults might experience allergic reactions to any plant-derived products such as mint (*Mentha* species) and chamomile (*Compositae* species).

Q Is zinc of any value in the treatment of colds?

A Zinc is an essential metal for good health, and zinc deficiencies can reduce immunocompetence. Zinc supplementation was recently found to improve the survival of infants who were small for their gestational age. Its value in the treatment of childhood upper respiratory tract infections has yet to be shown in carefully controlled studies.

Q Are over-the-counter herbs of any value in treating my child's colds?

A Many laboratory or animal-based studies of certain herbs, such as *Echinacea* or *Astragalus,* have shown them to have remarkable effects on the immune system. However, such results may not be extrapolated to necessarily imply a benefit in the management of the ill child. Investigations of the use of *Echinacea* to treat colds in a randomized controlled trial in children showed no benefit. Parents should be warned that some herbal remedies, such as camphor or eucalyptus oil, may be soothing if inhaled but also can have harmful effects, including seizures or coma, if ingested by children.

Resources

American Botanical Council
Web site: www.herbalgram.org

Center for Food Safety and Applied Nutrition
Web site: http://vm.cfsan.fda.gov/~dms/dietsupp.html

Consumer Federation of America
Web site: www.quackwatch.org

Dr Duke's Phytochemical and Ethnobotanical Databases
Web site: www.ars-grin.gov/duke

Drug Interactions Center
Web site: www.druginteractioncenter.org

Herb Research Foundation
Web site: www.herbs.org

National Center for Complementary and Alternative Medicine
Web site: www.nccam.nih.gov

National Certification Commission for Acupuncture and Oriental Medicine
Web site: www.nccaom.org

National Council Against Health Fraud
Web site: www.ncahf.org

Slone-Kettering Cancer Center
Web site: www.mskcc.org/aboutherbs

US Department of Agriculture Food & Nutrition Information Center:
Web site: www.nal.usda.gov/fnic

References

1. Dietary Supplement Health and Education Act of 1994. Available at: http://www.fda.gov/food/dietarysupplements/default.htm. Accessed March 7, 2011
2. Eisenberg DM, Davis RB, Ettner SL, et al. Trends in alternative medicine use in the United States, 1990–1997: results of a follow-up national survey. *JAMA.* 1998;280(18):1569–1575
3. Bardia A, Nisly NL, Zimmerman B, Gryzlak BM, Wallace RB. Use of herbs among adults based on evidence-based indications: findings from the National Health Interview Survey. *Mayo Clin Proc. 2007;82:361-366*
4. Spigelblatt L, Laine-Ammara G, Pless IB, Guyver A. The use of alternative medicine by children. *Pediatrics.* 1994;94(6 Pt 1):811–814
5. Ottolini MC, Hamburger EK, Loprieato JO, et al. Complementary and alternative medicine use among children in the Washington, DC area. *Ambul Pediatr.* 2001;1(2):122–125
6. Sawni-Sikand A, Schubiner H, Thomas RL. Use of complementary/alternative therapies among children in primary care pediatrics. *Ambulatory Pediatr.* 2002;2(2):99-103
7. Wilson KM, Klein JD, Sesselberg TS, et al. Use of complementary medicine and dietary supplements among U.S. adolescents. *J Adolesc Health.* 2006;38(4):385-394
8. Yussman SM, Wilson KM, Klein JD. Herbal products and their association with substance use in adolescents. *J Adolesc Health.* 2006;38(4):395-400
9. American Academy of Pediatrics, Committee on Children with Disabilities. Counseling families who choose complementary and alternative medicine for their child with chronic illness or disability. *Pediatrics.* 2001;107(3):598–601
10. Philen RM, Ortiz DI, Auerbach SB, Falk H. Survey of advertising for nutritional supplements in health and bodybuilding magazines. *JAMA.* 1992;268(8):1008–1011
11. Woolf A. Essential oil poisoning. *J Toxicol Clin Toxicol.* 1999;37(6):721–727
12. Angell M, Kassirer JP. Alternative medicine—the risks of untested and unregulated remedies. *N Engl J Med.* 1998;339(12):839–841
13. White NJ, Waller D, Crawley J, et al. Comparison of artemether and chloroquine for severe malaria in Gambian children. *Lancet.* 1992;339(8789):317–321
14. Zhao KS, Mancini C, Doria G. Enhancement of the immune response in mice by *Astragalus membranaceus* extracts. *Immunopharmacology.* 1990;20(3):225–233
15. Weizman Z, Alkrinawi S, Goldfarb D, Bitran C. Efficacy of herbal tea preparation in infantile colic. *J Pediatr.* 1993;122(4):650–652

16. Gardiner P, Riley DS. Herbs to homeopathy—medicinal products for children. *Pediatr Clin North Am.* 2007;54(6):859–874

17. Taylor JA, Weber W, Standish L, et al. Efficacy and safety of echinacea in treating upper respiratory tract infections in children: a randomized controlled trial. *JAMA.* 2003;290(21):2824-2830

18. Becker B, Kuhn U, Hardewig-Budny B. Double-blind, randomized evaluation of clinical efficacy and tolerability of an apple pectin-chamomile extract in children with unspecific diarrhea. *Arzneimittelforschung.* 2006;56(6):387-393

19. de la Motte S, Bose-O'Reilly S, Heinisch M, et al. [Double-blind comparison of an apple pectin-chamomile extract preparation with placebo in children with diarrhea]. [Article in German.] *Arzneimittelforschung.* 1997;47(11):1247-1249

20. Savino F, Cresi F, Castagno E, et al. A randomized double-blind placebo-controlled trial of a standardized extract of Matricariae recutita, Foeniculum vulgare and Melissa officinalis (ColiMil) in the treatment of breastfed colicky infants. *Phytother Res.* 2005;19(4):335-340

21. Paulsen E. Contact sensitization from Compositae-containing herbal remedies and cosmetics. *Contact Dermatitis.* 2002;47(4):189-198

22. Gardiner P. Complementary, holistic, and integrative medicine: chamomile. *Pediatr Rev.* 2007;28(4):e16

23. Chaiyakunapruk N, Kitikannakorn N, Nathisuwan S, Leeprakabboon K, Leelasettagool C. The efficacy of ginger for the prevention of postoperative nausea and vomiting: a meta-analysis. Am J Obstet Gynecol 2006; 194: 95-9.

24. Borrelli F, Capasso R, Aviello G, et al. Effectiveness and safety of ginger in the treatment of pregnancy-induced nausea and vomiting. *Obstet Gynecol.* 2005;105(4):849-856

25. Bent S, Padula A, Moore D, et al. Valerian for sleep: a systematic review and meta-analysis. *Am J Med.* 2006;119(12):1005-1012

26. Koetter U, Schrader E, Kaufeler R, et al. A randomized, double blind, placebo-controlled, prospective clinical study to demonstrate clinical efficacy of a fixed valerian hops extract combination (Ze 91019) in patients suffering from non-organic sleep disorder. *Phytother Res.* 2007;21(9):847-851

27. Muller SF, Klement S. A combination of valerian and lemon balm is effective in the treatment of restlessness and dyssomnia in children. *Phytomedicine.* 2006;13(6):383-387

28. Pachter LM. Culture and clinical care. Folk illness beliefs and behaviors and their implications for health care delivery. *JAMA.* 1994;271(9):690–694

29. Buchwald D, Panwala S, Hooton TM. Use of traditional health practices by Southeast Asian refugees in a primary care clinic. *West J Med.* 1992;156(5):507–511

30. Pachter LM, Cloutier MM, Bernstein BA. Ethnomedical (folk) remedies for childhood asthma in a mainland Puerto Rican community. *Arch Pediatr Adolesc Med.* 1995;149(9):982–988

31. Yeatman GW, Dang VV. Cao gio (coin rubbing). Vietnamese attitudes toward health care. *JAMA.* 1980;244(24):2748–2749

32. Forman J, Moline J, Cernichiari E, et al. A cluster of pediatric metallic mercury exposure cases treated with meso-2,3 dimercaptosuccinic acid (DMSA). *Environ Health Perspect.* 2000;108(6):575–577

33. Moore C, Adler R. Herbal vitamins: lead toxicity and developmental delay. *Pediatrics.* 2000;106(1):200–202

34. Risser A, Mazur LJ. Use of folk remedies in a Hispanic population. *Arch Pediatr Adolesc Med.* 1995;149(9):978–981

35. Centers for Disease Control and Prevention. Lead poisoning-associated death from Asian Indian folk remedies—Florida. *MMWR Morb Mortal Wkly Rep.* 1984;33(45):638–664

36. Kelly KJ, Neu J, Camitta BM, Honig GR. Methemoglobinemia in an infant treated with the folk remedy glycerited asafoetida. *Pediatrics.* 1984;73(5):717–719

37. Centers for Disease Control and Prevention. Folk remedy-associated lead poisoning in Hmong children—Minnesota. *MMWR Morb Mortal Wkly Rep.* 1983;32(42):555–556

38. Riley DM, Newby CA, Leal-Almeraz TO, Thomas VM. Assessing elemental mercury exposure from cultural and religious practices. *Environ Health Perspect.* 2001;109(8):779–784

39. Woolf AD, Hussain J, McCullough L, Petranovic M, Chomchai C. Infantile lead poisoning from an Asian tongue powder: a case report and subsequent public health inquiry. *Clin Toxicol (Phila).* 2008;46(9):841–844

40. Centers for Disease Control and Prevention. Water hemlock poisoning—Maine, 1992. *MMWR Morb Mortal Wkly Rep.* 1994;43(13):229–231

41. Benner MH, Lee HJ. Anaphylactic reaction to chamomile tea. *J Allergy Clin Immunol.* 1973;52(5):307–308

42. Grant KL, Boyer LV, Erdman BE. Chaparral-induced hepatotoxicity. *Integrative Med.* 1998;1:83–87

43. Centers for Disease Control and Prevention. Chaparral-induced toxic hepatitis—California and Texas. *MMWR Morb Mortal Wkly Rep.* 1992;41(43):812–814

44. Miller RL, Gould AR, Bernstein ML. Cinnamon-induced stomatitis venenata. Clinical and characteristic histopathologic features. *Oral Surg Oral Med Oral Pathol.* 1992;73(6):708–716

45. Perry PA, Dean BS, Krenzelok EP. Cinnamon oil abuse by adolescents. *Vet Hum Toxicol.* 1990;32(2):162–164

46. Huxtable RJ. Herbal teas and toxins: novel aspects of pyrrolizidine poisoning in the United States. *Perspect Biol Med.* 1980;24(1):1–14

47. Ridker PM, Ohkuma S, McDermott WV, Trey C, Huxtable RJ. Hepatic veno-occlusive disease associated with the consumption of pyrrolizidine-containing dietary supplements. *Gastroenterology.* 1985;88(4):1050–1054

48. Mattocks AR. Toxicity of pyrrolizidine alkaloids. *Nature.* 1968; 217(5130):723–728

49. Roulet M, Laurini R, Rivier L, Calame A. Hepatic veno-occlusive disease in the newborn infant of a woman drinking herbal tea. *J Pediatr.* 1988;112(3):433–436

50. Bach N, Thung SN, Schaffner F. Comfrey herb tea-induced hepatic veno-occlusive disease. *Am J Med.* 1989;87(1):97–99

51. Mullins RJ, Heddle R. Adverse reactions associated with echinacea: the Australian experience. *Ann Allergy Asthma Immunol.* 2002;88(1):42–51

52. Tibballs J. Clinical effects and management of eucalyptus oil ingestion in infants and young children. *Med J Aust.* 1995;163(4):177–180

53. Webb NJR, Pitt WR. Eucalyptus oil poisoning in childhood: 41 cases in south-east Queensland. *J Paediatr Child Health.* 1993;29(5):368–371

54. Tarty BZ. Garlic burns. *Pediatrics.* 1993;91(3):658–659

55. Larrey D, Vial T, Pauwels A, et al. Hepatitis after germander *(Teucrium chamaedrys)* administration: another instance of herbal medicine hepatotoxicity. *Ann Intern Med.* 1992;117(2):129–132

56. Siegel RK. Ginseng abuse syndrome. Problems with the panacea. *JAMA.* 1979;241(15):1614–1615

57. Centers for Disease Control and Prevention. Jin bu huan toxicity in children—Colorado 1993. *MMWR Morb Mortal Wkly Rep.* 1993;42(33):633–635

58. Horowitz RS, Feldhaus K, Dart RC, Stermitz FR, Beck JJ. The clinical spectrum of Jin Bu Huan toxicity. *Arch Int Med.* 1996;156(8):899–903

59. Russman S, Lauterburg BH, Helbling A. Kava hepatotoxicity. *Ann Intern Med.* 2001;135(1):68-69

60. Escher M, Desmeules J, Giostra E, Mentha G. Hepatitis associated with Kava, a herbal remedy for anxiety. *BMJ.* 2001;322(7279):139

61. Hall AH, Linden CH, Kulig KW, et al. Cyanide poisoning from laetrile ingestion: role of nitrite therapy. *Pediatrics.* 1986;78(2):269–272

62. Walker BR, Edwards CRW. Licorice-induced hypertension and syndromes of apparent mineralocorticoid excess. *Endocrinol Metab Clin North Am.* 1994;23(2):359–377

63. Samenuk D, Link MS, Homoud MK, et al. Adverse cardiovascular events temporally associated with Ma Huang, an herbal source of ephedrine. *Mayo Clin Proc.* 2002;77(1):12–16

64. Haller CA, Benowitz NL. Adverse cardiovascular and central nervous system events associated with dietary supplements containing ephedra alkaloids. *N Engl J Med.* 2000;343(25):1833–1838

65. Fatovich DM. Aconite: a lethal Chinese herb. *Ann Emerg Med.* 1992;21(3):309–311

66. Chan TYK, Tse LKK, Chan JCN, Chan WWM. Aconitine poisoning due to Chinese herbal medicines: a review. *Vet Human Toxicol.* 1994;36(5):452

67. Abernethy MK, Becker LB. Acute nutmeg intoxication. *Am J Emerg Med.* 1992;10(5):429–430

68. Brenner N, Frank OS, Knight E. Chronic nutmeg psychosis. *J Roy Soc Med.* 1993;86(3):179–180

69. Katz J, Prescott K, Woolf AD. Strychnine poisoning from a traditional Cambodian remedy. *Am J Emerg Med.* 1996;14(5):475–477

70. Sullivan JB Jr, Rumack BH, Thomas H Jr, Peterson RG, Bryson P. Pennyroyal oil poisoning and hepatotoxicity. *JAMA.* 1979;242(26):2873–2874

71. Anderson IB, Mullen WH, Meeker JE, et al. Pennyroyal toxicity: measurement of four metabolites in two cases and review of the literature. *Ann Intern Med.* 1996;124(8):726–734

72. Gordon WB, Forte AJ, McMurtry RJ, et al. Hepatotoxicity and pulmonary toxicity of pennyroyal oil and its constituent terpenes in the mouse. *Toxicol Appl Pharmacol.* 1982;65(3):413–424

73. Arnold WN. Vincent van Gogh and the thujone connection. *JAMA.* 1988;260(20):3042–3044

74. Weisbord SD, Soule JB, Kimmel PL. Poison on line-acute renal failure caused by oil of wormwood purchased through the Internet. *N Engl J Med.* 1997;337(12):825–827

75. Carson CF, Riley TV. Toxicity of the essential oil of *Melaleuca alternifolia* or tea tree oil. *J Toxicol Clin Toxicol.* 1995;33(2):193–194

76. Piscitelli SC, Burstein AH, Chaitt D, Alfaro RM, Falloon J. Indinavir concentrations and St John's wort. *Lancet.* 2000;355:547–548

77. Johne A, Brockmoller J, Bauer S, Maurer A, Langheinrich M, Roots I. Pharmacokinetic interaction of digoxin with an herbal extract from St John's wort (*Hypericum perforatum*). *Clin Pharmacol Ther.* 1999;66(4):338–345

78. Ruschitzka F, Meier PJ, Turina M, Luscher TF, Noll G. Acute heart transplant rejection due to Saint John's wort. *Lancet.* 2000;355(9203):548–549

79. Gardiner P, Phillips R, Shaughnessy AF. Herbal and dietary supplement-drug interactions in patients with chronic illnesses. *Am Fam Physician.* 2008;77(1):73-78

80. Woolf AD, Woolf NT. Childhood lead poisoning in two families associated with spices used in food preparation. *Pediatrics.* 2005;116(2):e314-e318

81. Saper RB, Kales SN, Paquin J, et al. Heavy metal content of Ayurvedic herbal medicine products. *JAMA.* 2004;292(23):2868-2873

82. Kaltsas HJ. Patent poisons. *Altern Med.* 1999;Nov:24–28

83. Toxic reactions to plant products sold in health food stores. *Med Lett Drugs Ther.* 1979;21(7):29–32

84. Saxe TG. Toxicity of medicinal herbal preparations. *Am Fam Physician.* 1987;35(5):135–142

85. Pecevski J, Savkovic D, Radivojevic D, Vuksanovic L. Effect of oil of nutmeg on the fertility and induction of meiotic chromosome rearrangements in mice and their first generation. *Toxicol Lett.* 1981;7(3):239–243

86. Pages N, Salazar M, Chamorro G, et al. Teratological evaluation of *Plectranthus fruticosus* leaf essential oil. *Planta Med.* 1988;54(4):296–298

87. Siegel R. Kola, ginseng, and mislabeled herbs. *JAMA.* 1978;237:25

88. Ang-Lee MK, Moss J, Yuan CS. Herbal medicines and perioperative care. *JAMA.* 2001;286(2): 208–216

89. Eisenberg DM. Advising patients who seek alternative medical therapies. *Ann Intern Med.* 1997;127(1):61–69

90. Wagner CL; Greer FR; American Academy of Pediatrics, Section on Breastfeeding and Committee on Nutrition. Clinical report—prevention of rickets and vitamin D deficiency in infants, children, and adolescents. *Pediatrics.* 2008;122(5):1142-1152

91. Institute of Medicine. *Dietary Reference Intakes for Calcium and Vitamin D.* Washington, DC: Institute of Medicine; November 30, 2010. Available at: http://iom.edu/Reports/2010/Dietary-Reference-Intakes-for-Calcium-and-Vitamin-D.aspx. Accessed June 2, 2011.

92. American Academy of Pediatrics, Committee on Nutrition. *Pediatric Nutrition Handbook.* Kleinman RE, ed. Elk Grove Village, IL: American Academy of Pediatrics; 2009

Chapter 20

Air Pollutants, Indoor

■ ■ ■ ■ ■ ■

Indoor air quality often affects children's health. There has been increasing concern in recent years as higher energy costs have led to building designs that reduce air exchanges. New synthetic materials have become more widely used in furnishings. Furthermore, children spend an estimated 80% to 90% of their time indoors at home, child care settings or at school. Indoor environments have a range of airborne pollutants, including particulate matter, gases, vapors, biological materials, and fibers that may have adverse effects on health. In the home, common sources of air pollutants include tobacco smoke, gas stoves and wood stoves, and furnishings and construction materials that may release organic gases and vapors. Allergens and biological agents include animal dander, fecal material from house-dust mites and other insects, mold spores, and bacteria (see Chapter 43). Pollutants such as particulate matter may be brought into the indoor environment from the outdoor air by natural and mechanical ventilation. Pesticides may be sprayed in the home to reduce insect infestations. This chapter describes indoor air pollution from combustion products, ammonia, volatile organic compounds (VOCs), and molds. Other chapters in the book focus on outdoor air pollution (Chapter 21), asbestos (Chapter 23), carbon monoxide (Chapter 25), radon (Chapter 39), and secondhand smoke (Chapter 40).

COMBUSTION POLLUTANTS

Route and Sources of Exposure

The route of exposure to combustion products is through inhalation. Combustion pollutants in the home arise primarily from gas ranges, particularly when they malfunction or are used as space heaters, and from improperly vented wood stoves and fireplaces.

Combustion of natural gas results in the emission of nitrogen dioxide (NO_2) and carbon monoxide (CO). Levels of NO_2 in the home generally are increased during the winter, when ventilation is reduced to conserve energy. During the winter, average indoor concentrations of NO_2 in homes with gas cooking stoves are as much as twice as high as outdoor levels. Some of the highest indoor NO_2 levels have been measured in homes in which ovens were used as space heaters. Residential levels of CO generally are low. Cooking or heating with wood results in the emission of liquids (suspended droplets), solids (suspended particles), and gases such as NO_2 and sulfur dioxide (SO_2). The aerosol mixture of very fine solid and liquid particles or "smoke" contains particles in the inhalable range, less than 10 μm in diameter. Measurements of wood smoke performed in indoor environments in the United States demonstrate that concentrations of inhalable particles are higher in homes with wood stoves, compared with homes without wood stoves. Depending on the frequency and duration of cooking or heating with wood and the adequacy of ventilation, the concentration of inhalable particles may exceed outdoor air standards. With adequate ventilation, however, operating a wood stove or fireplace may not adversely affect indoor air quality.

Systems Affected

The mucous membranes of the eyes, nose, throat, and respiratory tract are affected.

Clinical Effects

Clinical symptoms attributable to exposure are usually acute and short lived and generally cease with elimination of exposure. Exposure to high levels of NO_2 and SO_2 may result in acute mucocutaneous irritation and respiratory tract effects. The relatively low water solubility of NO_2 results in minimal mucous membrane irritation of the upper airway; the principal site of toxicity is the lower respiratory tract. If patients with asthma are exposed either simultaneously or sequentially to NO_2 and an aeroallergen, the risk of an exaggerated response to the allergen is increased.[1] The high water solubility of SO_2 makes it extremely irritating to the eyes and upper respiratory tract. Whether exposure to the relatively low levels of this gas attained in houses is associated with health effects remains to be determined.

Exposure to inhaled particles in wood smoke may result in irritation and inflammation of the upper and lower respiratory tract resulting in rhinitis, cough, wheezing, and worsening of asthma.[2]

Diagnostic Methods

If CO poisoning is suspected, the family should vacate the premises immediately, and carboxyhemoglobin levels should be measured promptly (see Chapter 25).

For an indoor air pollution-related respiratory illness, a specific etiology may be difficult to establish, because most respiratory signs and symptoms are nonspecific and may only occur in association with significant exposures. Effects of lower exposures may be milder and more vague. Furthermore, signs and symptoms in infants and children may be atypical. Multiple pollutants may be involved in a given situation. Establishing the environmental cause of a given respiratory illness is further complicated by the similarity of effects to those associated with allergies and respiratory infections. The clinician should ask whether anyone in smokes in the home, whether anyone else in the family is ill, and whether the child's symptoms clear when he is away from the home and recur when he returns. The clinician should also ask whether the family burns wood in a wood stove or fireplace. Use of space heaters, kerosene lamps or heaters, and gas ovens or ranges as home heating devices should raise concerns about exposure to combustion products, particularly if there is any indication that appliances may not be properly vented to the outside or that heating equipment may be in disrepair.

Prevention of Exposure

Measures that may help to minimize exposure include periodic professional inspection and maintenance of furnaces, gas water heaters, and clothes dryers; venting such equipment directly to the outdoors; and regular cleaning and inspection of fireplaces and wood stoves. Charcoal (in a hibachi or grill) should never be burned indoors or in a tent or camper.

Guidelines

Although there are no standards for indoor air quality in the United States, the World Health Organization (WHO) published a global update on air quality guidelines in 2005. The air quality guidelines in Table 20.1 are recommended to be achieved everywhere (indoors and outdoors) to significantly reduce the adverse health effects of pollution.[3]

AMMONIA

Ammonia is a major component of many common household cleaning products (eg, glass cleaners, toilet bowel cleaners, metal polishes, floor strippers, and wax removers).

Route and Sources of Exposure

The route of exposure to ammonia is through inhalation. People are frequently exposed to ammonia while using household products. Household ammonia solutions usually contain 5% to 10% ammonia in water. Ammonia is found in smelling salts and in swine confinement buildings. It is liberated during

Table 20.1: World Health Organization Air Quality Guidelines		
POLLUTANT	**AIR QUALITY GUIDELINE VALUE**	**AVERAGING TIME**
Carbon monoxide	100 mg/m³	15 minutes
	60 mg/m³	30 min
	30 mg/m³	1 hour
	10 mg/m³	8 hours
Nitrogen dioxide	200 µg/m³	1 hour
	40 µg/m³	Annual
Ozone	100 µg/m³	8 hour, daily maximum
Particulate matter		
PM$_{2.5}$	10 µg/m³	1 year
	25 µg/m³	24 hour
PM$_{10}$	20 µg/m³	1 year
	50 µg/m³	24 hour

PM$_{2.5}$ – particles < 2.5 µm in diameter.
PM$_{10}$ – particles < 10 µm in diameter.

combustion of nylon, silk, wood, and melamine, and used in the production of explosives, pharmaceuticals, pesticides, textiles, leather, flame retardants, plastics, pulp and paper, rubber, petroleum products, and cyanide. People who live near farms or cattle feedlots, poultry confinement buildings, or in the vicinity of other areas with high animal populations may be exposed to elevated ammonia levels. In enclosed animal confinement buildings, ammonia is adsorbed by dust particles that transport it more directly to small airways.

Systems Affected

The respiratory tract and eyes are affected.

Clinical Effects

Symptoms including rhinorrhea, scratchy throat, chest tightness, cough, dyspnea, and eye irritation usually subside within 24 to 48 hours. Symptoms have reportedly developed within minutes of entering animal confinement buildings. Typical environmental ammonia concentrations have not been reported to cause adverse health effects in the general population. However, low levels of ammonia may harm some people with asthma and other sensitive individuals.[4]

Diagnostic Methods

If the causes of the child's respiratory symptoms are not apparent, questions about the use of household products containing ammonia and exposures to animal confinement buildings should be included in the environmental history.

Prevention of Exposure

For household cleaning, a less toxic substitute for ammonia-containing household products is a vinegar and water solution or baking soda and water. If ammonia is used, it should never be mixed with bleach, because toxic chloramines can be released, which cause lung injury.

VOLATILE ORGANIC COMPOUNDS

Volatile organic compounds are chemicals that produce vapors readily at room temperature and normal atmospheric pressure.

Routes and Sources of Exposure

The route of exposure to volatile organic compounds occurs through inhalation and dermal contact with surfaces on which they are deposited. Many household furnishings and products release ("off-gas") volatile organic compounds. These chemicals include aliphatic and aromatic hydrocarbons (including chlorinated hydrocarbons), alcohols, and ketones in products such as finishes, rug and oven cleaners, paints and lacquers, and paint strippers.

Because product labels may not always specify the presence of organic compounds, the specific chemicals to which a product user may be exposed may be difficult to discern. Over the normal range of room temperatures, volatile organic compounds are released as gases or vapors from furnishings or consumer products. Table 20.2 lists some common volatile organic compounds, their uses, and sources of indoor exposure.

Measurements in residential and nonresidential buildings show that exposure to volatile organic compounds is widespread and highly variable. In general, levels of volatile organic compounds are likely to be higher in recently constructed or renovated buildings compared with older buildings. Off-gassing of volatile organic compounds is greatest when materials containing volatile organic compounds are new and decreases over time. Once building-related emissions decrease, consumer products (including cigarettes) are likely to remain the predominant source of exposure to volatile organic compounds. Concentrations of volatile organic compounds (measured using a personal monitor) are greater indoors than outdoors; breath levels correlate better with air exposures in a person's breathing zone than with outdoor air levels, and inhalation accounts for more than 99% of exposure for many volatile organic compounds.

Table 20.2: Common Volatile Organic Compounds (VOCs)

VOC	USES	SOURCES OF INDOOR EXPOSURE
1,1,1-Trichloroethane	As a dry-cleaning agent, a vapor degreasing agent, and a propellant	Wearing dry-cleaned clothes, using aerosol sprays and fabric protectors
1,3-Butadiene	Used to produce synthetic rubber	Breathing cigarette smoke, motor vehicle exhaust, or wood fire smoke
1,4-Dichlorobenzene	As an air deodorant and an insecticide	Using air fresheners, mothballs, and toilet-deodorizer blocks
2-Butanone	As a solvent, and in the surface coating industry, in manufacturing synthetic resins	Smoking cigarettes, using paints and glues, breathing motor vehicle exhaust
Acetone	As a solvent in the production of lubricating oils and as an intermediate in pharmaceuticals and pesticides	Using household chemicals, nail polish, and paint, breathing cigarette smoke
Acetaldehyde	In adhesives, coatings, lubricants, inks, nail polish remover, room air deodorizers	Breathing cigarette smoke; wood smoke; using room air deodorizers, nail polish remover, adhesives, coatings, lubricants, inks
Benzene	Constituent in motor fuels, solvent for fats, inks, oils, paints, plastics, and rubber; also used in the manufacturing of detergents, pharmaceuticals, explosives, and dyestuffs	Breathing cigarette smoke, motor vehicle exhaust
Carbon tetrachloride	Used to make refrigeration fluid and propellants for aerosol cans	Using industrial-strength cleansers
Chlorobenzene	Used in the manufacture of dyestuffs and pesticides	Living near a waste site containing chlorobenzene
Chloroform	As a solvent; widely distributed in atmosphere and water	Showering
Ethylbenzene	As a solvent and in the manufacture of styrene-related products; emitted vapors at filling stations and from motor vehicles	Breathing motor vehicle exhaust

Table 20.2: Common Volatile Organic Compounds (VOCs), *continued*

VOC	USES	SOURCES OF INDOOR EXPOSURE
Formaldehyde	In particleboard, insulation (UFFI), carpeting, mobile homes, temporary classrooms, and trailers	Breathing cigarette smoke, living in a mobile home or going to school in temporary classroom, using particleboard furniture
m-Xylene, p-Xylene, and o-Xylene	As solvents, constituents of paint, lacquers, varnishes, inks, dyes, adhesives, cement, and aviation fluids; also used in the manufacture of perfumes, insect repellants, pharmaceuticals, and the leather industry	Using paints, adhesives; breathing motor vehicle exhaust
Naphthalene	In mothballs and deodorant cakes. Comes from burning wood, tobacco, or fossil fuels.	Eating naphthalene mothballs or deodorant cakes or coming in close contact with clothing or blankets stored in naphthalene mothballs
Perchloroethylene	In dry cleaning	Wearing dry-cleaned clothes
Styrene	At high temperature, becomes a plastic; used in the manufacture of resins, polyesters, insulators, and drugs	Breathing motor vehicle exhaust, cigarette smoke; using photocopiers
Toluene	Used in the manufacture of benzene, as a solvent for paints and coatings, and as a component of car and aviation fuels	Using paints, breathing motor vehicle exhaust
Trichloroethylene	As a solvent in vapor degreasing, for extracting caffeine from coffee, as a dry-cleaning agent, and as an intermediate in production of pesticides, waxes, gums, resins, tars, and paints	Using wood stains, varnishes, finishes, lubricants, adhesives, typewriter correction fluid, paint removers, cleaners

Benzene

Benzene in indoor air comes primarily from cigarette smoking and consumer products, including off-gassing from particle board. Homes with attached garages have higher benzene levels than do homes with detached garages.

Formaldehyde

Formaldehyde is one of the most ubiquitous indoor air contaminants. It is found primarily in building materials and home furnishings. It is used in hundreds of products, such as urea-formaldehyde and phenol-formaldehyde resin (used to bond laminated wood products and to bind wood chips in particle board); as a carrier solvent in dyeing textiles and paper products; and as a stiffener and water repellent in floor coverings (eg, rugs and linoleum). Urea-formaldehyde foam insulation, one source of formaldehyde used in home construction until the early 1980s, is no longer used. The addition of new furniture to a home increases indoor formaldehyde concentrations. Mobile homes and classrooms, which have small enclosed spaces, low air exchange rates, and many particle board furnishings, may have much higher concentrations of formaldehyde than other types of homes and classrooms. Formaldehyde can also be released from the formaldehyde-releasing resins used to make stain- and wrinkle-resistant clothing. Cigarette smoke is an important source of formaldehyde and also of other volatile organic compounds including acrylonitrile, 1,3-butadiene, acrolein, and acetaldehyde.

Naphthalene

Naphthalene in the indoor air comes from moth balls, unvented kerosene heaters, and tobacco smoke.

Microbial Volatile Organic Compounds

Some fungi can give off volatile organic compounds; these are known as microbial volatile organic compounds.

Systems Affected

Exposure to volatile organic compounds leads mainly to respiratory, dermal, and mucocutaneous effects. Cancer may result from exposure to certain compounds.

Clinical Effects

Depending on the dominant compounds and route and level of exposure, signs and symptoms may include upper respiratory tract and eye irritation, rhinitis, nasal congestion, rash, pruritus, headache, nausea, and vomiting.[5] Symptoms are usually nonspecific and may be insufficient to permit identification of the offending compounds. Some volatile organic compounds (including benzene and formaldehyde) cause cancer in humans,[6,7] and others (1,3 butadiene, styrene, and naphthalene) cause cancer in animals and possibly cause cancer in humans.[8,9]

An association between household paint and solvent exposure and leukemia has been described[10-12] as well as an association between volatile organic compounds and pulmonary function deficits.[13] Clinical effects of some common volatile organic compounds are described in the following paragraphs. Microbial volatile organic compounds are further discussed under molds.

Benzene

The effects of exposure to benzene are described in Chapter 29. Both the International Agency for Research on Cancer (IARC) and the US Environmental Protection Agency (EPA) have assigned benzene their highest cancer classification, Group 1 ("is carcinogenic to humans")[6] and Category A ("known human carcinogen"),[14] respectively. Epidemiologic studies provide conclusive evidence of a causal association between benzene exposure and leukemia, acute nonlymphocytic leukemia, and also possibly chronic nonlymphocytic and chronic lymphocytic leukemias.[14] There have also been occasional reports of an increased risk in humans of other neoplastic changes in the blood or lymphatic system, including Hodgkin and non-Hodgkin lymphoma and myelodysplastic syndrome.[14]

Formaldehyde

Formaldehyde, which smells like pickles, can cause health effects even when an odor cannot be detected. Exposure to airborne formaldehyde may result in conjunctival and upper respiratory tract irritation (ie, burning or tingling sensations in eyes, nose, and throat); these symptoms are temporary and resolve with cessation of exposure.[15] Children may be more sensitive to formaldehyde-induced respiratory toxicity than adults are. Formaldehyde may exacerbate asthma in some infants and children.[16,17] In 2004, the International Agency for Research on Cancer determined that there was sufficient evidence to conclude that formaldehyde causes nasopharyngeal cancer in humans and reclassified it as a Group 1, known human carcinogen (previous classification: Group 2A – limited evidence of carcinogenicity in humans and sufficient evidence in animals).[7] The International Agency for Research on Cancer also reported there was limited evidence to conclude that formaldehyde exposure causes nasal cavity and para-nasal cavity cancer and "strong but not sufficient" evidence linking formaldehyde exposure to leukemia.[7,18]

Naphthalene

Exposure to large amounts of naphthalene may result in hemolytic anemia, resulting in jaundice and hemoglobinuria in children with glucose-6-phosphate dehydrogenase (G6PD) deficiency. Nausea, vomiting, and diarrhea also may occur. Newborn infants also appear to be susceptible to naphthalene-induced hemolysis, presumably because of a decreased ability to conjugate and excrete naphthalene metabolites. Naphthalene is possibly carcinogenic to humans

(Group 2B – limited evidence of carcinogenicity in humans and less than sufficient evidence in animals).[19,20]

Diagnostic Methods

When there is a respiratory symptom, several questions may help to identify potential exposure. Does anyone smoke in the home? Is there an attached garage? Does the family live in a mobile home or a new home with large amounts of pressed wood products? Is there new pressed wood furniture? Are mothballs being used? Have household members recently worked with crafts or graphic materials? Are chemical cleaners used extensively? Has remodeling recently been done? Has anyone recently used paints, solvents, or sprays in the home? Do the parents store paints or other chemicals in the home? Are soaked materials and solvents being disposed of properly? Do the child's symptoms clear when she is removed from the home and reappear when she returns? In addition to an evaluation for a potential environmental exposure, children with persistent respiratory symptoms also may require evaluation for possible infection, allergy, asthma, foreign body or other causes of respiratory symptoms.

Treatment

If volatile organic compounds are thought to be the cause of symptoms, the source should be identified and, if possible, removed. Measuring levels of volatile organic compounds in the air usually is not necessary.

Prevention of Exposure

The single most important step to reduce the concentrations of volatile organic compounds in the home is to prohibit smoking indoors. Another important prevention strategy is the modification of building codes to require detached garages. Attached garages should be isolated from living and working spaces by closing the doorways, sealing the structures and ensuring that there is a proper air pressure difference between the garage and other indoor spaces.

Homes or classrooms in which new materials have been installed or that have undergone renovation should receive increased outdoor air ventilation. In the initial months after building completion, the ventilation should operate 24 hours/day, 7 days/week. Installation of new products or renovation work should preferably occur when the space is unoccupied and will remain unoccupied until off-gassing of the strongest volatile organic compounds has occurred. Steps should be taken to reduce the relative humidity to 30% to 50% to reduce the growth of molds and microbial volatile organic compounds. Parents should avoid storing opened containers of unused paints and similar materials in the home and should dispose of soaked materials and solvents properly.

If it is not possible to remove the source of formaldehyde (ie, large amounts of pressed wood products), the exposure can be reduced by coating cabinets, paneling, and other furnishings with polyurethane or other nontoxic sealants and by increasing the amount of ventilation in the building. Formaldehyde concentrations decrease rapidly over the first year after a product is manufactured. Textiles that have been coated with formaldehyde resins (draperies and some permanent press clothes) should first be washed before using. Formaldehyde levels on treated fabrics greatly subside with each washing.

Infants should not be exposed to textiles (clothing/bedding) that have been stored for long periods with naphthalene-containing moth repellents. If families use naphthalene-containing moth repellents, the material should be enclosed in containers that prevent vapors from escaping and kept out of the reach of children. Blankets and clothing stored with naphthalene-containing moth repellents should be aired outdoors to remove naphthalene odors and washed before they are used.

Guidelines

The total of all volatile organic compounds measured in an air sample is called total volatile organic compounds. The concentration of total volatile organic compounds is expressed as $\mu g/m^3$ of air. The concentration of total volatile organic compounds in a building or home is a good indicator of whether or not there are elevated levels. On the basis of data from German homes, researchers have suggested that 300 $\mu g/m^3$ of total volatile organic compounds (the average value of the study) should not be exceeded.[21,22]

At present, there are no US standards for total volatile organic compounds. The European Community has prepared a target guideline value for total volatile organic compounds of 300 $\mu g/m^3$ in which no individual volatile organic compound should exceed 10% of the total volatile organic compound concentration.[22] Levels higher than this may result in irritation to some occupants. However, lower levels can also be an issue if a particularly toxic substance or odorant is present.[23] The INDEX project in the European Union proposed that indoor air concentrations of benzene and formaldehyde should be kept as low as reasonably achievable because of their known carcinogenicity. A long-term guideline value of 10 $\mu g/m^3$ for naphthalene was proposed.[24]

MOLDS

There are more than 200 000 species of fungi, including mold, yeast, and mushrooms. More than 100 000 mold species have been identified. Mildew is a kind of mold often found in bathroom tiles and on shower curtains.

Routes and Sources of Exposure

Exposure to molds occurs via inhalation of contaminated air and dermal contact with surfaces on which they are deposited. Molds are ubiquitous in the outdoor environment and can enter the home through doorways, windows, air conditioning systems, and heating and ventilation systems.

Molds proliferate in environments that contain excessive moisture, such as from leaks in plumbing, roofs, walls, and pet urine and plant pots. The most common molds found indoors are *Cladosporium, Penicillium, Aspergillus,* and *Alternaria* species.[25]

If a building is extremely wet for an extended period, other molds with higher water requirements, including *Stachybotrys* and *Trichoderma* species, can grow.[25]

Systems Affected

The eyes, nose, throat, and respiratory tract are affected by exposure to molds. Exposure to molds can also affect the skin and nervous system.

Clinical Effects

Exposure to molds may result in infectious, allergic, or toxic health effects. The American Academy of Pediatrics (AAP) *Red Book* provides guidance on fungal infections.[26] The Institute of Medicine and the AAP have published comprehensive reviews of the spectrum of health effects from dampness and molds.[27-29] Children's exposure to molds is associated with a higher risk of persistent upper respiratory tract symptoms such as rhinitis, sneezing, and eye irritation as well as lower respiratory tract symptoms, such as coughing and wheezing.[27-30] Both the Institute of Medicine and AAP concluded that moisture in buildings is associated with the exacerbation of asthma in children. A more recent guideline from the World Health Organization also found that there was sufficient evidence to conclude that there is an association between exposure to molds and the development of asthma.[31]

Toxic effects of molds may be attributable to inhalation of mycotoxins, lipid-soluble toxins readily absorbed by the airways.[32] Species of mycotoxin-producing molds include *Fusarium, Trichoderma,* and *Stachybotrys.* A single mold species may produce several different toxins, and a given mycotoxin may be produced by more than one species of mold. Furthermore, toxin-producing molds do not necessarily produce mycotoxins under all growth conditions, with production being dependent on the substrate, temperature, water content, and humidity.[33] Exposure to an extremely moldy home has been associated with multifocal choroiditis in an adult.[34]

Exposure to *Stachybotrys chartarum (atra)* and other molds has been associated with acute pulmonary hemorrhage among young infants in Cleveland, OH,[35-39] Kansas City, MO,[40] Delaware,[41] and New Zealand.[42] Exposure to *Trichoderma* species and other molds has been associated with acute pulmonary hemorrhage in a North Carolina infant.[43]

Studies of acute intratracheal exposure to the metabolites of *Stachybotrys* species in male rats demonstrate lung tissue injury. The studies concluded that lung cell damage was more likely attributable to toxins than fungal cell wall components.[44-47]

There have been a variety of neurologic symptoms associated with living in moldy environments, including fatigue, difficulty concentrating, and headaches.[32] Although few studies of children have been performed, it is biologically plausible that these symptoms could be associated with mold exposures. Many mycotoxins that have been isolated from spores, mold fragments, and dust from moldy areas are significantly toxic. In vitro and in vivo studies have demonstrated adverse effects, including immunotoxic, neurologic, respiratory, and dermal responses, after exposure to specific toxins, bacteria, molds, or their products. Many pure microbial toxins, such as the products of *Fusarium* species (fumonisin B_1, deoxynivalenol), *Stachybotrys* species (satratoxin G), *Aspergillus* species (ochratoxin A), and *Penicillium* species (ochratoxin A, verrucosidin), have been shown to be neurotoxic in vitro and in vivo.[48-53] In the indoor environment, various microbiological agents with diverse, fluctuating inflammatory and toxic potential are present simultaneously with other airborne compounds, inevitably resulting in interactions. Such interactions may lead to unexpected responses, even at low concentrations.[31]

Diagnostic Methods

Pediatricians must have a high index of suspicion, because mold is considered to be a "great masquerader."[54] Several key questions about the child's home environment may help to identify potential exposure to molds. These include: Has the home been flooded? Is there any water-damaged wood or cardboard in the house? Has there been a roof or plumbing leak? Have occupants seen any mold or noticed a musty smell? Has anyone else in the home been ill? Do the child's symptoms resolve when he is away from the home and recur when he returns? Guidance for clinicians on recognizing and managing health effects related to mold exposure and moisture indoors has been published by the University of Connecticut Health Center.[55] Table 20.3 lists sentinel health conditions that may suggest mold or moisture in the absence of an alternative explanation. The concept of a "sentinel condition" has great utility in the area of occupational and environmental health. The diagnosis of an individual with a "sentinel" illness associated with exposures in a particular environment may indicate that these exposures may also deleteriously affect others.[56,57] Intervention in the environment to limit such identified exposures is an opportunity for primary prevention.[55]

Testing the environment for specific molds usually is not necessary.[58,59] When testing is performed, the results may be difficult to interpret, because there are no

Table 20.3: Sentinel Conditions	
SYMPTOMS AND SYNDROMES THAT MAY SUGGEST MOLD OR MOISTURE IN THE ABSENCE OF AN ALTERNATIVE EXPLANATION	
CONDITIONS OF CONCERN	**PRECURSOR CONDITIONS**
New onset asthma	Mucosal irritation
Exacerbated asthma	Recurrent rhinitis/
Interstitial lung disease	sinusitis
Hypersensitivity pneumonitis	Recurrent hoarseness
Sarcoidosis	
Pulmonary hemorrhage in infants	

Reprinted with permission from the University of Connecticut Health Center, Farmington, CT, from *Guidance for Clinicians on the Recognition and Management of Health Effects Related to Mold Exposure and Moisture Indoors.* Available at: http://oehc.uchc.edu/CIEH.asp.

agreed-on standards. There are, however, some rules of thumb for assessing the number of mold spores found in the indoor air. Some investigators have categorized mean levels of culturable mold counts into 5 groups.[60]

Group 1: Low (<100 colony forming units [CFUs]/m^3)
Group 2: Medium (101–300 CFUs/m^3)
Group 3: High (301–1000 CFUs/m^3)
Group 4: Very high (1001–5000 CFUs/m^3)
Group 5: Extremely high (>5000 CFUs/m^3)

Tests to measure specific mycotoxins or mycotoxin adducts in urine have been developed for research purposes.[61,62] An adduct (from the Latin, adductus, "drawn towards"), is a species formed by the union of 2 species (usually molecules) held together by a coordinate covalent bond. There currently is no clinically available diagnostic test for mycotoxins in human tissue. Testing for antibodies to fungal antigens may not be helpful because of cross-reacting antigens from related organisms.

Microbial volatile organic compounds produced by molds are responsible for the characteristic odors produced by molds, often described as musty, earthy, or moldy. Microbial volatile organic compounds include certain aldehydes, alcohols, and ketones that are not typically found to emit from building materials. Frequently found microbial volatile organic compounds include geosmin, hexanone, and octanols. Some of these microbial volatile organic compounds have been found to be irritants to humans and contribute to sick building syndrome (see Chapter 11). Microbial volatile organic compounds can be easily measured in the air at very low levels, and their presence is an indication of mold contamination. Because mold is frequently found inside walls and other inaccessible areas, measurements of microbial volatile organic compound are sometimes used as a way of confirming and locating mold contamination.

Fireplace Safety

1. If possible, keep a window cracked open while the fire is burning.
2. Be certain the damper or flue is open before starting a fire. Keeping the damper or flue open until the fire is out will draw smoke out of the house. The damper can be checked by looking up into the chimney with a flashlight.
3. Use dry and well-aged wood. Wet or green wood causes more smoke and contributes to soot buildup in the chimney.
4. Smaller pieces of wood placed on a grate burn faster and produce less smoke.
5. Levels of ash at the base of the fireplace should be kept to 1 inch or less because a thicker layer restricts the air supply to logs, resulting in more smoke.
6. The chimney should be checked annually by a professional. Even if the chimney is not due for cleaning, it is important to check for animal nests or other blockages that could prevent smoke from escaping.

Prevention of Exposure

Prevention strategies include cleaning up water and removing all water-damaged items (including carpets) within 24 hours of a flood or leak. If this is performed, mold will not have the opportunity to grow. Interventions to reduce dampness and mold have been demonstrated to reduce asthma exacerbations among children.[63] Guidance on preventing mold exposure is available from the American Industrial Hygiene Association.[58]

GUIDELINES

The World Health Organization has produced Guidelines on Indoor Air Quality.[31]

Frequently Asked Questions

Q *What are the most important things I can do to protect my child from indoor air pollution?*

A Make sure you have a carbon monoxide detector on each sleeping level in your home and that each detector is in good working condition. Do not smoke and do not allow anyone to smoke in your home. Preventing children from being exposed to secondhand smoke is important. Keep your home dry and fix all water leaks promptly. If you have an attached garage, make sure that you keep the door between the garage and the house tightly closed to reduce the amount of benzene that comes in to the house. Wood stoves and fireplaces need to be checked yearly by a professional to make sure they are clean and running efficiently. Gas ovens should not be used to provide supplemental heat. Children should not come into contact with mothballs, because they contain dangerous chemicals. Air fresheners do not improve air quality and use artificial chemicals to provide scent.

Q *Are air fresheners hazardous?*

A There is limited information on the potential health effects of using air fresheners. One study has linked blood levels of 1,4-dichlorobenzene, a volatile organic compound often used in air fresheners, to reduced pulmonary function in adults. The long-term effects have not been studied. Scented candles also off-gas volatile organic compounds.

Q *My child has had a persistent runny nose. Could this be caused by the new carpet we installed last month?*

A The symptom could be caused by viruses, bacteria, allergies, or perhaps a foreign body in the nose. It also is possible that the symptoms relate to something in the child's environment, such as secondhand smoke or the chemical compounds released from a new carpet. Sometimes an exact diagnosis is difficult to determine. Symptoms from colds are temporary, and symptoms from environmental irritants tend to improve once exposure to the irritant is eliminated. If possible, have your child play and sleep in another room to see if symptoms improve. It may take some time to determine the cause of the child's symptoms.

Q *What are the effects of exposure to mothballs?*

A Two products, p-dichlorobenzene and naphthalene, are used as moth repellents. Reports of occupational exposure to the active ingredients of mothballs are available. Studies documenting health effects from residential exposure are limited. The active ingredient in mothballs usually is p-dichlorobenzene. Exposure to p-dichlorobenzene may cause irritation of the eyes, nose, and throat; swelling around the eyes; headache; and a runny nose, which usually subsides 24 hours after exposure ends. Prolonged occupational exposure to p-dichlorobenzene may result in loss of appetite, nausea, vomiting, weight loss, and liver damage. Consider replacing mothballs with cedar products.

Q *What can be done to reduce the levels of particulates from wood stoves and fireplaces?*

A Measures to reduce the levels of particulate matter from a wood stove include ensuring that the stove is placed in a room with adequate ventilation and properly vented directly to the outdoors. Newer stoves are designed to emit less particulate matter into the air. Information on improved wood stoves can be found at http://www.epa.gov/burnwise.

Q *What are ionizers and other ozone-generating air cleaners? Should they be used?*

A Ion generators act by charging the particles in a room so that they are attracted to walls, floors, tabletops, draperies, or occupants. Abrasion can result in resuspension of these particles into the air. In some cases, these devices contain a collector to attract the charged particles back to the unit. Although ion generators may remove small particles (eg, those in second-hand smoke), they do not remove gases or odors and may be relatively ineffective in removing large particles, such as pollen and house-dust allergens. Ozone generators are specifically designed to release ozone to purify the air.

Ozone is produced indirectly by ion generators and some electronic air cleaners and produced directly by ozone generators. Although indirect ozone production is of concern, there is even greater concern with the direct and purposeful introduction of ozone into indoor air. No difference exists, despite the claims of some marketers, between ozone in smog outdoors and ozone produced by ozone generators. Under certain conditions, these devices can produce levels of ozone high enough to be harmful to a child. Ozone-generating air cleaners may also contribute to indoor formaldehyde concentrations. They are not recommended for use in homes or schools.

Q *Can other air cleaners help?*

A Other air cleaners include mechanical filter, electronic (eg, electrostatic precipitators), and hybrid air cleaners using 2 or more techniques. The value of any air cleaner depends on its efficiency, proper selection for the pollutant to be removed, proper installation, and appropriate maintenance. Drawbacks include inadequate pollutant removal, redispersement of pollutants, deceptive masking of the pollutant rather than its removal, generation of ozone, and unacceptable noise levels. The EPA and Consumer Product Safety Commission have not taken a position either for or against the use of these devices.

Effective control at the source of a pollutant is key. Air cleaners are not a solution but are adjunct to source control and adequate ventilation. The state of California regulates air cleaners. The California Air Resources Board lists the models of air cleaners that have been certified by the Air Resources Board as meeting the testing and certification requirements of the state's air cleaner regulation. The certified air cleaner models may be viewed at http://www.arb.ca.gov/research/indoor/aircleaners/certified.htm.

Q *I am about to purchase a new vacuum cleaner for my home. Should I buy one with a HEPA filter?*

A HEPA (high efficiency particulate air) filters reduce dust by trapping small particles and not rereleasing them into the air as you vacuum. Although widely advertised for use in homes in which children with asthma or allergies are living, it is not clear whether HEPA filters reduce symptoms or medication use in children with asthma. The use of HEPA filters should not substitute for other allergen-reduction methods. Some vacuum cleaners advertise HEPA filters, but that does not necessarily mean they have an effective air filtration system. Unless the filter is contained in a sealed, airtight chamber, dirty air can still escape from the vacuum. Look for a system that is designated as "true HEPA," a term that indicates the entire system, not just the filter, meets HEPA standards.

Q   *When I bring clothes home from the dry cleaners, are the chemicals that are released from the clothes dangerous to my child?*

A   Perchloroethylene is the chemical most widely used in dry cleaning. In laboratory studies, it has been shown to cause cancer in animals. Recent studies indicate that people breathe low levels of this chemical both in homes where dry-cleaned goods are stored and as they wear dry-cleaned clothing. Dry cleaners recapture the perchloroethylene during the dry-cleaning process so they can save money by reusing it, and they remove more of the chemical during the pressing and finishing processes. Some dry cleaners, however, do not remove as much perchloroethylene as possible all of the time. Taking steps to minimize your exposure to this chemical is prudent. If dry-cleaned goods have a strong chemical odor when you pick them up, do not accept them until they have been properly dried. If goods with a chemical odor are returned to you on subsequent visits, try a different dry cleaner.

Of more concern is whether the home is located directly above or adjacent to a dry cleaning establishment. If so, the amount of daily exposure may be enough to cause adverse health effects.

Q   *Can exposure to chemicals from carpets make people sick?*

A   New carpet may emit volatile organic compounds, as do products such as adhesives and padding that accompany carpet installation. Some people report symptoms including eye, nose, and throat irritation; headaches; skin irritation; shortness of breath or cough; and fatigue, which may be associated with new carpet installation. Carpet also can act as a "sink" for chemical and biological pollutants including pesticides, dust mites, and molds.

Anyone seeking to purchase new carpet can ask retailers for information to help them select carpet, padding, and adhesives that emit lower amounts of volatile organic compounds. Before new carpet is installed, the retailer should unroll and air out the carpet in a clean, well-ventilated area. Opening doors and windows reduces the level of chemicals released. Ventilation systems should be in proper working order and operated during installation, and for 48 to 72 hours after the new carpet is installed.

Q *Can plants control indoor air pollution?*

A Reports in the media and promotions by representatives of the decorative houseplant industry characterize plants as "nature's clean air machine," claiming that research by the National Aeronautics and Space Administration shows that plants remove indoor air pollutants. Although it is true that plants remove carbon dioxide from the air, and the ability of plants to remove certain other pollutants from water is the basis for some pollution control methods, the ability of plants to control indoor air pollution is less well established. The only study of the use of plants to control indoor air pollutants in an actual building could not determine any benefit. As a practical means of pollution control, the plant removal mechanisms seem to be inconsequential when compared with common ventilation and air exchange rates. Overdamp planter soil conditions may promote growth of molds.

Q *How do I keep my fireplace safe?*

A The box lists measures to increase fireplace safety.

Q *Are there potential problems with incense burning?*

A Incense burning in homes can emit particulates, volatile organic compounds such as benzene, nitrogen dioxide, and carbon monoxide. Carbon monoxide levels from incense burning can reach a peak concentration of $9.6 \ mg/m^3$, which could exceed the EPAs National Ambient Air Quality Standard of $10 \ mg/m^3$ for an 8-hour average depending on the room volume, ventilation rate, and the amount of incense burned. Incense burning might be a significant contributor to indoor air pollution in cultures in which incense is burned frequently, for example when people use incense during religious rituals.

Q *What is your advice about disposing of solvents?*

A To avoid the problem of disposal, consider using safer alternatives, such as vinegar and water. If you purchase a hazardous material such as a solvent, buy a small amount so that it is more likely that you will use it up completely.

Read the label regarding the proper storage and disposal of the product. Always follow manufacturer's directions, not only for use but afterwards as well. There may be household hazardous product roundups in your community. Many local waste companies offer this service a couple of times a year. Consider contacting refuse companies found in the phone book or on the internet for more options. Leave the product in its original packaging and seal the container tightly. This will keep the hazardous material from contaminating anything else and always leave labels intact, even when throwing an empty container away. Check with neighbors and friends to see whether they have any use for any extra product that you may have, instead of disposing of the unused portion. To prevent unintentional poisoning, keep the product out of the reach of small children.

Resources

American Lung Association
Phone: 800-LUNG-USA.
Web site: www.lungusa.org

US Environmental Protection Agency
Indoor Air Quality Information Clearinghouse
Phone: 800-438-4318
Web site: www.epa.gov/iaq
Additional resources from the EPA include EPA regional offices and state and local departments of health and environmental quality. For regulation of specific pollutants, contact the EPA Toxic Substances Control Act Assistance Information Service: 202-554-1404.

Care for Your Air: A Guide to Indoor Air Quality
Understand indoor air in homes, schools, and offices.
Web site: www.epa.gov/iaq/pubs/careforyourair.html

Indoor Air Quality Scientific Findings Resource Bank
Web site: www.iaqscience.lbl.gov

US Consumer Product Safety Commission
Phone: 800-638-CPSC
Web site: www.cpsc.gov
Provides information on particular product hazards.

National Center for Healthy Housing, Pediatric Environmental Home Assessment
Web site: www.healthyhomestraining.org/Nurse/PEHA.htm

References

1. Hansel NN, Breysse PN, McCormack MC, et al. A longitudinal study of indoor nitrogen dioxide levels and respiratory symptoms in inner-city children with asthma. *Environ Health Perspect.* 2008;116(10):1428-1432
2. Robin LF, Less PS, Winget M, et al. Wood-burning stoves and lower respiratory illnesses in Navajo children. *Pediatr Infect Dis J.* 1996;15:859–865
3. World Health Organization. *Air Quality Guidelines: Global Update 2005.* Geneva, Switzerland: World Health Organization; 2006. Available at: http://www.euro.who.int/__data/assets/pdf_file/0005/78638/E90038.pdf. Accessed March 7, 2011
4. Agency for Toxic Substances and Disease Registry. *Toxicological Profile for Ammonia.* Atlanta, GA: Agency for Toxic Substances and Disease Registry; 2004. Available at: http://www.atsdr.cdc.gov/toxprofiles/tp.asp?id=11&tid=2. Accessed March 7, 2011
5. Mendell MJ. Indoor residential chemical emissions as risk factors for respiratory and allergic effects in children: a review. *Indoor Air.* 2007;17(4):259-277

6. International Agency for Research on Cancer. *IARC Monographs Supplement 7. Benzene.* 1987. Available at: http://monographs.iarc.fr/ENG/Monographs/suppl7/Suppl7-24.pdf

7. International Agency for Research on Cancer. *IARC Monograph on the Evaluation of Carcinogenic Risks to Humans.* Lyon, France: International Agency for Research on Cancer; 2006. Available at: http://monographs.iarc.fr/ENG/Monographs/vol88/index.php. Accessed March 7, 2011

8. International Agency for Research on Cancer. *IARC Monograph on the Evaluation of Carcinogenic Risks to Humans. Vol 82. Some traditional herbal medicines, some mycotoxins, naphthalene and styrene.* Lyon, France: International Agency for Research on Cancer; 2002. Available at: http://monographs.iarc.fr/ENG/Monographs/vol82/index.php. Accessed March 7, 2011

9. International Agency for Research on Cancer. *IARC Monograph on the Evaluation of Carcinogenic Risks to Humans. Vol 97. 1,3 butadiene, ethylene oxide and vinyl halides.* Lyon, France: International Agency for Research on Cancer; 2008. Available at: http://monographs.iarc.fr/ENG/Monographs/vol97/index.php. Accessed March 7, 2011

10. Freedman DM, Stewart P, Kleinerman RA, et al. Household solvent exposures and childhood acute lymphoblastic leukemia. *Am J Public Health.* 2001;91(4):564–567

11. Lowengart RA, Peters JM, Cicioni C, et al. Childhood leukemia and parents' occupational and home exposures. *J Natl Cancer Inst.* 1987;79(1):39–46

12. Scélo G, Metayer C , Zhang L, et al. Household exposure to paint and petroleum solvents, chromosomal translocations, and the risk of childhood leukemia. *Environ Health Perspect.* 2009;117(1):133-139

13. Elliott L, Longnecker MP, Kissling GE, London SJ. Volatile organic compounds and pulmonary function in the Third National Health and Nutrition Examination Survey, 1988–1994. *Environ Health Perspect.* 2006;114(8):1210-1214

14. US Environmental Protection Agency. *Integrated Risk Information System (IRIS) on Benzene.* Washington, DC: US Environmental Protection Agency, Center for Environmental Assessment, Office of Research and Development; 2002. Available at: http://www.epa.gov/iris/subst/0276.htm. Accessed March 7, 2011

15. Wantke F, Demmer CM, Tappler P, Gotz M, Jarisch R. Exposure to gaseous formaldehyde induces IgE-mediated sensitization to formaldehyde in school-children. *Clin Exp Allergy. 1996;26(3):276–280*

16. McGwin G, Lienert J, Kennedy JI. Formaldehyde exposure and asthma in children: a systematic review. *Environ Health Perspect.* 2009;118(3):313-317

17. Smedje G, Norback D, Edling C. Asthma among secondary school children in relation to the school environment. *Clin Exp Allergy.* 1997;27(11):1270–1278

18. Zhang L, Steinmaus C, Eastmond DA, Xin XK, Smith MT. Formaldehyde exposure and leukemia: A new meta-analysis and potential mechanisms. *Mutat Res.* 2009;681(2-3):150-168

19. Dobson CP, Neuwirth M, Frye RE, Gorman M. Index of suspicion. *Pediatr Rev.* 2006;27(1): 29-33

20. Athanasious M, Tsantali C, Trachana M, et al. Hemolytic anemia in a female newborn infant whose mother inhaled naphthalene before delivery. *J Pediatr.* 1995;130(4):680-681

21. Seifert B. Regulating indoor air. In: Walkinshaw DS, ed. *Indoor Air '90. Proceedings of the 5th International Conference on Indoor Air Quality and Climate.* Vol 5. Toronto, Canada, July 29-August 3, 1990:35-49

22. European Commission Joint Research Centre. *European Collaborative Action 'Indoor Air Quality and Its Impact on Man'. Total Volatile Organic Compounds (TVOC) in Indoor Air Quality Investigations.* Report No 19. EUR 17675 EN. Luxembourg: Office for Official Publications of the European Community; 1997

23. Health Canada. *Indoor Air Quality in Office Buildings: A Technical Guide. Available at:* http://www.hc-sc.gc.ca/ewh-semt/pubs/air/office_building-immeubles_bureaux/organic-organiques-eng.php. Accessed March 7, 2011

24. Kotzias D, Koistinen K, Kephalopoulos S, et al. *The INDEX Project. Critical Appraisal of the Setting and Implementation of Indoor Exposure Limits in the EU.* Ispra, Italy: European Commission, Institute for Health and Consumer Protection, Physical and Chemical Exposure Unit; 2005:1-50. Available at: http://ec.europa.eu/health/ph_projects/2002/pollution/fp_pollution_2002_frep_02.pdf. Accessed March 7, 2011

25. Centers for Disease Control and Prevention and US Department of Housing and Urban Development. *Healthy Housing Reference Manual.* Atlanta, GA: US Department of Health and Human Services; 2006

26. American Academy of Pediatrics. *Red Book: 2009 Report of the Committee on Infectious Diseases.* Pickering LK, Baker CJ, Kimberlin DW, Long SS, eds. 28th ed. Elk Grove Village, IL: American Academy of Pediatrics; 2009

27. Institute of Medicine. *Damp Indoor Spaces and Health.* Washington, DC: National Academy of Sciences; 2004

28. American Academy of Pediatrics, Committee on Environmental Health. Policy statement: spectrum of noninfectious health effects from molds. *Pediatrics.* 2006;118(6):2582-2586

29. Mazur LJ; Kim JJ; American Academy of Pediatrics, Committee on Environmental Health. Technical report: spectrum of noninfectious health effects from molds. *Pediatrics.* 2006;118(6):e1909-e1926

30. Antova T, Pattenden S, Brunekreef B, et al. Exposure to indoor mould and children's respiratory health in the PATY study. *J Epidemiol Community Health.* 2008;62(8):708-714

31. World Health Organization. *Guidelines for Indoor Air Quality: Dampness and Mold.* Copenhagen, Denmark: World Health Organization; 2009. Available at: http://www.euro.who.int/__data/assets/pdf_file/0017/43325/E92645.pdf. March 7, 2011

32. Croft WA, Jarvis BB, Yatawara CS. Airborne outbreak of trichothecene toxicosis. *Atmos Environ.* 1986;20(8):549–552

33. Burge HA, Ammann HA. Fungal toxins and B(1-3)-D-glucans. In: Macher J, ed. *Bioaerosols: Assessment and Control.* Cincinnati, OH: American Conference of Governmental and Industrial Hygienists; 1999:24-1–24-13

34. Rudich R, Santilli J, Rockwell WJ. Indoor mold exposure: a possible factor in the etiology of multifocal choroiditis. *Am J Ophthalmol.* 2003,135(3):402-404

35. Dearborn DG, Smith PG, Dahms BB, et al. Clinical profile of 30 infants with acute pulmonary hemorrhage in Cleveland. *Pediatrics.* 2002;110(3):627–637

36. Montaña E, Etzel RA, Allan T, Horgan TE, Dearborn DG. Environmental risk factors associated with pediatric idiopathic pulmonary hemorrhage and hemosiderosis in a Cleveland community. *Pediatrics.* 1997;99(1):e5

37. Etzel RA, Montaña E, Sorenson WG, et al. Acute pulmonary hemorrhage in infants associated with exposure to *Stachybotrys atra* and other fungi. *Arch Pediatr Adolesc Med.* 1998;152(8):757–762

38. Centers for Disease Control and Prevention. Update: pulmonary hemorrhage/hemosiderosis among infants—Cleveland, Ohio, 1993–1996. *MMWR Morb Mortal Wkly Rep.* 2000;49(9):180–184

39. Jarvis BB, Sorenson WG, Hintikka EL, et al. Study of toxin production by isolates of *Stachybotrys chartarum* and *Memnoniella echinata* isolated during a study of pulmonary hemosiderosis in infants. *Appl Environ Microbiol.* 1998;64(10):3620–3625

40. Flappan SM, Portnoy J, Jones P, Barnes C. Infant pulmonary hemorrhage in a suburban home with water damage and mold (*Stachybotrys atra*). *Environ Health Perspect*. 1999;107(11): 927–930

41. Weiss A, Chidekel AS. Acute pulmonary hemorrhage in a Delaware infant after exposure to *Stachybotrys atra*. *Del Med J*. 2002;74(9):363–368

42. Habiba A. Acute idiopathic pulmonary haemorrhage in infancy: case report and review of the literature. *J Paediatr Child Health*. 2005;41(9-10):532-533

43. Novotny WE, Dixit A. Pulmonary hemorrhage in an infant following two weeks of fungal exposure. *Arch Pediatr Adolesc Med*. 2000;154(3):271–275

44. Yike I, Rand T, Dearborn DG. The role of fungal proteinases in pathophysiology of *Stachybotrys chartarum*. *Mycopathologia*. 2007;164(4):171-181

45. McCrae KC, Rand TG, Shaw RA, et al. DNA fragmentation in developing lung fibroblasts exposed to *Stachybotrys chartarum (atra)* toxins. *Pediatr Pulmonol*. 2007;42(7):592-599

46. Kováciková Z, Tátrai E, Piecková E, et al. An in vitro study of the toxic effects of *Stachybotrys chartarum* metabolites on lung cells. *Altern Lab Anim*. 2007;35(1):47-52

47. Pieckova E, Hurbankova M, Cerna S, Pivovarova Z, Kovacikova Z. Pulmonary cytotoxicity of secondary metabolites of *Stachybotrys chartarum (Ehrenb) Hughes*. *Ann Agric Environ Med*. 2006;13(2):259-262

48. Rotter BA, Prelusky DB, Pestka JJ. Toxicology of deoxynivalenol (vomitoxin). *J Toxicol Environ Health*. 1996;48(1):1-34

49. Belmadani A, Steyn PS, Tramu G, Betbeder AM, Baudrimont I, Creppy EE. Selective toxicity of ochratoxin A in primary cultures from different brain regions. *Arch Toxicol*. 1999;73(2): 108-101

50. Kwon OS, Slikker W Jr, Davies DL. Biochemical and morphological effects of fumonisin B(1) on primary cultures of rat cerebrum. *Neurotoxicol Teratol*. 2000;22(4):565-567

51. Islam Z, Harkema JR, Pestka JJ. Satratoxin G from the black mold *Stachybotrys chartarum* evokes olfactory sensory neuron loss and inflammation in the murine nose and brain. *Environ Health Perspect*. 2006;114(7):1099-1107

52. Islam Z, Hegg CC, Bae HK, Pestka JJ. Satratoxin G-induced apoptosis in PC-12 neuronal cells is mediated by PKR and caspase independent. *Toxicol Sci*. 2008;105(1):142-152

53. Stockmann-Juvala H, Savolainen K. A review of the toxic effects and mechanisms of action of fumonisin B1. *Hum Exp Toxicol*. 2008;27(11):799-809

54. Etzel RA. What the primary care pediatrician should know about syndromes associated with exposures to mycotoxins. *Curr Probl Pediatr Adolesc Health Care*. 2006;36(8):282-305

55. Storey E, Dangman KH, Schenck P, et al. *Guidance for Clinicians on the Recognition and Management of Health Effects Related to Mold Exposure and Moisture Indoors*. Farmington, CT: University of Connecticut; 2004. Available at: http://oehc.uchc.edu/images/PDFs/MOLD%20 GUIDE.pdf. Accessed March 7, 2011

56. Rossman MD, Thompson B, Frederick M, et al. HLA and environmental interactions in sarcoidosis. ACCESS Group. *Sarcoidosis Vasc Diffuse Lung Dis*. 2008;25(2):125-132

57. Taskar V, Coultas D. Exposures and idiopathic lung disease. *Semin Respir Crit Care Med*. 2008;29(6):670-679

58. American Industrial Hygiene Association. *Recognition, Evaluation, and Control of Indoor Mold*. Prezant B, Weekes DM, Miller DM, eds. Fairfax, VA: American Industrial Hygiene Association; 2008

59. Government Accountability Office. *Indoor Mold*. Washington, DC: Government Accountability Office; September 2008

60. Platt SD, Martin CJ, Hunt SM, Lewis CW. Damp housing, mould growth, and symptomatic health state. *BMJ.* 1989;298(6689):1673-1678

61. Yike I, Distler AM, Ziady AG, Dearborn DG. Mycotoxin adducts on human serum albumin: biomarkers of exposure to *Stachybotrys chartarum. Environ Health Perspect.* 2006;114(8): 1221-1226

62. Hooper DG, Bolton VE, Guilford FT, Straus DS. Mycotoxin detection in human samples from patients exposed to environmental molds. *Int J Mol Sci.* 2009;10(4):1465-1475

63. Kercsmar CM, Dearborn DG, Schluchter M, et al. Reduction in asthma morbidity in children as a result of home remediation aimed at moisture sources. *Environ Health Perspect.* 2006;114(10):1574-1580

Chapter 21

Air Pollutants, Outdoor

■ ■ ■ ■ ■ ■

Outdoor air pollution consists of a complex mixture of pollutants found in ambient (outdoor) air.[1,2] Outdoor air pollutants can come from many sources, including large industrial facilities; smaller operations, such as dry cleaners and gas stations; natural sources, such as wildfires; highway vehicles; and other sources, such as aircraft, locomotives, and lawn mowers. The relative importance of these different sources varies from one community to another, depending on regional and nearby sources of pollution, time of day, and weather conditions. The potential for health risks posed by outdoor air pollution depends on the concentration and composition of the mixture, the duration of exposures, and the health status and genetic makeup of exposed individuals. The US Environmental Protection Agency (EPA) has established national ambient air quality standards for 6 principal pollutants, referred to as "criteria" pollutants: ozone, respirable particulate matter, lead, sulfur dioxide, carbon monoxide, and nitrogen oxides.[1,2] Additionally, the EPA monitors other toxic chemicals, or "hazardous air pollutants," released into the air by motor vehicles, industrial facilities, wood combustion, agricultural activities, and other sources. In the United States, a national monitoring network has been established for these criteria pollutants; fewer (approximately 300) monitoring sites across the country provide data on some other hazardous air pollutants. From 1980 to 2007, national average levels of the criteria pollutants showed general improvements in the nation's air quality.[1] However, air quality in some areas of the United States actually declined in recent years, and recent research suggests health effects at levels of some pollutants previously considered to be "safe."[2]

SPECIFIC AIR POLLUTANTS

Ozone

Ozone is one of the most pervasive outdoor air pollutants. Ozone and other photochemical oxidants, such as peroxyacetylnitrate, are secondary pollutants formed in the atmosphere from a chemical reaction between volatile organic compounds (VOCs) and nitrogen oxides in the presence of heat and sunlight. The primary sources of these precursor compounds include motor vehicle exhaust and power plants, although hydrocarbon emissions from chemical plants and refineries and evaporative emissions from gasoline and natural sources also can contribute to their formation. Atmospheric movement of these precursor pollutants may produce ozone hundreds of miles downwind from the sources of these pollutants. Ozone is the principal component of urban smog, the brownish haze often seen over cities in the summer. Concentrations of ozone generally are highest on hot, dry, stagnant summer days and increase to maximum concentrations in the late afternoon. Changes in weather patterns can contribute to differences in ozone concentrations from year to year. Indoor concentrations of ozone can vary from 10% to 80% of outdoor levels, depending on the amount of fresh air entering the building. Most personal exposure occurs in outdoor settings.

Particulate Matter

Particulate matter is a general term that refers to an airborne mixture of solid particles and liquid droplets. The term is applied to pollutants of varying chemical composition and physical properties. Particle size is the primary determinant of whether the particles will be deposited in the lower respiratory system. Particles larger than 10 μm in aerodynamic diameter are too large to be inhaled beyond the nasal passages. Children, however, frequently breathe through their mouths, thus bypassing the nasal clearance mechanism.

All particulate matter less than 10 μm in aerodynamic diameter is known as PM_{10}. Particles of this size cannot be seen with the naked eye, but their presence in the atmosphere can be seen as sooty clouds or general haze that impairs visibility. "Fine particles" are smaller than 2.5 μm in aerodynamic diameter and referred to as $PM_{2.5}$. Fine particles result from the combustion of fuels used in motor vehicles, power plants, and industrial operations as well as the combustion of organic material in fireplaces and wood stoves. Particles between 2.5 μm and 10 μm in aerodynamic diameter (or even larger) are referred to as "coarse" particles. Coarse particles include dusts that have been generated from the mechanical breakdown of solid matter (such as rocks, soil, and dust) and windblown dust. Compared with coarse particles, fine particles can remain suspended in the atmosphere for longer periods and be transported over longer distances. As a result, the concentration of fine particles tends to be more uniformly distributed over large urban areas, whereas the concentration of coarse particles tends to be more localized near particular sources. Although fine and coarse particles have been linked with adverse health effects, fine particles may have stronger respiratory effects in children than coarse particles.[2,3] Particulate matter easily moves from outdoors to indoors, and ambient measurements are good proxies for overall personal exposure.

Air quality standards have been established for fine and coarse particles. Additionally, scientists studying air pollution have recently focused on a subset of very small fine airborne particles called "ultrafine" particles (aerodynamic diameter ≤100 nanometers [nm]; 1 nm = 0.001 μm), which subsequently coalesce to form "fine" particles. Major sources of ultrafine particles include motor vehicle exhaust (especially diesel), power plants, and fires and wood stoves. Ultrafine particles are composed of numerous toxic compounds and reactive oxidant species that, when inhaled, can cause local and systemic inflammation.

Lead

Before the introduction of unleaded gasoline in the United States, leaded gasoline in motor vehicles was an important source of lead exposure for children. Today, paint and soil generally are the most common sources of lead exposure for US children (see Chapter 31); however, industrial operations, such as ferrous and nonferrous smelters, battery manufacturers, and other sources of lead emissions, can generate air emissions of lead that are potentially harmful for nearby communities. In a few countries, use of leaded gasoline continues (see Chapter 14).

Sulfur Compounds

Sulfur-containing compounds include sulfur dioxide, sulfuric acid (H_2SO4) aerosol, and sulfate particles. The primary source of sulfur dioxide is from the burning of coal and sulfur-containing oil; thus, major emitters of sulfur dioxide include coal-fired power plants, smelters, and pulp and paper mills. Sulfuric acid aerosol is formed in the atmosphere from the oxidation of sulfur dioxide in the presence of moisture. Facilities that either manufacture or use acids also can emit sulfuric acid aerosol. Sulfate particles are formed in the atmosphere from the chemical reaction of sulfuric acid with ammonia and may be measured as part of the fine particle fraction ($PM_{2.5}$ sulfate). In addition to adverse short- and long-term health effects on the respiratory system, sulfur dioxide contributes to the formation of acid rain.

Carbon Monoxide and Nitrogen Dioxide

In addition to fine particles and photochemical pollution, motor vehicle emissions also contribute to outdoor levels of carbon monoxide and nitrogen dioxide. Another important source of nitrogen oxides is fuel combustion from power plants. The emissions of nitrogen oxides that lead to nitrogen dioxide also contribute to the formation of ozone and nitrogen-bearing particles (nitrates and nitric acid). Outdoors, carbon monoxide occurs in areas of heavy traffic and is primarily a problem in cold weather. Indoor sources of nitrogen dioxide and carbon monoxide can generate higher levels indoors than those typically measured outdoors (see Chapters 20 and 25).

TOXIC AIR POLLUTANTS

Toxic air pollutants, also known as air toxics or hazardous air pollutants, represent a large group of substances, including volatile organic compounds, metals such as mercury, solvents, and combustion byproducts (such as dioxin), that are known or suspected to cause cancer or other serious health effects. There are currently 188 substances included on the list of hazardous air pollutants subject to emission regulations under the Clean Air Act. Some toxic air pollutants, such as benzene, 1,3-butadiene, and diesel exhaust, are emitted primarily from mobile sources, such as cars and trucks. Other toxic air pollutants come primarily from large, stationary industrial facilities. Smaller area sources (such as dry cleaners) and indoor sources also can release toxic air pollutants. Indoor concentrations of 11 prevalent volatile organic compounds often exceed outdoor concentrations, and obvious industrial sources (such as chemical plants) contribute a relatively small proportion to the average person's total exposure to many of these substances (see Chapter 20).

Traffic-Related Pollutants and Diesel Exhaust

In most urban areas, traffic-related emissions are a major source of air pollution. Concentrations of traffic-related pollutants are highest near and downwind of busy roads.[4] Traffic emissions contain numerous respiratory irritants and carcinogens, and laboratory and clinical studies have shown that constituents of traffic pollution can induce airway and systemic inflammation and increased airway responsiveness.[5] Over the last decade, numerous epidemiologic studies in the United States and Europe have found links between living near areas of high traffic density and increased respiratory symptoms (eg, wheezing, bronchitis), asthma symptoms, and asthma hospitalizations.[6-8] Additionally, longitudinal studies of children's respiratory health have found that children living near high-traffic roads had higher deficits in lung function and may have an increased risk of developing asthma compared with those living farther away from traffic.[9,10]

Because traffic pollution is a complex mixture, the components that have the strongest associations with health effects are not entirely clear. Several epidemiologic studies suggest that diesel exhaust may be particularly harmful to children.[7] Diesel exhaust particles may enhance allergic and inflammatory responses to antigen challenge and may facilitate development of new allergies.[11] Diesel exhaust exposure may worsen symptoms in children with allergic rhinitis or asthma. Most US school buses run on diesel fuel; a child riding in a school bus may be exposed to as much as 4 times the level of diesel exhaust as one riding in a car.[12] The EPA Clean School Bus Program (http://www.epa.gov/cleanschoolbus) includes grants to local school districts for retrofitting and replacing busses to reduce pollution.

Odors

The chemical identity of odors can sometimes be difficult to determine. Some common sources of odorous air pollution include sewage treatment plants, landfills, livestock feed lots, composts, pulp mills, geothermal plants, waste lagoons, tanneries, and petroleum refineries, among others. The odor of some compounds can be detected at levels below those generally recognized as posing a significant health risk. However, odors can negatively affect a person's quality of life and can exacerbate health problems among people who are particularly sensitive to odors.[13] Hydrogen sulfide, a fairly prevalent odorous air pollutant, is emitted as part of a variety of industrial processes, including oil refining, wood pulp production, and wastewater treatment as well as from concentrated animal feeding operations, geothermal plants, and landfills. Hydrogen sulfide, also known as sewer gas, has an odor similar to that of rotten eggs.

ROUTES OF EXPOSURE

The primary route of exposure to air pollution is through inhalation. Substances released into the atmosphere, however, can enter the hydrologic cycle as a result of atmospheric dispersion and precipitation and, thus, contaminate aquatic ecosystems. Similarly, deposition of suspended particulate matter occurs in soil. Thus, material that was originally released into the atmosphere can be ingested as a result of the subsequent contamination of water, soil, or vegetation or the consumption of fish from contaminated waters. Some toxic air pollutants (such as mercury, lead, polychlorinated biphenyls [PCBs], and dioxins) degrade very slowly or not at all and, thus, persist or accumulate in soil and the sediments of lakes and streams (see Chapters 17 and 18).

SYSTEMS AFFECTED

Most of the common outdoor air pollutants are recognized irritants to the respiratory system, with ozone being the most potent irritant. Some toxic air pollutants are known to have other systemic effects (eg, cancer and impaired neurologic development), and the specific health risks from many of these toxic compounds (lead, mercury, carbon monoxide, dioxins, volatile organic compounds) are addressed in other chapters.

CLINICAL EFFECTS

Children are considered especially vulnerable to outdoor air pollution for several reasons.[2] Because children tend to spend more time outside than adults do, often while being physically active, they have a greater opportunity for exposure to pollutants. While playing or at rest, children breathe more rapidly and inhale more pollutants per pound of body weight than do adults. In addition, because airway passages in children are narrower than those in adults, inflammation caused by air pollution can result in proportionally greater airway obstruction. Unlike adults, children may not cease vigorous outdoor activities when bronchospasm occurs.

From the viewpoint of toxicity, the key distinguishing features of outdoor air pollutants are their chemical and physical characteristics and concentration. Air pollutants may occur together; for example, on days when ozone levels are high, outdoor air levels of fine particles and acid aerosols also may be high. However, epidemiologic methods can be applied to try to tease out the relative contribution of the different pollutants. The combined effects of multiple pollutants are not completely understood but could produce synergistic effects.

In children, acute health effects associated with outdoor air pollution (including ozone and particulate matter) include increased respiratory symptoms, such as wheezing and cough, transient decrements in lung function, more serious lower respiratory tract infections, and increased school absenteeism because of respiratory illness.[2,14]

Because children with asthma have increased airway reactivity, the effects of air pollution on the respiratory system can be more serious for them. Increases in the number of hospital emergency department admissions have been observed when air pollution levels are elevated, which commonly occurs in major urban areas.[15,16] Children with asthma have been shown to experience more respiratory symptoms, use extra medication, and produce chronic phlegm following exposure to high levels of particulate pollution.[17,18] In addition, children with asthma whose condition is not well managed and who may have exposures to other pollutants also can be more vulnerable to asthma attacks because of poor air quality.

Most of the acute respiratory effects of outdoor air pollution, such as symptoms of cough, shortness of breath, or decrements in lung function, are thought to be reversible, but recent studies indicate that long-term exposure to outdoor air pollution (particulates and related copollutants and possibly ozone) has been associated with decrements in lung function among children.[19,20] Some of the increases in the prevalence of chronic obstructive lung disease in adults who live in more polluted areas could be the result of exposures that occurred during childhood. Particulate pollution has also been linked to low-birth weight, preterm birth, infant mortality,[21] and increased cardiovascular diseases in adults.[2,5]

Although extensive evidence shows that ambient air pollution exacerbates existing asthma, a link with the development of asthma has been difficult to establish, primarily because few prospective studies have been conducted with extensive exposure data. However, in the past few years, some limited data sets have emerged to support associations between air pollution or proximity to traffic and development of asthma.[5,10, 22]

The mechanisms by which air pollution can cause adverse effects are complex; gene-environment interactions are likely to be important. Ozone and ambient particulate matter are highly reactive oxidants, and there is emerging evidence that variants in genes that control the inflammatory and antioxidant response systems may increase a child's susceptibility to the adverse effects of air pollution.[23,24] Mechanistic, clinical, and epidemiologic studies suggest that antioxidants and nutritional status may modify the effect of air pollution on respiratory health.[25] Further studies are needed to address the role of supplementation strategies in the prevention of air pollution-related effects in children living in areas with high ambient air pollution.

TREATMENT OF CLINICAL SYMPTOMS

In addition to considering indoor air quality when evaluating triggers of a child's respiratory symptoms, it is also important for pediatricians to consider the effects of ambient air quality when assessing respiratory symptoms or function.

PREVENTION OF EXPOSURE

Under the Clean Air Act, the EPA has the authority to set standards for air pollutants that protect the health of people with specific sensitivities, including children and those with asthma (see Table 21.1).[26] Current US national ambient air quality standards are shown in Table 21.2. Although ambient concentrations of these 6 pollutants have decreased over the past decade, large numbers of people are still exposed to potentially unhealthful levels of these pollutants.

The EPA established the revised national ambient air quality standards for particulate matter and ozone in 2006 and 2008, respectively. For particulate matter, the new standards retain the current annual PM_{10} standard of 50 μg/m^3 but establish a new annual standard for $PM_{2.5}$ of 15 μg/m^3 and a new 24-hour standard (air measurement made for 24 hours) for $PM_{2.5}$ of 35 μg/m^3. For ozone, a new 8-hour standard of 0.075 parts per million was adopted. It should be noted that there are different averaging times used for each pollutant. The US Supreme Court upheld the scientific basis for the revised standards.

The Clean Air Act Amendments also give the EPA the authority to develop technology-based emission standards for 189 hazardous air pollutants. Although these standards are designed to protect public health, they are based on the available technology to control emissions.

Table 21.1: Clean Air Act Amendments[26]

Setting Guidelines for Criteria Air Pollutants

A few common air pollutants are regulated by first developing health-based criteria (science-based guidelines) as the basis for setting permissible levels. One set of limits (primary standard) protects health; another set of limits (secondary standard) is intended to prevent environmental and property damage. The criteria air pollutants are ozone, carbon monoxide, particulate matter, sulfur dioxide, lead, and nitrogen dioxide.

Regulating Nonattainment Areas

A nonattainment area is a geographic area whose air quality does not meet federal air quality standards designed to protect public health. Nonattainment areas are classified according to the severity of the area's air pollution problem. For ozone, these classifications are "marginal," "moderate," "serious," "severe," and "extreme." The EPA assigns each nonattainment area to 1 of these categories, thus triggering varying requirements the area must comply with to meet the ozone standard. Similar programs exist for areas that do not meet the federal health standards for carbon monoxide and particulate matter.

Regulating Mobile Sources

Cars and trucks are the sources for more than half of the pollutants that contribute to ozone and up to 90% of carbon monoxide emissions in urban areas. Tighter standards were established to reduce tail-pipe emissions and control fuel quality. Reformulated gasoline was required in the cities with the worst ozone problems, and oxygenated fuel was introduced in the winter months in areas that exceeded the carbon monoxide standard.

Reducing Toxic Air Pollutants

Toxic air pollutants are those pollutants that are hazardous to human health or the environment but are not specifically covered under another portion of the Clean Air Act. Emissions of toxic air pollutants are to be reduced through "maximum achievable control technology" standards for each major category of emissions sources.

Most large metropolitan areas are required to regularly monitor air quality for one or more of the national ambient air quality standards. The result of air quality monitoring is expressed as the Pollutant Standards Index, which also is commonly known as the Air Quality Index. The Air Quality Index converts the concentrations of 5 specific pollutants (ozone, carbon monoxide, nitrogen dioxide, sulfur dioxide, and particulate matter) into one number, scaled from 0 to 500. An Air Quality Index value of 100 corresponds to the short-term national ambient air quality standard; thus, an Air Quality Index value >100 indicates that the concentration of one or more pollutants exceeds its national standard. The descriptor terms associated with different Air Quality Index values are as follows: 0 to 50 = "good"; 51 to 100 = "moderate"; 101 to 150 = "unhealthy for sensitive groups"; 151 to 200 = "unhealthy"; 201 to 300 = "very unhealthy"; and 301 to 500 = "hazardous." Table 21.3 gives additional information about the Air Quality Index.[27]

Table 21.2: National Ambient Air Quality Standards

POLLUTANT	AMBIENT AIR LIMIT	AVERAGING TIME
Ozone	0.075 ppm	8 h
PM_{10}*	50 µg/m³ 150 µg/m³	Annual arithmetic mean 24 h
$PM_{2.5}$[†]	15 µg/m³ 35 µg/m³	Annual arithmetic mean 24 h
Sulfur dioxide	0.03 ppm 0.14 ppm	Annual arithmetic mean 24 h
Nitrogen dioxide	0.053 ppm	Annual arithmetic mean
Carbon monoxide	9 ppm (10 mg/m³) 35 ppm (40 mg/m³)	8 h 1 h
Lead	1.5 µg/m³	Quarterly

ppm indicates parts per million.
*Particles up to 10 µm in aerodynamic diameter.
[†] Particles up to 2.5 µm in aerodynamic diameter.

During periods of poor air quality, children's outdoor physical activity should be curtailed according to the guidelines provided in the Air Quality Index Table (See Table 21.3) (http://www.airnow.gov).

Finally, prevention of exposures to air pollution is an environmental justice issue. Children living near busy roads and industrial sources of pollution are more likely to be socially and economically disadvantaged.[28]

Table 21.3: Air Quality Index (AQI) and Associated General Health Effects and Cautionary Statements*[27]

INDEX VALUE	AQI DESCRIPTOR	GENERAL HEALTH EFFECTS	GENERAL CAUTIONARY STATEMENTS
0–50	Good	None for the general population.	None required.
51–100	Moderate	Few or none for the general population. Possibility of aggravation of heart or lung disease among persons with cardiopulmonary disease and the elderly with elevations of $PM_{2.5}$.[†]	Unusually sensitive people should consider limiting prolonged outdoor exertion.
101–150	Unhealthy for sensitive groups	Mild aggravation of respiratory symptoms among susceptible people.	Active children and adults and people with respiratory disease (such as asthma) and cardiopulmonary disease should avoid prolonged outdoor exertion.
151–200	Unhealthy	Significant aggravation of symptoms and decreased exercise tolerance in persons with heart or lung disease. Possible respiratory effects in the general population.	Active children and adults and people with respiratory and cardiovascular disease should avoid prolonged outdoor exertion. Everyone else, especially children, should limit prolonged outdoor exertion.
201–300	Very unhealthy	Increasingly severe symptoms and impaired breathing likely in sensitive groups. Increasing likelihood of respiratory effects in the general population.	Active children and adults and people with respiratory and cardiovascular disease should avoid all outdoor exertion. All others should limit outdoor exertion.
301–500	Hazardous	Severe respiratory effects and impaired breathing in sensitive groups, with serious risk of premature mortality in persons with cardiopulmonary disease and the elderly. Increasingly severe respiratory effects in the general population.	Elderly and persons with existing respiratory and cardiovascular diseases should stay indoors with the windows closed. Everyone should avoid outside physical exertion.

† Particles up to 2.5 μm in aerodynamic diameter.

Frequently Asked Questions

Q *How can I find out about the levels of air pollution in my community?*

A Information about the air quality in a community is often found on the Weather page of the local newspaper and is also available through http://www.airnow.gov.

Q *What can be done to protect my children from outdoor air pollution when they want and need to be able to play outdoors?*

A The potential harm posed by outdoor air pollution depends on the concentration of pollutants, which can vary from day to day, and even during the course of a day. Although exposure to outdoor air pollutants cannot be entirely prevented, it can be reduced by restricting the amount of time that children spend outdoors during periods of poor air quality, especially time spent engaged in strenuous physical activity. For example, ozone levels during the summer tend to be highest in the middle to late afternoon. On days when ozone levels are expected or reported to be high, outdoor activities could be restricted during the afternoon or rescheduled to the morning, particularly for children who have exhibited sensitivity to high levels of air pollution. In many areas, local radio stations, television news programs, and newspapers regularly provide information about air quality conditions.

Q *The recommendation to exercise in the early morning often conflicts with the reality of children's sports activity schedules. Should organized sports activities be canceled on days when air quality is poor?*

A Children should be encouraged to participate in physical activities because of the many health benefits associated with exercise. In most instances, the health benefits of physical activity likely outweigh the potential harm posed by intermittent or moderate levels of air pollution. However, on hot summer days when temperatures as well as smog levels are high, this balance could shift, and it may be advisable to shorten or cancel outdoor physical activities, especially for young children. When children have asthma, physicians and parents aim for optimal asthma control so that children can participate in normal outdoor sports activities, even on days with poor air quality. When asthma is unstable, children need to curtail their physical activities until their asthma becomes controlled again. Evidence suggests that children who exercise heavily (participating in 3 or more sports) and who live in communities with high levels of ozone pollution may experience a higher risk of developing asthma compared with children who do not play sports.[22]

Q *My family lives in an area that places them at risk of exposure to increased levels of outdoor air pollution. How can I help my child with asthma?*

A It is very appropriate for parents to discuss their concerns about air pollution and other possible asthma triggers with their child's physician. A child's entire environment, including the home, school, and playground, should be reviewed for possible asthma triggers. Improved medical management of the child's asthma and control of exposure to allergens and irritants in the child's home may be very effective in preventing asthma exacerbations. If a parent or a physician believes that emissions from a particular facility are harmful to a child with asthma, this information should be shared with the local or state environmental agencies that have authority over operating permits and enforcement actions.

Q *Would face dust masks be effective for protecting my children when air pollution levels are high?*

A Dust masks and other forms of respiratory protection, which are sized for adults and not children, are not recommended to protect against outdoor air pollution. Not only do poor fit and uncertain compliance limit any potential benefits, but most simple dust masks do not include the materials needed to filter out harmful volatile organic compounds or ozone.

Q *What is the relationship between ozone in urban smog and stratospheric ozone?*

A These issues are unrelated. Ozone in the troposphere, or ground level, is a major component of urban smog and a respiratory health hazard. The formation of ground-level ozone is independent of ozone in the upper atmosphere (the stratosphere). Stratospheric ozone provides a protective shield absorbing harmful ultraviolet (UV) radiation. Too little stratospheric ozone increases the risk of skin cancer and eye damage from ultraviolet rays.

Q *Why is asthma on the increase?*

A Scientists and public health officials are concerned by the apparent increase in the prevalence of asthma. The explanation for the increase has not been found but seems most likely to be related to a complex combination of factors, including increased exposure to environmental allergens and irritants indoors; increased exposure to complex environmental pollutants, such as secondhand tobacco smoke, diesel exhaust, and irritant gases during the early postnatal period of life; delayed maturation of immune responses because of changes in exposure to infection and infectious products; dietary factors; and psychosocial factors, such as stress and poverty.[29,30] Emerging evidence from scientific studies suggests that long-term exposures to air pollution and proximity to traffic may cause some cases of asthma, especially in those with genetic susceptibility.[10,15,22-24]

Q *Are odors from hog farms harmful to children?*

A Odors are an indicator of the presence of chemical emissions. Emissions from hog farms include volatile organic compounds, hydrogen sulfide, ammonia, endotoxins, and organic dusts. At sufficient concentrations over extended periods, there is ample evidence that these chemicals can cause disease. Whether the level and duration of exposures from emissions from hog farms is sufficient to cause harm to children through classic toxicological mechanisms is not known.[31] We do know, however, that odors can affect people through psychophysiological mechanisms, resulting in increased respiratory symptoms and other indicators of reduced quality of life.[13]

Q   If I live in an area with good air quality, is living next to a freeway still a concern? If so, what can I do to reduce my child's overall exposure to traffic pollution?

A   Levels of traffic pollution are highest when driving on a high traffic road, especially when there is stop-and-go traffic. Even if you living in an area with good regional air quality, pollution levels can be very high near a busy freeway, and high levels have been associated with increased risk of respiratory symptoms including asthma.[6-10] A multifaceted approach is needed to reduce children's overall exposures. Avoid standing near idling motor vehicles when possible. When walking or playing, choose areas away from traffic; even a distance of 100-200 meters (300-600 feet) will make a difference. Close windows and doors during peak traffic hours and place the air conditioner setting on recirculate. Encourage schools to enforce no idling rules at school pickup areas and advocate for switching school bus fleets to nondiesel fuel. Support federal and state efforts to reduce motor vehicle emissions. Some state and local governments have adopted laws to limit or require reduction strategies if schools or new residences are built close to busy roads. For other strategies see traffic fact sheets at: www.oehha.ca.gov/ http://www.oehha.ca.gov/public_info/public/kids/airkidshome.html.

Resources

American Lung Association
Phone: 212-315-8700
Local Associations phone: 800-LUNG-USA
Web site: www.lungusa.org

The Health Effects Institute
Phone: 617-886-9330
Fax: 617-886-9335
Web site: www.healtheffects.org

US Environmental Protection Agency,
Office of Air Quality Planning and Standards
Mail Code E143-03
Research Triangle Park, NC 27711
Fax: 919-541-0242
Web site: http://airnow.gov

References

1. US Environmental Protection Agency. *National Air Quality- Status and Trends through 2007*. Washington, DC: Office of Air Quality Planning and Standards, US Environmental Protection Agency; 2008. EPA Publication No. 454/R-08-006. Available at: www.epa.gov/air/ airtrends/2008/

2. American Academy of Pediatrics, Committee on Environmental Health. Ambient air pollution: health hazards to children. *Pediatrics*. 2004;114(6):1699-1707

3. Schwartz J, Neas LM. Fine particles are more strongly associated than coarse particles with acute respiratory health effects in school children. *Epidemiology*. 2000;11(1):6–10

4. Zhu Y, Hinds WC, Kim S, Sioutas C. Concentrations and size distribution of ultrafine particles near a major highway. *J Air Waste Manag Assoc*. 2002;52(9):1032-1042

5. Gilmour MI, Jaakkola MS, London SJ, Nel AE, Rogers CA. How exposure to environmental tobacco smoke, outdoor air pollutants, and increased pollen burdens influences the incidence of asthma .*Environ Health Perspect*. 2006;114(4):627-633

6. Delfino R. Epidemiologic evidence for asthma and exposure to air toxics: linkages between occupational, indoor, and community air pollution research. *Environ Health Perspect*. 2002;110(Suppl 4):573-589

7. Brunekreef B, Janssen NA, de Hartog J, Harssema H, Knape M, van Vliet P. Air pollution from truck traffic and lung function in children living near motorways. *Epidemiology*. 1997;8(3):298–303

8. Kim JJ, Huen K, Adams S, et al. Residential traffic and children's respiratory health. *Environ Health Perspect*. 2008;116(9):1274-1279

9. Gauderman WJ, Vora H, McConnell R, et al. Effect of exposure to traffic on lung development from 10 to 18 years of age: a cohort study. *Lancet*. 2007;369(9561):571-577

10. McConnell R, Berhane K, Yao L, et al. Traffic, susceptibility, and childhood asthma. *Environ Health Perspect*. 2006;114(5):766-772

11. Diaz-Sanchez D, Garcia MP, Wang M, Jyrala M, Saxon A. Nasal challenge with diesel exhaust particles can induce sensitization to a neoallergen in the human mucosa. *J Allergy Clin Immunol*. 1999;104(6):1183–1188

12. Natural Resources Defense Council. *No Breathing in the Aisles: Diesel Exhaust Inside School Buses*. San Francisco, CA. National Resources Defense Council; 2001

13. Shusterman D. Odor-associated health complaints: competing explanatory models. *Chem Senses*. 2001;26(3):339–343

14. Bates DV. The effects of air pollution on children. *Environ Health Perspect*. 1995;103(Suppl 6):49–53

15. Tolbert PE, Mulholland JA, MacIntosh DL, et al. Air quality and pediatric emergency room visits for asthma in Atlanta, Georgia USA. *Am J Epidemiol*. 2000;151(8):798–810

16. American Thoracic Society, Committee of the Environmental and Occupational Health Assembly. Health effects of outdoor air pollution. *Am J Respir Crit Care Med*. 1996;153(1):3–50

17. Ostro B, Lipsett M, Mann J, Braxton-Owens H, White M. Air pollution and exacerbation of asthma in African-American children in Los Angeles. *Epidemiology*. 2001;12(2):200–208

18. White MC, Etzel RA, Wilcox WD, Lloyd C. Exacerbations of childhood asthma and ozone pollution in Atlanta. *Environ Res*. 1994;65(1):56–68

19. Gauderman WJ, Gilliland GF, Vora H, et al. Association between air pollution and lung function growth in southern California children: results from a second cohort. *Am J Respir Crit Care Med*. 2002;166(1):76–84

20. Tager IB. Air pollution and lung function growth: is it ozone? *Am J Respir Crit Care Med*. 1999;160(2):387–389

21. Woodruff TJ, Parker JD, Schoendorf KC. Fine particulate matter ($PM_{2.5}$) air pollution and selected causes of post-neonatal infant mortality in California. *Environ Health Perspect.* 2006;114(5):786–790

22. McConnell R, Berhane K, Gilliland F, et al. Asthma in exercising children exposed to ozone: a cohort study. *Lancet.* 2002;359(9304):386–391

23. London SJ. Gene-air pollution interactions in asthma. *Proc Am Thorac Soc.* 2007;4(3):217-220

24. Salam MT, Gauderman WJ, McConnell R, et al. Transforming growth factor- 1 C-509T polymorphism, oxidant stress, and early-onset childhood asthma. *Am J Respir Crit Care Med.* 2007;176(12):1192-1199

25. Romieu I, Castro-Giner F, Kunzli N, Sunyer J. Air pollution, oxidative stress and dietary supplementation: a review. *Eur Respir J.* 2008;31(1):179-197

26. US Environmental Protection Agency, Office of Air Quality Planning and Standards. *The Plain English Guide to The Clean Air Act.* Washington, DC: Environmental Protection Agency; 2007. Publication No. EPA-456/K-07-001. Available at: http://www.epa.gov/air/peg/peg.pdf. Accessed March 9, 2011

27. US Environmental Protection Agency. *Air Quality Index: A Guide to Air Quality and Your Health.* Washington, DC: Environmental Protection Agency; August 2003. Publication No. EPA-454/K-03-002. Available at: http://airnow.gov/index.cfm?action=aqibroch.index. Accessed March 9, 2011

28. Jerrett M. Global geographies of injustice in traffic-related air pollution exposure. *Epidemiology.* 2009;20(2):231-233

29. Plopper CG, Fanucchi MV. Do urban environmental pollutants exacerbate childhood lung diseases? *Environ Health Perspect.* 2000;108(6):A252–A253

30. Gergen PJ. Remembering the patient. *Arch Pediatr Adolesc Med.* 2000;154(10):977–978

31. Merchant JA, Kline J, Donham KJ, Bundy DS, Hodne CJ. Human health effects. In: *Iowa Concentrated Animal Feeding Operation Air Quality Study, Final Report.* Ames, IA: Iowa State University and the University of Iowa Study Group; 2002:121–145. Available at: http://www.public-health.uiowa.edu/ehsrc/CAFOstudy.htm. Accessed March 9, 2011

Chapter 22

Arsenic

■ ■ ■ ■ ■ ■

Arsenic (As) is the 20th most abundant element in the earth's crust. A heavy metal—having a density >5 g/cm^3— this element has been recognized for centuries both as a valuable substance with many potential uses as well as a highly effective poison that is toxic to virtually all members of the animal kingdom, from insects to humans. In recent years, the scope of human exposure (and associated health consequences) has led to the passage of federal laws designed to protect the public from excessive exposure to arsenic.

Children may have greater exposure to arsenic than adults because of their smaller size and hand-to-mouth activities. Because many aspects of organogenesis and organ maturity take place during childhood, exposure to arsenic, which has antimetabolic and carcinogenic properties, may have greater impact on children.

Arsenic exists naturally in inorganic and organic forms. Inorganic arsenic is found in trivalent (arsenite) and pentavalent (arsenate) forms. Trivalent arsenic is substantially more toxic and carcinogenic than pentavalent. Most industrial uses of arsenic employ the trivalent form.

There are several forms of organic arsenic, including methylarsonic and dimethylarsinic acids.[1] Naturally occurring forms of organic arsenic are considered nontoxic, although organic arsenicals that have been developed as pesticides (eg, dimethylarsinic acid) are very toxic.

ROUTES OF EXPOSURE

Arsenic can be ingested or inhaled. There is no significant exposure through intact skin. Arsenic can be transmitted across the placenta.

SOURCES OF EXPOSURE

Natural

Arsenic is distributed in the earth in discrete locations or "veins." In the United States, higher concentrations are found in the southwestern states, eastern Michigan, and parts of New England.[2] Large veins of arsenic in bedrock can create contaminated earth adjacent to areas with little to no arsenic. Groundwater in contact with this earth can develop significant concentrations of arsenic, leading to contamination of well water. Arsenic in the earth's crust also leaches into ocean water, where it is ingested by marine life, thus entering the food chain (in the nontoxic, organic form).

Anthropogenic

Arsenic has been used industrially for many purposes, including pest control, and in the semiconductor, petroleum refining, and mining/smelting industries.[2] Its reliable toxicity contributed to arsenic's widespread use as a pesticide and antimicrobial. Before safer alternatives were found, arsenic was commonly administered to humans for treatment of syphilis, trypanosomiasis, and other infections[3] and for skin conditions (for which it was known as Fowler solution). As a pesticide for home use, arsenic was broadly used until the ban of most arsenical pesticides by the US Environmental Protection Agency (EPA) in 1991. Until the 1991 ban, sodium arsenate (Terro) was a common ant killer for home use. Of note, one arsenic-based pesticide that was exempt from this ban is chromated copper arsenate (CCA), a wood preservative (see Chapter 37). Until the use of chromated copper arsenate was discontinued in 2003, pressure-treated wood was impregnated with chromated copper arsenate to prevent termites and other pests from accelerating the decomposition of wood. Chromated copper arsenate contains 22% arsenic by weight; a 12-ft section of pressure-treated wood contains approximately 1 oz of arsenic.[4] Gallium arsenide, another form of arsenic, is a semiconductor that often is used in place of silicon.[1] Finally, arsenic may be found in alternative medications, including Chinese proprietary medicines and herbal remedies.[5]

As a result of anthropogenic use, arsenic is widely distributed in the environment. For example, it has been found at 1014 of the 1598 National Priorities List sites identified by the Agency for Toxic Substances and Disease Registry and the EPA.[6]

Because of arsenic's widespread presence in nature, along with extensive industrial uses, human exposure can be extensive. Industrial emissions, including incineration, can release arsenic into the atmosphere. Water, particularly unprocessed well water, may have significant inorganic arsenic contamination.[7] Many small water systems and private wells do not have arsenic treatment systems installed. Even treated water may be left with residual concentrations of arsenic, depending on the efficacy of the purification technique.

Foods, particularly seafood, can contain large quantities of organic arsenic; shellfish (eg, oysters and lobster) can have extremely large concentrations (as much as 120 parts per million [ppm] vs 2–8 parts per million in fish).[3] Such arsenic, however, is in the nontoxic form, so there is little concern about eating these foods.

Although arsenic pesticides have been almost completely banned, foods can still be contaminated with arsenic from past use, inadvertent use, or misuse of pesticides. Also, inorganic arsenical pesticides are still sometimes used in agriculture. For example, chickens may have small amounts of inorganic pesticide added to their feed as an anthelmintic. Foods containing inorganic arsenical pesticides can be very toxic, and such food could be unsafe for consumption, especially by children. The US Food and Drug Administration (FDA) estimates that a 6-year-old child consumes an average of 4.6 µg of inorganic arsenic daily in food. Exposure to inorganic arsenic in water, although highly variable, is estimated to be up to 4.5 µg daily.[4]

Soil contamination by arsenic (eg, from nearby mining, hazardous waste sites, and agricultural use) can expose children playing nearby and can contaminate clothes and be brought into the home. Children can be exposed to arsenic by sawing wood treated with chromated copper arsenate or burning it. There has been a case report of mild arsenic poisoning in a family of 8 exposed to the fumes from the burning of wood treated with chromated copper arsenate (see Chapter 37).[8]

TOXICOKINETICS, BIOLOGICAL FATE

Arsenic is well absorbed after its inhalation or ingestion. In animal models, gastrointestinal absorption of arsenic is increased in the presence of iron deficiency. Once absorbed, arsenic's half-life in blood is 10 hours. Circulating arsenic crosses the placenta and can result in elevated arsenic concentrations in the newborn and even fetal demise.[1] Humans are able to detoxify small amounts of absorbed inorganic arsenic by transforming it to organic species, including monomethylarsenate, dimethylarsenate, or trimethylarsenate forms. Children are less able than adults to methylate arsenic and, consequently, have more persistent concentrations of the toxic inorganic metal.[4]

Elimination of arsenic is almost exclusively renal; only 10% is excreted in bile. The average concentration of arsenic in urine is <25 µg/L. Within 2 to 4 weeks after exposure, the remaining body burden of arsenic is found in hair, skin, and nails.[1]

SYSTEMS AFFECTED

Arsenic affects every organ. Its primary action is as an antimetabolite. The mechanism of arsenic toxicity includes its replacement of phosphate molecules in adenosine triphosphate (arsenolysis) as well as potent inhibitory effects on key enzymes, including thiamine pyrophosphate. Arsenic has been shown to have endocrine-disrupting effects, inhibiting glucocorticoid-mediated transcription.[9] The clinical significance of this finding is unknown. Primary target organs for arsenic effects are the gastrointestinal tract and skin (because these are the most metabolically active tissues in the body). Arsenic exposure is associated with an increased risk of diabetes mellitus.[9]

CLINICAL EFFECTS

The characteristics of arsenic toxicity are different for acute versus chronic exposures. Acute, high-dose exposure to inorganic arsenic (>3–5 mg/kg) affects all major organs, including the gastrointestinal tract, brain, heart, kidneys, liver, bone marrow, skin, and peripheral nervous system. Severe ingestions lead within 30 minutes to gastrointestinal injury manifested by nausea, vomiting, hematemesis, diarrhea, and abdominal cramping. Intractable shock can ensue.[10] Lower-dose exposures result in a more protracted course: initial signs of gastrointestinal upset are followed by bone-marrow suppression with pancytopenia, hepatic dysfunction, myocardial depression with cardiac conduction disturbances, and a peripheral neuropathy.[11] The peripheral neuropathy of arsenic is of the sensorimotor type, typically involving the lower extremities more than upper extremities, and generally is stocking-glove in distribution. The early sign consists of ascending paresthesias, quickly followed by loss of proprioception, anesthesia, and weakness, a clinical picture that mimics Guillain-Barré syndrome. Severe central nervous system dysfunction is uncommon. Many of these effects can be permanent. A characteristic feature of acute arsenic exposure is the appearance of Mees lines (white, transverse creases across the fingernails that typically appear a few weeks after the poisoning event).

Chronic exposure may produce generalized fatigue and malaise. Bone-marrow depression, if present, is low grade. Other complications include malnutrition and inanition and increased risk of infections, particularly pneumonia.

Fetal and early childhood exposure to arsenic has been linked to bronchiectasis in early adulthood. Analysis of data from a historical cohort study conducted in Antofagasta, Chile, where arsenic-contaminated water was introduced into the municipal water supply as the population grew, revealed that birth cohorts with fetal and early childhood exposure to arsenic had dramatically increased standardized mortality ratios (the ratio of observed deaths to expected deaths) for lung cancer (6.1) and bronchiectasis (46.2) during adulthood (age 30-49 years).[12]

Arsenic can affect children's intellectual function,[13,14] hepatic function, and skin. Skin changes of arsenic poisoning include eczematoid eruptions, hyperkeratosis, and dyspigmentation. Alopecia also may occur.[1,3,6,11]

Arsenic is classified as a known human carcinogen by the National Toxicology Program[15] and the International Agency for Research on Cancer (IARC).[16] Chronic exposure is associated, in a dose-response relationship, with an increased risk of bladder, lung, and skin cancers.[15] Exposure to arsenic in drinking water during early childhood or in utero greatly increases subsequent mortality in young adults from lung cancer.[17] Arsenic also has been associated with an excess risk of acute myelogenous leukemia, aplastic anemia, and cancers of the kidney and liver.[18] The chronic consumption of water contaminated with arsenic in a concentration of 500 parts per million (1 part per million = 1 mg/L) is associated with an estimated risk of 1 in 10 people developing lung, bladder, or skin cancer. At a concentration of 50 parts per billion (ppb) (1 part per billion = 1 µg/L), cancer mortality is estimated to be in the range of 0.6 to 1.5 per 100, or approximately 1 in 100.[19] At 10 parts per billion, the EPA drinking water standard since 2006, the risk of bladder or lung cancer is 1 to 3 per 1000. Even arsenic concentrations of 3 parts per billion are associated with lifetime risk for bladder and lung cancer of 4 to 10 per 10 000.[15] Given that federal standards for environmental carcinogens historically have been set at concentrations that produce a cancer risk in the range of 1 in 1 million, the allowable amount of arsenic in drinking water confers an unusually high risk.

Because of transplacental transmission of arsenic, women chronically exposed to arsenic-contaminated water are at increased risk for spontaneous abortion, stillbirth, and preterm birth.[20] Although inorganic arsenic is teratogenic in animals, it has not been clearly shown to have teratogenicity in humans.[1]

DIAGNOSTIC METHODS

Because most arsenic is excreted in urine, the diagnostic test of choice is a urine collection.[11] In adult patients, the concentration of arsenic in a single urine specimen is commonly measured, adjusting the concentration to the concentration of urinary creatinine. Such "spot" urine tests for arsenic have not been well validated in children and are generally not recommended. Rather, a timed urinary collection for 8 to 24 hours is preferred. The method most commonly used for arsenic measurement in urine does not distinguish organic from more toxic inorganic forms. Therefore, in circumstances in which it is important to determine the form of arsenic, the pediatrician should request that the urinary arsenic be speciated. Alternatively, to establish a diagnosis of intoxication by inorganic arsenic, patients should abstain from ingestion of all seafood for at least 5 days prior to conducting the urine collection. Because the half-life of arsenic in blood is short, its measurement in blood is not recommended.

Hair and fingernail analyses have been used for the diagnosis of arsenic exposure. However, like hair analysis for most other environmental agents, the validity of this test has not been established.[11] Although techniques including segmental analysis and use of pubic hair may improve the reliability of hair analysis, hair should not be the sole specimen analyzed for the diagnosis of arsenic poisoning. Similarly, fingernail analysis is not sufficiently sensitive to establish the diagnosis of arsenic poisoning. Therefore, neither hair nor nail analysis is recommended.[1,21]

TREATMENT

If a diagnosis of significant arsenic exposure is established, chelation therapy may be indicated. Chelators that have been demonstrated to be effective in accelerating arsenic clearance are dimercaprol (BAL), d-penicillamine, and succimer.[7] As with all metal intoxications, chelation therapy should be undertaken only in consultation with a toxicologist.

PREVENTION OF EXPOSURE

Public health policies primarily have focused on control of arsenic in water. The EPA, through the Safe Drinking Water Act, is required to regulate the concentration of water contaminants, including arsenic. Since 1947, the maximum contaminant level of arsenic in water has been 50 parts per billion. Following recommendations by the Institute of Medicine to lower the acceptable standard to 10 parts per billion, the EPA changed it to 10 parts per billion. There have been recommendations to reduce the standard to 3 parts per billion, although even at 3 parts per billion, cancer mortality risk exceeds 1 in 10 000.[19] However, concentrations of arsenic in water lower than 3 parts per billion currently are not achievable by municipal systems at reasonable cost with existing technology.

The World Health Organization (WHO) recommends a water standard of 10 parts per billion.[2] Other guidelines to the public include the recommendation that all drinking water wells be tested for arsenic.[7] In areas with large water systems, water will be tested for arsenic by the water company or provider. Water providers are required to inform consumers when water fails to meet drinking water standards. In areas with elevated levels of arsenic in drinking water, home water treatment devices are available; however, these have varying efficacy at removing arsenic. Using bottled water is an option. Boiling water and filtering water through charcoal filters will not remove arsenic.

The use of chromated copper arsenate in pressure-treated wood in the United States for residential uses ended in 2003, as a result of an agreement between the manufacturers and EPA. However, existing structures will continue to be potential sources of concern, and chromated copper arsenate-treated wood manufactured prior to that date still may be available for sale.

Frequently Asked Questions

Q *What precautions should I take about my young children's exposure to the pressure-treated wood on my deck and playground structure?*

A Chromated copper arsenate is a pesticide used in pressure-treated wood to prolong its useful life. Treated wood commonly is used for decking, poles that are sunk in the ground, raised beds for gardens, and playground play structures. With aging of the wood and exposure to water, arsenic may be leached out and be present on the wood surface and in soil under decks or in garden beds made of chromated copper arsenate-treated lumber. Touching treated wood or contaminated soils and then engaging in hand-to-mouth activities may result in children having significant exposure to arsenic, a known human carcinogen.[22,23] In several countries that have banned or severely restricted the use of chromated copper arsenate, alternative treatments are available. Currently, there is limited availability of lumber treated with these chemicals in the United States.[24] Coating treated wood with a sealant at least every year (in accordance with wood manufacturers' recommendations) will reduce arsenic leaching.[25] Steps to reduce children's exposure include:

1. When possible, use alternatives to chromated copper arsenate-treated wood for new outdoor structures, including rot-resistant woods.
2. Keep children and pets out from under deck areas where arsenic may have leached.
3. Do not use chromated copper arsenate-treated wood for raised gardens, and do not grow vegetables near chromated copper arsenate-treated decks.
4. Never burn chromated copper arsenate-treated wood.
5. Make sure that children wash their hands after playing on chromated copper arsenate-treated surfaces, particularly before eating.
6. Cover picnic tables that are made with treated wood with a plastic cover before placing food on the table.

Q *What types of coatings are most effective to reduce leaching of arsenic from chromated copper arsenate-treated wood?*

A Some studies suggest that applying certain penetrating coatings (eg, oil-based, semitransparent stains) on a regular basis (once per year or every other year, depending on wear and weathering) may reduce the migration of wood preservative chemicals from chromated copper arsenate-treated wood. In selecting a finish, consumers should be aware that, in some cases, "film-forming," nonpenetrating stains (eg, latex semitransparent, latex opaque, and oil-based opaque stains) on outdoor surfaces such as decks and fences are not recommended, because they are less durable. Talk with a hardware or paint store about appropriate coatings in your area.

Q *My child's child care center, which has a large play structure built from pressure-treated wood, was recently found to have soil arsenic concentrations of 80 parts per million. Should I be concerned?*

A Cleanup standards for arsenic in soil are established by federal (EPA) and state guidelines. State guidelines are highly variable, depending on background concentrations of arsenic in soil, and range from 10 to 1000 parts per million. On the basis of conservative risk estimates, remediation should be considered when the soil arsenic concentration in areas where children routinely play exceeds 20 to 40 parts per million. Options, depending on concentration, include placement of a ground cover (eg, additional soil) or removal. If the source of arsenic is determined to be the structure, and not background activity, the child care center also should develop a plan for frequent application of a wood sealant or other barrier while plans for the structure's eventual removal are developed.

Q *Do I need to limit my child's seafood consumption because of possible arsenic contamination? Are there ever fish advisories about arsenic like there are for mercury and polychlorinated biphenyls?*

A The arsenic in seafood is organic, a form that has not been associated with toxicity. Therefore, there is no reason to limit your child's consumption of seafood as an arsenic avoidance measure.

References

1. Dart R. Arsenic. In: Sullivan J, Krieger G, eds. *Hazardous Materials Toxicology: Clinical Principles of Environmental Health.* Baltimore, MD: Williams & Wilkins; 1992:818-824

2. Breslin K. Safer sips: removing arsenic from drinking water. *Environ Health Perspect.* 1998;106(11):A548-A550

3. Malachowski M. An Update on arsenic. *Clin Lab Med.* 1990;10(3):459-472

4. Environmental Working Group. *Poisoned Playgrounds.* Washington, DC: Environmental Working Group; 2001. Available from: http://www.ewg.org/reports/poisonedplaygrounds. Accessed March 21, 2011

5. Espinoza E, Mann M, Bleasdell B. Arsenic and mercury in traditional Chinese herbal ball. *N Engl J Med.* 1995;333(12):803-804

6. Agency for Toxic Substances and Disease Registry. *Arsenic.* Atlanta, GA: Agency for Toxic Substances and Disease Registry; 2001

7. Franzblau A, Lilis R. Acute arsenic intoxication from environmental arsenic exposure. *Arch Environ Health.* 1989;44(6):385-390

8. Peters H, Croft WA, Woolson EA, Darcey BA, Olson MA. Seasonal arsenic exposure from burning chromium-copper-arsenate-treated wood. *JAMA.* 1984;251(18):2393-2396

9. Kaltreider R, Davis AM, Lariviere JP, Hamilton JW. Arsenic alters the function of the glucocorticoid receptor as a transcription factor. *Environ Health Perspect.* 2001;109(3):245-251

10. Levin-Scherz J, Patrick JD, Weber FH, Garabedian C Jr. Acute arsenic ingestion. *Ann Emerg Med.* 1987;16(6):702-704

11. Landrigan P. Arsenic—state of the art. *Am J Ind Med.* 1981;2(1):5-14

12. Smith AH, Marshall G, Yuan Y, et al. Increased mortality from lung cancer and bronchiectasis in young adults after exposure to arsenic in utero and in early childhood. *Environ Health Perspect*. 2006;114(8):1293-1296

13. von Ehrenstein OS, Poddar S, Yuan Y, et al. Children's intellectual function in relation to arsenic exposure. *Epidemiology*. 2007;18(1):44-51

14. Wang SX, Wang ZH, Cheng XT, et al. Arsenic and fluoride exposure in drinking water: children's IQ and growth in Shanyin county, Shanxi province, China. *Environ Health Perspect*. 2007;115(4):643-647

15. National Toxicology Program. *10th Report on Carcinogenics*. Research Triangle Park, NC: National Toxicology Program; 2002. Available at: http://ehp.niehs.nih.gov/roc/toc10.html. Accessed March 21, 2011

16. International Agency for Research on Cancer. *Overall Evaluations of Carcinogenicity*. International Agency for Research on Cancer. Vol Suppl 7. Lyon, France: International Agency for Research on Cancer; 1987

17. Liaw J, Marshall G, Yuan Y, Ferreccio C, Steinmaus C, Smith AH. Increased childhood liver cancer mortality and arsenic in drinking water in northern Chile. *Cancer Epidemiol Biomarkers Prev*. 2008;17(8):1982-1987

18. Khan MM, Sakauchi F, Sonoda T, Washio M, Mori M. Magnitude of arsenic toxicity in tube-well drinking water in Bangladesh and its adverse effects on human health including cancer: evidence from a review of the literature. *Asian Pac J Cancer Prev*. 2003;4(1):7-14

19. National Research Council. *Arsenic in Drinking Water: 2001 Update*. Washington, DC: National Academies Press; 2001. Available at: http://www.nap.edu/books/0309076293/html/. Accessed March 21, 2011

20. Ahmad SA, Sayed MH, Barua S, et al. Arsenic in drinking water and pregnancy outcomes. *Environ Health Perspect*. 2001;109(6):629-631

21. Hall A. Arsenic and arsine. In: Shannon MW, Borron SW, Burns M, eds. *Haddad and Winchester's Clinical Management of Poisoning and Drug Overdose*. New York, NY: Elsevier Inc; 2007:1024-1027

22. California Department of Health Services. *Evaluation of Hazards Posed by the Use of Wood Preservatives on Playground Equipments*. Sacramento, CA: California Department of Health Services, Office of Environmental Health Hazard Assesment; 1987

23. Stilwell D, Gorny K. Contamination of soil with copper, chromium, and arsenic under decks built from pressure treated wood. *Bull Environ Contam Toxicol*. 1997;58(1):22-29

24. Fields S. Caution—children at play: how dangerous is CCA? *Environ Health Perspect*. 2001;109(6):A262-A269

25. Consumer Reports. Exterior deck treatments test: all decked out. *Consumer Reports*. 1998;63:32-34

Chapter 23

Asbestos

■ ■ ■ ■ ■ ■

Asbestos is a fibrous mineral product and includes 6 minerals: amosite, chryso-tile, crocidolite, and the fibrous varieties of tremolite, actinolite, and anthophyl-lite. Asbestos occurs naturally in rock formations in certain areas of the world and is mined and refined for its commercial use. It can also be found in small amounts in other rock formations, including marble and vermiculite ore, which are mined and processed for other purposes. Asbestos fibers vary in length; they may be straight or curled; they can be carded, woven, and spun into cloth; and they can be used in bulk or mixed with materials such as asphalt or cement.

Asbestos is virtually indestructible. It resists heat, fire, and acid. Because of these properties, asbestos has been used in a wide range of manufactured goods, including insulation; roofing shingles; ceiling and floor tiles; paper products; asbestos cement; clutches, brakes, and transmission parts; textiles; packaging; gaskets; and coatings. Between the 1920s and the early 1970s, millions of tons of asbestos were used in the construction of homes, schools, and public buildings in the United States, mainly for insulation and fireproofing.

Products contaminated with asbestos can be found in many settings. Today in the United States, use of asbestos in new construction has come to almost a complete halt. However, large amounts of asbestos remain in place in older buildings, especially in schools, posing a potential hazard to children, adolescents, and adults now and in the future. Large amounts of asbestos are still used in new construction in other nations, especially in certain developing countries. A major challenge to pediatricians, public health officials, and school authorities in the United States has been to develop a systematic and rational approach to dealing with asbestos in schools and other buildings to protect the health of children.

In 1980 (the last time that national statistics were compiled), the US Environmental Protection Agency (EPA) estimated that more than 8500 schools nationwide contained deteriorated asbestos and that approximately 3 million students (as well as more than 250 000 teachers, personnel, and staff) were at risk of exposure.[1] Subsequent field studies have found that approximately 10% of the asbestos in schools is deteriorating and/or accessible to children and, thus, poses an immediate threat to health. The remaining 90% is not deteriorating or accessible to children and, therefore, does not pose an immediate hazard.[2]

ROUTES OF EXPOSURE

Inhalation of microscopic airborne asbestos fibers is the most concerning route of exposure. Asbestos becomes a health hazard when fibers become airborne.[3] Asbestos that is tightly contained within building materials (such as in insulation or ceiling tiles) or behind barriers poses no immediate hazard. However, when asbestos fibers are liberated into the air through deterioration, destruction, or repair/renovation of asbestos-containing materials, children and adults are at risk of inhaling airborne fibers.

Children can be exposed to asbestos if they live in areas where mining or refining of asbestos-containing ore occurs. From 1924 through 1990, vermiculite ore was mined and milled from Zonolite Mountain in Libby, MT. The vermiculite was used widely in the community at residential and commercial locations. It was also disbursed across the country to as many as 245 processing sites. The ore from Libby was contaminated with asbestos, and radiologic evidence of adverse health effects has been noted in workers employed in Libby at the mine, mill, and refining plant. Workers in the mine and their families have experienced increased rates of asbestos-related diseases, including mesothelioma.[4,5] In 2002, the Agency for Toxic Substances and Disease Registry (ATSDR) reported that asbestosis mortality rates in the Libby community were 40 to 80 times higher than expected and that lung cancer mortality was 20% to 30% higher than expected.[6] Most of these cases were in workers or their household contacts. Children can also be exposed to asbestos from living in areas where there are naturally occurring deposits of ore that contains asbestos. A case-control study in California found that residential proximity to naturally occurring asbestos showed a dose-response association with mesothelioma, independent of occupational asbestos exposure.[7]

Gastrointestinal exposure to asbestos occurs rarely, usually in circumstances in which drinking water is transferred through deteriorating asbestos-containing concrete pipes. Asbestos fibers also can enter drinking water that passes through rock formations that contain naturally occurring asbestiform fibers.

SYSTEMS AFFECTED

Asbestos can cause cancer in the lungs, throat, larynx, and gastrointestinal tract. Malignancies caused by asbestos also are seen in the pleura, pericardium, and peritoneum. High-dose occupational exposure (an unlikely exposure situation in children) can cause asbestosis, a fibrotic disease of the lungs and/or pleura.

CLINICAL EFFECTS

Asbestos produces no acute toxicity. Workers who have been heavily exposed to asbestos in industry may develop asbestosis. The effects of long-term exposure to asbestos typically do not manifest until at least 20 to 30 years after initial exposure. In its earlier stages, asbestosis neither causes symptoms nor impairs lung function. In later stages, asbestosis presents with cough and exertional dyspnea. Patients with advanced disease develop extensive pulmonary fibrosis. Asbestosis is not seen in children because of their much lower levels of exposure.

The main risk of asbestos to children lies in its capacity to cause cancer many years after exposure. The 2 most important cancers caused by asbestos are lung cancer and malignant mesothelioma, a cancer that can occur in the pleura, pericardium, or peritoneum. Symptoms of mesothelioma include chest pain under the rib cage, painful coughing, shortness of breath, and unexplained weight loss. Asbestos also has been observed to cause cancer of the throat, larynx, and gastrointestinal tract among adults heavily exposed in industry. There appears to be a link between low-level exposure to asbestos in the community and cancer of the ovary.[8]

The relationship between asbestos and cancer was first recognized among workers exposed occupationally as miners, shipbuilders, and insulation workers.[9] Thousands of cases of mesothelioma and lung cancer have occurred in these men and women, and cases resulting from past exposures will continue to develop. An estimated 300 000 US workers will eventually die of asbestos-related diseases,[10] and it is projected that 250 000 workers will die over the next 35 years in western Europe, where adoption of protective measures was delayed.[11] Mesothelioma cases in the United States peaked in males in the mid 1990s and are now slowly declining. Deaths are not expected to come down to background rates until 2055, 80 years after widespread use in the United States ceased.[12] Ongoing exposures in developing nations will produce a further toll of disease and death that has not yet been quantified.

Lung Cancer

Asbestos exposure can by itself cause lung cancer. Additionally, a strongly synergistic interaction has been found between asbestos and cigarette smoking, resulting in lung cancer.[13] Adults who are exposed to asbestos but who do not smoke have 5 times the background rate of lung cancer. In contrast, adults who are exposed to asbestos and who also smoke have more than 50 times the background rate of lung cancer. This powerful synergistic association is one more reason why pediatricians should urge parents, children, and adolescents not to smoke.

Mesothelioma

Malignant mesothelioma seems to occur solely as a result of exposure to asbestos. No interaction is evident between asbestos and smoking in the causation of mesothelioma. Mesothelioma is the form of cancer that is of greatest concern for children exposed to asbestos in homes and schools, because it can be caused by low levels of exposure and can appear as late as 5 decades after exposure. Women who were former residents of an asbestos mining and milling town who did not work in the asbestos industry but were exposed to asbestos in their environment or in their home were found to have excess cancer mortality.[8]

DOSE-RESPONSE

The degree of cancer risk associated with asbestos is dose related, and the greater the cumulative exposure, the greater the risk.[14] Families of children with brief, low-level exposures to airborne asbestos should be reassured that their risk of cancer resulting from the asbestos exposure is very low. However, any exposure to asbestos involves some risk of cancer; no safe threshold level of exposure has been established. For example, mesotheliomas have been observed decades after exposure in the spouses and children of asbestos workers who brought asbestos fibers home on their work clothing, in nonsmoking women who were never employed in the asbestos industry but lived their entire lives in the asbestos mining area of Quebec,[15] and in people who lived in a town near an asbestos-cement factory in Italy.[16]

Some scientists and industry representatives have claimed that the form of asbestos used most commonly in buildings in North America (Canadian chrysotile) is harmless. However, extensive clinical, epidemiologic, and toxicologic data have consistently documented that chrysotile asbestos is carcinogenic in experimental animals and that it can cause lung cancer and mesothelioma in humans.[17] All forms of asbestos are hazardous and carcinogenic. Exposure to all forms of asbestos must be kept to a minimum.[18]

DIAGNOSTIC METHODS

There is no reliable method of detecting past asbestos exposure except through obtaining a history of exposure. Chest x-rays are not indicated for children exposed or potentially exposed to asbestos, because acute radiographs provide no information on whether exposure has occurred. The radiographic findings of pleural plaques—raised fibrous plaques that are sometimes calcified—that occur within the pleura or pericardium are evidence of past exposure to asbestos. The latency period from first exposure to the development of pleural plaques ranges from 10 to more than 40 years in heavily occupationally exposed adults.[19] Such plaques were seen in 6.4% of US males and 1.7% of US females 35 to 74 years of age examined between 1976 and 1980 in the Second National Health and

Nutrition Examination Survey (NHANES). No comparable data are available for children.[20]

To determine whether children are at risk of asbestos exposure or have been exposed, an environmental inspection may be undertaken by a properly certified inspector in schools and other buildings where children live, work, and play. Bulk samples of insulation or other suspicious materials should be obtained and examined by electron microscopy in a certified laboratory. Children may be at risk of exposure if asbestos in a building is deteriorating or it is within reach or renovations are taking place. Air sampling is of little value in assessing a potential asbestos hazard to children in a school, because airborne releases of asbestos fibers are typically intermittent and likely to be missed.

TREATMENT

Because asbestos exposure does not produce acute symptoms, there is no treatment for acute exposure. There also is no treatment that removes asbestos fibers from the lungs once they are inhaled. It is important to discuss the risk of developing health problems if there has been asbestos exposure (see Chapter 45). Although no exposure is completely free of risk, parents and exposed children may be assured that the risk associated with brief, low-level exposure to asbestos is minimal.[21] The context of such a discussion provides an important "teachable moment" in which a pediatrician can reinforce information about the need to avoid tobacco smoking. Cigarette smoking causes more than 400 000 deaths in the United States every year (see Chapter 40).

PREVENTION OF EXPOSURE

The best way to prevent asbestos exposure is to use less hazardous materials in building construction and renovation. This approach is now followed almost universally in the United States, Canada, and western Europe, where use of asbestos in new construction is severely restricted. The Collegium Ramazzini, an independent group of experts in environmental and occupational medicine, has issued a call for an international ban on all new uses of asbestos, especially in developing nations, where asbestos is still widely used.[22]

The removal or renovation of existing structural asbestos may aerosolize fibers and significantly increase its hazard to health. Small areas of fraying asbestos insulation can be contained by carefully wrapping it in duct tape. Loose vermiculite attic insulation is a pebble-like, lightweight, brown or gold colored product that can contain varying amounts of asbestos and should particularly not be disturbed. If more than minor repairs are needed or if asbestos is to be removed, a certified asbestos contractor always should be hired and full EPA and state regulations should be obeyed. Because asbestos may not be obvious in the home, families considering remodeling should educate themselves about items that may contain asbestos that could be liberated by renovation work. "Do-it-yourself" removal of asbestos is never recommended.

In schools, preventing asbestos exposure requires full compliance with the provisions of the federal Asbestos Hazard Emergency Response Act (AHERA) of 1986. This act requires periodic inspection of every school—public, private, and parochial—by a certified inspector, and it establishes criteria specifying when asbestos must be removed and when it can be safely managed in place. Removal, when needed, must proceed in full compliance with state and federal laws. The results of all inspections conducted under AHERA must be made available to the public by school authorities (see also Chapter 11).

Frequently Asked Questions

Q *How will I know if there are asbestos materials in my house?*

A Asbestos is not found as commonly in private homes in the United States as in schools, apartment buildings, and public buildings. Nevertheless, asbestos is present in many homes, especially those built prior to the 1970s.

The following are locations in homes where asbestos may be found:

— Insulation around pipes, stoves, and furnaces (the most common locations)

— Insulation in walls and ceilings, such as sprayed-on or troweled-on material or vermiculite attic insulation (see http://www.epa.gov/asbestos/pubs/insulation.html)

— Patching and spackling compounds and textured paint

— Roofing shingles and siding

— Older appliances, such as washers and dryers

— Older asbestos-containing floor tiles

To determine whether your home contains asbestos, you can take the following steps:

— Evaluate appliances and other consumer products by examining the label or the invoices to obtain the product name, model number, and year of manufacture. If this information is available, the manufacturer can supply information about asbestos content.

— Evaluate building materials. A professional asbestos manager with qualifications similar to those of managers employed in school districts may be hired. This person can inspect your home to determine whether asbestos is present and give advice on its proper management.

— Test for asbestos. State and local health departments as well as regional EPA offices have lists of individuals and laboratories certified to analyze a home for asbestos and test samples for the presence of asbestos (see Resources).

Q *If there is asbestos in my home, what should I do?*

A If asbestos-containing materials are found in your home, the same options exist for dealing with these materials as in a school. In most cases, asbestos-containing materials in a home are best left alone. If materials such as insulation, tiling, and flooring are in good condition and out of the reach of children, there is no need to worry. However, if materials containing asbestos are deteriorating or if you are planning renovations and the materials will be disturbed, it is best to find out whether the materials contain asbestos before renovations begin and, if necessary, have the materials properly removed. Improper removal of asbestos may cause serious contamination by dispersing fibers throughout the area. Any asbestos removal in a home must be performed by properly accredited and certified contractors. A listing of certified contractors in your area may be obtained from state or local health departments or from the regional office of the EPA (see Resources). Many contractors who advertise themselves as asbestos experts have not been trained properly. Only contractors who have been certified by the EPA or by a state-approved training school should be hired. The contractor should provide written proof of up-to-date certification.

Children should not be permitted to play in areas where there are friable asbestos-containing materials.

To obtain additional information about asbestos in the home, you can read more on the EPA Web site (http://www.epa.gov/asbestos/pubs/ashome.html) or write to the EPA for the booklet "Asbestos in Your Home," which can be obtained from the Toxic Substances Control Act Assistance Information Service, Mail Code 7408M, 1200 Pennsylvania Ave NW, Washington, DC 20460; phone: 202-554-1404; e-mail: tsca-hotline@epamail.epa.gov. State or local health departments will have additional information about asbestos (see Resources).

Q *Is there asbestos in hair dryers?*

A In the past, asbestos was used in some electrical appliances, including hair dryers. However, hair dryers containing asbestos were recalled by the US Consumer Product Safety Commission (CPSC) in 1980, and currently, manufacturers of household appliances in the United States are not allowed to use asbestos.

Q *Is there asbestos in talc?*

A Talc, like asbestos, is a mineral product. Talc from some mines contains asbestos-like fibers, and these fibers are present in talcum powder made from that talc. Because talcum powder is not required to carry a label indicating whether it contains asbestos-like fibers, parents should not use talc-containing products for infant and child care. A further reason to avoid talcum powder in the nursery is to prevent talc pneumoconiosis, which can result from accidental inhalation of bulk powder if a can should tip over into a baby's face. Talc pneumoconiosis has been associated with a number of infant fatalities.

Q *Is there asbestos in play sand?*

A Play sand that comes from naturally occurring sand deposits, such as sand dunes or beaches, generally does not contain asbestos. However, some commercially available play sand is produced by crushing quarried rock, and this sand has been shown to contain asbestos-like fibers. The CPSC does not require that the label on play sand indicate the source of the sand. The label on sand is not required to carry any information on whether it contains asbestos-like fibers. For these reasons, pediatricians are advised to warn parents against the use of play sand unless the source of the sand can be verified or the sand is certified as asbestos free.

Q *My spouse works with asbestos. Is there danger to my child?*

A Any family member who works in an occupation potentially involving contact with asbestos (or similar fibers such as fiberglass or reactive ceramic fibers) may bring home fibers on clothing, shoes, hair, skin, and in the car. These fibers can contaminate the home environment and become a source of exposure to children.[23]

Studies conducted in the homes of asbestos workers have shown that the dust in these homes can be heavily contaminated by asbestos fibers. Mesothelioma, lung cancer, and asbestosis all have been observed in the

---

Many jobs involve potential occupational exposure to asbestos.

These include:

- Asbestos mining and milling

- Asbestos product manufacture

- Construction trades, including sheet metal work, carpentry, plumbing, insulation work, air-conditioning, rewiring, cable installation, spackling, drywall work, and demolition work

- Shipyard work
- Asbestos removal
- Fire fighting
- Custodial and janitorial work
- Brake repair

family members of asbestos workers. In many cases, these diseases occurred years or even decades after the exposure.

Preventing household exposure is essential. People who work with asbestos (eg, construction and demolition workers and workers who repair brakes) must scrupulously shower, change clothing, and change shoes before getting into a car and returning home. These procedures are mandated by the federal Occupational Safety and Health Act but often are not enforced. Workers often are not aware of their exposure. Exposure is prevented only if employees leave contaminated shoes and clothing at the workplace.

Q Is there a risk of asbestos exposure from the events of September 11, 2001?
A The risk to children associated with low levels of exposure to asbestos or with brief encounters lasting only a few days or weeks such as occurred in September 2001 in communities near the World Trade Center in New York City is not nil. However, the risk associated with such exposure is certainly much lower than the risk that results from continuing exposure, such as occurs among adults in industry who have been exposed for many years.[24]

Resources

Agency for Toxic Substances and Disease Registry
Phone: 888-422-8737
Web site: www.atsdr.cdc.gov/Asbestos

US Environmental Protection Agency
Phone: 202-272-0167
Web site: www.epa.gov/asbestos/index.html

State and local health departments also can provide information about asbestos.

References

1. American Academy of Pediatrics, Committee on Environmental Hazards. Asbestos exposure in schools. *Pediatrics.* 1987;7(2):301–305
2. US Environmental Protection Agency. Asbestos-containing materials in schools: final rule and notice. *Fed Regist.* 1987;52:41826–41903
3. American Academy of Pediatrics, Committee on Injury and Poison Prevention. *Handbook of Common Poisonings in Children.* Rodgers GC Jr, ed. 3rd ed. Elk Grove Village, IL: American Academy of Pediatrics; 1994
4. Agency for Toxic Substances and Disease Registry. *Asbestos Exposure in Libby, Montana, Medical Testing and Results Atlanta, GA: Agency for Toxic Substances and Disease Registry. Available at:* http://www.atsdr.cdc.gov/asbestos/sites/libby_montana/medical_testing.html. Accessed August 10, 2010
5. Sullivan PA. Vermiculite, respiratory disease, and asbestos exposure in Libby, Montana: update of a cohort mortality study. *Environ Health Perspect.* 2007;115(4):579-585

6. Agency for Toxic Substances and Disease Registry. *Summary Report: Exposure to Asbestos-Containing Vermiculite from Libby, Montana, at 28 Processing Sites in the United States.* Atlanta, GA: Agency for Toxic Substances and Disease Registry. Available at: http://www.atsdr.cdc.gov/asbestos/sites/national_map/Summary_Report_102908.pdf. Accessed August 10, 2010

7. Pan et al. Residential proximity to naturally occurring asbestos and mesothelioma risk in California. *Am J Respir Crit Care Med.* 2005;172(8):1019-1025

8. Reid A, Heyworth J, de Klerk N, Musk AW. The mortality of women exposed environmentally and domestically to blue asbestos at Wittenoom, Western Australia. *Occup Environ Med.* 2008; 65(11):743-749

9. Selikoff IJ, Churg J, Hammond EC. Asbestos exposure and neoplasia. *JAMA.* 1964;188:22–26

10. Nicholson WJ, Perkel G, Selikoff IJ. Occupational exposure to asbestos: population at risk and projected mortality—1980–2030. *Am J Ind Med.* 1982;3(3):259–311

11. Peto J, Decarli A, LaVecchia C, Levi F, Negri R. The European mesothelioma epidemic. *Br J Cancer.* 1999;79(3-4):666–672

12. Price et al. Mesothelioma trends in the United States: an update based on surveillance, epidemiology, and end results program data for 1973 through 2003. *Am J Epidemiol. 2004;159(2):107-112*

13. Selikoff IJ, Hammond EC, Churg J. Asbestos exposure, smoking and neoplasia. *JAMA.* 1968;204(2):106–112

14. Agency for Toxic Substances and Disease Registry. *Toxicological Profile on Asbestos.* Atlanta, GA: Agency for Toxic Substances and Disease Registry; 2001

15. Camus M, Siemiatycki J, Meek B. Nonoccupational exposure to chrysotile asbestos and the risk of lung cancer. *N Engl J Med.* 1998;338(22):1565–1571

16. Magnani C, Dalmasso P, Biggeri A, Ivaldi C, Mirabelli D, Terracini B. Increased risk of malignant mesothelioma of the pleura after residential or domestic exposure to asbestos: a case-control study in Casale Monferrato, Italy. *Environ Health Perspect.* 2001;109(9):915–919

17. International Agency for Research on Cancer. *The Evaluation of Carcinogenic Risks to Humans.* IARC Monographs. Lyon, France: International Agency for Research on Cancer; 1987;Suppl 7:106–116

18. Landrigan PJ. Asbestos—still a carcinogen. *N Engl J Med.* 1998;338(22):1618–1619

19. Epler, GR, McLoud, TC, Gaensler, EA. Prevalence and incidence of benign asbestos pleural effusion in a working population. *JAMA. 1982;247(5):617-622*

20. Rogan WJ, Ragan NB, Dinse GE. X-ray evidence of increased asbestos exposure in the US population from NHANES I and NHANES II 1973–1978. National Health Examination Survey. *Cancer Causes Control.* 2000;11(5):441–449

21. Needleman HL, Landrigan PJ. *Raising Children Toxic Free: How to Keep Your Child Safe From Lead, Asbestos, Pesticides, and Other Environmental Hazards.* New York, NY: Farrar, Straus and Giroux; 1994

22. Landrigan PJ, Soffritti M. Collegium Ramazzini call for an international ban on asbestos. *Am J Ind Med.* 2005;47(6):471-474

23. Chisolm JJ Jr. Fouling one's own nest. *Pediatrics.* 1978;62(4):614–617

24. Landrigan PJ, Lioy PJ, Thurston G, et al. Health and environmental consequences of the world trade center disaster. NIEHS World Trade Center Working Group. *Environ Health Perspect.* 2004;112(6):731-739

Chapter 24

Cadmium, Chromium, Manganese, and Nickel

■ ■ ■ ■ ■ ■

This chapter discusses cadmium, chromium, manganese, and nickel, metallic elements from which health effects are increasingly being understood.

CADMIUM

Cadmium (Cd) is a heavy metal found in the earth's crust. It is disseminated in the environment by natural processes (erosion of rocks, forest fires, eruption of volcanoes) and by human activities (mining; smelting; disposal of products containing cadmium, such as batteries; waste incineration).[1] Cadmium can be taken up by plants (in particular, "root" plants, such as potatoes or onions) or animals (in particular, in the liver and kidneys), thereby entering the food chain. Airborne cadmium pollution from hazardous waste sites and/or industry may create inhalational exposures. Cadmium is a common industrial chemical, and its fume is generated by use of gold and silver solder during jewelry fabrication. Cigarette smoke is a well-known source of cadmium, because tobacco plants take up cadmium found in soil. Cadmium has been found in children's jewelry.[2]

Routes of Exposure

Cadmium can be ingested or inhaled. The primary route of exposure in children is via ingestion of food. A child may be exposed after swallowing a piece of cadmium-containing jewelry. Exposure may also occur from biting, sucking, or mouthing cadmium-containing jewelry or from hand-to-mouth contact after handling a jewelry piece.[2] Secondhand tobacco smoke (SHS) is a source of inhaled cadmium. Dermal absorption is negligible.

Sources of Exposure

Significant potential sources of cadmium exposure for humans include foods (leafy vegetables, potatoes, grains, and liver/kidney meats), cigarette smoke, and occupational exposures. Areas with very high levels of cadmium in soil can lead to significant exposure through locally grown food.

Biological Fate

Absorption of cadmium depends on the route of exposure. After inhalation, cadmium is well absorbed in the lungs. A cigarette contains approximately 2.0 µg of cadmium, 2% to 10% of which is transferred to primary cigarette smoke.[3] Of the cadmium in the primary inhaled cigarette smoke, nearly 50% is absorbed from the lungs into the systemic circulation during active smoking.[3-5] Smokers typically have cadmium blood concentrations much higher than those of nonsmokers.[6] Physicians should be aware that smokers (and children exposed to secondhand smoke) also have higher urinary cadmium concentrations.[7] Gastrointestinal tract absorption is less efficient, and adults absorb approximately 1% to 10% of ingested cadmium.[8] However, nutritional deficiencies, such as iron deficiency, will increase cadmium absorption.[7]

Cadmium bioaccumulates in the liver and kidneys, with approximately 50% of total cadmium body stores found in these 2 organs. Bone is a third depot for cadmium, and bone toxicity can be direct (through incorporation into the bone matrix) and indirect (via renal disease and subsequent disturbances in calcium excretion and vitamin D metabolism). The half-life of cadmium in these tissues is on the order of 10 to 20 years. The primary route of excretion is through the urine. The rate of excretion is low, in part because cadmium binds tightly to metallothionein, a transport and storage protein synthesized in response to cadmium and zinc exposure, preventing excretion into the tubules. In addition, the majority of filtered cadmium is reabsorbed in the renal tubules. Cadmium concentration in blood reflects recent exposure; urinary cadmium concentration more closely reflects total body burden. However, the kidney is also a prime target of cadmium toxicity, and if renal damage from cadmium exposure occurs, the excretion rate may increase sharply, and urinary cadmium concentrations will no longer reflect body burden.

Systems Affected

Exposure to cadmium may affect organs including the lungs, nervous system, bones, and kidneys. The route of exposure in some cases may determine the site of toxicity (ie, inhalation and lung toxicity). The property of bioaccumulation tends to increase the risks from chronic toxicity.

Clinical Effects

Acute and Short-Term Effects

Acute exposure via inhalation can lead to severe pneumonitis. In humans, several fatal inhalation exposures have occurred through occupational accidents. High-dose inhaled cadmium is particularly toxic to the lungs and produces a well-described pneumonitis with fever and significant radiographic changes. During the acute inhalation, symptoms are relatively mild, but within a few days following exposure, severe pulmonary edema and chemical pneumonitis develop, sometimes causing death as a result of respiratory failure. Exposures to environmental contaminants (eg, cadmium in secondhand smoke) have little acute toxicity, but bioaccumulation of cadmium is a concern for chronic health effects, given cadmium's half–life, which is measured in years.

Large oral exposure can produce renal toxicity. A tragic episode of industrial dumping of cadmium into the environment occurred in the Jinzu and Kakehashi river basins in Japan, leading to contamination of locally grown rice. This event produced widespread human exposure and a syndrome of renal disease coupled with brittle bones referred to as "Itai-itai" (ouch-ouch) disease. The disease was particularly common among women,[8,9] perhaps because of their higher prevalence of iron deficiency and, therefore, greater cadmium absorption.

Chronic Toxicity

Cadmium is well recognized as a toxicant in occupational exposures. Chronic occupational exposures most commonly produce renal toxicity; microproteinuria is one of the earliest signs. Chronic exposure effects also include decreased bone mass/osteoporosis and lung cancer.[10] The US Environmental Protection Agency (EPA) has classified cadmium as a group B1 or "probable" human carcinogen; the International Agency for Research on Cancer (IARC) and the US National Toxicology Program have classified cadmium as a known human carcinogen.[11]

Some epidemiologic studies have suggested that cadmium exposure may be associated with adverse neurodevelopmental outcomes in children. Associations have been reported between hair cadmium concentrations and mental retardation[12] as well as lower verbal IQ scores,[13] although 2 small studies failed to detect significant associations between hair cadmium concentrations and IQ[14] and dentine cadmium and mental retardation.[15] Epidemiologic studies have also reported associations between higher hair cadmium concentrations and learning disability[16] and poor reading performance.[17]

Diagnosis

Cadmium can be measured in whole blood or urine. Urine cadmium concentrations are considered the gold standard measure of cumulative exposure, because cadmium accumulates in the kidney; urine concentrations, thus, reflect long-term exposure. Twenty-four–hour urine collections are standard, but spot urine measures in conjunction with urinary creatinine to adjust for urine volume can also be used to assess exposure. Twenty-four–hour urinary excretion in adults should be <10 µg/g of creatinine; there is no child-specific standard to determine cadmium toxicity. The geometric mean urinary cadmium concentration in children 6 to 11 years of age on the basis of data from the National Health and Nutrition Examination Survey (NHANES) is 0.075 µg/g of creatinine. From occupational monitoring studies, the first signs of renal abnormalities in adults typically occur at 2 µg/g of creatinine and include microscopic proteinuria—in particular, β_2-microglobulin and α_1-microglobulin are spilled. Each can also be measured directly. At urinary cadmium concentrations of 4 µg/g of creatinine, enzymes such as N-acetyl-B-glucosaminidase are found in urine; signs of more significant glomerular damage (such as albumin in the urine and decreases in glomerular filtration rate) are seen. In the final stages of cadmium nephropathy, glycosuria, wasting of calcium and phosphate, and altered calcium metabolism with secondary effects on the skeleton of osteoporosis and osteomalacia are seen, in part resulting from the effects on the kidneys and bone.[18]

Prevention of Exposure

Because there is no effective treatment for cadmium toxicity or exposure, prevention of exposure is key. Chelation therapy has been shown to mobilize tissue cadmium and increase renal cadmium concentrations, increasing renal toxicity. Children younger than 6 years should not be given or allowed to play with inexpensive metal jewelry.[2] Cadmium should also not be used in consumer products unless absolutely necessary, particularly not in products designed to be used by or with children. Reducing children's exposure to secondhand smoke has obvious health benefits beyond reducing cadmium exposure. Consumption of liver and kidney from exposed animals are potential sources of high dietary cadmium. Exposure to environmental cadmium can be prevented by reducing environmental levels in soil, in water used to irrigate food crops, and by reducing drinking water levels of cadmium. Cadmium concentrations in drinking water supplies are typically less than 1 µg/L (1 part per billion [ppb, equivalent to µg/L]). The EPA has established a reference dose (RfD [the maximum acceptable oral dose of a toxic substance]) of 5×10^{-4} mg/kg/day in water. The EPA has set the maximum contaminant level (MCL) for cadmium in water at 0.005 mg/L or 5 parts per billion.

CHROMIUM

Chromium (Cr) is an element found in the earth, in plants, and in animals, including humans. The most common forms are elemental (metallic) chromium (0), trivalent chromium (III), and hexavalent chromium (IV).[19] Chromium (III), the naturally occurring form, is an essential nutrient. Chromium stimulates fatty acid and cholesterol synthesis and is important in insulin metabolism.[20] Hexavalent chromium (chromate) is a toxic form of chromium.

Chromium can be found in many consumer products, including leather tanned with chromic sulfate and stainless steel cookware. Chromated copper arsenate (CCA) was used in the past as a wood preservative. Pressure-treated lumber containing chromated copper arsenate may still be present in outdoor playgrounds and other structures (see chapter 22). Wood is now sometimes treated with copper dichromate. Chromium is used in industrial processes, such as corrosion inhibition, chrome plating, and pigments, and can be released into the environment intentionally or accidentally. Chromium is present in tobacco smoke.[19]

Routes of Exposure

Chromium can be ingested, inhaled, and absorbed through the skin. Hexavalent chromium crosses the placenta and passes into human milk.

Sources of Exposure

Chromium is naturally found in many foods and beverages (eg, meat, cheese, whole grains, eggs, and some fruits and vegetables). The Adequate Intake (AI [a dietary recommendation made by the Food and Nutrition Board of the Institute of Medicine]) for chromium ranges from 0.2 µg/day for infants to 35 µg/day for adolescent males to 45 µg/day for lactating women.

Chromium enters the soil, air, and water primarily as a result of industrial emissions of the trivalent and hexavalent forms. Typical chromium concentrations in soil are 400 parts per million (ppm [equivalent to mg/kg])[21] but can range from 1 to 2000 parts per million.[22] Because of its widespread use, chromium is a contaminant found in more than half of all National Priorities List Superfund hazardous waste sites and in many landfills.[21] Chromium in air is found as fine dust particles, which can settle in soil and water.[21] Most atmospheric chromium results from fossil fuel combustion and steel production.[22] Chromium concentrations in the atmosphere are estimated at 0.01 µg/m³ in rural areas and 0.01 to 0.03 µg/m³ in urban areas.[21] Chromium contamination of water can be extensive; about one third of drinking water supplies in California have detectable levels of chromium (VI).[23] In water, chromium can move to areas distant from the original site of contamination.[21] Typical concentrations of chromium in tap water are 0.4 to 8.0 parts per billion and those in rivers and lakes typically fall between 1 and 30 parts per billion.[22] In the infamous Pacific Gas and Electric Company mass exposure (popularized by the movie *Erin Brockovich*), concentrations of hexavalent chromium in water were 580 parts per billion, far in excess of the state limit of 50 parts per billion.[21]

Childhood exposure to hexavalent chromium most commonly occurs via ingestion of contaminated water or play near a hazardous waste site.[19] Chromium-laden dust can be found in house dust in areas where there is significant local contamination. Adults who work in industries using chromium can bring significant amounts of it, along with other hazardous materials, into the home on their clothing and shoes. When children play on structures made of wood preserved with chromated copper arsenate, chromium and arsenic are detectable on their hands. There is no report in the literature to indicate that this chromium enters the blood. The exposure to chromium from the burning or demolition of wood treated with chromated copper arsenate appears to be small.[24]

Biological Fate

Absorption of chromium depends on the route of exposure and the form of the element. After inhalation, elemental and trivalent chromium are poorly absorbed; in contrast, the hexavalent form, because it is more water soluble, is well absorbed from the lungs. After ingestion, trivalent chromium salts are poorly absorbed (<2%), but up to 50% of the hexavalent form can be absorbed from the gastrointestinal tract. A significant proportion of ingested hexavalent chromium, however, is converted to the less soluble trivalent form in the gut, considerably limiting its absorption. After dermal contact, chromium (III) and (IV) are both absorbed; the amount depends on the condition of the skin and the particular compound.[19]

Chromium is stored in all body tissues, although retention does not seem to be prolonged; the kidneys excrete approximately 60% of a chromium dose within 8 hours of ingestion.[22] An estimated 80% of chromium is excreted by the kidneys; bile and sweat are minor routes of excretion.

Systems Affected

Acute exposure to chromium may affect organs including the skin, gastro-intestinal tract, kidneys, and lungs.

Clinical Effects

Acute and Short-Term Effects

Hexavalent chromium, the most toxic of the 3 forms of chromium, can have immediate and long-term effects. Even short-term skin exposure can result in significant irritation and sensitization, producing allergic contact dermatitis with subsequent exposures. Chromium is considered second only to nickel in being the most allergenic metal to which humans are regularly exposed.[21] Once found in significant concentration in detergents and bleaches, chromium was thought to be the cause of the once common "housewives' eczema."[21] "Blackjack disease" was a term describing the eczematous dermatitis found in card players exposed to chromium in felt. Ingestion of high-dose hexavalent chromium produces gastrointestinal symptoms (nausea, vomiting, hematemesis), which can be severe. Large ingestions can produce acute renal failure. High-dose inhalation can produce acute pneumonitis. Other acute toxicities include effects on the nasal mucosa, with runny nose, sneezing, nosebleeds, and with repeated exposures, nasal septum ulcers.[19]

Chronic/Long-Term Effects

Chronic inhalation of hexavalent chromium is associated with increased risks of nasal and lung cancers in adults,[19] including in people who work in industries using chromium.[21] The International Agency for Research on Cancer, the US National Toxicology Program, the World Health Organization (WHO), and the EPA have concluded that hexavalent chromium is a human carcinogen.[19] The risk of lung cancer increases with the duration of exposure, with latency periods ranging from 13 to 30 years (although cases have appeared following as few as 5 years of exposure).[22] Declines in the incidence of cancer as exposures fall among chromium workers suggest a threshold effect for the carcinogenic potential of hexavalent chromium.[22] Carcinogenicity has not been observed from exposure to elemental or trivalent chromium salts.

Although there is evidence to suggest that hexavalent chromium increases the risk of other cancers in adults (cancers of bone, stomach, and prostate; lymphoma, and leukemia), there are insufficient data to confirm this.

Hexavalent chromium has other toxicities. Low birth weight, birth defects, and other reproductive toxicities have been observed in experimental animal models of chronic hexavalent chromium exposure.[21] Exposure to chromium significantly disturbs spermatogenesis in animals.[22]

Type IV hypersensitivity skin reactions with contact dermatitis or eczema are common consequences of long-term dermal exposure. For example, chromium sensitivity occurs in as many as 8% to 9% of cement workers; among workers exposed to chromium in the automotive repair industry, sensitivity has been reported in as many as 24%.[22] Chronic inhalational exposure can produce chronic lung disease (pneumoconiosis).

Diagnosis

Chromium can be measured in serum or urine. Normal serum concentrations have been reported as 0.052 to 0.156 µg/L. Because only hexavalent chromium penetrates erythrocytes, red cell chromium may be a better indicator of exposure to hexavalent chromium rather than serum chromium, which reflects exposure to all chromium species.[22] Urine measurement of chromium generally reflects absorption over the previous 1 to 3 days; the typical range of concentration in urine is 0 to 40 µg/L. Chromium also can be measured in hair, although reference values are not available. Samples of human milk may have an average concentration of 0.3 parts per billion of chromium. These analyses are not useful in the clinical setting. Because of species interconversion, no biological specimen has sufficient sensitivity to identify exposure to one particular form (eg, hexavalent).[21] Diagnosis of toxicity, therefore, relies largely on historical evidence and environmental documentation of exposure, supplemented by biological monitoring.

Treatment

Any treatment of chromium (as well as manganese and nickel) exposure should be conducted in consultation with an expert in pediatric environmental health and/or occupational health. There are no known chelators of chromium. However, given its rapid and apparently complete elimination, chelation should not be needed. Ascorbic acid (vitamin C) is considered a valuable treatment after hexavalent chromium ingestion because of its ability to reduce hexavalent chromium to the less soluble trivalent chromium.

Prevention of Exposure

Exposure to chromium can be prevented by fencing hazardous land sites and prohibiting children from playing in soils near sites where chromium may have been discarded. Because of possible chromium contamination of well water, analysis for chromium in well water should be considered before that water is consumed. The EPA has set a limit of 100 parts per billion total chromium (not hexavalent specifically) in water.[25] Chromium concentrations in air are not regulated, although control measures are being enacted; environmental rules that help to reduce exposure from ambient atmospheric pollution are needed.

Ingestions of chromium also should be minimized. Reference (maximum recommended) doses for chromium are 1 mg/kg per day for trivalent chromium and 5 µg/kg per day for hexavalent chromium.[22]

MANGANESE

Manganese (Mn) is a metal known for its light weight and durability. Uses of inorganic manganese include production of steel alloys, batteries, glass and ceramics, incendiaries, fungicides, and as a catalyst for the chlorination of organic compounds. Permanganates (manganese oxides) are used as disinfectants and in metal cleaning, bleaching, flower preservation, and photography. Organic manganese compounds are used as gasoline and fuel oil additives and as fungicides.[26,27] Manganese may be an essential human nutrient. It is involved in the formation of bone and in the metabolism of amino acids, lipids, and carbohydrates. Manganese is required in a number of different enzymes: hexokinase, xanthine oxidase, pyruvate carboxylase, arginase, manganese superoxide dismutase, and the neuron-specific enzyme glutamine synthetase.

Manganese is present in the environment in inorganic and organic forms. There are 7 species of inorganic forms, ranging in valence from 0 to 7+; heptavalent manganese includes the permanganates, which are potent oxidizing agents. The primary organomanganese compound of concern is methylcyclopentadienyl manganese tricarbonyl (MMT), an antiknock gasoline additive.

Routes of Exposure

Manganese can be ingested and inhaled. Manganese crosses the placenta and passes into human milk.

Sources of Exposure

Foods and beverages are significant sources of manganese, providing daily intakes ranging from 2 to 9 mg. Dietary intake is much higher among vegetarians, approaching 20 mg daily.[26] Foods high in manganese include whole barley, rye, and wheat; pecans; almonds; and leafy green vegetables. The highest amounts are found in nuts. Tea is a high-source beverage. Manganese concentration in human milk is very low (4-8 µg/L) and varies with month of lactation. Cow milk and cow milk-based formulas have concentrations of 30 to 60 µg/L, and soy formulas have concentrations 50 to 75 times higher than human milk. Absorption is greater from human milk. Soy and rice "milks" that are not formulas and not intended to be ingested by infants may contain even more manganese and result in intakes that exceed the upper limit for children 1 to 3 years of age.[28-30] Dietary supplements and alternative medicines can contain significant amounts of manganese; cases of manganese toxicity from the use of a Chinese herbal remedy have been reported.[31]

Major sources of nondietary manganese exposure in children result from pollution of air, water, and soil.[27] Average levels of manganese in outdoor air (0.02 µg/m^3)[32] are generally higher in urban areas and have decreased over time. Sources of atmospheric manganese include combustion of fossil fuels (20%) and industrial emissions (80%).

Methylcyclopentadienyl manganese tricarbonyl (25.2% manganese) was introduced into gasoline in the 1970s, replacing lead as an antiknock compound. It is rarely used today (see Chapter 29).

Water contamination is another potential source of excess manganese. Freshwater typically contains manganese in a range of 1 to 200 µg/L. Well water contamination from natural and anthropogenic sources is relatively common, with concentrations up to an order of magnitude greater (up to 2000 µg/L).

Soil can contain high manganese concentrations occurring naturally and from surface pollution. Concentrations of manganese in soil average 40 to 900 parts per million, with an average of 330 ppm; concentrations near industry can approach 7000 parts per million.[26] In a pattern similar to that observed when lead was added to gasoline, the concentration of manganese in soil decreases with the distance from heavily traveled roads.[33]

Biological Fate

Manganese absorption from the gut is highly regulated via homeostatic mechanisms. Iron and manganese share the same mucosal transport system. Very little manganese is absorbed from the gastrointestinal tract; the average absorption of dietary manganese averages 3% to 5%.[26] Children have less well developed homeostatic mechanisms for regulating manganese absorption and elimination. Iron deficiency and low protein intake are associated with increased oral manganese absorption, and high dietary calcium or phosphate decrease its absorption. There also seems to be extensive genetic modulation of manganese absorption from the gut, mediated by the highly prevalent hemochromatosis gene. Women typically absorb more manganese than men, presumably because of their lower iron stores. Once absorbed, manganese is transported by plasma proteins (including the β-1 globulin transmanganin)[34] and within the erythrocyte. Plasma protein transferrin also is important in manganese transport. Excretion of manganese is primarily though the bile; renal excretion of the metal is negligible. The biological half-life of manganese is approximately 40 days. Data from studies in animals suggest that the elimination of manganese from the central nervous system (CNS) is slower than from other tissues.

Unlike ingested manganese, inhaled manganese is completely absorbed; through this route, it can be transported directly to the CNS without hepatic first-pass clearance.[35]

Systems Affected

Acute exposure to manganese can affect the lungs and skin. Chronic exposure may result in neurotoxicity, pulmonary disease, and reproductive toxicity.

Clinical Effects

Acute Effects

Acute exposure to manganese oxides can produce a syndrome known as "metal fume fever" or manganese pneumonitis.[27] This syndrome includes flulike symptoms, such as fever, cough, congestion, and malaise. This illness most commonly occurs in the industrial setting with processes such as welding or metal cutting. Permanganate solutions can be extremely corrosive. Another significant consequence of acute manganese poisoning is hepatic injury.[26] There is no reported acute CNS toxicity from manganese; CNS symptoms require long-term exposure.

Chronic/Long-Term Effects

Central nervous system effects of manganese were first described in the 1800s, when the term "manganese madness" was first coined.[26] Initial symptoms of manganese toxicity are psychiatric, characterized by emotional lability, hallucinations, asthenia, irritability, and insomnia. Chronic manganese intoxication (manganism) is best known for inducing neurological injury that mimics Parkinson disease, with masklike facies, cogwheel rigidity, tremor, and clumsiness. This syndrome typically appears after 2 to 25 years of excess manganese exposure but also has been observed within several months of heavy exposure.[26] Manganese-induced neurotoxicity can be progressive and can worsen after exposure has ended.[26] The cellular mechanism of neurotoxicity is unclear. Manganese can displace iron from transferrin; the neurotoxicity of manganese may, therefore, be related to increases in iron-induced oxidative injury to neurons.[36] Experimental studies in animals suggest that neonates have greater transport of manganese into the CNS, a lower threshold for manganese-induced neurotoxicity, and greater retention of manganese in the brain compared with older animals.[28] Iron deficiency is associated with increased CNS concentrations of manganese. Therefore, infants, children, and menstruating women are at greater risk of manganese neurotoxicity. Iron excess also increases the risk of manganese neurotoxicity. Pathologic changes include deterioration of the globus pallidus and corpus striatum as well as decreased activity of catecholamines (particularly dopamine) and serotonin in the corpus striatum.[34] Unlike Parkinson disease, manganese toxicity is associated with preservation of nigro-striatal dopaminergic pathways.[28] Although manganese-induced neurotoxicity is most commonly found after chronic inhalation, ingestion of manganese-contaminated water also has been associated with neurotoxicity. Cohort studies in which contaminated well water (containing 0.08–14 mg/L) was ingested have reported neurodevelopmental injury.[34] In one study in children, long-term manganese exposure in drinking water was associated with poor school performance and decrements in neurobehavioral performance.[37] Recent data have associated manganese exposure with diminished intellectual function.[38] In animal studies, prenatal manganese exposure is associated with significant neurotoxicity among progeny.

Chronic inhalation of manganese dust can lead to pulmonary disease, manifested by chronic respiratory tract inflammation.[27]

Reproductive toxicities in males can occur with chronic manganese exposure. Decreased spermatogenesis occurs in animals; epidemiologic studies have shown a significant decrease in the number of children born to workers exposed to manganese dust.[39] Stillbirths and birth defects, including cleft lip, imperforate anus, cardiac defects, and deafness, have been reported in populations chronically exposed to excessive manganese.[27]

Diagnosis

Normal ranges of manganese concentrations are approximately 4 to 15 μg/L in blood, 1 to 8 μg/L in urine, and 0.4 to 0.85 μg/L in serum. Biological monitoring for manganese exposure is very difficult.[20,27] Manganese is bound to red blood cells, making serum concentrations very low and subject to contamination by hemolysis. Moreover, whole blood manganese concentrations are so variable that they may not be useful as clinical indicators of magnesium status. Urinary measurements, similarly, do not reflect past exposure to manganese. Human milk concentrations of manganese vary widely (6.2 μg /L to 17.6 μg /L) depending on the time postpartum that that sample is taken and, presumably, other factors.[27]

Treatment

Treatment of excess manganese exposure may include chelation therapy. Calcium disodium edetate ($CaNa_2EDTA$) increases urinary excretion and may result in clinical improvement in selected cases of severe manganese intoxication.

Prevention of Exposure

Prevention of manganese exposure includes taking environmental actions to reduce outdoor air pollution and ensuring that water supplies, particularly well water, are closely monitored. The EPA has calculated a reference ambient air concentration (an estimate of a continuous inhalation exposure to humans [including sensitive subgroups] that is likely to be without an appreciable risk of deleterious effects during a lifetime) of manganese on the basis of changes in neuropsychological function in adults, to equal 0.05 μg/m³.[40] The current EPA limit for manganese in water is 50 μg/L. Because this is not a health-based standard and is set for aesthetic or cosmetic reasons to avoid stains on plumbing and laundered clothes, all efforts should be made to ensure that concentrations of manganese in drinking water remain below this concentration. Recommended daily intakes from diet include an EPA reference dose of 0.14 mg/kg per day, based on the risk of the appearance of neurobehavioral toxicity in adults. The Institute of Medicine's adequate intake recommendations for manganese range from 3 μg/day in infants to 2.2 mg/day in adolescent males.[20] Methylcyclopentadienyl manganese tricarbonyl should not be used in gasoline.

NICKEL

Nickel (Ni) is a white magnetic metal commonly used in alloys with copper, chromium, iron, and zinc. These alloys are used in fuel production, making jewelry, clothing fasteners, metallic coins, domestic utensils, medical prostheses, heat exchangers, valves, and magnets. Nickel salts are used in electroplating, in pigments, in ceramics, in batteries, and as a catalyst in food production. Nickel compounds, especially nickel carbonyl ($Ni[CO]_4$), a potent carcinogen, are present in secondhand smoke.

Nickel occurs naturally in the earth's crust and may be emitted from volcanoes and in rock dust. It is a natural constituent of soil and is transported in streams and waterways.[41,42] Nickel has been reported in Montreal snow at 200 to 300 parts per billion.[43] Anthropogenic emissions include industrial sources from mining and recycling, steel production, and municipal incineration.[44] Power plants fueled by peat, coal, natural gas, and oil are sources of nickel compound emissions. Nickel accumulates along roadways from abrasion of metal parts of vehicles and the use of gasoline containing nickel. Industrial waste has been disposed of by land spreading, land filling, ocean dumping, and incineration. Emissions by aerosols can be transported far from the source.[44,45]

Routes of Exposure

Nickel can enter the body through inhalation, ingestion, or the skin.

Sources of Exposure

Children are exposed to nickel through air, especially when it contains second-hand smoke. They are exposed through food, possibly through drinking water, and by dermal absorption. There is a potential for iatrogenic exposure through dialysis and through dental and surgical prostheses.[42] Nickel has been found to leach from stainless steel cookware, especially in mildly acidic conditions at boiling temperatures.[44,46]

Natural food sources of nickel include cocoa, nuts, soybean, and oatmeal. Oysters and salmon may accumulate high levels when fished from water with increased concentrations of nickel. Nickel may be present in higher concentrations in vegetables such as peas, beans, cabbage, spinach, and lettuce. Certain plants and bacteria have been found to carry nickel-containing enzymes. Nickel, however, has not been shown to be an essential nutrient in humans.[41] Nickel deficiency has been induced in rats, chicks, cows, and goats. Decreasing growth and abnormal morphology and oxidative metabolisms in the liver have been noted in these animals. Nickel may act as a ligand cofactor facilitating the gastrointestinal absorption of ferric irons.[47]

Biological Fate

After nickel enters the body, soluble ions of nickel may be absorbed directly, whereas insoluble compounds may be phagocytosed. Nickel bisulfide (Ni_3S_2) and nickel oxide (NiO) are relatively insoluble; however, they play an important role in carcinogenesis when phagocytosed by cells lining the respiratory tract. Soluble nickel compounds may be absorbed through the gastrointestinal tract from water and food, however, a large percentage of this nickel is excreted in feces. Soluble nickel that enters the bloodstream may accumulate in the kidneys and be excreted in the urine.[41,42] Nickel may be dermally absorbed by direct contact.

Clinical Effects

Workers in nickel refinery and processing industries exposed by inhalation have a higher incidence of respiratory cancers of the lung, larynx, and nasopharyngeal passages.[41,48] Nickel carbonyl inhalation in workers has been described to cause adrenal, hepatic, and renal damage leading to death. Inhaled nickel sulfate has been known to cause asthma.[49] Occupational exposure is associated with a higher incidence of spontaneous abortions, congenital structural malformations,[50] and chromosomal aberrations.[51]

The most common adverse health effect in children from nickel is the development of allergies. An estimated 10% to 20% of the population is sensitive to nickel.[41] Nickel is one of the most common causes of contact dermatitis from jewelry, white gold, wrist watches, metal clothing fasteners, and dental prostheses. A nickel allergy may be induced on the ears by ear piercing, on the abdomen by snaps in the waistband of pants where the component of a snap in the waistband of pants rubs against the skin, and on wrists and necks by jewelry.[52,53] Nickel dermatitis has been described in infants.[54]

A 2-year-old child who accidentally ingested nickel sulfate ($NiSO_4$) crystals (570 mg of nickel/kg) died from cardiac arrest 8 hours after exposure.[41]

Diagnosis

A urine nickel concentration of 5 µg/dL in an individual with acute exposure is considered to be at the upper limits of normal. Acute poisoning is diagnosed at higher concentrations.

Treatment

Acute toxicity may be treated with chelating agents especially diethyl-dithiocarbamate. Disulphiram, which is metabolized to diethyl-dithiocarbamate, may be effective. Penicillamine has been used in treating acute toxic effects of nickel compounds.[41]

Regulations

The EPA has designated nickel and its compounds as toxic pollutants. The EPA recommends that drinking water should contain no more than 0.1 mg/L.

The WHO has classified nickel compounds as group I carcinogens (human carcinogens) and metallic nickel as a group IIB carcinogen (possible human carcinogen).[41] In 1996, the European Union announced a directive to restrict the use of nickel to reduce the prevalence of nickel allergy. The directive prohibits the use of nickel in jewelry, especially earrings, for pierced ears, wristwatches, and clothing that may be in direct contact with the skin for prolonged periods.[55]

Prevention of Exposure

Because the incidence of nickel dermatitis is high and many people develop sensitization to nickel, it is prudent to educate the public about its widespread use in jewelry and clothes fasteners and to alert people with sensitivity to avoid exposing their skin to nickel. People who are sensitive to nickel and those who have atopic tendencies may also want to avoid nickel-containing stainless steel cookware.

Frequently Asked Questions

Q   *Should I worry about the nickel in coins, cookware, jewelry, and clothes fasteners? Can my child develop cancer from nickel?*

A   Metallic nickel has not been shown to produce cancer in children. Contact with metallic nickel can cause allergic dermatitis generally if the metal is in contact with the skin for prolonged periods. Workers in nickel refineries who inhaled large quantities of nickel salts were found to have a higher risk of cancers of the nasopharynx and lungs. Children are generally not exposed to such high levels from nickel in the outdoor air.

Q   *My child is overweight and has acanthosis nigricans with marked elevation in her serum insulin. Do you think she is deficient in chromium? Should her level be measured?*

A   There is no known correlation between chromium deficiency and insulin resistance; therefore, there is no need to measure a chromium level. This is, however, an active area of research.

References

1. Agency for Toxic Substances and Disease Registry. *Case Studies in Environmental Medicine: Cadmium Toxicity.* Atlanta, GA: Agency for Toxic Substances and Disease Registry; 1990

2. New York State Department of Health. *Cadmium in Children's Jewelry.* Available at: http://www.health.state.ny.us/environmental/chemicals/cadmium/cadmium_jewelry.htm. Accessed March 21, 2011

3. Mannino D, Holguin F, et al. Urinary cadmium levels predict lower lung function in current and former smokers: data from the Third National Health and Nutrition Examination Survey. *Thorax.* 2004;59(3):194-198

4. Satarug S, Baker JR, Urbenjapol S, et al. A global perspective on cadmium pollution and toxicity in non-occupationally exposed population. *Toxicol Lett.* 2003;137(1-2):65-83

5. Satarug S, Moore M. Adverse health effects of chronic exposure to low-level cadmium in foodstuffs and cigarette smoke. *Environ Health Perspect.* 2004;121(10):1099-1103

6. Jarup L, Hellstrom L, Carlsson MD, et al. Low level exposure to cadmium and early kidney damage: the OSCAR study. *Occup Environ Med.* 2000;57(10):668-672

7. Eltzer HM, Brantsaeter AL, Borch-Iohnsen B, et al. Low iron stores are related to higher blood concentrations of manganese, cobalt and cadmium in non-smoking, Norwegian women in the HUNT 2 study. *Environ Res.* 2010;110(5):497-504

8. Horiguchi H, Oguma E, Sasaki S, et al. Comprehensive study of the effects of age, iron deficiency, diabetes mellitus, and cadmium burden on dietary cadmium absorption in cadmium-exposed female Japanese farmers. *Toxicol Appl Pharmacol*. 2004;196(1):114-123

9. Kobayashi E, Suwazono Y, Uetani M, et al. Estimation of benchmark dose as the threshold levels of urinary cadmium, based on excretion of total protein, β2-microglobulin and N-acetyl-β-D-glucosaminidase in cadmium nonpolluted regions in Japan. *Environ Res*. 2006;101(3): 401-406

10. Waalkes M. Cadmium carcinogenesis. *Mutat Res*. 2003;533(1-2):107-120

11. Agency for Toxic Substances and Disease Registry. *Case Studies in Environmental Medicine (CSEM). Cadmium Toxicity. How Does Cadmium Induce Pathogenic Changes?* Atlanta, GA: US Department of Health and Human Services, 2008. Available at: http://www.atsdr.cdc.gov/csem/cadmium/cdpathogenic_changes.html. Accessed March 21, 2011

12. Jiang HM, Han GA, He ZL. Clinical significance of hair cadmium content in the diagnosis of mental retardation of children. *Chin Med J (Engl)*. 1990;103(4):331-334

13. Thatcher RW, Lester ML, McAlaster R, Horst R. Effects of low levels of cadmium and lead on cognitive functioning in children. *Arch Environ Health*. 1982;37(3):159-166

14. Wright RO, Amarasiriwardena C, Woolf AD, Jim R, Bellinger DC. Neuropsychological correlates of hair arsenic, manganese, and cadmium levels in school-age children residing near a hazardous waste site. *Neurotoxicology*. 2006;27(2):210-216

15. Gillberg C, Noren JG, Wahlstrom J, Rasmussen P. Heavy metals and neuropsychiatric disorders in six-year-old children. Aspects of dental lead and cadmium. *Acta Paedopsychiatr*. 1982;48(5):253-263

16. Pihl RO, Parkes M. Hair element content in learning disabled children. *Science*. 1997;198(4313):204-206

17. Thatcher RW, McAlaster R, Lester ML, Cantor DS. Comparisons among EEG, hair minerals and diet predictions of reading performance in children. *Ann N Y Acad Sci*. 1984b;433:87-96

18. Roels HA, Hoet P, Lison D. Usefulness of biomarkers of exposure to inorganic mercury, lead, or cadmium in controlling occupation and environmental risks of nephrotoxicity. *Ren Fail*. 1999;21(3-4):251-262

19. Agency for Toxic Substances and Disease Registry. *Draft Toxicological Profile for Chromium*. Atlanta, GA. Agency for Toxic Substances and Disease Registry; 2008. Available at: http://www.atsdr.cdc.gov/ToxProfiles/tp7.pdf. Accessed March 21, 2011

20. Institute of Medicine, Food and Nutrition Board. *Dietary Reference Intakes for Vitamin A, Vitamin K, Arsenic, Boron, Chromium, Copper, Iodine, Iron, Manganese, Molybdenum, Nickel, Silicon, Vanadium, and Zinc*. Washington, DC: National Academies Press; 2000. Available at: http://www.nap.edu/catalog.php?record_id=10026. Accessed March 21, 2011

21. Pellerin C, Booker SM. Reflections on hexavalent chromium: health hazards of an industrial heavyweight. *Environ Health Perspect*. 2000;108(9):A402–A407

22. Barceloux DG. Chromium. *J Toxicol Clin Toxicol*. 1999;37(2):173–194

23. Sedman RM, Beaumont J, McDonald TA, Reynolds S, Krowech G, Howd R. Review of the evidence regarding the carcinogenicity of hexavalent chromium in drinking water. *J Environ Sci Health C Environ Carcinog Ecotoxicol Rev*. 2006;24(1):155-182

24. Wasson SJ, Linak WP, Gullett BK, et al. Emissions of chromium, copper, arsenic, and PCDDs/Fs from open burning of CCA-treated wood. *Environ Sci Technol*. 2005;39(22): 8865-8876

25. US Environmental Protection Agency. Basic Information about Chromium in Drinking Water. Available at: http://water.epa.gov/drink/contaminants/basicinformation/chromium.cfm. Accessed March 21, 2011

26. Barceloux DG. Manganese. *J Toxicol Clin Toxicol*. 1999;37(2):293–307

27. Agency for Toxic Substances and Disease Registry. *Toxicological Profile for Manganese.* Washington, DC: US Department of Health and Human Services, Public Health Service; 2000

28. Aschner M. Manganese: brain transport and emerging research needs. *Environ Health Perspect.* 2000;108(Suppl 3):429–432

29. American Academy of Pediatrics, Committee on Nutrition. *Pediatric Nutrition Handbook.* Kleinman RE, ed. Elk Grove Village, IL: American Academy of Pediatrics; 2009

30. Dobson AW, Erikson KM, Aschner M. Manganese neurotoxicity. *Ann N Y Acad Sci.* 2004;101(2):115-128

31. Pal PK, Samii A, Calne DB. Manganese neurotoxicity: a review of clinical features, imaging and pathology. *Neurotoxicology.* 1999;20:227–238

32. National Air Toxics Program. Integrated Urban Strategy. Report to Congress. Available at: http://www.epa.gov/airtoxics/urban/natpapp.pdf. Accessed March 21, 2011

33. McMillan DE. A brief history of the neurobehavioral toxicity of manganese: some unanswered questions. *Neurotoxicology.* 1999;20(2-3):499–507

34. Gilmore DA, Bronstein AC. Manganese and magnesium. In: Sullivan JB, Krieger GR, eds. *Hazardous Materials Toxicology—Clinical Principles of Environmental Health.* Baltimore, MD: Williams & Wilkins; 1992:896–902

35. Davis JM. Methylcyclopentadienyl manganese tricarbonyl: health risk uncertainties and research directions. *Environ Health Perspect.* 1998;106(Suppl 1):191-201

36. Verity MA. Manganese neurotoxicity: a mechanistic hypothesis. *Neurotoxicology.* 1999; 20(2-3):489–497

37. Zhang G, Liu D, He P. [Effects of manganese on learning abilities in school children.] *Zhonghua Yu Fang Yi Xue Za Zhi.* 1995;29(3):156–158

38. Szpir M. New thinking on neurodevelopment. *Environ Health Perspect.* 2006;114(2): A100-A107

39. Lauwerys R, Roels H, Genet P, Toussaint G, Bouckaert A, De Cooman S. Fertility of male workers exposed to mercury vapor or to manganese dust: a questionnaire study. *Am J Ind Med.* 1985;7(2):171–176

40. US Environmental Protection Agency. Manganese. Integrated Risk Information System IRIS. Available at: http://www.epa.gov/iris/subst/0373.htm. Accessed March 21, 2011

41. Agency for Toxic Substances and Disease Registry. *Toxicological Profile for Nickel (update).* Washington, DC: US Department of Health and Human Services, Public Health Service; 1997

42. Snow ET, Costa M. Nickel toxicity and carcinogenesis. In: Rom WN, ed. *Environmental and Occupational Medicine.* 3rd ed. Philadelphia, PA: Lippincott-Raven Publishers; 1998:1057–1062

43. Landsberger S, Jervis RE, Kajrys G, Monaro S. Characterization of trace elemental pollutants in urban snow using proton induced x-ray emission and instrumental neutron activation analysis. *Intern J Environ Anal Chem.* 1983;16:95–130

44. Australian Department of the Environment and Heritage. *Nickel & Compounds: Overview.* Canberra, ACT, Australia: Australian Department of the Environment and Heritage; 2006. Available at: http://www.npi.gov.au/substances/nickel/index.html. Accessed March 21, 2011

45. Bennett BG. 1984. Environmental nickel pathways in man. In: Sunderman FW Jr, ed. *Nickel in the Human Environment. Proceedings of a Joint Symposium.* Lyon, France: International Agency for Research on Cancer; March 8–11, 1983:487–495. IARC Scientific Publication No. 53

46. Kuligowski J, Halperin KM. Stainless steel cookware as a significant source of nickel, chromium, and iron. *Arch Environ Contam Toxicol.* 1992;23(2):211–215

47. Nielsen FH, Shuler TR, McLeod TG, Zimmerman TJ. Nickel influences iron metabolism through physiologic, pharmacologic and toxicologic mechanisms in the rat. *J Nutr.* 1984;114(7):1280–1288

48. Goldberg M, Goldberg P, Leclerc A, et al. Epidemiology of respiratory cancers related to nickel mining and refining in New Caledonia (1978–1984). *Int J Cancer.* 1987;40(3):300–304

49. McConnell LH, Fink JN, Schleuter DP, Schmidt MG Jr. Asthma caused by nickel sensitivity. *Ann Intern Med.* 1973;78(6):888–890

50. Chashschin VP, Artunina GP, Norseth T. Congenital defects, abortion and other health effects in nickel refinery workers. *Sci Total Environ.* 1994;148(2-3):287–291

51. Elias Z, Mur JM, Pierre F, et al. Chromosome aberrations in peripheral blood lymphocytes of welders and characterization of their exposure by biological samples analysis. *J Occup Med.* 1989;31(5):477–483

52. Larsson-Stymne B, Widstrom L. Ear piercing—cause of nickel allergy in schoolgirls? *Contact Dermatitis.* 1985;13(5):289–293

53. Rencic A, Cohen BA. Prominent pruritic periumbilical papules: a diagnostic sign in pediatric atopic dermatitis. *Pediatr Dermatol.* 1999;16(6):436–438

54. Ho VC, Johnston MM. Nickel dermatitis in infants. *Contact Dermatitis.* 1986;15(5):270–273

55. Delescluse J, Dinet Y. Nickel allergy in Europe: the new European legislation. *Dermatology.* 1994;189(Suppl 2):56–57

Chapter 25

Carbon Monoxide

∎ ∎ ∎ ∎ ∎ ∎

Carbon monoxide (CO) is a colorless, odorless, tasteless toxic gas that is a
product of the incomplete combustion of carbon-based fuels. Carbon monoxide
has a vapor density slightly less than that of air. The health effects from acute
CO exposure range from nonspecific flulike symptoms, such as headache,
dizziness, nausea, vomiting, weakness, and confusion, to coma and death from
prolonged or intense exposure. Fetuses, infants, pregnant women, elderly people,
and people with anemia or with a history of cardiac or respiratory disease
may be particularly sensitive to CO. Evidence of delayed neuropsychological
health effects and slow resolution of these sequelae from CO exposures are
documented in the literature, although no definitive diagnostic or therapeutic
approaches have been established. The effects of long-term, low-level exposure
is another area of CO poisoning that lacks a definitive approach for diagnosis
and treatment.[1,2]

Unintentional CO poisonings accounted for approximately 400 to 500 deaths
(all ages) and more than 15 000 emergency department visits in the United
States annually between 1999 and 2004.[3] During the same period, the number
of calls to poison control centers increased significantly, indicating a possible
increase in the number of nonfatal CO poisonings.[4] The most recently available
data estimate that there are 4383 annual hospital discharges for CO-related
conditions.[5] In a study of 3034 poisoning deaths among 10- to 19-year-olds,
38.2% were attributable to CO inhalation, of which 65.1% were categorized as
suicide and 34.9% as unintentional. Motor vehicle exhaust accounted for 84.4%
of the CO-related suicides and 65.6% of the unintentional fatal CO poisonings.[6]
Death rates from fire-related CO poisoning are higher for children younger
than 15 years and for the elderly than for other age groups.[7] The prevalence

of unintentional nonfatal CO poisonings is difficult to estimate, because the nonspecific clinical presentation of mild and severe poisoning poses a diagnostic challenge.[2,8-11] Often, the presentation can mimic influenza. In a study of 46 children presenting during winter months to the emergency department for flulike symptoms, more than half had carboxyhemoglobin (COHb) concentrations that exceeded 2%, and 6 of these children had COHb concentrations that exceeded 10%.[8]

ROUTE AND SOURCES OF EXPOSURE

The route of exposure to CO is through inhalation. Unintentional exposure to CO can be largely attributed to smoke inhalation from fires, motor vehicle exhaust, faulty or improperly vented gas-fueled (natural or liquified petroleum) appliances (including heating appliances), solid fuel appliances (such as wood burning stoves), and tobacco smoke. Confined, poorly ventilated spaces such as garages, campers, tents, and boats also are susceptible to elevated, often lethal, levels of CO.[1] Common sources of CO exposure are listed in Table 25.1. Exposure to CO may occur in and around motor vehicles when there is inadequate combustion resulting from substandard vehicle maintenance and poor ventilation. Exposure also may occur when gasoline-powered equipment, such as generators, lawn mowers, snow blowers, leaf blowers, and ice rink resurfacing machines, are used in poorly ventilated spaces.[1,7,12]

The risk from CO poisoning increases after disasters, when gasoline-powered generators may be more frequently used to supply power. After Hurricane Ike, generators were used to supply electricity used to watch television or power

---

Table 25.1: Sources of Carbon Monoxide Exposure

Motor vehicle exhaust

Motorboats

Unvented kerosene and propane gas space heaters

Leaking chimneys and furnaces

Backdrafting from furnaces

Woodstoves and fireplaces

Charcoal or propane grills

Gas appliances: stoves, dryers, water heaters

Gasoline-powered generators

Gasoline-powered equipment: ice rink resurfacers, lawnmowers, leaf blowers, floor polishers, snowblowers, pressure washers

Tobacco smoke

video games, resulting in the CO poisoning death of one child and the poisoning injuries of 15 other children.[13]

SYSTEMS AFFECTED

CO is inhaled, diffuses across the alveolar-capillary membrane, and is measurable in the bloodstream as COHb. The relative affinity of CO for hemoglobin is approximately 240 to 270 times greater than that of oxygen, resulting in decreased oxygen-carrying capacity of the blood when CO concentrations are elevated. CO in the bloodstream causes a leftward shift of the oxyhemoglobin dissociation curve, resulting in decreased oxygen delivery to the tissues. Removal from the source of CO exposure leads to dissociation of the COHb complex, resulting in excretion of CO by the lungs.[14,15]

Infants and children have an increased susceptibility to CO toxicity because of their higher metabolic rates. Fetuses are especially vulnerable. Maternal CO diffuses across the placenta and increases the levels of CO in the fetus. Fetal hemoglobin has a higher affinity for CO than does adult hemoglobin, and the elimination half-life of COHb is longer in the fetus than in the adult. The leftward shift in the normal oxyhemoglobin dissociation curve caused by CO results in a substantial decrease in oxygen delivery to the placenta and ultimately to fetal tissues.[16,17] Children with existing pulmonary or hematologic illness (eg, anemia) that compromise oxygen delivery also are more susceptible to adverse effects at lower levels of CO exposures than are healthy individuals.[1]

Poisoning from exposure to CO results in tissue hypoxia affecting multiple organ systems. Systems with high metabolic rates and high oxygen demand are preferentially affected, with the central nervous and cardiovascular systems being primary targets.[1,2,18] Typical pathologic changes found on neuroimaging studies, when present, include bilateral necrosis in the basal ganglia, including the caudate, globus pallidus, and putamen. Imaging can also demonstrate diffuse homogenous demyelination of the white matter of the cerebral hemispheres.[19,20] Cardiac toxicity can be manifested by ischemia on electrocardiography, arrhythmia, and infarction.[18]

Recent research has focused on investigating the possible mechanisms of toxicity from CO. Mechanisms include tissue hypoxia attributable to decreased oxygen-carrying capacity but also attributable to decreased cardiac output secondary to myocardial dysfunction. Other mechanisms of interest that are being investigated include the production of hydroxyl radicals and nitric oxide radicals.[2]

CLINICAL EFFECTS

The clinical presentation of CO poisoning is highly variable, and the severity of the symptoms correlates poorly with the level of exposure (parts per million [ppm] of CO over time) and clinical laboratory determination of poisoning (blood COHb concentrations). This important phenomenon is explained in part by the fact that within the body, CO can be found in 4 distinct states. In addition to binding to hemoglobin, CO also binds to myoglobin and the cytochrome p450 system and exists in its free state in the plasma at a low concentration, the latter of which is thought to play an important role in clinical toxicity. This is illustrated by animal studies that showed no clinical symptoms in animals transfused with blood containing highly saturated COHb but minimal free CO. Low concentrations of COHb may be present in cases of severe poisoning.[2,8,10,14]

Symptoms of CO poisoning include headache, dizziness, fatigue, lethargy, weakness, drowsiness, nausea, vomiting, skin pallor, dyspnea on exertion, palpitations, confusion, irritability, irrational behavior, loss of consciousness, coma, and death. Severity of symptoms ranges from mild to very severe (coma, respiratory depression) and is not correlated with the magnitude of COHb concentrations.[18] In a series of pediatric patients treated for CO poisoning, lethargy and syncope were reported more frequently than in adult series. These symptoms also occurred at lower COHb concentrations than usually reported for adults.[10] Delayed neuropsychological sequelae following CO exposure have been reported in adults and children. Sequelae can occur as early as 24 hours after exposure, with impairment in memory, attention, and executive functioning.[21] Other impairments can include cognitive and personality changes, parkinsonism, dementia, and psychosis.[10,1618,22] The incidence of delayed neuropsychiatric sequelae varies widely but has been estimated to occur in 10% to 30% of victims.[18] Neuropsychiatric testing is only completed on a small proportion of patients being treated for CO poisoning.[22]

DIAGNOSIS

A thorough history and physical examination and a high index of clinical suspicion are necessary to diagnose CO poisoning. Physicians should consider CO exposure when members of the same household present with similar nonspecific symptoms. Clinical examination is often without findings suggestive of CO poisoning, other than the nonspecific signs and symptoms described in the previous section.

Measurement of oxygen saturation by pulse oximetry and arterial blood gas determination is not helpful in the diagnosis of CO poisoning. The pulse oximeter typically misinterprets COHb as oxyhemoglobin, resulting in an elevated oxygen saturation reading by this device.[23] Arterial oxygen tension (PaO_2) is typically normal in CO poisoning, because PaO_2 measures the amount of oxygen dissolved in plasma, which is unaffected in this condition. However, the blood gas determination will demonstrate metabolic acidosis in significant CO poisoning.

The measurement of blood COHb may help to establish whether exposure to CO has occurred. An elevated concentration confirms the diagnosis of CO poisoning. Low and moderately increased concentrations must be interpreted with caution, because the COHb concentration does not indicate severity of illness. Delay between exposure and laboratory measurement, treatment with oxygen, and complicating factors, such as exposure to tobacco smoke, should be considered when interpreting COHb results. Background concentrations of COHb range from 1% to 3% in nonsmokers.[18] Baseline COHb concentrations in smokers typically range from 3% to 8%, although higher values have been reported.[18,24,25]

TREATMENT

Patients who have been exposed to CO should be removed from the source immediately. Therapy consists of supplemental oxygen, ventilatory support, and monitoring for cardiac dysrhythmias. The elimination half-life of COHb is approximately 4 hours in room air. Administering 100% oxygen as the antidote will effectively reduce the elimination half-life of COHb to approximately 1 hour. Administration of hyperbaric oxygen decreases the half-life to approximately 20 to 30 minutes.[14,15,18]

The use of hyperbaric oxygen remains controversial.[26-28] Six randomized controlled trials were included in the most recent Cochrane Database of Systematic Reviews, 2 of which showed a benefit. In terms of methodologic quality, only 2 trials received the highest scores. They are the only trials that received a blinded control with a sham treatment in the hyperbaric oxygen chamber.[29] One trial of patients 16 years and older poisoned by CO showed fewer cognitive sequelae following 3 hyperbaric oxygen treatments within a 24-hour period.[28] This randomized trial did not enroll children younger than 16 years, so it is not known whether the results can be generalized to children. The other trial failed to show benefit from this intervention.[26] After a pooled analysis of all the data, the Cochrane review concluded there was insufficient evidence to conclude that hyperbaric oxygen therapy reduced the incidence of neurologic sequelae.[29] However, it appears that the use of hyperbaric oxygen for the treatment of CO poisoning in the United States has remained the same since 1992.[4]

If hyperbaric oxygen therapy is being considered, the following have been used as criteria: (1) COHb concentration ≥25%; (2) anginal pain or ischemia on electrocardiogram; or (3) measurable neurologic impairment.[15] The choice of treatment modalities is tailored to the patient on the basis of the severity of the poisoning, as determined by the observed clinical manifestations. An additional consideration for using hyperbaric oxygen therapy should be the location of the nearest center with a hyperbaric chamber and whether such a transfer may delay treatment. When the patient poisoned by CO is cared for, consultation with a pediatric critical care specialist familiar with treatment options, including hyperbaric oxygen therapy, is suggested. In addition, because treatment with hyperbaric oxygen needs to be individualized, providers should also consult with the poison control center or the Divers Alert Network (www.diversalertnetwork.org).

PREVENTION OF EXPOSURE

Primary prevention of CO poisoning requires limiting exposure to known sources. Proper installation, maintenance, and use of combustion appliances can help to reduce excessive CO emissions. Table 25.2 provides suggestions to prevent CO poisoning.[12]

The US Environmental Protection Agency (EPA) has set significant harm levels of 50 parts per million (8-hour average), 75 parts per million (4-hour average), and 125 parts per million (1-hour average). Exposure under these conditions could result in COHb concentrations of 5% to 10% and cause significant health effects in sensitive individuals. The current ambient (outdoor) air quality standards for CO (9 parts per million for 8 hours and 35 parts per million for 1 hour) are intended to keep COHb concentrations below 2.1% to protect the most sensitive members of the general population (ie, individuals with coronary artery disease).[1]

Smoke detectors and CO detectors, when used properly, may provide early detection and warning and may prevent unintentional CO-related deaths. CO detectors are designed to alarm before potentially life-threatening levels of CO are reached. CO detectors measure the amount of CO (parts per million) that has accumulated over time and should alarm within 189 minutes when CO in the air reaches 70 parts per million,[30] corresponding to a concentration of approximately 5% COHb in the blood. This is based on relationships between CO levels measured in air and corresponding blood COHb concentrations in adults. Significant exposure to children may have occurred before the CO alarm sounds.[30]

The US Consumer Product Safety Commission (CPSC) recommends installation of a CO detector in the hallway near every separate sleeping area of the home. A residential CO detector should meet the requirements of the most recent revision of Underwriters Laboratories (UL) Standard 2034.[31] Because electric heating and cooking appliances shut down during a power failure, battery-operated detectors are recommended when gas appliances or auxiliary heating sources (eg, fireplaces) are used during periods when electrical service is disrupted. The effectiveness of CO detectors in preventing CO poisoning has not been evaluated.

Table 25.2: Preventing Problems With CO in the Home and Other Environments

FUEL-BURNING APPLIANCES

- Forced-air furnaces should be checked by a professional once a year or as recommended by the manufacturer. Pilot lights can produce CO and should be kept in good working order.

- All fuel-burning appliances (eg, gas water heaters, gas stoves, gas clothes dryers) should be checked professionally once a year or as recommended by the manufacturer.

- Gas cooking stove tops and ovens should not be used for supplemental heat.

FIREPLACES AND WOODSTOVES

- Fireplaces and woodstoves should be checked professionally once a year or as recommended by the manufacturer. Check to ensure the flue is open during operation. Proper use, inspection, and maintenance of vent-free fireplaces (and space heaters) are recommended.

SPACE HEATERS

- Fuel-burning space heaters should be checked professionally once a year or as recommended by the manufacturer.

- Space heaters should be properly vented during use, according to the manufacturer's specifications.

BARBECUE GRILLS/HIBACHIS

- Barbecue grills and hibachis should never be used indoors.

- Barbecue grills and hibachis should never be used in poorly ventilated spaces such as garages, campers, and tents.

AUTOMOBILES/OTHER MOTOR VEHICLES

- Regular inspection and maintenance of the vehicle exhaust system are recommended. Many states have vehicle inspection programs to ensure this practice.

- Never leave an automobile running in the garage or other enclosed space; CO can accumulate even when a garage door is open.

GENERATORS/OTHER FUEL-POWERED EQUIPMENT

- Follow the manufacturer's recommendations when operating generators and other fuel-powered equipment.

- Never operate a generator indoors.

continued on page 374

continued from page 373

Table 25.2: Preventing Problems With CO in the Home and Other Environments, *continued*

BOATS

- Be aware that carbon monoxide poisoning can mimic symptoms of sea sickness.

- Schedule regular engine and exhaust system maintenance.

- Consider installing a CO detector in the accommodation space on the boat.

- Never swim under the back deck or swim platform as carbon monoxide builds up near exhaust vents.

Frequently Asked Questions

Q   What sort of things can I do to help limit my family's exposure to CO?

A   Table 25.2 lists recommendations for preventing CO problems in the home and other environments.[12]

Q   Is using a CO detector a good way to prevent CO poisoning?

A   CO detectors are widely available in stores, and you may want to consider buying one as a backup but not as a replacement for proper use and maintenance of fuel-burning appliances (see Table 25.2). The technology of CO detectors is still developing. There are several types on the market, and they are not generally considered to be as reliable as the smoke detectors found in homes today. Some CO detectors have been laboratory tested, and their performance varied. Some performed well, others failed to alarm even at very high CO levels, and still others alarmed even at very low levels that do not pose any immediate health risk. With smoke detectors, you can easily confirm the cause of the alarm, but because CO is invisible and odorless, it is harder to tell whether an alarm is false or a real emergency.

Organizations such as Consumers Union (publisher of *Consumer Reports*), the American Gas Association, and Underwriters Laboratories have published guidance for consumers. Look for Underwriters Laboratories certification on any CO detector. CO detectors always have been and still are designed to alarm before potentially life-threatening levels of CO are reached. The Underwriters Laboratories Standard 2034 (1998 revision) has stricter requirements that the detector/alarm must meet before it can sound. As a result, the possibility of nuisance alarms is decreased.

Q   Should I purchase a CO detector for my motor home or other recreational vehicles?

A   The CPSC notes that CO detectors are available for boats and recreational vehicles and that they should be used, and that the Recreational Vehicle
Industry Association requires CO detectors in motor homes and in towable
recreational vehicles that have a generator or are prepped for a generator.

Q   What do I do if my CO detector alarms?

A   Never ignore an alarming CO detector/alarm. If the CO detector goes off:
— Make sure it is your CO detector and not your smoke detector.
— Check to see if any member of the household is experiencing symptoms
of poisoning.
— If they are, get them out of the house immediately and call 911. Seek
medical attention at an emergency department. Tell the doctor that you
suspect CO poisoning.
— If no one is feeling symptoms, ventilate the home with fresh air, turn off
all potential sources of CO, including oil or gas furnace, gas water heater,
gas range, oven, gas dryer, gas or kerosene space heater, and any vehicle or
small engine.
— Have a qualified technician inspect your fuel-burning appliances and
chimneys to make sure they are operating correctly and that there
is nothing blocking the fumes from being vented out of the house.
Checking appliances and other possible CO sources should be done
before they are turned back on.

*Q   I recently found out that my furnace has been leaking CO, even though I feel fine.
Are there any long-term effects?*

A   There are no data that show that chronic CO exposure produces any long-
term sequelae. The long-term effects, such as the neuropsychiatric sequelae,
only have been described in patients who have had documented evidence of
a severe, acute CO poisoning. Even though you feel fine, it is imperative that
you and your family vacate the premises and have the furnace problem evaluated and fixed immediately. Ignoring this problem could prove fatal to you
and your family.

Q   Are carbon monoxide detectors required in my home?

A   Many states or municipalities have enacted laws requiring the use of CO
detectors in rental units and other residences. The specific requirements vary
by state and town.

Resources

Divers Alert Network
Web site: www.diversalertnetwork.org

Undersea and Hyperbaric Medical Society
Phone: 301-942-2980
Web site: http://uhms.org

Underwriters Laboratories
Phone: 847-272-8800
Web site: www.ul.com

US Consumer Product Safety Commission
Phone: 800-638-2772
Web site: www.cpsc.gov

**US Environmental Protection Agency Indoor Air Quality
Information Clearinghouse**
Phone: 800-438-4318
Web site: www.epa.gov/iaq/iaqinfo.html

References

1. US Environmental Protection Agency. *Air Quality Criteria for Carbon Monoxide.* Research Triangle Park, NC: Office of Health and Environmental Assessment, Office of Research and Development; 2000. EPA Publication 600/P-99/001F. Available at: http://www.epa.gov/NCEA/pdfs/coaqcd.pdf. Accessed August 10, 2010
2. Raub JA, Mathieu-Nolf M, Hampson NB, Thom SR. Carbon monoxide poisoning—a public health perspective. *Toxicology.* 2000;145(1):1–14
3. Centers for Disease Control and Prevention. Carbon monoxide-related deaths—United States, 1999-2004. *MMWR Morb Mortal Wkly Rep.* 2007;56(50):1309-1312
4. Hampson NB. Trends in the incidence of carbon monoxide poisoning in the United States. *Am J Emerg Med.* 2005;23(7):838-841
5. Ball LB, MacDonald SC, Mott JA, Etzel RA. Carbon monoxide- related injury estimation using ICD-coded data: Methodologic implications for public health surveillance. *Arch Environ Occup Health.* 2005;60(3):119-127
6. Shepherd G, Klein-Schwartz W. Accidental and suicidal adolescent poisoning deaths in the United States, 1979–1994. *Arch Pediatr Adolesc Med.* 1998;152(12):1181–1185
7. Cobb N, Etzel RA. Unintentional carbon monoxide-related deaths in the United States, 1979 through 1988. *JAMA.* 1991;266(5):659–663
8. Baker MD, Henretig FM, Ludwig S. Carboxyhemoglobin levels in children with nonspecific flu-like symptoms. *J Pediatr.* 1988;113(3):501–504
9. Heckerling PS, Leikin JB, Terzian CG, Maturen A. Occult carbon monoxide poisoning in patients with neurologic illness. *J Toxicol Clin Toxicol.* 1990;28(1):29–44
10. Crocker PJ, Walker JS. Pediatric carbon monoxide toxicity. *J Emerg Med.* 1985;3(6):443–448
11. Weaver LK. Carbon monoxide poisoning. *N Engl J Med.* 2009;360(12):1217-1225

12. American Thoracic Society. Environmental controls and lung disease. *Am Rev Respir Dis.* 1990;142(4):915–939

13. Fife CE, Smith LA, Maus EA, et al. Dying to play video games: carbon monoxide poisoning from electrical generators used after Hurricane Ike. *Pediatrics.* 2009;123(6):e1035-e1038

14. Vreman HJ, Mahoney JJ, Stevenson DK. Carbon monoxide and carboxyhemoglobin. *Adv Pediatr.* 1995;42:303–334

15. Piantadosi CA. Diagnosis and treatment of carbon monoxide poisoning. *Respir Care Clin North Am.* 1999;5(2):183–202

16. Koren G, Sharev T, Pastuszak A, et al. A multicenter prospective study of fetal outcome following accidental carbon monoxide poisoning in pregnancy. *Reprod Toxicol.* 1991;5(5):397–404

17. Kopelman AE, Plaut TA. Fetal compromise caused by maternal carbon monoxide poisoning. *J Perinatol.* 1998;18(1):74–77

18. Ernst A, Zibrak JD. Carbon monoxide poisoning. *N Engl J Med.* 1998;339(22):1603–1608

19. Bianco F, Floris R. MRI appearances consistent with haemorrhagic infarction as an early manifestation of carbon monoxide poisoning. *Neuroradiology.* 1996;38(Suppl 1):S70–S72

20. Hopkins RO, Fearing MA, Weaver LK, Foley JF. Basal ganglia lesions following carbon monoxide poisoning. *Brain Injury.* 2006;20(3):273-281

21. Porter SS, Hopkins RO, Weaver LK, et al. Corpus callosum atrophy and neuropsychological outcome following carbon monoxide poisoning. *Arch Clin Neuropsychol.* 2002;17(2):195-204

22. Seger D, Welch L. Carbon monoxide controversies: neuropsychologic testing, mechanism of toxicity, and hyperbaric oxygen. *Ann Emerg Med.* 1994;24(2):242–248

23. Buckley RG, Aks SE, Eshom JL, Rydman R, Schaider J, Shayne P. The pulse oximetry gap in carbon monoxide intoxication. *Ann Emerg Med.* 1994;24(2):252–255

24. Hausberg M, Somers VK. Neural circulatory responses to carbon monoxide in healthy humans. *Hypertension.* 1997;29(5):1114–1118

25. Hee J, Callais F, Momas I, et al. Smokers' behaviour and exposure according to cigarette yield and smoking experience. *Pharmacol Biochem Behav.* 1995;52(1):195–203

26. Scheinkestel CD, Bailey M, Myles PS, et al. Hyperbaric or normobaric oxygen for acute carbon monoxide poisoning: a randomized controlled clinical trial. *Med J Aust.* 1999;170(5):203–210

27. Juurlink DN, Stanbrook MB, McGuigan MA. Hyperbaric oxygen for carbon monoxide poisoning. *Cochrane Database Syst Rev.* 2000;(2):CD002041

28. Weaver LK, Hopkins RO, Chan KJ, et al. Hyperbaric oxygen for acute carbon monoxide poisoning. *N Engl J Med.* 2002;347(14):1057–1067

29. Judge BS, Brown MD. To dive or not to dive? Use of hyperbaric oxygen therapy to prevent neurologic sequellae in patients acutely poisoned with carbon monoxide. *Ann Emerg Med.* 2005;46(5):462-464

30. Etzel RA. Indoor air pollutants in homes and schools. *Pediatr Clin North Am.* 2001;48(5):1153–1165

31. Underwriters Laboratories. *UL2034: Standard for Single and Multiple Station Carbon Monoxide Detectors.* Northbrook, IL: Underwriters Laboratories; 1992. Revised Standard 2034. Available at: http://ulstandardsinfonet.ul.com/scopes/2034.html and http://www.protechsafety.com/standard/ul2034.pdf. Accessed August 10, 2010

Chapter 26

Cold and Heat

■ ■ ■ ■ ■ ■

Heat and cold stress are environmental hazards. Because of their unique physiology, children are more susceptible to temperature extremes and their health effects. Optimal body function requires a body temperature of approximately 98.6°F (37°C). As homeotherms (organisms that generate heat to maintain body temperature, typically above the temperature of surroundings [also known as endotherms]), humans have extensive mechanisms for maintaining body temperature in a narrow range. These mechanisms, which emanate from the hypothalamic temperature-regulating center, include vasodilation and sweating (with heat stress) and piloerection and shivering (with cold stress). Changes in behavior that may not occur at a conscious level (eg, the decision to wear cool or warm clothing) can be important in temperature control.[1] Children are less able to thermoregulate compared with adults.[2] As a result, children are more likely to develop significant health effects when they are exposed to environmental temperature extremes.

Four physical properties—convection, conduction, radiation, and evaporation—determine the interaction between ambient and body temperature. Convection is a mechanism of heat exchange through a medium such as air or water. Air is a relatively inefficient medium; exposure to cold air must take place over several hours for a human to develop hypothermia. Water is a medium that transmits energy more efficiently; cold-water immersion can change body temperature in minutes. Conduction is the transfer of heat between 2 bodies in contact (eg, skin-to-skin contact). Radiation is the process by which the body gains heat from surrounding hot objects, such as hot pipes, and loses heat to cold objects, such as chilled metallic surfaces, without any direct contact.

Environmental temperature extremes result from natural or manmade causes. Natural causes include heat waves, unseasonably cold weather, and winter storms.

Table 26.1: Physiologic Effects and Clinical Manifestations of Cold

CORE BODY TEMPERATURE	PHYSIOLOGIC RESPONSE
Mild (90°F–95°F; 32°C–35°C)	Shivering Tachycardia or bradycardia Confusion
Moderate (82.4°F–90°F; 28°C–32°C)	Loss of shivering Loss of deep tendon reflexes; peripheral anesthesia Bradycardia, hypotension Central nervous system depression
Severe (<82.4°F; <28°C)	Severe bradycardia Cardiac arrhythmias Coma

Manmade events can result from inadequate home heating or cooling, extended exposure to temperature extremes without proper gear, and overheated indoor environments, such as automobiles. Climate change appears to have a significant role in recent changes in the pattern of heat and cold injury.[3,4] Current evidence suggests that anthropogenic activities are important contributors to these climatic changes and that an increase in natural disasters involving cold and heat can be anticipated.

The public health consequences of cold and heat extremes are substantial. These have been most evident in the effects of heat waves that have occurred over the last several years.[2,5] In a summer heat wave in Europe in 2003, an estimated 15 000 people were killed.[2,6] In the southwest United States, where in recent summers ambient temperatures have been greater than 110°F (46°C) for extended periods, numerous deaths have been reported. Predictions are that heat waves are likely to increase.[2,7]

COLD

Humans are less able to compensate for cold stress compared with heat stress.[8] Because they are less able to thermoregulate than adults, children can quickly become hypothermic (defined as a core body temperature <95°F [35°C]) when exposed to cold. Children are also more susceptible to hypothermia because of their large body surface area-to-mass ratio, which predisposes them to rapid heat loss.[9] Newborn infants are highly prone to hypothermia because of their large body surface area, small amount of subcutaneous fat, and decreased ability to shiver. Risk factors for developing hypothermia in children include hypothyroidism, hypoglycemia, and taking ethanol or certain medications (eg, opioids, phenothiazines). Hypothermia can be classified as mild, moderate, or severe (Table 26.1).

Table 26.2: Physiologic Effects of Extreme Cold and Heat		
BODY SYSTEM	**COLD**	**HEAT**
Neurologic	Delirium Central nervous system depression	Coma Seizures
Cardiovascular	Bradycardia Cardiac arrest	Tachycardia, cardiovascular collapse
Musculoskeletal	Shivering	Rhabdomyolysis
Metabolic	Hyperglycemia	Metabolic acidosis
Respiratory	Depressed respirations	Tachypnea

There are several specific causes of cold exposure. Winter storms can occur unpredictably, leading to sudden and prolonged periods of cold temperatures. If the storm produces a power failure, the interior of a home can become dangerously cold. Direct contact with water is another important cause of cold exposure; cold-water immersion can produce hypothermia in minutes because of water's efficient conductive ability. Wet clothing can increase heat loss fivefold.[9]

An associated hazard resulting from cold extremes is the use of potentially dangerous heating sources. Families may use gas stoves, fireplaces, wood stoves, space heaters, and propane heaters as supplements or alternatives to home heating or during power outages. These heat sources carry the threat of fire hazard, production of indoor air pollutants (in the case of poorly maintained fireplaces and wood stoves), and carbon monoxide poisoning (with improper use of propane heaters and generators [see Chapter 25]).

Children and adults respond to cold extremes in the same way (Tables 26.1 and 26.2).[10] As core body temperature falls, metabolic rate increases to create more heat. At body temperatures of 90°F to 95°F (32°C-35°C), patients develop shivering, "goose bumps," lethargy, and bradycardia. With moderate hypothermia (82.4°F-90°F [28°C-32°C]), shivering ends; disorientation, and stupor occur. Severe hypothermia (<82.4°F [28°C]) produces profound bradycardia and cardiac arrhythmias. Slowed nerve conduction velocity contributes to the development of numbness (anesthesia). Disorientation can occur. An electrocardiogram will display a J-wave (Osborn wave), characteristic of severe hypothermia.

An unusual compensatory mechanism for extreme cold is known as the diving reflex. When immersed in cold water, which produces rapid hypothermia, the body begins to preferentially divert blood from organs such as the gastrointestinal tract and kidneys to the brain and heart. As a result, there is remarkable preservation of the central nervous system for extended periods of oxygen deprivation. In reported cases, humans who were immersed for as long as 2 hours have had recovery with completely intact neurologic function. Children have a more robust diving reflex than adults, suggesting that it is an immature reflex.

Cold injuries can be mild or severe and transient or permanent. Frostnip is the mildest form of cold injury, consisting of pain and pallor of the cold-exposed area. It is commonly found among skiers, sledders, skaters, and other outdoor sports enthusiasts.[8] Frostnip is treated by warming the affected area. Recovery is complete. Chronic cold injury, just above freezing, can produce an uncommon condition known as chilblain (trench foot). In contrast to frostnip and chilblain, frostbite is severe and results in permanent tissue injury. Tissue destruction by cold can result in loss of the affected area, particularly the digits, ears, and nose. During an initial evaluation, it is often not possible to determine whether a cold injury is frostnip or frostbite.

Treatment of cold injury consists of rewarming. The child's affected body part should be placed against another individual's body part. If hands are involved, the affected individual may place the hands in his or her axillae. If that is not possible, the exposed body part can be placed near a heat source or in warm water as soon as possible. Care should be taken to avoid burning the area. It is also important not to rub the affected area; rather, the affected area (such as hands) should be placed under water and soaked, not rubbed together. Rewarming should only be initiated when there is no chance of additional cold exposure; the rewarming of injured tissue followed by additional cold exposure can produce greater injury to the affected body part. Victims of significant cold injury should be evaluated by a pediatrician or in an emergency department, particularly if they have a significant change in behavior or a body part that appears cold, stiff, and pale.

Prevention

Preventing cold extremes and their consequences consists of several interventions:
- Wearing proper cold-weather gear;
- Carefully selecting timed periods of cold exposure;
- Avoiding severe cold;
- Finding alternate shelter if the home or residence has lost its heat; and
- Using safe indoor heating sources.

HEAT

As with cold extremes, heat extremes have changed in pattern and prevalence over recent years. This has been associated in part with climate change, particularly the greenhouse effect.[5] Carbon dioxide, produced primarily by fuel combustion, creates an atmospheric blanket that traps solar energy that is naturally reflected from the earth's surface (see Chapter 54).

A heat wave is defined as more than 3 consecutive days with ambient temperatures greater than 90°F (32.2°C).[1] Over the last decade, heat waves have increased in prevalence around the globe. An important secondary consequence of heat extremes is the increased production of smog and other ambient pollutants and the development of wildfires and power failures.[2]

Manmade events have also resulted in a greater prevalence of heat injury. Events include siting of homes in areas known to have heat extremes and inadequate supervision of children or the elderly, who might be unable to signal for help or to escape the heat threat without help.

Children spend more time outdoors than adults, during play, sports, and work activities. For example, adolescents may spend extended periods outdoors working in landscaping or agriculture. Outdoor workers can develop severe or even fatal heat-related injuries.[11]

The human body has mechanisms, including vasodilation and sweating, for maintaining normal temperature across a wide range of ambient temperatures.[1] Vasodilation results in simple radiant loss from hot skin; this can account for up to 60% of the body's cooling ability. Sweating and its evaporation account for 25% of heat-reducing capacity.[2] High humidity prevents evaporative loss, leading to decreased cooling ability and a greater risk of hyperthermia.[1] Children sweat less than adults, which limits their heat-reduction capacity.[4]

Other risk factors for heat-associated illness in children include chronic diseases (eg, diabetes, obesity, cystic fibrosis), medications (eg, anticholinergics, stimulant medications, opioids, phenothiazines), and reduced mobility (infants, children with physical disabilities).

Heat extremes can produce several health effects in children, the most common of which is dehydration. Dehydration occurs from the combination of insensible water losses through exhaled air and sweating. Children generally sweat at a rate of 1 L/hour/m². In unacclimatized adolescents, 1 to 4 L of fluid can be lost in a single hour of exertion, accompanied by the loss of several grams of salt.

When the body is no longer able to compensate for temperature extremes, core temperature rises, producing pyrexia (fever). Core body temperatures of 100°F to 106°F (37.8°C-41.1°C) can lead to sweating, tachycardia, and disorientation. Body temperatures greater than 106°F (41.1°C) are associated with agitation, seizures, tachycardia, ventricular irritability, and metabolic acidosis. Body temperatures greater than 110°F (43.3°C) can quickly lead to cardiovascular collapse.

Types of Heat Injury

Injuries resulting from heat extremes include heat exhaustion, heat cramps, and heat stroke. These often occur in a continuum when early signs of heat injury are not addressed.[12]

Heat exhaustion typically results from the combination of sustained heat and dehydration. Children can develop faintness, extreme tiredness, and headache; there may be fever and intense thirst.[12] Other signs and symptoms include nausea, vomiting, hyperventilation, and paresthesias. Heat exhaustion is treated with rest, fluids, and hydration with electrolyte-containing drinks.

Heat cramps most commonly occur in children who are participating in outdoor sports, work, or play; cramps typically occur in conditioned children who have been drinking water but have not been adequately replacing salt losses. Heat cramps usually start during relaxation and can be triggered by cold.[1] Children complain of muscle aches with the lower extremities more commonly affected than the upper extremities. Pain may be severe and may result from muscle spasms. The cause of the pain of heat cramps is unclear but has been attributed in part to electrolyte disturbances and accumulation of lactic acid in muscles. The treatment for heat cramps is rest, cooling, and hydration with electrolyte-containing drinks. Although the loss of electrolytes appears to be a risk factor, there is no role for salt tablets.

Heat stroke is an emergency that occurs independently of hydration. It is typically categorized as exertional and nonexertional. Exertional heat stroke tends to occur in highly motivated athletes, soldiers, and laborers[12]; it remains one of the most common causes of death in US high school athletes.[1,12] Nonexertional heat stroke occurs in the absence of physical activity. In children, nonexertional heat stroke is most often the result of children being left unattended in vehicles.[12] Children with heat stroke develop stupor or coma, tachycardia, hypertension, or hypotension. Severe rhabdomyolysis can occur, resulting in myoglobinuria and acute renal failure, complications that are often fatal. Victims of heat stroke have, by definition, lost the ability to sweat. Sweating is the primary mechanism for body cooling; without sweating, the core body temperature of heat stroke victims can increase to >115°F. Children with evidence of heat stroke should immediately be taken to a hospital where aggressive cooling techniques can be initiated to bring the temperature back to normal. Intravenous hydration and fluid monitoring are needed. There is no role for antipyretics, such as acetaminophen or ibuprofen, in pyrexia caused by heat exposure.

Prevention

Because children are more susceptible to heat illness, preventing heat extremes is especially important in children.[13] Preventive measures include:

1. Families without reliable access to air conditioning should make plans for home cooling or alternate shelters in the event of a heat wave.
2. Parents and caregivers should never leave children unattended in vehicles, particularly on hot days. Automobile cabins can reach temperatures greater than 158°F (70°C). The temperature increase in automobile cabins reaches

80% of its peak within 30 minutes; cracking the window does not significantly change the rate of increase.[14]

3. There should be a well-outlined program of conditioning for athletes that includes adequate access to water and periods of rest.

4. For those who work outdoors, heat-stress management programs should be created by the employer.[11] These should provide:

   a. training of supervisors and employees in the prevention, recognition, and treatment of heat illness;

   b. creation and implementation of a heat-acclimatization program;

   c. availability of proper amounts and types of fluids;

   d. creation of work/rest schedules appropriate for the heat index;

   e. access to shade or cooling areas;

   f. monitoring of the environment and of workers during hot conditions; and

   g. prompt medical attention to workers who show signs of heat illness.

Similar recommendations have been created for team sports during heat extremes (Table 26.3). Athletes should wear light clothing. Garments that restrict sweat loss (eg, waterproof outfits) are extremely dangerous and should never be used in hot environments.[12] Finally, communities should establish heat-wave plans. Campaigns should be initiated every summer to advise citizens of plans for management of heat extremes.[2] Warning systems for heat avoidance should be established. Such recommendations may differ for artificial turf and natural grass surfaces because artificial turf absorbs heat making those surfaces

Table 26.3: Recommended Restraints on Activities at Different Temperature Levels

WET BULB GLOBE TEMPERATURE		RESTRAINTS ON ACTIVITIES
°C	°F	
<24	<75	All activities allowed, but be alert for prodromal symptoms and signs of heat-related illness during prolonged events
24.0–25.9	75.0–78.6	Longer rest periods in the shade; enforce drinking every 15 minutes
26–29	79–84	Stop activity of unacclimatized persons and other persons with high risk; limit activities of all others (disallow long-distance races, cut down further duration of other activities)
>29	>85	Cancel all athletic activities

Reprinted from the American Academy of Pediatrics.[4]
Wet bulb globe temperature is a composite temperature used to estimate the effect of temperature, humidity, and solar radiation on humans.

hotter than natural grass surfaces when subject to the same environmental conditions.[15] Finally, local public health authorities should develop a system for identifying and contacting high-risk individuals; this is best coordinated with social services, visiting nurses, and volunteer agencies.[2]

Frequently Asked Questions

Q *What are recommendations for hydration in excessive heat?*

A Recommendations for athletic activities during heat have been published by the American Academy of Pediatrics (Table 26.3).[4] During the activity, periodic drinking should be enforced (ie, for each 20 minutes, a child weighing 40 kg [88 lb] should consume 150 mL [5 oz] of cold tap water or a flavored sports electrolyte beverage, and an adolescent weighing 60 kg [132 lb] should consume 250 mL [9 oz], even if the child does not feel thirsty).

Q *Is there a certain temperature at which I should not let my child play outdoors?*

A Heat indices have been created to identify the health threats arising from the combined influence of temperature and humidity. Air quality indices may be included in the determination of whether to avoid outdoor play (see Chapter 21). These are typically printed in newspapers, broadcast on television or radio, or found on the Internet. Along similar lines, cold indices typically combine multiple factors, including ambient temperature and wind chill factor; these can also be obtained from local weather sources.

Resources

Centers for Disease Control and Prevention

Heat-Related Illness Web site:
www.bt.cdc.gov/disasters/extremeheat/faq.asp

Hypothermia Web site:
www.bt.cdc.gov/disasters/winter/staysafe/hypothermia.asp

References

1. Ewald M, Baum C. Environmental emergencies. In: Fleisher G, Ludwig S, eds. *Textbook of Pediatric Emergency Medicine*. Philadelphia, PA: Lippincott Williams & Wilkins; 2006:1017-1021

2. Kovats R, Hajat S. Heat stress and public health: a critical review. *Annu Rev Public Health*. 2008;29:41-55

3. Davis R, et al. Changing heat-related mortality in the United States. *Environ Health Perspect*. 2003;111(14):1712-1718

4. American Academy of Pediatrics, Committee on Sports Medicine and Fitness. Climatic heat stress and the exercising child and adolescent. *Pediatrics*. 2000;106(1 Pt 1):158-159

5. American Academy of Pediatrics, Committee on Environmental Health. Global climate change and children's health. *Pediatrics*. 2007;120(5):1149-1152

6. Bouchama A. The 2003 European heat wave. *Intens Care Med*. 2004;30(1):1-3

7. O'Neill M, Ebi K. Temperature extremes and health: impacts of climate variability and change in the United States. *J Occup Environ Med.* 2009;51:13-25

8. Jurkovich G. Environmental cold-induced injury. *Surg Clin North Am.* 2007;87(1):247-267

9. Kazenbach T, Dexter W. Cold injuries. Protecting your patients from the dangers of hypothermia and frostbite. *Postgrad Med.* 1999;105(1):72-80

10. Centers for Disease Control and Prevention. Winter Weather: Hypothermia. Available at: http://www.bt.cdc.gov/disasters/winter/staysafe/hypothermia.asp. March 21, 2011

11. Centers for Disease Control and Prevention. Heat-related deaths among crop workers— United States, 1992-2006. *MMWR Morb Mortal Wkly Rep.* 2008;57(24):649-653

12. Jardine D. Heat illness and heat stroke. *Pediatr Rev.* 2007;28(7):249-258

13. Centers for Disease Control and Prevention. Frequently Asked Questions About Extreme Heat. Available at: http://www.bt.cdc.gov/disasters/extremeheat/faq.asp. Accessed March 21, 2011

14. McLaren C, Null J, Quinn J. Heat stress from enclosed vehicles: moderate ambient temperatures cause significant temperature rise in enclosed vehicles. *Pediatrics.* 2003;116(1):e109-e112

15. Claudio L. Synthetic turf: Health debate takes root. *Environ Health Perspect.* 2008;116(3): A116–A122

Chapter 27

Electric and Magnetic Fields

■ ■ ■ ■ ■ ■

Electric and magnetic fields (EMFs) are invisible lines of force created by electric charges that surround power lines, electrical appliances, and other electrical equipment. Humans have always been exposed to electric and magnetic fields from natural sources, including the earth's magnetic field. Electric and magnetic fields also are emitted by living organisms, including humans. The widespread use of electricity began in the late 1800s and led to expanding usage for heating, lighting, communications, and other uses.[1]

The most common form of electricity is alternating current (AC), which reverses direction 60 times per second in the United States.[2] The unit that denotes the frequency of alternation is called a hertz (Hz). Electrical charges create electric fields when the charges stand still and magnetic fields when the charges are in motion. The strength or intensity of magnetic fields is commonly measured in units called gauss (1 gauss = 1000 milligauss) or tesla. One tesla equals 1 million microtesla; 1 milligauss is the same as 0.1 microtesla.

The electric and magnetic fields associated with electric power are extremely low-frequency or power-frequency (50 Hz or 60 Hz, respectively) field levels. Cellular telephones and towers emit and receive radio-frequency and microwave-frequency electric and magnetic fields, involving a much higher frequency range (800–900 and 1800–1900 megahertz [MHz; 1 MHz = 1 million Hz]) than power lines or many electrical appliances.[2]

SOURCES OF EXPOSURE

Residential Exposures

Electricity is produced from coal or other sources at power plants, then sent through long-distance high-power transmission lines to substations, where the current is stepped down.[2] The lower levels of electrical current are then transmitted to homes, schools, workplaces, and other locations via distribution lines. It is estimated that only approximately 1% of children reside near high-voltage power lines.[3] The primary sources of extremely low-frequency exposure for all children is at home via electrical wiring and appliances held close to the body (including hair dryers, heating pads, and electric blankets) and others to which children are exposed at varying distances (including televisions, microwave ovens, computer monitors, and cellular phones).[2] Children are also exposed at varying levels at school and during transportation to and from activities. Electric and magnetic field levels are reduced dramatically by increasing distance from the source, with magnetic field levels reduced to background levels at distances as short as a few feet from most electrical appliances (see Table 27.1), approximately 100 ft from a distribution line and 300 ft to 500 ft from a transmission line.[2]

Typical median magnetic fields in homes measure between 0.05 and 0.1 microtesla on the basis of studies of children who carried computerized meters that took measurements every 30 seconds while at home or away from home over the course of 24 hours.[3,4] Population surveys confirm the results from measurement studies of children. The sources of children's electric and magnetic field exposure vary with age. Exposure to appliances is estimated to represent 30% of total electric and magnetic field exposure. Most of the magnetic field exposure to younger children is related to power lines near their homes and, to a much lesser extent, exposures away from home, whereas only approximately 40% of the exposure to older children comes from power lines near their homes and 60% comes from other sources away from home.[3,5]

Wireless Technologies

The primary sources of radio-frequency and microwave-frequency exposures to children have typically been from microwave ovens and handheld cellular telephones.[6,7] These exposures have significantly changed with the advent of wireless in-house communications, such as wireless monitors used in or near cribs/beds, cordless phones, wireless computer technology, and cellular phone use by someone in close proximity to children and by children themselves.[3] At present, radio-frequency exposures have been less well-characterized than the extremely low frequency magnetic fields associated with household appliances. The rapid evolution of these technologies[8] and difficulties in measuring radio-frequency exposures contribute to the challenges in studying these exposures and child health.

To date, children's typical exposure to radio-frequency fields has not been measured using meters as described previously for power-frequency exposures. The average number of years of exposure to radio-frequency field sources and the mean number of minutes of exposure to children by day, week, month, or

Table 27.1: Median 60-Hz Magnetic Field Exposure Level (in Microtesla) From Household Appliances According to Distance From the Appliance

MAJOR CATEGORY	SPECIFIC TYPE	DISTANCE			
		6 in	1 ft	2 ft	4 ft
Bathroom	Hair dryer	30	0.1	—	—
	Electric shaver	10	2	—	—
Kitchen	Blender	7	1	0.2	—
	Can opener	60	15	2	0.2
	Coffee maker	0.7	—	—	—
	Dishwasher	2	1	0.4	—
	Food processor	3	0.6	0.2	—
	Microwave oven[a]	20	0.4	1	0.2
	Mixer	10	1	0.1	—
	Electric oven	0.9	0.4	—	—
	Refrigerator	0.2	0.2	0.1	—
	Toaster	1	0.3	—	—
Living/family room	Ceiling fan	NM[b]	0.3	—	—
	Window air conditioner	NM	0.3	0.1	—
	Color TV	NM	0.7	0.2	—
	Black/white TV	NM	0.3	—	—
Laundry/utility room	Electric dryer	0.3	0.2	—	—
	Washing machine	2	0.7	0.1	—
	Iron	0.8	0.1	—	—
	Vacuum cleaner	30	6	1	0.1
Bedroom	Digital clock	NM	0.1	—	—
	Analogue (dial-face) clock	NM	1.5	0.2	—
	Baby monitor	0.6	0.1	—	—

continued on page 392

continued from page 391

Table 27.1: Median 60-Hz Magnetic Field Exposure Level (in Microtesla) From Household Appliances According to Distance From the Appliance, *continued*

MAJOR CATEGORY	SPECIFIC TYPE	DISTANCE			
		6 in	1 ft	2 ft	4 ft
Workshop	Battery charger	3	0.3	—	—
	Drill	15	3	0.4	—
	Power saw	20	4	0.5	—
Office	Video display terminal (color monitor)	1.4	0.5	0.2	—
	Electric pencil sharpener	20	7	2	0.2
	Fluorescent lights	4	0.6	0.2	—
	Fax machine	0.6	—	—	—
	Copy machine	9	2	0.7	0.1
	Air cleaner	18	3.5	0.5	0.1

— indicates magnetic field levels at background level or lower.

[a] For microwave ovens, the range of 60-Hz magnetic field levels (in microtesla) according to distance are: at 6 in: 10–30; at 1 ft: 0.1–20; at 2 ft: 0.1–3; and at 4 ft: 0–2.

[b] NM, not measured.

year have not been examined. It is important to note that modern children will experience a longer period of exposure to radio-frequency fields from cellular phone use than will adults, because they started using cellular phones at earlier ages and will have a longer lifetime exposure to them.

EFFECTS OF EXPOSURE TO ELECTRIC AND MAGNETIC FIELDS

The 60-Hz extremely low-frequency fields deliver low "packets" of energy not strong enough to break chemical bonds to cause irreversible changes to molecules, such as DNA, or to body tissue.[2] The low-energy packets from microwaves cannot break up DNA, but the electric charges on water molecules "wiggle" in response to the oscillations of the microwaves.[6,7] The friction generated by the wiggling generates heat by the same basic principle that allows microwave ovens to heat food. Radio-frequency fields from radio and television transmitters or cellular telephones alternate millions of times per second, compared with extremely low-frequency or power-frequency fields that alternate only 60 times per second.[1,6,7] At high power levels, microwave- or radio-frequency radiation can heat body tissues or create electric currents that might interfere with a cardiac pacemaker or the normal cardiac conduction system when a person is very near the source. Suggested exposure limits have been derived to avoid the adverse biological effects at high power levels, such as heating of body tissues or creation of electric currents that can interfere with pacemakers.

The World Health Organization (WHO) evaluated childhood exposure to electric and magnetic fields in a 2004 meeting that addressed exposures and outcomes and made recommendations for further study, including laboratory and epidemiologic studies of electric and magnetic fields and childhood leukemia, investigations on the exposures and outcomes of cellular telephone use in children and adolescents, and improved electric and magnetic field measurement methods.[3] There are no federal standards limiting occupational or residential exposure to 60-Hz electric and magnetic fields, but several states have set standards for transmission line electric fields.[2] Interference with cardiac pacemakers and implantable defibrillators from sources producing lower-frequency exposures (such as power lines, rail transportation, and welding equipment), as well as higher-frequency sources (such as cellular telephones, paging transmitters, citizen band radios, wireless computer links, microwave signals, and radio and television transmitters) is currently an area of active research. Although a federal radio-frequency protection guide for workers was issued in 1971, it was advisory and not regulatory. The radio-frequency exposure safety limits adopted by the Federal Communications Commission in 1996 are based on criteria quantified according to the specific absorption rate, a measure of the rate at which the body absorbs radio-frequency energy.[7]

Power levels associated with handheld cellular telephones are low, and it is unlikely that such exposures cause consequential heating of brain tissue.[8,9] Similarly, the exposure to the general public from radio waves emanating from cellular transmitting towers is very low at distances greater than several meters from the antenna.[7] The 60-Hz fields, similarly, do not have enough energy to break chemical bonds or to heat body tissues.[2] Some physicists have indicated that the weak electric currents produced in the human body by 60-Hz alternating current magnetic fields in a typical living room are thousands of times weaker than the physiological currents occurring in normal nerve cells.[9,10] Even fields 10 to 50 times stronger than that would deposit energies equivalent to a whisper in the "hurricane of Brownian molecular movement" in the body. For this reason, many physicists have argued that physiological or pathological effects of AC magnetic fields below 10 microtesla are theoretically impossible.[9-11] Other physicists, however, have argued that there may be an array of molecules or interconnected cells that could sort out the weak "signal" from the "noise."

EPIDEMIOLOGIC STUDIES OF EXPOSURE

Extremely Low-Frequency Magnetic Field Exposures

Magnetic fields have been studied as a risk factor for childhood leukemia since the late 1970s. Since then, more than 20 epidemiologic studies have been conducted to evaluate this potential risk. It was on the basis of these studies that, in 2002, the International Agency for Research on Cancer (IARC) classified extremely low-frequency magnetic fields as a possible carcinogen.[11,12] This classification was based on epidemiologic studies that investigated the relationship of exposure to residential magnetic fields and the risk of childhood leukemia.[12,13]

Early studies suggested an association between occupational exposures to magnetic fields and breast cancer in men (a very rare condition),[13-15] adult leukemia,[15,16] and adult brain cancer.[16,17] Little evidence of an association of residential magnetic field exposures and childhood brain tumors[17-19] was found in a review of approximately 20 epidemiologic studies conducted between 1979 and 2000.

More than 20 studies have evaluated childhood leukemia risk and exposure to residential magnetic field exposures. These studies have been pooled in 2 separate meta-analyses. One of these studies found a combined relative risk estimate for leukemia of 1.7 in children exposed to average magnetic fields >0.3 microtesla compared with those exposed to <0.1 microtesla. The second meta-analysis, which used more specific inclusion criteria, reported a risk estimate of 2.0 for exposures ≥0.4 microtesla compared with exposures <0.1 microtesla.

Epidemiologic studies suggesting an association between residential magnetic field exposures and childhood leukemia estimated exposure in a variety of ways, including (1) distance of residences from power lines; (2) "wire codes," a system of classification based on type of power line (transmission lines or distribution lines) and distance from the lines; (3) measurements (including spot or 30-second measurements, 24- and 48-hour residential measurements, and personal measurements) of children's estimated exposure to the magnetic field obtained after diagnosis; and (4) estimates of the magnetic field around the time of diagnosis on the basis of historical records of current flows and the distance of the lines from the home.[1] It is important to note that these studies have been predominately retrospective and are limited by challenges in measuring actual exposure and selection and recall bias. In addition, there are other factors, such as traffic density, pesticide use near power lines, and other potential exposures that make absolute interpretation of the potential risk conferred by residential magnetic field exposures difficult.

Five studies have evaluated risks of childhood leukemia or brain and nervous system tumors associated with use of electrical appliances.[1] Associations with childhood leukemia have been observed in 2 or 3 of these studies, including small increases in risk linked with prenatal and postnatal use of electric blankets, hair dryers, and televisions. An extensive body of literature evaluating adult occupational (but not residential) exposures to extremely low-frequency magnetic field exposures suggests that there may be modest increases in risk of brain tumors and chronic lymphocytic leukemia.[1,19-21] Some epidemiologic evidence has suggested that male, and to a lesser extent female, breast cancer may be linked with occupational (but not residential) exposure to extremely low-frequency electric and magnetic fields, but the evidence is inconsistent.[1,13-15] Several studies have evaluated the relationship of residential electric and magnetic field exposures and occurrence of adult brain tumors, leukemia, and breast cancer; there is no consistent evidence of association.[1,3]

In summary, a twofold excess risk of childhood leukemia is associated with residential magnetic field exposures of 0.4 microtesla or higher, but risks of childhood leukemia are not increased with lower magnetic field levels, nor are risks of brain tumors linked with residential magnetic fields on the basis of results of a pooled analysis of major studies. Reasons are unknown for the elevated risk of childhood leukemia in relation to high residential magnetic field exposures.[19,20] Findings have been inconsistent for childhood leukemia and brain tumors in relation to prenatal or postnatal exposures to electrical appliances.

Radio-Frequency and Microwave-Frequency Exposures

There have been no epidemiologic studies assessing the relationship between radio-frequency or microwave-frequency exposures and serious childhood diseases. A comprehensive and critical review of epidemiologic studies of radio-frequency exposures and human cancers published in 1999 reported that a few positive associations have been identified, but the results are inconsistent and no type of cancer has been consistently found to be increased.[21,22] Four additional case-control studies have shown no clear evidence of significantly elevated risk overall or a dose-response relationship between the use of handheld cellular telephones and occurrence of brain tumors in adults.[22,23] More recently, a nation-wide cohort of 420 095 cellular telephone users in Denmark who had been followed for up to 21 years (mean of 8.5 years) did not identify an association between tumor risk and cellular telephone use.[23,24] This study, which evaluated adults only, did not find increased risk of brain tumors, acoustic neuromas, salivary gland tumors, eye tumors, leukemia, or overall cancers.

Cellular phone use by mothers was studied in the Danish National Birth Cohort, which enrolled mothers who had children between 1996 and 2002.[25] A questionnaire was administered when the children reached 7 years of age and included questions on behavior and pre- and postnatal cellular phone use. A higher overall risk of behavioral problems was found in the children with the highest exposure to pre- and postnatal maternal cellular phone use. However, the authors urged caution in the interpretation of their results, because there is no known biological mechanism to explain these results. They also noted that the findings may not be causal because of unmeasured confounding factors.

The Interphone study (conducted among adults in Australia, Canada, Denmark, Finland, France, Germany, Israel, Italy, Japan, New Zealand, Norway, Sweden, and the United Kingdom) assessed whether exposure from cell phones was associated with an increased risk of malignant or benign brain tumors and other head and neck tumors. Among all cell phone users, the study showed no increased risk for glioma or meningioma. Among the small proportion of study participants who reported spending the most total time on cell phone calls, however, there was some increased risk of glioma.[26] The International Agency for Research on Cancer has classified radiofrequency electromagnetic fields as possibly carcinogenic to humans (Group 2B), on the basis of the increased risk of glioma associated with wireless phone use.[27]

LABORATORY STUDIES

Extremely Low-Frequency Magnetic Field Exposures

Because the 60-Hz and radio-frequency fields usually present in the environment do not ionize molecules or heat tissues, it was believed that they have no effect on biological systems.[9,10] During the mid-1970s, a variety of laboratory studies on cell cultures and animals demonstrated that biological changes could be produced by these fields when applied in intensities of hundreds or thousands of microtesla. A series of comprehensive studies reported during 1997 to 2001 showed no consistent evidence of an association between extremely low-frequency magnetic field exposures and risk of leukemia or lymphoma in rodents on the basis of long-term (up to 2.5 years) bioassays, initiation/promotion studies, investigations in transgenic models, and tumor growth studies. Three large-scale chronic bioassays of carcinogenesis in rats or mice exposed to magnetic fields for 2 years revealed no increase in mammary cancer, resulting in a general consensus that power-frequency magnetic fields do not act as a complete carcinogen in the rodent.[10,11]

Inconsistent findings from one laboratory suggesting that magnetic fields may stimulate mammary carcinogenesis in rats treated with a chemical carcinogen could not be replicated in 2 other laboratories.[10,11] A specific concern in relation to breast cancer was that extremely low-frequency magnetic field exposures might mediate occurrence of breast cancer through the melatonin pathway.[28,29] To date, the experimental literature has shown relatively little support for this hypothesis.[28,29]

In studies undertaken to investigate alterations in cellular processes associated with magnetic field exposures previously reported in the literature, regional electric and magnetic field exposure facilities established to investigate these reports, which were provided with experimental protocols, cell lines, and relevant experiment details, generally found no effects of magnetic fields on gene expression, particularly those genes that may be involved in cancer; killing of cells cultured from patients with ataxia-telangiectasia, which are highly sensitive to genotoxic chemicals; gap junction intercellular communication; the influx of calcium ions across the plasma membrane of cells or the intracellular calcium concentration; activity of ornithine decarboxylase (an enzyme implicated in tumor promotion); or other in vitro processes that may be related to carcinogenesis.[10,11] In a review of 63 laboratory-based studies published between 1990 and 2003, the conclusions from 29 investigations did not identify increased cytogenetic damage following electric and magnetic field exposure, whereas 14 studies suggested a genotoxic potential of electric and magnetic field exposure. The observations in 20 other reports were inconclusive.[28,30] Therefore, the preponderance of the evidence suggests that electric and magnetic fields are not genotoxic or carcinogenic.[10,11,28,30]

Radio-Frequency and Microwave-Frequency Exposures

Radio-frequency field sources in the home include microwave ovens, cellular telephones, burglar alarms, computer terminals, and television sets. Although some experimental studies suggest that radio-frequency fields may accelerate the development of certain tumors, including one demonstrating an increase in lymphoma incidence in transgenic mice,[29,31] overall data from more than 100 studies conducted in frequency ranges from 800 to 3000 MHz indicate that these exposures are not directly mutagenic, nor do they act as cancer initiators. Adverse effects from exposure of organisms to high radio-frequency exposure levels are predominantly the result of hyperthermia, although some studies suggest an effect on intracellular levels of ornithine decarboxylase.[30-33]

Frequently Asked Questions

Q *I am about to buy a house, but there is a power line (or transformer) near the home. Should I buy it?*

A This is a decision only a parent can make. It is important to consider that there remains some degree of uncertainty in the literature on electric and magnetic field exposure and cancer risk. This uncertainty should be considered in the context of the low individual risk and the comparable environmental risks (eg, traffic hazards) in other locations. Obtaining magnetic field measurements in the home sometimes will show that field levels are at approximately the average level despite proximity to the power line.

Q *Our child has leukemia and was exposed to power lines or an electric appliance. Could this have caused the leukemia?*

A It is important to find out why the parents suspect the power lines as the cause of leukemia and whether they may be blaming themselves for the exposure or may be considering litigation. From an objective viewpoint, pinpointing the cause of a particular case of childhood leukemia is currently beyond the ability of science. Even when there is scientific consensus that a factor such as ionizing radiation can cause childhood leukemia, it is impossible to be certain whether a particular case of leukemia was caused by radiation. It is even more problematic for electric and magnetic fields, for which evidence of an association is weak.

Q *Have any states or countries set standards for electric and magnetic fields?*

A Lack of knowledge has prevented scientists from strongly recommending any health-based regulations. The International Agency for Research on Cancer recommends that policy makers establish guidelines for electric and magnetic field exposures for both the general public and workers and that low-cost measures of reducing exposure be considered. Several states have adopted regulations governing transmission line-generated 60-Hz fields. The initial concern was the risk of electric shock from strong electric fields (measured in kilovolts [kV] per meter). Some states, such as Florida and New York, have adopted regulations that preclude new lines from exceeding the fields at the edge of the current right of way. These standards are in the hundreds of milligauss. The California Department of Education requires that new schools be built at certain distances from transmission lines. These distances, 100 ft for 100-kV lines and 250 ft for 345-kV power lines, were chosen on the basis of the estimate that electric fields would have reached the background level at these distances. All of the current regulations relate to transmission lines, and no state has adopted regulations that govern distribution lines, substations, appliances, or other sources of electric and magnetic fields.

Q *Is it all right for my child or teenager to use a cellular telephone?*

A Epidemiologic studies have not been conducted to assess the risk of cellular telephone use by children. The level of energy absorption in children while using cellular telephones is comparable to the levels in adults; however, because of the larger number of ions contained in the tissue of children, the specific tissue absorption rate may be higher. Experts in some countries have suggested that widespread use of cellular telephones by children be discouraged.[3,32,34] Because modern children will experience a longer period of exposure to cellular telephones than current adults, additional research in this area is needed. In the interim, exposures can be reduced by encouraging children to use text messaging when possible, make only short and essential calls on cellular phones, use hands free kits and wired headsets, and maintain the cellular phone an inch or more away from the head. Talking on a cell phone while driving or texting while driving result in distraction and increase the risk of automobile crashes with resulting injuries and fatalities. Teenagers and others should not talk on the phone or text while driving.

Q *I understand the uncertainty in the science, but I believe that it is prudent to avoid magnetic fields when possible. What low- and no-cost measures of avoidance can I take?*

A For most people, their highest magnetic field exposures come from using household appliances with motors, transformers, or heaters. The easily avoidable exposures would come from these appliances. If a parent is concerned about electric and magnetic field exposure from appliances, the major sources of exposure could be identified and the parent could limit the child's time near such appliances.[2] Manufacturers have reduced magnetic field exposures from electric blankets (since 1990) and from computers (since the early 1990s). Because magnetic fields decline rapidly with increasing distance, an easy measure is to increase the distance between the child and the appliance.

Q *What are the concerns about cell phone use among pregnant women?*

A Three studies on this topic from the Danish National Birth Cohort have been published. Two studies demonstrated that cell phone use prenatally was associated with behavioral difficulties, such as emotional and hyperactivity problems, around the age of school entry.[25,35] A third study of cell phone use during pregnancy did not identify delays in developmental milestones among offspring up to 18 months of age.[36] Additional research is needed to clarify this issue.

Resources

National Institute of Environmental Health Sciences
  Phone: 919-541-3345
  Web site: www.niehs.nih.gov
  Available publications include *Questions and Answers About EMF and Assessment of Health Effects from Exposure to Power-Line Frequency Electric and Magnetic Fields,* both available at http://www.niehs.nih.gov/emfrapid/booklet/home.htm.

National Research Council
  Phone: 800-624-6242
  Web site: www.nationalacademies.org/nrc/index.html
  Available publications include *Possible Health Effects of Exposure to Residential Electric and Magnetic Fields.*

National Cancer Institute
  FactSheets: *Magnetic Field Exposure and Cancer: Questions and Answers and Cellular Telephone Use and Cancer: Questions and Answers* are both available at www.cancer.gov/cancertopics.

US Federal Communications Commission (FCC)

Web site: www.fcc.gov

The FCC licenses communications systems that use radio-frequency and microwave-frequency EMF (available at: http://www.fcc.gov/oet/info/documents/bulletins/#56).

US Food and Drug Administration (FDA)

Phone: 888-INFO-FDA (888-463-6332)

Web site: www.fda.gov

Information about cellular telephones can be found at: http://www.fda.gov/cellphones.

World Health Organization

Monograph No. 238, and Fact Sheet No. 322, available at http://www.who.int/peh-emf/en

References

1. Feychting M, Ahlbom A, Kheifets L. EMF and health. *Annu Rev Public Health*. 2005;26: 165-189
2. EMF RAPID Program. Electric and Magnetic Fields. Research Triangle Park, NC: National Institute of Environmental Health Sciences, National Institutes of Health; 2002. Available at: http://www.niehs.nih.gov/emfrapid/booklet/home.htm. Accessed August 19, 2010
3. Kheifets L, Repacholi M, Saunders R, van Deventer E. The sensitivity of children to electromagnetic fields. *Pediatrics*. 2005;116(2):e303-e313
4. Friedman DR, Hatch EE, Tarone R. Childhood exposure to magnetic fields: residential area measurements compared to personal dosimetry. *Epidemiology*. 1996;7(2):151-155
5. Zaffanella L. *Survey of Residential Magnetic Field Sources: Volumes 1 and 2*. Palo Alto, CA: Electric Power Research Institute; 1993. Available at: http://my.epri.com/portal/server.pt?space =CommunityPage&cached=true&parentname=ObjMgr&parentid=2&control=SetCommunity &CommunityID=404&RaiseDocID=TR-102759-V1&RaiseDocType=Abstract_id. Accessed August 19, 2010
6. World Health Organization. Electromagnetic fields (300 Hz to 300 GHz). Geneva, Switzerland: World Health Organization; 1993. Environmental Health Criteria No. 137
7. Cleveland RF Jr, Ulcek JL. *Questions and Answers About Biological Effects and Potential Hazards of Radiofrequency Electromagnetic Fields*. 4th ed. Washington, DC: Federal Communications Commission; 1999. OET Bulletin No. 56
8. International Commission on Non-Ionizing Radiation Protection. ICNIRP statement on EMF-emitting new technologies. *Health Phys*. 2008;94(4):376-392
9. Dimbylow PJ, Mann SM. SAR calculations in an anatomically realistic model of the head for mobile communication transceivers at 900 MHz and 1.8 GHz. *Phys Med Biol*. 1994;39(10):1537-1553
10. American Physical Society. APS council adopts statement on EMFs and public health. *APS News Online*. 1995;4(7). Reaffirmed 2008. Available at: http://www.aps.org/publications/apsnews/199507/council.cfm. Accessed August 19, 2010
11. Moulder JE. The electric and magnetic fields research and public information dissemination (EMF-RAPID) program. *Radiat Res*. 2000;153(5 Pt 2):613-616

12. International Agency for Research on Cancer. *IARC Monographs on the Evaluation of Carcinogenic Risks to Humans. Volume 80. Non-Ionizing Radiation, Part 1: Static and Extremely Low-Frequency (ELF) Electric and Magnetic Fields*. Lyon, France: International Agency for Research on Cancer; 2002

13. Schuz J. Implications from epidemiologic studies on magnetic fields and the risk of childhood leukemia on protection guidelines. *Health Phys*. 2007;92(6):642-648

14. Tynes T, Andersen A. Electromagnetic fields and male breast cancer. *Lancet*. 1990;336(8730):1596

15. Matanoski GM, Breysse PN, Elliott EA. Electromagnetic field exposure and male breast cancer. *Lancet*. 1991;337(8743):737

16. Kheifets LI, Afifi AA, Buffler PA, Zhang ZW, Matkin CC. Occupational electric and magnetic field exposure and leukemia. A meta-analysis. *J Occup Environ Med*. 1997;39(11):1074-1091

17. Kheifets LI, Afifi AA, Buffler PA, Zhang ZW. Occupational electric and magnetic field exposure and brain cancer: a meta-analysis. *J Occup Environ Med*. 1995;37(12):1327-1341

18. Ahlbom IC, Cardis E, Green A, Linet M, Savitz D, Swerdlow A. Review of the epidemiologic literature on EMF and health. *Environ Health Perspect*. 2001;109(Suppl 6):911-933

19. Greenland S, Sheppard AR, Kaune WT, Poole C, Kelsh MA. A pooled analysis of magnetic fields, wire codes, and childhood leukemia. Childhood Leukemia-EMF Study Group. *Epidemiology*. 2000;11(6):624-634

20. Kheifets L, Shimkhada R. Childhood leukemia and EMF: review of the epidemiologic evidence. *Bioelectromagnetics*. 2005;(Suppl 7):S51-S59

21. Kheifets LI. Electric and magnetic field exposure and brain cancer: a review. *Bioelectromagnetics*. 2001;(Suppl 5):S120-S131

22. Elwood JM. A critical review of epidemiologic studies of radiofrequency exposure and human cancers. *Environ Health Perspect*. 1999;107(Suppl 1):155-168

23. Frumkin H, Jacobson A, Gansler T, Thun MJ. Cellular phones and risk of brain tumors. *CA Cancer J Clin*. 2001;51(2):137-141

24. Schuz J, Jacobsen R, Olsen JH, Boice JD Jr, McLaughlin JK, Johansen C. Cellular telephone use and cancer risk: update of a nationwide Danish cohort. *J Natl Cancer Inst*. 2006;98(23): 1707-1713

25. Divan HA, Kheifets L, Obel C, Olsen J. Prenatal and postnatal exposure to cell phone use and behavioral problems in children. *Epidemiology*. 2008;19(4):523-529

26. INTERPHONE Study Group. Brain tumour risk in relation to mobile telephone use: results of the INTERPHONE international case-control study. *Int J Epidemiol*. 2010;39(3): 675-694

27. International Agency for Research on Cancer. IARC classifies radiofrequency electromagnetic fields as possibly carcinogenic to humans [press release]. Lyon, France: International Agency for Research on Cancer; May 31, 2011. Available at: http://www.iarc.fr/en/media-centre/pr/2011/pdfs/pr208_E.pdf. Accessed July 14, 2011

28. Brainard GC, Kavet R, Kheifets LI. The relationship between electromagnetic field and light exposures to melatonin and breast cancer risk: a review of the relevant literature. *J Pineal Res*. 1999;26(2):65-100

29. Davis S, Mirick DK, Stevens RG. Residential magnetic fields and the risk of breast cancer. *Am J Epidemiol*. 2002;155(5):446-454

30. Vijayalaxmi, Obe G. Controversial cytogenetic observations in mammalian somatic cells exposed to extremely low frequency electromagnetic radiation: a review and future research recommendations. *Bioelectromagnetics*. 2005;26(5):412-430

31. Repacholi MH, Basten A, Gebski V, Noonan D, Finnie J, Harris AW. Lymphomas in E mu-Pim1 transgenic mice exposed to pulsed 900 MHZ electromagnetic fields. *Radiat Res.* 1997;147(5):631-640

32. Brusick D, Albertini R, McRee D. Genotoxicity of radiofrequency radiation. DNA/Genetox Expert Panel. *Environ Mol Mutagen.* 1998;32(1):1-16

33. Repacholi MH. Health risks from the use of mobile phones. *Toxicol Lett.* 2001;120(1-3): 323-331

34. Independent Expert Group on Mobile Phones. *Mobile Phones and Health.* Available at: http://www.iegmp.org.uk/report/text.htm. Accessed August 19, 2010

35. Divan HA, Kheifets L, Obel C, Olsen J. Cell phone use and behavioural problems in young children. *J Epidemiol Community Health.* Epub ahead of print December 7, 2010

36. Divan HA, Kheifets L, Olsen J. Prenatal cell phone use and developmental milestone delays among infants. *Scand J Work Environ Health.* Epub ahead of print March 14, 2011. doi: 10.5271/sjweh.3157

Chapter 28

Endocrine Disrupters

■ ■ ■ ■ ■ ■

Endocrine disrupters are exogenous synthetic or natural chemicals that can mimic or modify the action of endogenous hormones. Although initially applied to substances with estrogenic effects, the term has widened to include those that interfere with thyroid hormone, insulin, and androgen activity and complex processes involving multiple hormones, such as pubertal growth and development.

The idea that pesticides could interfere with endocrine processes in vertebrates goes back to the observation that dichlorodiphenyltrichloroethane (DDT) decreased the hatchability of the eggs of pelagic birds (those that live in the open sea rather than in coastal or inland waters).[1] DDT and other pesticides, such as methoxychlor and chlordecone,[2] as well as industrial chemicals, such as specific polychlorinated biphenyls (PCBs), can act as estrogens in laboratory assays.

In addition to the synthetic chemicals, phytoestrogens in plants can occur at sufficiently high concentrations to be active as estrogens in animals consuming them (see Chapter 16).

ROUTES OF EXPOSURE

The primary route of exposure is ingestion, including through breastfeeding; the fetus may be exposed transplacentally.

SYSTEMS AFFECTED AND CLINICAL EFFECTS

A wide variety of chemicals have estrogenic activity in some biological system. The most widely used test system is a yeast with a human estrogen receptor and a reporter gene. If the chemical being tested occupies and activates the receptor, then the reporter gene product, usually a phosphorescent protein, is synthesized and can be easily measured. Similar assays exist for other kinds of hormonal activity. Other hormone actions have been reported for environmental chemicals. One form of DDT is an anti-androgen,[3] some pesticides and congeners of PCBs can occupy thyroid hormone receptors,[4] and other agents produce symptoms (such as infertility in workers in contact with chlordecone and dibromochloropropane) that are plausibly the result of interference with normal endocrine function, even if a hormonal basis has yet to be established.

Secular trends in sperm counts (reviewed recently[5]); rates of testicular cancer,[6] undescended testicles,[7] and hypospadias[8]; and the decreased ratio of male to female births in the general population[9] have been attributed to synthetic environmental agents. Although DDT has been studied and does not appear to produce hypospadias or undescended testicles in children[10] or breast cancer in adults,[11] few studies are available in which the specific outcome and the responsible chemical have been measured in the same individuals or groups; thus, these associations in general are not well supported (see Rogan and Ragan[12] for a review). Table 28.1 shows pediatric studies of plausible endocrine outcomes in which an environmental chemical has been measured or in which exposure can be reasonably inferred.

In the United States (North Carolina), at background exposures to PCBs and dichlorodiphenyldichloroethylene (DDE), the higher the prenatal exposure to DDE, the taller and heavier boys were at 14 years of age.[13] There was no effect on the ages at which pubertal stages were attained. Postnatal (ie, lactational) exposures to DDE had no apparent effects; neither did exposure to PCBs. This large effect of DDE was not confirmed in another prospective study of 304 adolescent boys.[14] Girls with the highest transplacental PCB exposures were 5.4 kg heavier for their height than were other girls by 14 years of age, but the difference was significant only if the analysis was restricted to white subjects. Although there was some evidence that the girls with the highest PCB exposure reached the early stages of puberty sooner, the numbers were small, and age at menarche seemed unaffected.[13] Neither of these findings have been replicated.

Several other agents, including lead and phthalate plasticizers, have been studied for effects on puberty.[12] Higher blood lead concentrations have been associated with later puberty in several studies, but this effect is consistent with a decrease in blood lead caused by increased bone mass in puberty. Phthalate plasticizers were much higher in the blood of girls with premature thelarche in Puerto Rico,[15] but no confirmation of this strong effect has been reported. Maternal exposure to phthalates was associated with shorter anogenital index in male children in one study (see Chapter 38).[16] Anogenital distance is a sexually dimorphic trait commonly used in rodent experiments to evaluate androgen antagonists. A Danish study of boys with cryptorchidism measured endogenous sex hormones in breastfed male infants at 3 months as well as phthalates in their mothers' milk. Although there was no difference in phthalate exposure between

Table 28.1: Listing of Pediatric Studies

CHEMICAL	OUTCOME	AGE/ROUTE OF EXPOSURE	SELECTED STUDIES
Polychlorinated biphenyls	Increased weight in adolescent females and/or early puberty	Prenatal	Inconsistent results from multiple studies[13,34,35]
	Changes in thyroid economy	Mostly prenatal	Inconsistent results from multiple studies[36]
Dichlorodiphenyl-trichloroethane (DDT)	Increased weight in adolescent males; no effect on pubertal development	Prenatal	Present in one study,[13] not in another[14]
	Decreased duration of lactation	Maternal exposure to food supply in United States and Mexico	Inconsistent results from multiple studies[23,26,37]
Polychlorinated biphenyls/ polychlorinated dibenzofurans at high dose	Decreased penis size at adolescence	Prenatal-maternal poisoning from contaminated cooking oil	Prospective study, 25 males, 104 females[38]
	Decreased height in adolescent females		
	Decreased sperm motility		Prospective study, 12 exposed males[28]
Dioxin (TCDD) or polychlorinated dibenzofurans at high dose	Decrease in number of male births	Preconception, to the father, from an industrial explosion	Historical cohort— 239 males, 298 female parents with 328 males, 346 female children[29] Retrospective study, 50 male, 81 female children[30]
Soy isoflavones	Altered cholesterol metabolism in infants	Infant formula	Clinical trial, 7 infants[39]
	Minor menstrual irregularities in 20- to 34-year-olds		Follow-up of a clinical trial, 128 females[33]
Polybrominated biphenyls	Early menarche	Prenatal	Survey of 327 5- to 24- year-old female offspring of participants in an exposure registry[40]

continued on page 406

continued from page 405

Table 28.1: Listing of Pediatric Studies, *continued*			
CHEMICAL	**OUTCOME**	**AGE/ROUTE OF EXPOSURE**	**SELECTED STUDIES**
Phthalate esters	Early thelarche	Concurrent body burden	Case-control study with 41 cases[15]
	Decreased anogenital index	Maternal exposure	Cross sectional study of 134 male infants[16]
	Decreased sex hormones in 3-month-old males	Breastfeeding	Case control study of cryptorchidism with 62 cases[17]

the boys with cryptorchism and controls, boys whose mothers had higher concentrations of certain phthalates in milk had lower serum concentrations of testosterone and higher luteinizing hormone concentrations.[17]

In 2 studies of background exposure to PCBs and child development, hypotonia at birth was related to prenatal exposure to PCBs[18] or to a history of consuming PCB-contaminated fish.[19] The finding of hypotonia suggested an effect on thyroid hormone. PCBs were known to be toxic to the developing thyroid gland.[20] Subsequently, hypotonia was shown to be accompanied by higher thyroid-stimulating hormone concentrations in one study,[21] and now there are comparable data from multiple studies (reviewed by Hagmar[22]). In general, associations among a variety of measures of thyroid hormone status have been weak, inconsistent, or absent. The hypothesis has a very reasonable basis in laboratory evidence, however, and is probably worth further innovative study.

An estrogen-like effect of DDE (ie, shortened duration of lactation) was seen in 2 studies, one in North Carolina and the other in Mexico.[23] Although a similar effect was seen among Michigan women,[24] a study in upstate New York[25] and another Mexican study[26] showed no association between DDE and weaning.

In Taiwan, adolescent males who had been exposed in utero to high levels of PCBs and polychlorinated dibenzofurans when their mothers were poisoned (see Chapter 35) had normal progression through the Tanner stages but smaller penises than a comparison group. Puberty in girls was unaffected.[27] This is a complicated effect, not obviously an estrogenic one, and its mechanism is unknown. In a different study of the same cohort, the prenatally exposed adolescents had decreased sperm motility compared with a comparison group.[28]

There was a clear excess of female births in the Seveso region of Italy, where an explosion had released large quantities of 2,3,7,8-tetrachlorodibenzo-*p*-dioxin (TCDD), a toxic halogenated hydrocarbon, but the effect was seen only when the father was exposed.[29] A similar deficiency in male births was seen in a

Taiwanese study of people with high exposures to PCBs and polychlorinated dibenzofurans, but again, only when the father was exposed.[30] This finding was without laboratory confirmation until recently, when a Japanese group was able to produce it in TCDD-exposed mice.[31] Males exposed to TCDD in Seveso had changes in sperm counts and motility; the effects were different depending on when exposure had taken place, and the clinical significance is not yet known.[32]

Soybeans and, thus, soy-based infant formula, contain estrogenic isoflavones. Soy formula is discussed in detail in Chapter 16. The only follow-up study available is one of 128 women fed soy formula as infants who filled out a mailed questionnaire at 20 to 34 years old; the only differences plausibly related to estrogenicity of their formula are longer duration of menstrual bleeding and more pain with their menstrual periods.[33] This study is useful but small, and more work is needed in this area.

What role, if any, environmental chemicals have in morbidity attributable to endocrine disruption remains unclear. Many studies of endometriosis, testicular cancer, puberty, neonatal estrogenization, and other plausible end points are underway. Currently, however, endocrine disruption of humans by environmental pollution still is mainly extrapolation of laboratory evidence. Although there are now many more studies of children and the area is under active investigation, few findings have been replicated in multiple studies, and new findings from any one study have to be regarded as provisional.

REGULATION

The Food Quality Protection Act of 1996 requires testing chemicals that will be released into the environment for their potential to be endocrine disrupters, and the US Environmental Protection Agency (EPA) is now designing a testing protocol. Progress toward implementation can be checked at the EPA Endocrine Disrupter Web site (http://www.epa.gov/endo). Most likely, such testing would serve to select agents for more intense study. It would not replace more traditional tests for general toxicity and carcinogenicity.

Frequently Asked Questions

Q   *Could my child's undescended testicle or hypospadias be due to my exposure to a pollutant chemical during pregnancy?*

A   No controlled studies show such associations. Some evidence exists that these conditions have been increasing, but even if they are increasing, the cause of such an increase is unclear.

Q   *My daughter started her menstrual period when she was 10 years old. Could this be because of chemical exposure?*

A   Since about 1840, menarche has been starting earlier among white, northern European girls, perhaps due to better nutrition. There has been no abrupt change in age at menarche in the United States recently, although the standards have been changed to reflect the inclusion of black girls and their generally younger age at menarche. An expert panel's recent opinion is that that puberty is occurring earlier in girls, but there is, as yet, insufficient evidence that it is earlier in boys. Increasing obesity clearly plays a role in earlier maturation, but whether environmental chemicals are an important cause is not yet known.[41]

Q *If a chemical like bisphenol A is an endocrine disrupter in laboratory tests, why is it still allowed in packaging?*

A Carcinogens are the only toxicologically defined class of compounds with zero tolerance. The Delaney clause, first introduced into the Food and Drug Amendments of 1958, required zero tolerance for any food additives shown to be human or animal carcinogens at any dose. There is no such legislation requiring a zero-dose standard for endocrine disrupters. They are, therefore, regulated like any other potential toxicant, through some form of weight-of-evidence approach. This approach considers all data available and may not result in a ban of a substance because it has endocrine activity in some test system. In the case of bisphenol A, the laboratory findings are complex and, to some degree, controversial. Although there are data showing that humans are exposed, there are none showing unequivocal toxicity. Even though there is uncertainty, Canada recently banned baby bottles made of plastics containing bisphenol A.

References

1. Fry DM. Reproductive effects in birds exposed to pesticides and industrial chemicals. *Environ Health Perspect*. 1995;103(Suppl 7):165-171

2. Boylan JJ, Egle JL, Guzelian PS. Cholestyramine: use as a new therapeutic approach for chlordecone (kepone) poisoning. *Science*. 1978;199(4331):893-895

3. Kelce WR, Stone CR, Laws SC, Gray LE, Kemppainen JA, Wilson EM. Persistent DDT metabolite p,p-DDE is a potent androgen receptor antagonist. *Nature*. 1995;375(6532):581-584

4. Rickenbacher U, McKinney JD, Oatley SJ, Blake CC. Structurally specific binding of halogenated biphenyls to thyroxine transport proteins. *J Med Chem*. 1986;29(3):641-648

5. Hauser R. The environment and male fertility: recent research on emerging chemicals and semen quality. *Semin Reprod Med*. 2006;24(3):156-167

6. Liu S, Semenciw R, Waters C, Wen SW, Mery LS, Mao Y. Clues to the aetiological heterogeneity of testicular seminomas and non-seminomas: time trends and age-period-cohort effects. *Int J Epidemiol*. 2000;29(5):826-831

7. James WH. Secular trends in monitors of reproductive hazard. *Hum Reprod*. 1997;12(3):417-421

8. Paulozzi LJ, Erickson JD, Jackson RJ. Hypospadias trends in two US surveillance systems. *Pediatrics*. 1997;100(5):831-834

9. Davis DL, Gottlieb MB, Stampnitzky JR. Reduced ratio of male to female births in several industrial countries: a sentinel health indicator? *JAMA*. 1998;279(13):1018-1023

10. Longnecker MP, Klebanoff M, Brock JW, et al. Maternal serum level of 1,1-dichloro-2, 2-bis(p-chlorophenyl)ethylene and risk of cryptorchidism, hypospadias, and polythelia among male offspring. *Am J Epidemiol*. 2002;155(4):313-322

11. Laden F, Collman GW, Iwamoto K, et al. 1,1-Dichloro-2,2-bis(p-chlorophenyl)ethylene and polychlorinated biphenyls and breast cancer: combined analysis of five U.S. studies. *JNCI.* 2001;93(10):768-775

12. Rogan WJ, Ragan NB. Some evidence of effects of environmental chemical on the endocrine system in children. *Int J Hyg Environ Health.* 2007;210(5):659-667

13. Gladen BC, Ragan NB, Rogan WJ. Pubertal growth and development and prenatal and lactational exposure to polychlorinated biphenyls and dichlorodiphenyl dichloroethene. *J Pediatr.* 2000;136(4):490-496

14. Gladen BC, Klebanoff M, Hediger ML, Katz SH, Barr DB, Davis MD, et al. Prenatal DDT exposure in relation to anthropometric and pubertal measures in adolescent males. *Environ Health Perspect.* 2004;112(17):1761-1767

15. Colón I, Caro D, Bourdony CJ, Rosario O. Identification of phthalate esters in the serum of young Puerto Rican girls with premature breast development. *Environ Health Perspect.* 2000;108(9):895-900

16. Swan S, Main KM, Liu F, Stewart SL, Kruse RL, Calafat AM, et al. Decrease in anogenital distance among male infants with prenatal phthalate exposure. *Environ Health Perspect.* 2005;113(8):1056-1061

17. Main KM, Mortensen GK, Kaleva MM, Boisen KA, Damgaard IN, Chellakooty M, et al. Human breast milk contamination with phthalates and alterations of endogenous reproductive hormones in infants three months of age. *Environ Health Perspect.* 2006;114(2):270-276

18. Rogan WJ, Gladen BC, McKinney JD, Carreras N, Hardy P, Thullen JD, et al. Neonatal effects of transplacental exposure to PCBs and DDE. *J Pediatr.* 1986;109(2):335-341

19. Jacobson JL, Jacobson SW, Fein GG, Schwartz PM, Dowler JK. Prenatal exposure to an environmental toxin: a test of the multiple effects model. *Dev Psychol.* 1984;20:523-532

20. Collins WT, Capen CC. Fine structural lesions and hormonal alterations in thyroid glands of perinatal rats exposed *in utero* and by the milk to polychlorinated biphenyls. *Am J Pathol.* 1980;99(1):125-142

21. Koopman-Esseboom C, Morse DC, Weisglas-Kuperus N, Lutkeschipholt IJ, Van der Paauw CG, Tuinstra LG, et al. Effects of dioxins and polychlorinated biphenyls on thyroid hormone status of pregnant women and their infants. *Pediatr Res.* 1994;36(4):468-473

22. Hagmar L. Polychlorinated biphenyls and thyroid status in humans: a review. *Thyroid.* 2003;13(11):1021-1028

23. Gladen BC, Rogan WJ. DDE and shortened duration of lactation in a Northern Mexican town. *Am J Public Health.* 1995;85(4):504-508

24. Karmaus W, Davis S, Fussman C, Brooks K. Maternal concentration of dichlordiphenyl dichloroethylene (DDE) and initiation and duration of breast feeding. *Paediatr Perinat Epidemiol.* 2005;19(5):388-398

25. McGuiness B, Vena JE, Buck GM, et al. The effects of DDE on the duration of lactation among women in the New York State Angler Cohort. *Epidemiology.* 1999;10:359

26. Cupul-Uicab LA, Gladen BC, Hernandez-Avila M, Weber JP, Longnecker MP. DDE, a degradation product of DDT, and duration of lactation in a highly exposed area of Mexico. *Environ Health Perspect.* 2008;116(2):179-183

27. Chen YC, Guo YL, Yu ML, Lai TJ, Hsu CC. Physical and cognitive development of Yu-Cheng children born after year 1985. In: Fiedler H, Frank H, Hutzinger O, Parzefall W, Riss A, Safe S, eds. *Organohalogen Compounds.* 14th ed. Vienna, Austria: Federal Environmental Agency; 1993:261-262

28. Guo YL, Hsu PC, Hsu CC, Lambert GH. Semen quality after exposure to polychlorinated biphenyls and dibenzofurans. *Lancet.* 2000;356(9237):1240-1241

29. Mocarelli P, Gerthoux PM, Ferrari E, et al. Paternal concentration of dioxin and sex ratio of offspring. *Lancet.* 2000;355(9218):1858-1863

30. Gomez I, Marshall T, Tsai P, Shao YS, Guo YL. Number of boys born to men exposed to polychlorinated biphenyls. *Lancet.* 2002;360(9327):143-144

31. Ishihara K, Warita K, Tanida T, Sugawara T, Kitagawa H, Hoshi N. Does paternal exposure to 2,3,7,8-tetrachlorodibenzo-p-dioxin (TCDD) affect the sex ratio of offspring? *J Vet Med Sci.* 2007;69(4):347-352

32. Mocarelli P, Gerthoux PM, Patterson DG, et al. Dioxin exposure, from infancy through puberty, produces endocrine disruption and affects human semen quality. *Environ Health Perspect.* 2008;116(1):70-77

33. Strom BL, Schinnar R, Ziegler EE, et al. Exposure to soy-based formula in infancy and endocrinological and reproductive outcomes in young adulthood. *JAMA.* 2001;286(7):807-814

34. Vasiliu O, Muttineni J, Karmaus W. In utero exposure to organochlorines and age at menarche. *Hum Reprod.* 2004;19(7):1506-1512

35. Denham M, Schell L, Deane G, Gallo MV, Ravenscroft J, DeCaprio AP. Relationship of lead, mercury, mirex, dichlorodiphenyldichloroethylene, hexachlorobenzene, and polychlorinated biphenyls to timing of menarche among Akwesasne Mohawk girls. *Pediatrics.* 2005;115(2):e127-e134

36. Brouwer A, Longnecker M, Birnbaum L, et al. Characterization of potential endocrine-related health effects at low-dose levels of exposure to PCBs. *Environ Health Perspect.* 1999; 107(Suppl 4):639-649

37. Rogan WJ, Gladen BC, McKinney JD, et al. Polychlorinated biphenyls (PCBs) and dichlorodiphenyl dichloroethene (DDE) in human milk: effects on growth, morbidity, and duration of lactation. *Am J Public Health.* 1987;77(10):1294-1297

38. Guo YL, Lai TJ, Ju SH, Chen YC, Hsu CC. Sexual developments and biological findings in Yucheng children. In: Fiedler H, Frank H, Hutzinger O, Parzefall W, Riss A, Safe S, eds. *Organohalogen Compounds.* 14th ed. Vienna, Austria: Federal Environmental Agency; 1993: 235-238

39. Cruz ML, Wong WW, Mimouni F, Hachey DL, Setchell KD, Klein PD, et al. Effects of infant nutrition on cholesterol synthesis. *Pediatr Res.* 1994;35(2):135-140

40. Blanck HM, Marcus M, Tolbert PE, et al. Age at menarche and tanner stage in girls exposed in utero and postnatally to polybrominated biphenyl. *Epidemiology.* 2000;11(6):641-647

41. Golub MS, Collman GW, Foster PMD, et al. Public health implications of altered puberty timing. *Pediatrics.* 2008;121(Suppl 3):S218-S230

Chapter 29

Gasoline and Its Additives

■ ■ ■ ■ ■ ■

Gasoline is a complex mixture of volatile hydrocarbons derived by distillation from crude petroleum. Gasoline contains as many as 1000 different chemical substances,[1] including alkanes, alkenes, and aromatics. The composition of gasoline varies depending on the source of crude oil, refining process, geographic region, season of the year, and performance requirements (octane rating). More than 170 billion gallons of gasoline were consumed in the United States in 2005 (a 25% increase over 10 years).[2] In 2006, the United States accounted for approximately 43% of gasoline consumption worldwide.[3] Gasoline combustion is an important contributor to ambient air pollution and global climate change.[4] Gasoline frequently contaminates drinking water in the United States.[5] This chapter reviews the health effects of gasoline and its additives. The hazards associated with exposure to automotive exhaust, including diesel exhaust, are considered in Chapter 21.

Toxic and carcinogenic constituents of gasoline include benzene, 1,3-butadiene, 1,2-dibromoethane, toluene, ethyl benzene, antiknock agents, and oxygenates.[1] Benzene, a polycyclic aromatic hydrocarbon that causes leukemia and probably causes multiple myeloma,[6-8] constitutes up to 4% of gasoline by weight, except in Alaska, where it is 5% of gasoline by weight.[6]

Tetraethyl lead was the principal antiknock agent used in gasoline in the United States until it was phased out between 1976 and 1990, resulting in a 90% reduction in children's blood lead concentrations.[9] Tetraethyl lead is used in gasoline in an ever-decreasing number of nations. As of 2010, the United Nations Environmental Programme (UNEP) reported that only 9 nations were still using leaded gasoline.[10] Average blood lead concentrations among children in nations that use leaded gasoline are 10 to 15 μg/dL higher than those in US children.[11] Further discussion of these issues is found in Chapter 31.

Methylcyclopentadienyl manganese tricarbonyl (MMT) has been proposed as a replacement for tetraethyl lead as an antiknock agent.[12] Occupational exposure to manganese is a known cause of parkinsonism.[13] Available data suggest that community exposures to manganese resulting from combustion of MMT in gasoline may be associated with subclinical neurologic impairment.[13-15] A further discussion of MMT and manganese can be found in Chapter 24.

Oxygenates are added to gasoline, especially in the winter months, to reduce carbon monoxide emissions.[16,17] Methyl tertiary butyl ether (MTBE) was the oxygenate that was most widely used in the United States and was added to gasoline at concentrations up to 15% by volume.[18] Combustion of MTBE produces acrid emissions, including formaldehyde, and has been linked to respiratory irritation and asthma attacks in children.[16,19] It has leaked into groundwater in many areas of the United States and is one of the most frequently detected volatile organic compounds (VOCs) found in drinking water sources in the United States.[5] At concentrations as low as 20 parts per billion (ppb), MTBE can create an unpleasant taste that can render water undrinkable. In California, a maximum contaminant level of 5 parts per billion was set for MTBE in drinking water based on taste and odor.[20] MTBE was not subjected to toxicologic testing before its commercial introduction.[21] It subsequently has been shown in experimental animal studies to cause lymphatic tumors and testicular cancer.[22] In 1999, in view of these findings, the governor of California issued the first state order in the United States to completely phase out MTBE from gasoline by December 31, 2002.[23] As of 2009, 25 states mandated a complete or partial MTBE ban.[24]

Ethanol also is used as an oxygenate in the United States and is added at concentrations of up to 10% by volume. People are briefly exposed to low levels of known carcinogens and other potentially toxic compounds while pumping gasoline, regardless of whether the gasoline is oxygenated.[25,26]

ROUTES AND SOURCES OF EXPOSURE

Inhalation

Children can inhale volatile gasoline vapors at service stations, along highways, and in communities near petroleum-processing and gasoline-transfer facilities. Children can inhale gasoline engine exhaust. Engine exhaust includes uncombusted gasoline and toxic gasoline combustion products, such as polyaromatic hydrocarbons.[27] If tetraethyl lead or MMT have been added to gasoline, exhaust will contain lead or manganese. Exposure to components of gasoline exhaust, such as carbon monoxide, oxides of nitrogen, and respirable particulates can cause health problems. These issues are considered in detail in Chapters 21 and Chapter 25. Children can be exposed acutely to high doses of gasoline vapor through intentional gasoline "sniffing," a form of inhalant abuse.[28,29]

Dermal Absorption

Gasoline is lipophilic and can be absorbed through the skin.

Ingestion

Children can inadvertently ingest gasoline. A common scenario is that a child swallows gasoline that has been stored in a container usually containing a food or beverage, such as a soda bottle. Severe toxicity can result. Children can be exposed to certain components of gasoline, such as MTBE and benzene, through consumption of contaminated water and through showering. Large ingestions are uncommon in toddlers but may be seen in adolescents. In the 1970s, the practice of gasoline siphoning from parked cars was commonplace and was a potential source of exposure among teenagers. Gasoline is poorly absorbed via the gastrointestinal tract, so toxicity is typically mild if aspiration does not occur.

SYSTEMS AFFECTED

Ingestion of large amounts of gasoline can result in any or all of 3 acute systemic syndromes: (1) pneumonitis; (2) central nervous system (CNS) toxicity; or (3) visceral involvement, which may include hepatotoxicity, cardiomyopathy, renal toxicity, or hepatosplenomegaly.[30] The widespread contamination of drinking water supplies with low concentrations of gasoline and its additives, such as MTBE, raises concern about the potential health effects of chronic low-level exposure. Chronic exposure to gasoline and certain components, such as benzene, may be carcinogenic at high levels of exposure. There are no data in humans about the carcinogenicity of MTBE in drinking water or from chronic environmental exposure to MBTE in gasoline.

Lungs

Ingestion of liquid gasoline is followed by chemical pneumonitis.[31,32] Aspiration seems to be the principal route of pulmonary exposure, and therefore, vomiting should not be induced following gasoline ingestion, except in special circumstances (see Treatment). Symptoms of dyspnea, gagging, and fever may appear within 30 minutes of exposure, but symptoms can be delayed up to 4 hours. Cyanosis appears in 2% to 3% of patients. Symptoms typically worsen over 48 to 72 hours after ingestion but then resolve in 5 days to 1 week. Death occurs in fewer than 2% of cases.

Pathologic changes in the lungs in gasoline pneumonitis include interstitial inflammation, edema, and intra-alveolar hemorrhage. The pathophysiology is incompletely understood but probably involves direct injury to pulmonary tissue as well as disruption of the surfactant layer.[32] Radiographic changes include increased perihilar markings, basilar infiltrates, and consolidation; these changes appear in 50% to 90% of patients. Radiographs, which may be normal initially, do not correlate well with severity of clinical symptoms or with the clinical examination. Radiographic changes can persist for many weeks after resolution of symptoms. Long-term follow-up of survivors shows occasional cases of bronchiectasis and pulmonary fibrosis and a high prevalence (82%) of asymptomatic minor abnormalities on pulmonary function tests.[33]

Central Nervous System

The lipophilic nature of gasoline allows it to cross the blood-brain barrier; however, gasoline is poorly absorbed from the gastrointestinal tract, so ingestion does not typically lead to CNS symptoms. Acute inhalational exposure to gasoline vapors in high concentrations is narcotic and can produce dizziness, excitement, anesthesia, and loss of consciousness.[34] Seizures and coma are reported in a small percentage of cases. Dementia and brainstem dysfunction have been documented.

Cardiovascular System

Sudden sniffing death syndrome, resulting from arrhythmias or cardiac dysfunction can follow exposure to high concentrations of gasoline vapors for periods as brief as 5 minutes.[29] It is the leading cause of fatality related to inhalant abuse. Cardiomyopathy can occur after chronic gasoline sniffing but is uncommon.

Liver

High-dose exposure can cause hepatocellular damage and hepatosplenomegaly.[6,20]

Kidneys

High-dose exposure can cause renal tubular injury.[6,20]

Carcinogenicity

Chronic occupational exposure to gasoline seems to be associated with renal cell carcinoma and nasal cancer.[1,35] This may be an important public health concern, given the widespread exposure to gasoline vapors in retail service stations and rising rates of kidney cancer in the United States. An association between gasoline exposure and kidney cancer also is seen in animal studies.[1,36] Several components of gasoline are proven or probable carcinogens (Table 29.1).

It is important to note the inherent limitations of epidemiologic studies examining the human carcinogenicity of gasoline and its components. These limitations include (1) the absence of complete information on past exposure levels to gasoline vapor or on concurrent exposures to other substances such as gasoline or diesel engine exhaust; (2) the constantly changing composition of gasoline; and (3) the long latency period, frequently many years, between exposure to a constituent of gasoline and the subsequent appearance of disease.

Table 29.1: Carcinogens in Gasoline		
CHEMICAL	ASSOCIATED CANCERS	CERTAINTY OF CAUSAL ASSOCIATION
Benzene	Leukemia, multiple myeloma	Leukemia proven, myeloma probable[7,8]
1,3-Butadiene	Lymphoma, leukemia, myeloid metaplasia	Probable[37]
MTBE	Testicular, lymphatic cancers	Strongly positive in animal studies[22]; no data in humans

For these reasons, epidemiologic studies tend to underestimate the strength of associations between toxic exposures and disease. Toxicologic studies in experimental animals can complement epidemiologic investigations, just as epidemiologic studies complement experimental animal studies.

DIAGNOSIS

Acute, high-dose exposure to gasoline is diagnosed by history and by detecting the odor of gasoline on exhaled breath. Although MTBE and its breakdown product, butyl alcohol, can be measured in exhaled air, blood, and urine, the availability and clinical utility of these measures currently are limited. Benzene can be measured in exhaled air and blood. Certain metabolites of benzene, such as phenol, can be measured in urine. However, this test is not a quantitative indicator of the level of benzene exposure, because phenol is present in urine from other sources, such as diet.[38] The tests for the metabolites of MTBE and benzene are most appropriately used in the context of epidemiologic studies and are generally not available in clinical settings. Diagnosis is typically made via history of exposure.

Assessment of levels of exposure to gasoline and its constituents in community air or in groundwater requires expert air or water sampling by a certified environmental scientist or government agency, such as a state or county health department or department of environmental protection. An important source of data on community exposures is the US Environmental Protection Agency (EPA)'s Toxic Release Inventory (www.scorecard.org).

TREATMENT

Treatment of chemical pneumonitis caused by acute high-dose exposure to gasoline begins with clinical assessment of the severity of illness and evaluation of the amount of gasoline ingested. Many children who ingest a small amount of gasoline never become symptomatic. When such children present for medical evaluation, observation for 4 hours after ingestion can identify those who can safely discharged. Because most cases involve only small amounts of gasoline, outpatient evaluation with close follow-up (depending on the reliability of the family) is usually sufficient if the child is asymptomatic 4 hours after ingestion. Children who are even mildly symptomatic (ie, with coughing, tachypnea, wheezing, or hypoxia) should be admitted for observation because of risk of disease progression. More severe cases require hospital admission, possibly to the pediatric intensive care unit.

Whether to use gastric emptying was the subject of long-standing debate. At present, gastric emptying via ipecac or gastric lavage is contraindicated because of the danger of aspiration.[32,39] Steroids offer little benefit in gasoline pneumonitis. Antibiotics are indicated if bacterial superinfection develops. Debate about whether prophylactic antibiotics are warranted is long-standing and unresolved.

In the most severe cases with advanced respiratory distress, mechanical ventilation may be required. Positive end-expiratory pressure (PEEP) ventilation has been used, as well as high-frequency jet ventilation using very high respiratory rates (220–260 breaths/min). Extracorporeal membrane oxygenation has been used when other options have failed.[32]

PREVENTION OF EXPOSURE

Exposure of children and adolescents to gasoline and its vapors should be minimized to prevent occurrence of delayed health consequences, especially cancer. Young children should not pump gasoline or work in retail service stations.

Gasoline should never be stored in a bottle or other container that normally contains a food or beverage and is accessible and attractive to young children.

Community exposures to gasoline vapors near refineries, transfer stations, and other petroleum-handling facilities may require concerted community action for their amelioration, including the development of partnerships among community residents, pediatricians, and environmental agencies.

Prevention of exposures to gasoline and its additives in groundwater requires either installation of activated charcoal filters at the tap or switching to bottled water. Prevention of exposure to the most toxic additives to gasoline, such as tetraethyl lead, MMT, MTBE, or benzene, is best achieved by governmental regulation or phasing out of these compounds.[9,23]

Frequently Asked Questions

Q *What is the risk to a child of brief exposure to gasoline vapors when a parent takes the family car to a service station for fueling?*

A The risk is minimal, but exposure should be kept as brief as possible to minimize risk of delayed consequences, especially leukemia caused by inhalation of benzene vapor. Closing the windows is recommended. Mothers fueling vehicles should not hold infants. Although learning to fuel a car is a necessary life skill, this practice is not recommended for preadolescent children. Some states regulate the age at which children can fuel cars, with age limits typically 16 years of age or older.

Q *What is the responsibility of a pediatrician who lives in a community where the leaking underground storage tank of a gasoline station is contaminating ground water?*

A Strong state and federal regulations developed in recent years require monitoring and abatement of leaking underground storage tanks. A pediatrician should inform the state environmental agency and/or US EPA if such a problem is identified. Families who may drink water from a gasoline-contaminated source should be advised to install activated charcoal filters to their water tap or switch to bottled water. These measures should be taken when there is an unknown source of contamination, when contaminant levels are rising (even though levels still may be below drinking water standards), or when levels of contaminants are steady but higher than drinking water standards (See Chapter 17 for drinking water standards).

Q *A family's water supply has measurable amounts of some gasoline components that are below the EPA standard. Their community water authority says that the water meets standards and that for further advice they should contact their pediatrician. What do I tell them?*

A The EPA sets an "enforceable standard" or maximum contaminant level (MCL) based on both their best estimate of health risk and the "ability of public water systems to detect and remove contaminants using suitable treatment technologies."[40] Water that meets EPA standards confers minimal to no health risk. If a family is concerned anyway, activated charcoal filtration will remove benzene and other aromatic components that make up most of gasoline. All filtration systems require care and maintenance. Community water supplies may transiently exceed standards. If the water is in violation of standards, filtration is a short-term solution, but documenting the efficacy of the filter is a problem. A private well that is contaminated with gasoline poses a serious remediation problem, because such contamination often represents widespread contamination of groundwater beyond the control of the homeowner. Activated charcoal filtration or a reverse osmosis filtration may be necessary, but it may be difficult or impossible to make the water potable.

Q *What are the long-term risks of gasoline sniffing to children and adolescents?*

A Mental deterioration and chronic injury to the nervous system are the principal health dangers of chronic abuse of solvents, including gasoline.[28,41] This leads to trouble with attention, memory, and problem-solving as well as muscle weakness, tremor, and balance problems. The chronic user's mood changes as dementia develops. Renal effects are nephritis and tubular necrosis. Chronic gasoline sniffing also causes certain cancers. Gasoline sniffing is a marker that a child or teenager is at very high risk of trying or already using other drugs.

Q *Should pediatricians be concerned about proposals to add MMT to gasoline as antiknock agents?*

A Yes. Manganese is a known neurotoxicant. It is not used currently in US gasoline. MMT use in Canada to improve octane rating and as an antiknock agent began in 1976. A few other countries, such as Australia and South Africa, were still using MMT as of this writing. Neurotoxic effects have been seen at high- and low-dose exposures and span the range from overt symptomatic parkinsonism at high exposures to subclinical neurobehavioral impairment. Permitting the addition of MMT to the US gasoline supply would not be prudent. This could increase risk of widespread subclinical neurotoxicity (see Chapter 50).

Q *What can pediatricians do to reduce gasoline consumption and help combat global climate change?*

A Pediatricians should support campaigns to develop safe, efficient mass transportation that will reduce atmospheric emissions and risk of automotive injury to children. Children should be encouraged, where possible, to walk or bike to school and to play activities, and pediatricians should take the lead in encouraging construction of community walkways and bikeways. Reduction of obesity among children will be an added benefit of this strategy. In their communities, pediatricians should advocate for land-use planning that results in reduced dependence on driving and that fosters walking, bicycle riding, and use of mass transportation.

References

1. Dement JM, Hensley L, Gitelman A. Carcinogenicity of gasoline: a review of epidemiological evidence. *Ann NY Acad Sci.* 1997;837:53–76
2. Research and Innovative Technology Administration, Bureau of Transportation Statistics. Fuel Consumption by Mode of Transportation in Physical Units. Available at: http://www.bts.gov/publications/national_transportation_statistics/html/table_04_05.html. Accessed September 29, 2010
3. US Energy Information Administration. Petroleum Consumption by Type of Refined Petroleum Product: All Countries, Year 2005 for the International Energy Annual 2006. Available at: http://www.eia.doe.gov/emeu/international/oilconsumption.html. Accessed September 29, 2010
4. Intergovernmental Panel on Climate Change. *Climate Change 2007: Synthesis Report.* Geneva, Switzerland: Intergovernmental Panel on Climate Change; 2007. Available at: http://www.ipcc.ch/pdf/assessment-report/ar4/syr/ar4_syr.pdf. Accessed September 29, 2010
5. Carter JM, Grady SJ, Delzer GC, Koch B, Zogorski JS. Occurrence of MTBE and other gasoline oxygenates in CWS source waters. *American Water Works Association Journal.* Apr 2006;98(4):91

6. Agency for Toxic Substances and Disease Registry. *Toxicological Profile for Benzene, August 2007.* Available at: http://www.atsdr.cdc.gov/toxprofiles/tp3.html. Accessed September 29, 2010

7. Rinsky RA, Smith AB, Hornung R, et al. Benzene and leukemia. An epidemiologic risk assessment. *N Engl J Med.* 1987;316(17):1044–1050

8. International Agency for Research on Cancer. *The Evaluation of Carcinogenic Risk to Humans: Occupational Exposures in Petroleum Refining: Crude Oil and Major Petroleum Fuels.* IARC Monographs. Vol. 45. Lyon, France: International Agency for Research on Cancer; 1989

9. Centers for Disease Control and Prevention. Update: blood lead levels—United States, 1991–1994. *MMWR Morb Mortal Wkly Rep.* 1997;46(7):141–146

10. United Nations Environmental Programme. *The Global Campaign to Eliminate Leaded Gasoline:* Available at: http://www.unep.org/pcfv/PDF/LeadReport.pdf. Accessed September 29, 2010

11. Landrigan PJ, Boffetta P, Apostoli P. The reproductive toxicity and carcinogenicity of lead: a critical review. *Am J Ind Med.* 2000;38(3):231–243

12. Needleman HL, Landrigan PJ. Toxins at the pump. *New York Times.* March 13, 1996:A19

13. Gorell JM, Johnson CC, Rybicki BA, et al. Occupational exposures to metals as risk factors for Parkinson's disease. *Neurology.* 1997;48(3):650–658

14. Mergler D. Neurotoxic effects of low level exposure to manganese in human population. *Environ Res.* 1999;80(2 Pt 1):99–102

15. Mergler D, Baldwin M, Belanger S, et al. Manganese neurotoxicity, a continuum of dysfunction: results from a community based study. *Neurotoxicology.* 1999;20(2-3):327–342

16. Mehlman MA. Dangerous and cancer-causing properties of products and chemicals in the oil refining and petrochemical industry—Part XXII: health hazards from exposure to gasoline containing methyl tertiary butyl ether: study of New Jersey residents. *Toxicol Ind Health.* 1996;12(5):613–627

17. Mannino DM, Etzel RA. Are oxygenated fuels effective? An evaluation of ambient carbon monoxide concentrations in 11 Western states, 1986 to 1992. *J Air Waste Manage Assoc.* 1996;6:20-24

18. Ahmed FE. Toxicology and human health effects following exposure to oxygenated or reformulated fuel. *Toxicol Lett.* 2001;123(2-3):89–113

19. Joseph PM, Weiner MG. Visits to physicians after the oxygenation of gasoline in Philadelphia. *Arch Environ Health.* 2002;57(2):137–154

20. *Office of Environmental Health Hazard Assessment.* Water—Public Health Goals [memorandum]. Available at: http://www.oehha.org/water/phg/399MTBEa.html. Accessed September 29, 2010

21. Mehlman MA. MTBE toxicity. *Environ Health Perspect.* 1996;104(8):808

22. Belpoggi F, Soffritti M, Maltoni C. Methyl-tertiary-butyl ether (MTBE)—a gasoline additive—causes testicular and lymphohaematopoietic cancers in rats. *Toxicol Ind Health.* 1995;11(2):119–149

23. Schremp G. Staff Findings: Timetable for the Phaseout of MTBE From California's Gasoline Supply. California Energy Commission; 1999

24. US Environmental Protection Agency. *State Actions Banning MTBE (Statewide).* EPA420-B-07-013. August 2007. Available at: http://www.epa.gov/mtbe/420b07013.pdf. Accessed September 29, 2010

25. Backer LC, Egeland GM, Ashley DL, et al. Exposure to regular gasoline and ethanol oxyfuel during refueling in Alaska. *Environ Health Perspect.* 1997;105(8):850–855

26. Moolenaar RL, Hefflin BJ, Ashley DL, Middaugh JP, Etzel RA. Blood benzene concentration in workers exposed to oxygenated fuel in Fairbanks, Alaska. *Int Arch Occup Environ Health.* 1997;69(2):139–143

27. International Agency for Research on Cancer. *Diesel and Gasoline Engine Exhausts and Some Nitroarenes.* IARC Monographs. Vol 46. Lyon, France: International Agency for Research on Cancer; 1989

28. Cairney S, Maruff P, Burns C, Currie B. The neurobehavioural consequences of petrol (gasoline) sniffing. *Neurosci Biobehav Rev.* 2002;26(1):81–89

29. Williams JF, Storck M, and the Committee on Substance Abuse and the Committee on Native American Child Health. Inhalant abuse. *Pediatrics.* 2007;119(5):1009-1017

30. Reese E, Kimbrough RD. Acute toxicity of gasoline and some additives. *Environ Health Perspect.* 1993;101(Suppl 6):115–131

31. Eade NR, Taussig LM, Marks MI. Hydrocarbon pneumonitis. *Pediatrics.* 1974;54(3):351–357

32. Shih RD. Hydrocarbons. In: Goldfrank L, ed. *Goldfrank's Toxicologic Emergencies.* 6th ed. Stamford, CT: Appleton & Lange; 1998:1383–1398

33. Gurwitz D, Kattan M, Levinson H, Culham JA. Pulmonary function abnormalities in asymptomatic children after hydrocarbon pneumonitis. *Pediatrics.* 1978;62(5):789–794

34. Burbacher TM. Neurotoxic effects of gasoline and gasoline constituents. *Environ Health Perspect.* 1993;101(Suppl 6):133–141

35. Lynge E, Andersen A, Nilsson R, et al. Risk of cancer and exposure to gasoline vapors. *Am J Epidemiol.* 1997;145(5):449–458

36. Mehlman MA. Dangerous and cancer-causing properties of products and chemicals in the oil refining and petrochemical industry: part I. Carcinogenicity of motor fuels: gasoline. *Toxicol Ind Health.* 1991;7(5-6):143–152

37. Landrigan PJ. Critical assessment of epidemiological studies on the carcinogenicity of 1,3-butadiene and styrene. In: Sorsa M, Peltonen K, Vainio H, Hemminki K, eds. *Butadine and Styrene: Assessment of Health Hazards.* Lyon, France: International Agency for Research on Cancer; 1993:375–388. IARC Scientific Publication No. 127

38. Agency for Toxic Substances and Disease Registry. *ToxFAQs.* Available at: http://www.atsdr.cdc.gov/toxfaqs/index.asp. Accessed September 29, 2010

39. Vale JA; Kulig K; American Academy of Clinical Toxicology; European Association of Poisons Centres and Clinical Toxicologists. Position paper: gastric lavage. *J Toxicol Clin Toxicol. 2004;42(7):933-943*

40. US Environmental Protection Agency. *Consumer Factsheet on: Benzene.* Available at: http://www.epa.gov/ogwdw/contaminants/dw_contamfs/benzene.html. Accessed September 29, 2010

41. Burns TM, Shneker BF, Juel VC. Gasoline sniffing multifocal neuropathy. *Pediatr Neurol.* 2001;25(5):419–421

Chapter 30

Ionizing Radiation (Excluding Radon)

■ ■ ■ ■ ■ ■

Radiation includes energy transmitted by waves through space or some type of medium, such as light seen as colors, infrared rays perceived as heat, and audible radio waves amplified through radio and television. We cannot similarly perceive radiation with shorter wavelengths: ultraviolet rays, x-rays, and gamma rays. Radiation with the shortest wavelengths, x-rays and gamma rays, possess immense quantities of energy and penetrate solid objects. This energy may cause ionization in tissue, which drives outer electrons from their orbits around atoms. The free electrons created can react with other molecules in living organisms and cause tissue damage. Fig 30.1 shows wavelengths for different types of radiation.[1]

ROUTES OF EXPOSURE

People may be exposed to ionizing radiation by inhalation, by ingestion, and through the skin. People may also be exposed through injection of radioisotopes for medical indications. The fetus may be exposed if the mother is exposed. There may be exposure through human milk.

SOURCES OF EXPOSURE

Radiation exposures are derived from external sources, such as background cosmic radiation, radon, or medical x-rays, as well as internal sources, such as radioactive fallout or medical radioisotopes. These exposures can be from natural or man-made sources. The energy in ionizing radiation is high enough to cause displacement of electrons from atoms and breaks in chemical bonds. This

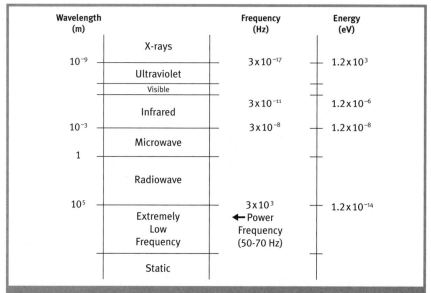

Figure 30.1: Approximate Range of Wavelength, Frequency, and Energy for Different Types of Electromagnetic Radiation or Fields. Hz indicates Hertz; eV, electronvolts.

transfer of energy in sufficient doses from the environment to individuals can adversely affect their health.[1,2] X-rays transfer energy along thin paths, whereas neutrons have greater mass and transfer energy along wider paths.

There are different ways (ie, direct or indirect) and units used to measure radiation. Direct measurement is the measurement of radiation on a patient. The dose of absorbed radiation per unit of mass, previously measured as "radiation absorbed dose" (rad) is now measured in Gray (Gy); 1 Gy = 100 rad. One Gy delivers 1 joule (J) of energy per kg of matter. These measurements have several problems: different types of radiation differ in their ability to produce effects (eg, alpha particles are more effective per unit of absorbed dose than are x-rays in producing chromosomal abnormalities), and different tissues and organs in a body have different probabilities and severities of harm.

This is why *equivalent and effective doses* were introduced. Equivalent dose is the product of absorbed dose and a weight factor. The unit of equivalent dose is named the sievert (Sv). The equivalent dose was previously measured as roentgen equivalent man (rem); 1 Sv = 100 rem. Equivalent dose refers to the radiation energy deposited in a specific organ and effective dose corresponds to the sum of the dose to a number of tissues as if the whole body had been exposed. For every tissue, there is a weight factor depending on its sensitivity to radiation induced effects (Fig 30.2).

On average, the annual effective dose equivalent of ionizing radiation to the population in the United States is 0.006 Sv (0.6 rem), 37% of which is from

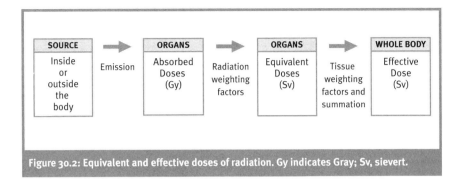

Figure 30.2: Equivalent and effective doses of radiation. Gy indicates Gray; Sv, sievert.

radon, 13% from other natural sources, 24% from computerized tomography, 12% from nuclear medicine, 7% from interventional fluoroscopy, 5% from medical x-rays, and 2% from other man-made sources.[2]

Radiation exposure may be instantaneous (atomic bomb), chronic (uranium miners), fractionated (radiotherapy), or partial-body. For a given dose, whole-body exposure is generally more harmful than partial-body exposure. Radioisotopes decay with time into stable elements and have physical half-lives of various lengths, from fractions of a second to millions of years. They also have biological half-lives related to the rate at which they are excreted from the body.

SYSTEM(S) AFFECTED AND BIOLOGICAL PROCESSES

Atoms or molecules that become ionized attain stability by forming substances that may alter molecular processes within a cell or its environment. Ionizing radiation, when it collides with a cell, is capable of introducing DNA strand breaks and gene mutations. If this damage is not repaired, the cell may die or be transformed into a malignant cell.

Acute Effects

Ionizing radiation produces the same reactions regardless of the type of particle or ray emitted. Differences are quantitative, not qualitative. The effects of overexposure may occur within hours to days and include acute radiation sickness (nausea, vomiting, diarrhea, declining white blood cell count, and thrombocytopenia), epilation (loss of hair), and death. Table 30.1 shows the doses at which these effects typically occur.

Delayed Effects

In general, the best estimates of dose-related delayed effects of ionizing radiation come from studies of the Japanese atomic bomb survivors who experienced a single, instantaneous whole-body exposure; this was possibly complicated by other adverse influences, such as malnutrition in war-torn Japan. Delayed effects largely are attributable to mutagenesis, teratogenesis, and carcinogenesis.

Table 30.1: Estimated Threshold Doses for Effects Following Acute Radiation Exposure*			
		ABSORBED DOSE	
HEALTH EFFECT	ORGAN	rad	Gy
Temporary sterility	Testes	15	0.15
Reduced production of blood cells	Bone marrow	50	0.50
Nausea and vomiting in 10% of people within 48 hours	Gastrointestinal	100	1
Permanent sterility, female	Ovaries	250-600	2.5-6
Temporary alopecia	Hair follicles	300-500	3-5
Permanent sterility, male	Testes	350	3.5
Erythema	Skin	500-600	5-6

*From the National Council on Radiation Protection and Measurements.[3] Gy indicates Gray.

The smaller the exposure, the less likely that late effects will be found. It is also important to note that there may be a latency period between the exposure to ionizing radiation and the clinical manifestations, especially in the carcinogenic process (see Carcinogenesis).

Children are more vulnerable and at higher risk of deleterious radiation-induced effects than are adults.[4,5] Their tissues are more radiosensitive and have longer life expectancy, resulting in a greater potential for manifestation. Female infants have almost double the risk as male infants.[6]

Mutagenesis

The harmful effects of ionizing radiation are attributable to its ability to induce DNA damage. This results in genotoxicity in the form of DNA mutations, DNA strand breaks, and whole chromosome breaks. These chromosome breaks in somatic cells (eg, lymphocytes and skin fibroblasts) are detectable decades after exposure[7] and presumably account for the increased rates of cancer observed after exposure in childhood or adulthood. The magnitude of the genotoxic effect depends on the degree of exposure and the concentration of ions induced by the absorption of the energy emitted by the ionizing radiation source.

Studies of children who were conceived after one or both parents were exposed to the atomic bomb have as yet shown no excess of direct genetic effects. The studies started with clinical observations and then included cytogenetic, biochemical, and molecular studies. Scientists evaluated chromosome damage in individuals who were in utero during the atomic bomb detonations in Japan and

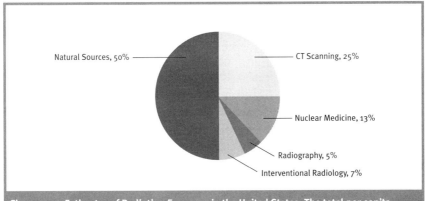

Figure 30.3: Estimates of Radiation Exposure in the United States. The total per capita average radiation dose is estimated at 6 mSv. The figure and percentages were derived from Mettler et al.[18] mSv indicates millisievert.

older than 40 years of age at the time of study.[8] They found that frequency of chromosomal translocations did not increase with the in utero radiation dose. In another study, children exposed to ionizing radiation after the Chernobyl accident in 1986 were found to have above average levels of genome damage.[9] It is possible that the fetus receives lower exposures to ionizing radiation.

Teratogenesis

The effect of a potential teratogen is dependent on the gestational age at the time of exposure as well as the dose absorbed. Much of the information on the effects of acute exposure to ionizing radiation and teratogenesis has been obtained from studies carried out on the survivors of the atomic bomb detonations of Hiroshima and Nagasaki.[10,11] Intrauterine exposure to ionizing radiation was associated with small head size alone or with severe mental retardation. Susceptibility to severe mental retardation was greatest at 8 to 15 weeks of gestational age, with some occurring during the 16th to 25th week of gestation. The lowest dose that caused severe mental retardation from atomic bomb exposure was 0.6 Sv. The lowest dose associated with small head size but no mental retardation was 0.10 to 0.19 Sv among fetuses exposed at 4 to 17 weeks of gestational age. Mental retardation resulting from radiation exposure may be attributable to interruption in the proliferation and migration of neurons from near the cerebral ventricles to the cortex.

Carcinogenesis

Atomic Bomb Exposure

In the years immediately following the atomic bomb detonations in Hiroshima and Nagasaki, leukemia appeared early and was one of the most striking evident somatic effects of radiation in atomic bomb survivors.[12] Approximately 30 years after the detonation, the rates of leukemia returned to baseline.

After childhood exposure to ionizing radiation, increased frequencies of cancers in adulthood are expected if the exposure and sample size are large enough. A significant time period of observation is also required to assess effects of childhood radiation exposure and cancer risk. Among all atomic bomb survivors, the lowest dose at which an excess of cancer was found was 0.05 Sv (5 rem).[13] Initial studies of the 807 Japanese atomic bomb survivors exposed in utero suggested that there was no excess of childhood cancer.[11]

However, a subsequent study of solid cancer incidence in 2452 adult subjects exposed in utero to the atomic bomb in Japan identified 94 cancers, an increase over the expected number.[14] This effect was identified 50 years after the exposure to the atomic bomb detonation. This study also evaluated 15 388 adult subjects who were younger than 6 years at the time of the detonation and found increased solid tumor risk.[14] Epidemiologic studies revealed the longer term sequelae of this type of childhood radiation exposure. An excess of thyroid cancer, a very rare childhood cancer, occurred in children exposed to the atomic bomb beginning at 11 years of age.[14] Increased rates of breast cancer after childhood exposure were identified after the cohort became 30 years old (ie, the usual age for early-onset breast cancer in the general population).[15]

Nuclear Power Plant Accidents

When a nuclear power plant does not function properly (as occurred in March 2011, when the nuclear power plant near Fukushima, Japan, was damaged by a major earthquake and resulting tsunami), individuals, land, and structures in the vicinity of the plant can be exposed to a mixture of radioactive products generated inside the reactor, also known as "nuclear fission products." The main radionuclides representing health risk are radioactive cesium and radioactive iodine.

After the 1986 Chernobyl nuclear power plant disaster, populations of Ukraine, Belarus, and Russia were exposed to a wide spectrum of radioactive isotopes. In addition to the acute exposure, individuals were further exposed through food, milk, and water supplies. Significantly increased rates of thyroid cancer in children and adults have been found in several studies.[16] Adults can experience increase in thyroid cancer as late as 20 years after the initial exposure. Increased rates of leukemia following the accident have not been observed in children or power plant workers involved in the clean-up,[17] although statistical power is limited in these studies. About 200 000 people from the highly contaminated regions have emigrated to New York City, and a National Tumor Registry to follow their health was launched in New York City in 2008 (http://www.projectchernobyl.org).

Diagnostic Radiation

In recent years, radiation exposure from medical diagnostic and therapeutic radiologic procedures has become greater than the environmental radiation exposures. In 1980, the estimated per capita medical radiation exposure in the United States was 0.54 millisievert (mSv = 0.001 Sv). This exposure increased by nearly 600% to 3 mSv between 1982 and 2006.[18] It is now estimated that medical radiation accounts for half of the total radiation exposure in the United States (Fig 30.3).

The risk factors for most childhood cancers are not known, but radiation exposure is postulated to contribute to childhood cancer risk because of its ability to induce DNA damage (see also Chapter 45). Studies that began more than 50 years ago suggested a 1.6-fold excess of almost every type of cancer in children younger than 10 years after maternal exposure to diagnostic abdominal x-rays during pregnancy.[5] Subsequent epidemiologic studies confirmed these findings, but others did not.[19,20] The concerns raised by these studies led to the near-elimination of diagnostic x-rays during pregnancy.

The potential carcinogenic effects of postnatal diagnostic radiation exposure have been much less studied.[20] Large-scale data collection on pediatric exposure to diagnostic medical radiation began in the mid-1990s. To date, there is very little evidence that postnatal exposure to diagnostic radiation increases childhood cancer risk. A potential exception is the association of increased breast cancer risk later in life in adolescents with repeated exposure to diagnostic examinations for scoliosis.[21,22]

The use of computed tomography (CT) scans in pediatric patients for the diagnosis of a variety of conditions has been increasing. CT scanning exposes patients to much higher levels of ionizing radiation than conventional radiography.[23] Pediatric interventional and fluoroscopic imaging modalities also potentially expose children to high doses of diagnostic radiation. To date, there are no definitive findings that multiple CT scans or fluoroscopic procedures increase childhood increase cancer risk. However, large-scale studies have not yet been conducted, and it is prudent to reduce exposure to diagnostic radiation whenever possible.[24-29]

SPECIAL SUSCEPTIBILITY AND EPIDEMICS

Special Susceptibility

Children with genetic syndromes attributable to defects in DNA repair mechanisms have increased susceptibility to ionizing radiation. Ataxia-telangiectasia (AT) is caused by mutations in the ATM gene that results in abnormal DNA repair. These patients have severe, progressive ataxia and are prone to the development of lymphoma. When treated with conventional doses of radiotherapy for lymphoma, they suffer an acute radiation reaction that may result in death.[30,31] Multiple mutations have been documented among patients with Fanconi anemia, another inherited DNA repair disorder. These patients are especially sensitive to DNA damaging agents, including ionizing radiation and chemotherapy.[32]

Epidemics

Gamma rays (external radiation) and radioisotopes (internal emitters) in fallout have caused epidemics of delayed radiation effects after in utero or childhood exposure. Developmental effects and cancer were caused by exposure to the atomic bombs, thyroid ablation in 2 infants and thyroid neoplasia in Marshall Islanders were attributable to fallout from nuclear weapons tests,[33] and hundreds of cases of thyroid cancer in children in the Ukraine and Belarus were attributed to fallout from the Chernobyl accident.[34]

DIAGNOSTIC METHODS

Radiation-induced diseases are indistinguishable from their counterparts that occur in the general population. The role of radiation can be implicated only by epidemiologic studies (1) that show a dose-response effect; (2) after alternative explanations have been excluded (eg, cigarette smoking); and (3) that show the link between exposure and the effect is biologically plausible. In clinical practice, if there is suspicion for significant exposure to ionizing radiation (ie, accidental release), biodosimetry may be conducted through a clinical consultation from a radiation specialist. Biodosimetry typically does not measure radioactivity directly; it measures clinical or laboratory surrogate endpoints and correlates them with a radiation dose estimated to have produced the effect. Knowing radiation dose is clinically useful, because it can help the clinician select appropriate prophylactic and therapeutic measures; estimate prognosis, which is especially useful in mass casualty situations when resources may be limited; and transfer appropriate patients to facilities with the expertise to manage severe acute radiation syndrome. Biological dosimetry can estimate exposures above 0.2 Gy (20 rad) by studies of chromosomal translocations and tests of glycophorin A somatic mutations in red blood cells.

TREATMENT OF CLINICAL SYMPTOMS

For acute radiation sickness caused by the Chernobyl accident, blood counts of those affected were sustained through the use of combined treatment with cytokines, such as granulocyte colony-stimulating factor and erythropoietin. These cytokines are useful in supporting white and red blood cells, but their use should be limited to severely affected individuals. Otherwise treatment after such accidents is symptomatic. For delayed radiation effects, treatment of the disease is generally the same as that when radiation exposure was not involved. Drugs to prevent radiation sickness have substantial adverse effects or are not yet known to be safe or effective.[35,36] The Radiation Injury Treatment Network, a voluntary consortium of bone marrow transplant centers, donor centers, and umbilical cord blood banks, was established to develop plans for radiation event response.[37]

PREVENTION OF EXPOSURE

Fallout (Internal Emitters)

Radioisotopes may be released after a power plant malfunction, nuclear weapon detonation, or terrorist event. These radioisotopes can be inhaled or ingested. People in exposed areas should avoid drinking fresh milk in particular. Foods are edible if they were harvested or prepared before the fallout occurred and were not exposed to it.

Radioiodine is a radioisotope that would be released after one of these events. Prompt treatment with potassium iodide (KI) can be quite effective in protecting the thyroid. The Nuclear Regulatory Commission (NRC) recommends that state and local governments provide KI to all citizens living within 10 miles of a nuclear power plant as a supplement to plans for evacuation and sheltering.[38,39] In December 2001, the NRC wrote to the 31 states that had or were within 10 miles of a plant to offer 2 KI pills for every person living within the 10-mile radius. The US Food and Drug Administration (FDA) has also issued recommendations for the use of KI in radiation emergencies.[40,41] The guidance is aimed at federal agencies and state and local governments responsible for radiation emergencies. It is based primarily on data accumulated after the accident at the Chernobyl nuclear power plant in 1986. That disaster resulted in the massive release of ^{131}I and other radioiodines, some with very short half-lives. The short-lived radioiodines are believed to increase the risk of thyroid cancer in children more than [131]I.

The protective effect of KI lasts about 24 hours and daily dosing provides optimum prophylaxis until a significant risk from inhalation or ingestion no longer exists. Early action is crucial; KI optimally should be administered before exposure, on notification of an emergency.[42] It may also have a protective effect even if taken 3 to 4 hours after exposure.

The FDA issued guidelines and instructions on how to prepare KI tablets as a fluid for infants and children[41] (see Tables 30.2 and 30.3). Three KI products are approved by the FDA for over-the-counter use as a thyroid-blocking agent in radiation emergencies. These are Thyro-Block (MedPointe Inc, Somerset, NJ), IOSAT (Anbex Inc, Palm Harbor, FL), and ThyroSafe (Recip US, Honey Brook, PA). IOSAT can be obtained by calling 866-283-3986 and through the Internet at www.nukepills.com; Thyro-Block can be obtained by calling 800-804-4147 and at www.nitro-pak.com; and Thyro-Safe can be obtained by calling 610-942-8972 and at www.thyrosafe.com. Potassium iodide also can be

Table 30.2: Guidelines for Potassium Iodide (KI) Administration*†

PATIENT	EXPOSURE, Gy (rad)	KI DOSE (mg)
>40 years of age	>5 (500)	130
18 through 40 years of age	≥0.1 (10)	130
Adolescents 12 through 17 years of age‡	≥0.05 (5)	65
Children 4 through 11 years of age	≥0.05 (5)	65
Children 1 month through 3 years of age§	≥0.05 (5)	32
Birth through 1 month of age	≥0.05 (5)	16
Pregnant or lactating women	≥0.05 (5)	130

Gy indicates Gray.

*From US Food and Drug Administration, Center for Drug Evaluation and Research.[40]

† KI is useful for exposure to a radioiodine only. KI is given once only to pregnant women and neonates unless other protective measures (evacuation, sheltering, and control of the food supply) are unavailable. Repeat dosing should be on the advice of public health authorities.

‡ Adolescents weighing more than 70 kg should receive the adult dose (130 mg).

§ KI from tablets or as a freshly saturated solution may be diluted in water and mixed with milk, formula, juice, soda, or syrup. Raspberry syrup disguises the taste of KI the best. KI mixed with low-fat chocolate milk, orange juice, or flat soda (eg, cola) has an acceptable taste. Low-fat white milk and water did not hide the salty taste of KI.

ordered from Anbex Inc by calling 727-784-3483 and at www.anbex.com. It is approved by the FDA and is also carried by some pharmacies. Detailed information about radiation disasters can be found in the 2003 American Academy of Pediatrics policy statement "Radiation Disasters and Children."[43]

DIAGNOSTIC RADIATION

The risk of cancer associated with most diagnostic radiation is low, and use of radiation should not be restricted when needed for correct diagnosis. Any medical procedure has a risk, and diagnostic radiography is no exception. Limitation of radiation; shielding sensitive body parts, such as the thyroid and gonads; and ensuring a nonpregnant state are components of good medical practice.[21] For decades, pediatric radiologists have strongly endorsed the "as low as reasonably achievable" (ALARA) principle in diagnostic imaging. In the past several years, ALARA has taken on even greater meaning with the significant increases in use of CT and other diagnostic radiology modalities.[24] Efforts to encourage judicious uses of radiation ("Image Gently") have been published.[24-29]

CT scans require radiation exposures that one report suggests could result in increased cancer rates later in life: potentially 500 cancer cases among an estimated 600 000 children exposed annually.[44] More active reduction in CT exposure settings was recommended. Table 30.4 shows estimated radiation doses from several procedures.

Table 30.3: Guidelines for Home Preparation of Potassium Iodide (KI) Solution.*

Two tablet sizes are available, 130 mg and 65 mg.

- Put one **130-mg** KI tablet in a small bowl and grind into a fine powder with the back of a spoon. The powder should not have any large pieces.

- Add 4 tsp (20 mL) of water to the KI powder. Use a spoon to mix them together until the KI powder is dissolved in the water.

- Add 4 tsp (20 mL) of milk, juice, soda, or syrup (eg, raspberry) to the KI/water mixture. The resulting mixture is 16.25 mg of KI per teaspoon (5 mL).

- Age-based dosing guidelines

  — Newborn through 1 month of age: 1 tsp

  — 1 month through 3 years of age: 2 tsp

  — 4 years through 17 years of age: 4 tsp
  (if child weighs more than 70 kg, give one 130-mg tablet)

- Put one **65-mg** KI tablet in a small bowl and grind into a fine powder with the back of a spoon. The powder should not have any large pieces.

- Add 4 tsp (20 mL) of water to the KI powder. Use a spoon to mix them together until the KI powder is dissolved in the water.

- Add 4 tsp (20 mL) of milk, juice, soda, or syrup (eg, raspberry) to the KI/water mixture. The resulting mixture is 8.125 mg of KI per teaspoon (5 mL)

- Age-based dosing guidelines

  — Newborn through 1 month of age: 2 tsp

  — 1 month through 3 years of age: 4 tsp

  — 4 years through 17 years of age: 8 tsp or one 65-mg tablet
  (if child weighs more than 70 kg, give two 65-mg tablets)

HOW TO STORE THE PREPARED KI MIXTURE

- Potassium iodide mixed with any of the recommended drinks will keep for up to 7 days in the refrigerator.

- The US Food and Drug Administration recommends that the KI drink mixtures be prepared fresh weekly; unused portions should be discarded.

*Adapted from US Food and Drug Administration, Center for Drug Evaluation and Research.[41]

Estimates of the radiation dose to the embryo/fetus from maternal diagnostic examinations have been compiled and have been shown to be quite variable. This is because of differences in the imaging modality, body area evaluated, and gestational age. Because previous studies have suggested increased cancer risk in the offspring of women undergoing diagnostic radiologic procedures during pregnancy, alternative imaging modalities, such as ultrasound, should be considered when clinically feasible.[24,29]

Table 30.4: Estimates of Radiation Dose to Children From Diagnostic Radiology

TYPE OF EXAMINATION	DOSE QUANTITY	DOSE TO CHILDREN BY AGE AT EXPOSURE		
		1 YEAR	5 YEARS	ADULT
Radiography				
Skull AP	ESD (mGy)	0.60	1.25	2.3
Skull LAT	ESD (mGy)	0.34	0.58	1.2
Chest PA	ESD (mGy)	0.08	0.11	0.15
Abdomen AP	ESD (mGy)	0.34	0.59	4.7
Pelvis AP	ESD (mGy)	0.35	0.51	3.6
Dental radiography				
Intra oral	PED (mGy)		1.15*	1.85
Panoramic	DAP (mGy/cm²)		70*	70
Diagnostic fluoroscopy procedures				
Micturating cystourethrography	DAP (mGy/cm²)	483	740	9260
Barium swallow	DAP (mGy/cm²)	863	858	6350
Computed tomography				
Brain	ED (mSv)	2.2	1.9	1.9
Facial bone/sinuses	ED (mSv)	0.5	0.5	0.9
Chest	ED (mSv)	2.2	2.5	5.9
Entire abdomen	ED (mSv)	4.8	5.4	10.4
Spine	ED (mSv)	11.4	8	10.1
Diagnostic nuclear medicine				
[123]I sodium iodide (thyroid uptake)	ED (mSv)	19	16	7.2
[99]Tcm – DMSA (with normal renal function)*	ED (mSv)	0.7	0.8	0.8

mSv indicates millisievert; mGy, milligray (1 mGy = 0.001 Gy).
Data were derived from Linet et al,[20] in which details of dose estimates at differing ages were reviewed.
ESD indicates entrance surface dose; PED, patient entrance dose; DAP, dose area product; ED, effective dose.
*Derived from Gadd et al.[45]

Special populations, such as infants with extremely low birth weight, may undergo multiple radiological examinations during a short period. Fluoroscopy and CT scan should be used sparingly for preterm infants, particularly when other imaging techniques are available. Limiting exposures will keep the cumulative dose low. Pediatricians should make sure that the most conservative procedures are used.

REGULATIONS

Recommendations concerning radiation protection are made by the National Commission on Radiation Protection and Measurements and the International Commission on Radiological Protection. The Nuclear Regulatory Commission regulates and monitors nuclear facilities and the medical/research uses of radioisotopes.

Frequenty Asked Questions

Q   *How many x-rays are safe for my child?*

A   As many as your child's physicians think necessary for diagnosis and follow-up, taking into account the benefit weighed against the (very small) risk. Because the radiation doses from certain diagnostic procedures (eg, CT scans) are high, pediatricians are urged to request radiologic procedures only when necessary and to check to ensure that CT operators use settings appropriate for children (see also Table 30.4).

Q   *Will x-ray examinations of my child affect future grandchildren?*

A   It is highly unlikely that an individual's x-ray examinations would affect their future children or grandchildren. No genetic effects of radiation from the atomic bombs in Japan have been demonstrated. In evaluating the feasibility of studying the offspring of military veterans, an expert committee of the Institute of Medicine noted that exposures of fathers to fallout from weapons tests, as in the South Pacific, seldom exceeded 0.005 rem (0.5 Sv).[46] The committee noted that at the maximum relative risk (0.2% increase in adverse reproductive outcomes) a sample size of 212 million exposed children would be needed to detect a statistically significant excess compared with unexposed children. Or, the frequency of such effects among the 500 000 children of veterans exposed to the atomic bomb would have to be increased 150-fold to be detected.

Q   *Is my child's leukemia attributable to past radiation exposures?*

A   There is no way to determine this for an individual patient. Illnesses induced by radiation cannot be distinguished from illnesses in the general population. The relationship can only be established by large epidemiologic studies showing a higher incidence in a radiated group (such as atomic bomb survivors) supported by other evidence.

Q *Is there a risk of later recurrence in children exposed to the Chernobyl accident who have had thyroidectomies for thyroid cancer?*

A Yes, there is a risk of later recurrence, especially in adolescents who have had thyroid cancer. Long-term follow up is critically important. Young patients who have undergone thyroidectomy should have an ultrasound of the neck, thyroid function tests, and thyroglobulin and anti-thyroglobulin antibodies measured once yearly. If all results are normal after 2 years, less-frequent follow up visits can be scheduled.[47] Patients should be managed in consultation with experts in thyroid cancer.

Q *We live close to a nuclear power plant. Should I be concerned and should I take special precautions?*

A Nuclear power plants are designed and built with public safety as a priority. Emissions from the plant should not require protective actions on your part. However, if you live within 10 miles of a nuclear power plant, you may be issued potassium iodide (KI) tablets. In the event of a release of radioactive iodine, these tablets can prevent radioiodine from concentrating in your thyroid. These should be taken only if instructed by local emergency management directors. KI tablets will only protect you from radioactive iodine and not from other radioactive substances.

Resources

National Cancer Institute, Radiation Epidemiology Branch
Web site: http://dceg.cancer.gov/reb
Phone: 301-496-6600

National Cancer Institute, Pediatric CT scan information
Web site: www.cancer.gov/cancertopics/causes/radiation-risks-pediatric-CT

National Council on Radiation Protection
Web site: www.ncrponline.org
Phone: 301-657-2652

Environmental Protection Agency, RadTown USA
Web site: www.epa.gov/radtown/index.html
This site has a wide-variety of topics related to all types of radiation.

RadiologyInfo: Radiology information resource for patients
Web site: www.radiologyinfo.org

American College of Preventive Medicine, Radiation Exposure from Iodine-131
Web site: www.iodine131.org

References

1. Mettler FA Jr, Upton AC. *Medical Effects of Ionizing Radiation.* 2nd ed. Philadelphia, PA: WB Saunders Co; 1995

2. Institute of Medicine, Committee to Assess Health Risks from Exposure to Low Levels of Ionizing Radiation, National Research Council. *Health Risks from Exposure to Low Levels of Ionizing Radiation: BEIR VII – Phase 2.* Washington, DC: National Academies Press; 2006

3. National Council on Radiation Protection and Measurements. *Management of Terrorist Events Involving Radioactive Material.* Bethesda, MD: National Council on Radiation Protection and Measurements; 2001. NCRP Report No. 138

4. Preston RJ. Children as a sensitive subpopulation for the risk assessment process. *Toxicol Appl Pharmacol.* 2004;199(2):132-141

5. Bithell JF, Stewart AM. Pre-natal irradiation and childhood malignancy: a review of British data from the Oxford Survey. *Br J Cancer.* 1975;31(3):271-287

6. Delongchamp RR, Mabuchi K, Yoshimoto Y, Preston DL. Cancer mortality among atomic bomb survivors exposed in utero or as young children. *Radiat Res.* 1997;147(3):385-395

7. Kodama Y, Pawel D, Nakamura N, et al. Stable chromosome aberrations in atomic bomb survivors: results from 25 years of investigation. *Radiat Res.* 2001;156(4):337-346

8. Ohtaki K, Kodama Y, Nakano M, et al. Human fetuses do not register chromosome damage inflicted by radiation exposure in lymphoid precursor cells except for a small but significant effect at low doses. *Radiat Res.* 2004;161(4):373-379

9. Fucic A, Brunborg G, Lasan R, Jezek D, Knudsen LE, Merlo DF. Genomic damage in children accidentally exposed to ionizing radiation: a review of the literature. *Mutat Res.* 2008;658(1-2):111-123

10. De Santis M, Di Gianantonio E, Straface G, et al. Ionizing radiations in pregnancy and teratogenesis: a review of literature. *Reprod Toxicol.* 2005;20(3):323-329

11. Miller RW. Discussion: severe mental retardation and cancer among atomic bomb survivors exposed in utero. *Teratology.* 1999;59(4):234-235

12. Ichimaru M, Ishimaru T. Review of thirty years study of Hiroshima and Nagasaki atomic bomb survivors. II. Biological effects. D. Leukemia and related disorders. *J Radiat Res (Tokyo).* 1975;(16 Suppl):89-96

13. Preston DL, Shimizu Y, Pierce DA, Suyama A, Mabuchi K. Studies of mortality of atomic bomb survivors. Report 13: Solid cancer and noncancer disease mortality: 1950-1997. *Radiat Res.* 2003;160(4):381-407

14. Preston DL, Cullings H, Suyama A, et al. Solid cancer incidence in atomic bomb survivors exposed in utero or as young children. *J Natl Cancer Inst.* 2008;100(6):428-436

15. Land CE, Tokunaga M, Koyama K, et al. Incidence of female breast cancer among atomic bomb survivors, Hiroshima and Nagasaki, 1950-1990. *Radiat Res.* 2003;160(6):707-717

16. Ron E. Thyroid cancer incidence among people living in areas contaminated by radiation from the Chernobyl accident. *Health Phys.* 2007;93(5):502-511

17. Howe GR. Leukemia following the Chernobyl accident. *Health Phys.* 2007;93(5):512-515

18. Mettler FA Jr, Thomadsen BR, Bhargavan M, et al. Medical radiation exposure in the U.S. in 2006: preliminary results. *Health Phys.* 2008;95(5):502-507

19. Schulze-Rath R, Hammer GP, Blettner M. Are pre- or postnatal diagnostic X-rays a risk factor for childhood cancer? A systematic review. *Radiat Environ Biophys* 2008;47(3):301-312

20. Linet MS, Kim KP, Rajaraman P. Children's exposure to diagnostic medical radiation and cancer risk: epidemiologic and dosimetric considerations. *Pediatr Radiol.* 2009;39(Suppl 1):S4-S26

21. Hoffman DA, Lonstein JE, Morin MM, Visscher W, Harris BS, III, Boice JD Jr. Breast cancer in women with scoliosis exposed to multiple diagnostic x rays. *J Natl Cancer Inst.* 1989;81(17):1307-1312

22. Ronckers CM, Doody MM, Lonstein JE, Stovall M, Land CE. Multiple diagnostic X-rays for spine deformities and risk of breast cancer. *Cancer Epidemiol Biomarkers Prev.* 2008;17(3): 605-613

23. Brody AS, Frush DP, Huda W, Brent RL. Radiation risk to children from computed tomography. *Pediatrics.* 2007;120(3):677-682

24. Goske MJ, Applegate KE, Boylan J, et al. The 'Image Gently' campaign: increasing CT radiation dose awareness through a national education and awareness program. *Pediatr Radiol.* 2008;38(3):265-269

25. Strauss KJ, Kaste SC. ALARA in pediatric interventional and fluoroscopic imaging: striving to keep radiation doses as low as possible during fluoroscopy of pediatric patients—a white paper executive summary. *J Am Coll Radiol.* 2006;3(9):686-688

26. Strauss KJ, Goske MJ, Kaste SC, et al. Image gently: Ten steps you can take to optimize image quality and lower CT dose for pediatric patients. *AJR Am J Roentgenol.* 2010;194(4):868-873

27. Goske MJ, Applegate KE, Bell C, et al. Image Gently: providing practical educational tools and advocacy to accelerate radiation protection for children worldwide. *Semin Ultrasound CT MR.* 2010;31(1):57-63

28. Applegate KE, Amis ES Jr, Schauer DA. Radiation exposure from medical imaging procedures. *N Engl J Med.* 2009;361(23):2289

29. Bulas DI, Goske MJ, Applegate KE, Wood BP. Image Gently: why we should talk to parents about CT in children. *AJR Am J Roentgenol.* 2009;192(5):1176-1178

30. Perlman S, Becker-Catania S, Gatti RA. Ataxia-telangiectasia: diagnosis and treatment. *Semin Pediatr Neurol.* 2003;10(3):173-182

31. Becker-Catania SG, Gatti RA. Ataxia-telangiectasia. *Adv Exp Med Biol.* 2001;495:191-198

32. Alter BP. Radiosensitivity in Fanconi's anemia patients. *Radiother Oncol.* 2002;62(3):345-347

33. Conard RA, Rall JE, Sutow WW. Thyroid nodules as a late sequela of radioactive fallout, in a Marshall Island population exposed in 1954. *N Engl J Med.* 1966;274(25):1391-1399

34. Tronko MD, Bogdanova TI, Komissarenko IV, et al. Thyroid carcinoma in children and adolescents in Ukraine after the Chernobyl nuclear accident: statistical data and clinicomorphologic characteristics. *Cancer.* 1999;86(1):149-156

35. Mettler FA Jr, Voelz GL. Major radiation exposure—what to expect and how to respond. *N Engl J Med.* 2002;346(20):1554-1561

36. Moulder JE. Report on an interagency workshop on the radiobiology of nuclear terrorism. Molecular and cellular biology dose (1-10 Sv) radiation and potential mechanisms of radiation protection (Bethesda, Maryland, December 17-18, 2001). *Radiat Res.* 2002;158(1):118-124

37. Weinstock DM, Case C Jr, Bader JL, et al. Radiologic and nuclear events: contingency planning for hematologists/oncologists. *Blood.* 2008;111(12):5440-5445

38. US Nuclear Regulatory Commission. *Frequently Asked Questions about Potassium Iodide.* Washington, DC: US Nuclear Regulatory Commission; 2002. Available at: http://www.nrc.gov/what-we-do/regulatory/emer-resp/emer-prep/ki-faq.html. Accessed March 15, 2011

39. American Thyroid Association. *American Thyroid Association Endorses Potassium Iodide for Radiation Emergencies.* Falls Church, VA: American Thyroid Association; 2002. Available at: http://www.thyroid.org/professionals/publications/statements/ki/02_04_09_ki_endrse.html. Accessed March 15, 2011

40. US Food and Drug Administration, Center for Drug Evaluation and Research. *Guidance Document Potassium Iodide as a Thyroid Blocking Agent in Radiation Emergencies.* Rockville, MD: US Food and Drug Administration; Drug Information Branch; 2001. HFD-210. Available at: http://www.fda.gov/cder/guidance/4825fnl.htm. Accessed March 15, 2011

41. US Food and Drug Administration, Center for Drug Evaluation and Research. *Home Preparation Procedure for Emergency Administration of Potassium Iodide Tablets for Infants and Small Children.* 2006. Available at: http://www.fda.gov/cder/drugprepare/kiprep.htm. Accessed March 15, 2011

42. Christodouleas JP, Forrest RD, Ainsley CG, et al. Short-term and long-term health risks of nuclear-power-plant accidents. *N Engl J Med.* 2011;364(24):2334-2341

43. American Academy of Pediatrics, Committee on Environmental Health. Radiation disasters and children. *Pediatrics.* 2003;111(6 Pt 1):1455-1466

44. Brenner D, Elliston C, Hall E, Berdon W. Estimated risks of radiation-induced fatal cancer from pediatric CT. *AJR Am J Roentgenol.* 2001;176(2):289-296

45. Gadd R, Mountford PJ, Oxtoby JW. Effective dose to children and adolescents from radiopharmaceuticals. *Nucl Med Commun.* 1999;20(6):569-573

46. Institute of Medicine, Committee to Study the Feasibility of, and Need for, Epidemiologic Studies of Adverse Reproductive Outcomes in Families of Atomic Veterans. *Adverse Reproductive Outcomes in Families of Atomic Veterans: The Feasibility of Epidemiologic Studies.* Washington, DC: National Academies Press; 1995

47. Tuttle RM, Leboeuf R. Follow up approaches in thyroid cancer: a risk adapted paradigm. *Endocrinol Metab Clin North Am.* 2008;37(2):419-435

Chapter 31

Lead

■ ■ ■ ■ ■ ■

Childhood lead toxicity has been recognized for at least 100 years. As recently as the 1940s, many believed that children with lead poisoning who did not die during the acute toxic episode had no residual effects. After it was recognized that learning and behavior disorders occurred in children who recovered from acute toxicity, many believed that only children with frank symptoms suffered neurobehavioral deficits. In the 1970s and 1980s, however, studies worldwide demonstrated that asymptomatic children with higher levels of lead had lower IQ scores,[1,2] more language difficulties,[3] attention problems, and behavior disorders.[4,5] With better epidemiologic studies, the definition of a harmful level of lead has changed markedly. As recently as 1968, children were discharged from the hospital when the blood lead level decreased to 60 µg/dL,[6] and through the 1970s,[7] children with blood lead levels up to 29 µg/dL were thought to have inconsequential lead exposure. Over subsequent years, however, effects were seen at lower and lower levels. There is, as yet, no reliable threshold for these long-lasting effects of lead exposure on cognitive test scores. In 2 independent meta-analyses conducted in the 1990s of prospective studies from several countries,[1,2] damage was documented beginning at a blood lead level of 10 µg/dL. More recent studies have demonstrated a relationship between blood lead level at the time of testing and decreased scores on reading and arithmetic tests that is apparent even in children 6 to 16 years of age, including those whose blood lead levels by then are less than 5 µg/dL.[8] Canfield et al[9] reported that among 172 children followed prospectively with measurements of blood lead level, 101 had never had a blood lead level greater than 10 µg/dL, and there was still a strong negative relationship between blood lead level and IQ when the children were 3 to 5 years of age, a result subsequently confirmed by Bellinger and Needleman.[10]

Since lead was removed from gasoline and paint more than 3 decades ago, fatal lead encephalopathy has all but disappeared and symptomatic lead poisoning is now rare. The continued exposure, however, of thousands of children to lead-laden dust in deteriorating housing mars what would otherwise be a public health triumph. Such low-level lead exposure produces cognitive impairment without identifiable clinical symptoms, and it is this asymptomatic cognitive impairment that constitutes most lead poisoning in the United States. The focus has, thus, shifted from the care of symptomatic children to primary prevention of lead exposures and reduction of exposures for children with elevated levels and subclinical effects. Although much of the management of children at risk of lead poisoning is nonclinical, pediatricians commonly find themselves participating in or even directing these activities.[11]

ROUTES AND SOURCES OF EXPOSURE

Children most often are exposed to lead through the unintentional ingestion of lead-containing particles, such as dust from paint or soil, or from water or foreign bodies. Lead can be absorbed from the pulmonary tract if inhaled as fumes or respirable particles.

Lead (Pb) is an element and occurs naturally, but blood lead levels are low in the absence of industrial activities.[12] In the United States, there have been 2 major sources of industrially derived lead for children: airborne lead, mostly from the combustion of gasoline containing tetraethyl lead, and leaded chips and dust, mostly from deteriorating lead paint.

The years since 1980 have witnessed a substantial decrease in childhood exposure to airborne lead in the United States. Federal legislation in the 1970s removed lead from gasoline and reduced smokestack emissions from smelters and other sources, causing blood lead levels in children to decrease. From 1976 to 1980, before the regulations had their full impact, US children 1 to 5 years of age had a median blood lead level of 15 µg/dL; 88% of them had levels at or above 10 µg/dL.[13] From 1999 to 2004, the most recent data available, only 1.4% of children 1 to 5 years of age had blood lead levels at or above 10 µg/dL.[14] Although levels have decreased in all children, black children and poor children continue to have relatively high blood lead levels. Airborne lead should no longer be a source of exposure in most US communities. However, residual lead in the soil in areas heavily affected by airborne lead, such as around smelters, continues to be a problem even decades after closure of the worst sites.[15]

The source for most lead-poisoned children now is the dust and chips from deteriorating lead paint on interior surfaces. Children living in homes with deteriorating lead paint can achieve blood lead levels of at least 20 µg/dL without frank pica.[16] This exposure commonly arises from normal, developmentally-appropriate hand-to-mouth behavior in an environment that is contaminated with lead dust. Children can ingest lead-laden dust with their cereal, for example, by dropping dry cereal on the floor at mealtime and then hunting it down and eating it later, or with their banana by squishing the fruit through their dust-laden hands in preparation for consumption.[17] Children can ingest lead from mouthing contaminated toys.

The use of heavily leaded paint on interior surfaces ceased in the United States by 1978. However, in 1998, of the 16.4 million homes with 1 child or more younger than 6 years, 27% still had significant lead paint hazards (lead-based paint in such a deteriorated condition that exposure is likely).[18] Dust also is a final resting place for old airborne lead from gasoline, and lead in urban soils can recontaminate cleaned houses.[19]

Individual children may be exposed to lead fumes or respirable dust resulting from sanding or heating old paint, burning or melting automobile batteries, or melting lead for use in a hobby or craft. Some toy jewelry is made of lead, and a child who ingested a lead charm died of lead poisoning in 2006.[20] Some old toys made in the United States and some imported toys were painted with lead-based paint, and some plastic toys and vinyl have lead added as a softener. The US Consumer Product Safety Commission (CPSC) has required recalls of some of these toys and is working with importers and manufacturers to prevent further importation of products containing unsafe amounts of lead. Although individual children could chew on or ingest these products and, thus, absorb lead from them, it is still not clear how much toys and plastics are contributing to the exposure of most children.

Lead plumbing (Latin "plumbus" means lead) has contaminated drinking water for centuries. In 2003-2004, some tap water in Washington, DC, was found to exceed US Environmental Protection Agency (EPA) regulations. This was thought to be caused by a change in water disinfection procedures, which increased the water's ability to leach lead from connector pipes between the water mains and interior plumbing in old houses. The extent of this problem in Washington and other cities is not yet known. It was recommended that affected families drink filtered or bottled water until the pipes can be replaced. Uncommon sources of exposure include cosmetics, folk remedies, pottery glaze, old or imported cans with soldered seams, and contaminated vitamin supplements.

Table 31.1 lists risk factors for lead poisoning and prevention strategies.

SYSTEMS AFFECTED

For lead exposure now seen in the United States, subclinical effects on the central nervous system (CNS) are the most common effects. The best-studied effect is cognitive impairment, measured by IQ tests. The strength of this association and its time course are characteristic and have been similar in

Table 31.1: Risk Factors for Lead Exposure and Prevention Strategies

RISK FACTOR	PREVENTION STRATEGY
Environmental	
Paint	Identify, evaluate, and remediate
Dust	Control sources
Soil	Restrict play in area, plant groundcover
Drinking water	Check with local authorities about morning flush of water from faucet; use cold water for cooking and drinking, especially if tap water used for preparing formula
Folk remedies	Avoid use
Some imported cosmetics (eg, kohl or surma)	Avoid use
Old ceramic or pewter cookware, old urns/kettles, decorative pottery from Mexico and ceramics from China	Avoid use
Some imported toys, crayons	Avoid use
Parental occupations (painter, lead-paint abatement, etc)	Shower and remove work clothing and shoes before leaving work
Hobbies	Proper use, storage, and ventilation
Home renovation	Proper containment, ventilation; pregnant women and young children should vacate premises while work is done and not reenter until premises certified as lead-safe
Buying or renting a new home	Inquire about lead hazards, look for deteriorated paint before occupancy, hire certified lead risk assessor to evaluate hazard and recommend control options
Host	
Hand-to-mouth activity (or pica)	Control sources; frequent hand washing
Inadequate nutrition	Adequate iron and calcium
Developmental disabilities	Enrichment programs as available

multiple studies in several countries.[21] In most countries, including the United States, blood lead levels peak at approximately 2 years of age and then decrease without intervention. Although there is some relationship between peak blood lead level and IQ tested later, it is now clear that contemporaneous blood lead, even though it is lower, is more strongly associated with school-aged IQ.[21,22] The Centers for Disease Control and Prevention (CDC)[23] and American Academy of Pediatrics (AAP)[11] currently use 10 μg/dL as the level that should prompt public health action.[24] A blood lead level of 10 μg/dL should not be interpreted as a threshold; no threshold for effects has been identified.[24,25] Although lead is a risk factor for developmental and behavioral problems, its impact has significant individual variability, which may be modulated by the psychosocial environment and educational experiences of the developing child.[24] Many factors affect cognition and behavior.

Other aspects of CNS function also may be affected by lead, but they are less well documented. Subclinical effects on hearing[26] and balance[27] may occur at commonly encountered blood lead levels. Some studies have measured tooth or bone lead levels, which are thought to represent integrated, possibly lifetime, exposure. Teachers reported that students with elevated tooth lead levels were more inattentive, hyperactive, disorganized, and less able to follow directions.[3,28] Further follow-up in 1 of the studies[3] showed higher rates of failure to graduate from high school, reading disabilities, and greater absenteeism in the final year of high school.[29] Elevated bone lead levels were associated with increased attentional dysfunction, aggression, and delinquency.[30]

Although there are reasonable animal models of low-dose lead exposure and cognition and behavior,[31] the mechanisms by which lead affects CNS function are not known. Lead alters very basic nervous system functions, like calcium-modulated signaling, at very low concentrations in vitro.[32] The age of 2 years, when lead levels peak, is the same age at which a major reduction in dendrite connections occurs, among other events crucial to development. It is, thus, plausible that lead exposure at that time interferes with a critical development process in the CNS, but what that process is has not been identified. Brain imaging studies in adults with elevated blood lead levels in childhood have demonstrated region-specific reductions in gray matter volume,[33] alterations of white matter microstructure,[34] and a significant impact of lead on brain reorganization associated with language function.[35]

Lead also has important nonneurodevelopmental effects. The kidneys are a primary target organ; children exposed to lead are at significantly greater risk of becoming hypertensive adults. Another renal effect of lead in children is impaired 1-d-hydroxylation of vitamin D, a necessary step towards activating this vitamin. Lead interferes with heme synthesis beginning at blood lead levels of approximately 25 μg/dL.[36] Both d-aminolevulinate dehydratase, an early-step enzyme, and ferrochelatase, which closes the heme ring, are inhibited. Ferrochelatase inhibition is the basis of an erstwhile screening test for lead poisoning that measured erythrocyte protoporphyrin, the immediate heme precursor. Because it is insensitive to the lower levels of blood lead that are of concern now, the test is now obsolete for that use. A recent cross-sectional study suggests that environmental exposure to lead may delay growth and pubertal development in black and Mexican-American girls.[37] Finally, episodes of severe lead poisoning can cause growth arrest of the long bones, producing "lead lines."

CLINICAL EFFECTS

Some children with blood lead levels greater than 60 μg/dL may complain of headaches, abdominal pain, loss of appetite, or constipation or may be asymptomatic. Children displaying clumsiness, agitation, or decreased activity and somnolence are presenting with premonitory symptoms of CNS involvement that may rapidly proceed to vomiting, stupor, and convulsions.[6] Symptomatic lead toxicity should be treated as an emergency. Although lead can cause abdominal colic, peripheral neuropathy, and renal disease in adults with occupational exposures, these are rare in children.

DIAGNOSTIC MEASURES

The diagnosis of lead poisoning or increased lead absorption depends on the measurement of a blood lead level. This is best performed on a venous sample, but finger-stick samples can be used if care is taken to avoid contamination. Most initial blood lead measurements are now performed as screening tests, because children meet some general eligibility criteria or because of parental concern rather than because children have symptoms suggestive of lead poisoning.

Screening

Until 1997, the AAP and CDC recommended that virtually all children have at least one measurement of blood lead beginning at 12 months of age, with a retest at 24 months of age, if possible. Because the prevalence of elevated blood lead levels has decreased substantially, the CDC in 1997 recommended that health departments determine a lead screening strategy for their jurisdictions on the basis of prevalence of housing risks and children with blood lead levels ≥10 mg/dL. However, regardless of the local recommendation, federal policy requires that all children enrolled in Medicaid receive screening blood lead tests at ages 12 and 24 months and that blood lead screening be performed for children 36 to 72 months of age who have not been screened previously.[38] Most children with elevated blood lead levels are Medicaid eligible. The CDC Advisory Committee on Childhood Lead Poisoning Prevention has proposed criteria by which a state might become exempt from this requirement,[39] but they have not yet been implemented.

Blood lead screening and assessments of risks for exposures to lead vary considerably by locale from universal blood lead screening to application of targeted blood lead testing determined by risk assessment tools. Clinicians should consult city, county, or state health departments to determine the appropriate recommendations for their jurisdiction. This information is available for most states on the CDC Web site (http://www.cdc.gov/nceh/lead/programs. htm). Children not on Medicaid and residing in states with no screening policy should have blood lead testing in accordance with Medicaid guidelines. The sensitivities of personal risk questionnaires and other substitutes for measuring blood lead levels vary by population assessed and often are unacceptably low.

Children of all ages who are recent immigrants, refugees, or adoptees have an increased prevalence of elevated—sometimes very elevated—blood lead levels and, thus, should be screened at the earliest opportunity. Those 6 months to 6 years of age and older children, as warranted, should be tested again 3 to 6 months after moving into permanent residences.[25] These children may have had lead exposure in their native country, but it is also possible that their exposure occurred in unsuitable housing once they arrived in the United States. The CDC Web site has a toolkit that discusses risks for these children.

Because of lead's effects on the developing fetus, some states have developed lead screening guidelines for pregnant women. The CDC recently published guidelines on the screening of pregnant women for lead, medical and environmental management, and follow-up of mothers and infants when maternal lead levels are ≥5 µg/dL.[40] Care of the infant includes measuring cord or neonatal blood lead to establish a baseline; further management guidelines depend on baseline blood lead level. Lead is transmitted in human milk. However, because breastfeeding is an optimal source of infant nutrition and is associated with many beneficial aspects of growth and development, the guideline calls for an interruption of breastfeeding only if the maternal blood lead level is ≥40 µg/dL; above this level, women should pump and discard their milk until after their blood lead level decreases below 40 µg/dL. These breastfeeding infants require repeated blood lead evaluations and potentially other medical and environmental evaluations to ensure that their blood lead levels are not increasing excessively.

Diagnostic Testing

Some experienced clinicians measure the blood lead level in children with growth retardation, speech or language dysfunction, anemia, and attentional or behavioral disorders, especially if the parents have a specific interest in lead or in health effects from environmental chemicals. However, persistent elevation of blood lead levels into school age is unusual, even if peak blood lead level at 2 years of age was high and the child's housing has not been abated. Thus, a relatively low blood lead level in a school-aged child does not rule out earlier lead poisoning. If the question of current lead poisoning arises, however, the only reliable way to make a diagnosis is with blood lead measurement. Hair[41] or urine lead levels give no useful information and should not be performed.

MANAGEMENT OF CLINICAL AND LOW-LEVEL LEAD TOXICITY

Management should be provided to all children with a blood lead level of 10 µg/dL or greater[24] (see Table 31.2). Proper management includes finding and eliminating the source of the lead, instruction in proper hygienic measures (personal and household), optimizing the child's diet and nutritional status, and close follow-up (see Tables 31.3 and 31.4). Because most children with higher blood lead levels live in or visit regularly a home with deteriorating lead paint, successful therapy depends on eliminating the child's exposure. Any treatment regimen that does not control environmental exposure to lead is considered inadequate. Pediatricians should refer poisoned children to local public health offices for environmental assessment of the child's residence(s). Public health staff should conduct a thorough investigation of the child's environment and family lifestyle for sources of lead.

Deteriorated lead paint is the most common source of exposure. However, other sources that should be considered include tableware, cosmetics such as surma and kohl, home remedies, dietary supplements of calcium, tap water, and parental occupation. Some children will have persistently elevated blood lead levels without access to lead paint. Their exposure may come from any of the sources listed in Table 31.1. Blood lead levels should decrease as the child passes the age of 2 years or so, and a stable or increasing blood lead level past that age is likely to be attributable to ongoing exposure. In children who have spent prolonged periods in a leaded environment, blood lead levels will decrease more slowly after exposure ceases,[42] probably because bone stores are greater.

The CDC Advisory Committee on Childhood Lead Poisoning Prevention issued case management guidelines for children with lead poisoning in March 2002.[43] These guidelines should be consulted as needed.

Although there are no studies that have identified effective strategies to reduce blood lead levels <10 µg/dL, guidelines for potential strategies for managing blood lead levels <10 µg/dL have been published by the CDC Advisory Committee on Childhood Lead Poisoning Prevention.[24] Because nutritional deficiencies can influence lead absorption and may have their own associations with health outcomes independent of lead exposures, specific attention should be paid to identifying and treating iron deficiency and ensuring adequate calcium and zinc intake.

Chelation therapy for children with blood lead levels of 20 to 44 µg/dL can be expected to lower blood lead levels but has not been shown to reverse or

Table 31.2: Recommended Follow-up Actions, According to Blood Lead Level (BLL)*	
BLL (µg/dL)	**ACTIONS**
<10	Continued surveillance For a child whose BLL is approaching 10 µg/dL, more frequent blood lead screening (ie, more than annually) might be appropriate, particularly if the child is aged <2 years old, was tested at the start of warm weather when BLLs tend to increase, or is at high risk of lead exposures[24]
10–14	Obtain a confirmatory venous BLL within 1 month; if still within this range: ■ Provide education to decrease lead exposure ■ Repeat BLL test within 3 months
15–19	Obtain a confirmatory venous BLL within 1 month; if still within this range: ■ Take a careful environmental history ■ Provide education to decrease lead exposure and to decrease lead absorption ■ Repeat BLL test within 2 months
20–44	Obtain a confirmatory venous BLL within 1 week; if still within this range: ■ Conduct a complete medical history (including an environmental evaluation and nutritional assessment) and physical examination ■ Provide education to decrease lead exposure and lead absorption ■ Refer the patient to the local health department or provide case management that should include a detailed environmental investigation with lead hazard reduction and appropriate referrals for support services ■ Chelation not currently recommended for BLLs <45 µg/dL
45–69	Obtain a confirmatory venous BLL within 2 days; if still within this range: ■ Conduct a complete medical history (including an environmental evaluation and nutritional assessment) and a physical examination ■ Provide education to decrease lead exposure and lead absorption ■ Refer the patient to the local health department or provide case management that should include a detailed environmental investigation with lead hazard reduction and appropriate referrals for support services ■ Begin chelation therapy in consultation with clinicians experienced in lead toxicity therapy
≥70	Hospitalize the patient and begin medical treatment, including parenteral chelation therapy, immediately in consultation with clinicians experienced in lead toxicity therapy ■ Obtain a confirmatory BLL immediately ■ The rest of the management should be as noted for management of children with BLLs between 45 and 69 µg/dL

*Adapted from Centers for Disease Control and Prevention.[43]

Table 31.3: Clinical Evaluation*

Medical History

Ask about

- Symptoms
- Developmental history
- Mouthing activities
- Pica
- Previous blood lead level measurements
- Family/maternal history of exposures to lead

Environmental History

Paint and soil exposure

- What is the age and general condition of the residence?
- Is there evidence of chewed or peeling paint on woodwork, furniture, or toys?
- How long has the family lived at that residence?
- Have there been recent renovations or repairs in the house?
- Are there other sites where the child spends significant amounts of time?
- What is the character of indoor play areas?
- Do outdoor play areas contain bare soil that may be contaminated?
- How does the family attempt to control dust/dirt?

Relevant Behavioral Characteristics of the Child

- To what degree does the child exhibit hand-to-mouth activity?
- Does the child exhibit pica?
- Are the child's hands washed before meals and snacks?

Exposures to and Behaviors of Household Members

- What are the occupations of adult household members?
- What are the hobbies of household members? (Fishing, working with ceramics or stained glass, and hunting are examples of hobbies that involve risk for lead exposure)
- Are painted materials or unusual materials burned in household fireplaces?

Miscellaneous Questions

- Does the home contain vinyl miniblinds made overseas and purchased before 1997?
- Does the child receive or have access to imported food, cosmetics, or folk remedies?
- Is food prepared or stored in imported pottery or metal vessels?

Nutritional History

- Take a dietary history
- Evaluate the child's iron status using appropriate laboratory tests
- Ask about history of food stamps or Special Supplemental Nutrition Program for Women, Infants, and Children program (WIC) participation

Physical Examination

- Pay particular attention to the neurologic examination and to the child's psychosocial and language development

*Adapted from Centers for Disease Control and Prevention.[43]

Table 31.4: Schedule for Follow-up Blood Lead Level (BLL) Testing*

VENOUS BLL (μg/dL)	EARLY FOLLOW-UP (FIRST 2–4 TESTS AFTER IDENTIFICATION)	LATE FOLLOW-UP (AFTER BLL BEGINS TO DECLINE)
10–14	3 months	6–9 months
15–19	1–3 months	3–6 months
20–24	1–3 months	1–3 months
25–44	2 weeks–1 month	1 month
≥45	As soon as possible	Chelation with subsequent follow-up

*Adapted from Centers for Disease Control and Prevention.[43]
Note: Seasonal variation of BLLs exists and may be more apparent in colder climate areas. Greater exposure in the summer months may necessitate more frequent follow-up. Some clinicians may choose to repeat blood lead tests on all new patients within a month to see whether their BLL is increasing more quickly than anticipated.

diminish cognitive impairment or other behavioral or neuropsychological effects of lead.[44]

If the blood lead level is greater than 45 μg/dL and the exposure has been controlled, treatment should begin. A pediatrician experienced in managing children with lead poisoning should be consulted—these can be found through the AAP Council on Environmental Health, at hospitals that participated in the clinical trial of succimer,[44] at Pediatric Environmental Health Specialty Units, or through lead programs at state health departments (http://www.cdc.gov/nceh/lead/grants/contacts/CLPPP%20Map.htm). Detailed treatment guidelines were published by the AAP in 1995.[45]

Frequently Asked Questions

Q   I'm worried that my child has any detectable lead in his blood. How can I eliminate exposure?

A   In children with low blood lead levels, recommended interventions have to be not only effective but also very safe. Generally, applicable recommendations include taking an environmental history to identify potential sources for lead exposure, testing the child for iron deficiency and correcting it if it is found, testing drinking water, inspecting any older building in which the child spends time for evidence of deteriorating paint, and then following US Department of Housing and Urban Development guidelines for necessary household renovation. Having a child with a blood lead level of 5 or 10 μg/dL may be a source of concern, but no specific drug therapies have been tested and shown to be safe and effective at these low levels.

Q *We have imported ceramic dishes. Is it safe to use them?*

A Some imported ceramics contain lead. Of particular concern have been pottery from Mexico and ceramic ware from China. At the dishes wear, become chipped or cracked, lead can leach from the dishes into foods. Some imported dishes labeled as "lead-free," have been found to contain unsafe amounts of lead. There are many safe alternatives, so using such dishes should be avoided. The US Food and Drug Administration began regulating lead in glazes used on dishes made in the United States in the 1980s and further strengthened regulations in the 1990s. Dishes made in the United States before these regulations took effect may contain lead.

Q *We have vinyl miniblinds. Should I get rid of them?*

A In the mid-1990s, some imported, nonglossy vinyl miniblinds were found to contain lead. Children who touch these miniblinds and put their fingers in their mouths may ingest small amounts of lead. Sunlight and heat can break down the blinds, causing release of lead-contaminated dust. If you purchase new miniblinds, look for products with labels that say "new formulation" or "nonleaded formula." Older ones must be discarded if they have begun to chalk or deteriorate.

Q *Is there still lead in canned food?*

A Cans with soldered seams can add lead to foods. In the United States, soldered cans have been replaced by seamless aluminum containers, but some imported canned products still have lead-soldered seams.

Q *What about testing for lead in water?*

A If you are using tap water to reconstitute infant formula or juice or there has been local concern, you may want to have your water tested. To help determine whether your water might contain lead, call the EPA Safe Drinking Water Hotline at 800-426-4791 or your local health department to find out about testing your water. Well water should be tested for lead when the well is new and tested again when a pregnant woman, infant or child less than 18 years of age moves into the home; for a discussion of well water for infants, see the AAP policy statement on drinking water from private wells.[46] Most water filters remove lead.

Q *How can I tell if a toy has lead paint or is made of lead?*

A Toys are not all routinely tested for lead. Many toys are imported from countries with poorly enforced safety rules by companies that do not test the toys before selling them. The AAP advises parents to monitor the Consumer Product Safety Commission Web site for notices of recalls and to avoid nonbrand toys and toys from discount shops and private vendors. Old and used toys should be examined for damage and clues to the origin of the toy. If the toy is damaged or worn or from a country with a history of poor monitoring of manufacturing practices, the safest action is to remove it from use. Be particularly attentive to costume jewelry and other small metal pieces that can be swallowed.

Q What is the correct procedure to follow when a child is witnessed ingesting a piece of lead-containing paint?

A A diagnostic lead level is indicated when a parent expresses concern about ingestion of potential lead-containing substances. Such a test should be done right away, because it is likely that the child ingested similar substances even before someone identified it as a problem. With ingestions, blood lead levels rise rapidly (within hours to days) and can continue to rise during bowel transit of the object. Once the object has been excreted, the blood level falls to a new body equilibrium over the next month. An abdominal x-ray to assess presence of lead-containing substances is indicated if a child's lead level is 45 µg/dL or higher. X-rays of long bones to assess "lead lines" (ie, dense metaphyseal lines of growth arrest) are not indicated.

This might be a good occasion to also assess the child's iron status, because iron deficiency is associated with more efficient absorption of lead from the gut, and pica behavior has sometimes been associated with iron-deficient status. Low ferritin, even in the absence anemia, low mean corpuscular volume (MCV), or elevated red cell distribution width (RDW), should be treated with therapeutic doses of iron.

It would also be wise to check the paint to see whether lead is present. In homes built before 1978, paint chips should be assumed to contain lead unless tested and proven otherwise. Your local or state health department can answer your questions about obtaining a home inspection to check for lead.

Basophilic stippling may be seen, but generally at lead levels much higher than are common today. Also consider vitamin B_{12} and folate deficiencies as causes of basophilic stippling.

Q Should iron be prescribed for patients with lead levels between 10 and 20 µg/dL?

A Not unless they are iron deficient. Theoretically, iron could affect absorption of lead from the gut. Lead is taken up by the iron absorption machinery and secondarily blocks iron through competitive inhibition. There are no supporting research data to demonstrate the efficacy of prescribing therapeutic iron to all children with elevated lead. Iron therapy should not be prescribed unless iron status is deficient (low ferritin or another indicator).

Resources

National Lead Information Center
422 South Clinton Avenue
Rochester, NY 14620
Phone: 1-800-424-LEAD
Fax: (585) 232-3111

Office of Healthy Homes and Lead Hazard Control, Department of Housing and Urban Development

Web site: www.hud.gov/offices/lead

US Environmental Protection Agency Federal Plan for Eliminating Childhood Lead Poisoning

Web site: http://yosemite.epa.gov/ochp/ochpweb.nsf/content/whatwe_tf_proj.htm

References

1. Schwartz J. Low-level lead exposure and children's IQ: a meta-analysis and search for a threshold. *Environ Res.* 1994;65(1):42-55

2. Pocock SJ, Smith M, Baghurst P. Environmental lead and children's intelligence: a systematic review of the epidemiological evidence. *BMJ.* 1994;309(6963):1189-1197

3. Needleman HL, Gunnoe C, Leviton A, et al. Deficits in psychologic and classroom performance of children with elevated dentine lead levels. *N Engl J Med.* 1979;300(13):689-695

4. Bellinger D, Needleman HL, Bromfield R, Mintz M. A followup study of the academic attainment and classroom behavior of children with elevated dentine lead levels. *Bio Trace Element Res.* 1984;6:207-223

5. Chen AM, Cai B, Dietrich KN, Radcliffe J, Rogan WJ. Lead exposure, IQ, and behavior in urban 5- to 7-year-olds: does lead affect behavior only by lowering IQ? *Pediatrics.* 2007;119(3):e650-e658

6. Chisolm JJ Jr, Kaplan E. Lead poisoning in childhood—comprehensive management and prevention. *J Pediatr.* 1968;73(6):942-950

7. Centers for Disease Control. *Preventing Lead Poisoning in Young Children.* Washington, DC: US Department of Health, Education, and Welfare; 1978

8. Lanphear BP, Dietrich KN, Auinger P, Cox C. Cognitive deficits associated with blood lead concentrations of <10 μg/dL in US children and adolescents. *Public Health Rep.* 2000;115(6):521-529

9. Canfield RL, Henderson CR, Cory-Slechta DA, Cox C, Jusko TA, Lanphear BP. Intellectual impairment in children with blood lead concentrations below 10 μg per deciliter. *N Engl J Med.* 2003;348(16):1517-1526

10. Bellinger DC, Needleman HL. Intellectual impairment and blood lead levels. *N Engl J Med.* 2003;349(5):500-502

11. American Academy of Pediatrics, Committee on Environmental Health. Screening for elevated blood lead levels. *Pediatrics.* 1998;101(6):1072-1078

12. Patterson CC. *Natural Levels of Lead in Humans.* Chapel Hill, NC: Institute for Environmental Studies, University of North Carolina at Chapel Hill; 1982

13. Pirkle JL, Brody DJ, Gunter EW, et al. The decline in blood lead levels in the United States. The National Health and Nutrition Examination Surveys (NHANES). *JAMA.* 1994;272(4):284-291

14. Jones RL, Homa DM, Meyer PA, et al. Trends in blood lead levels and blood lead testing among US children aged 1 to 5 years, 1988–2004. *Pediatrics.* 2009;123(3):e376-e385

15. von Lindern I, Spalinger S, Petroysan V, von Braun M. Assessing remedial effectiveness through the blood lead:soil/dust lead relationship at the Bunker Hill Superfund Site in the Silver Valley of Idaho. *Sci Total Environ.* 2003;303(1-2):139-170

16. Charney E, Sayre J, Coulter M. Increased lead absorption in inner city children: where does the lead come from? *Pediatrics.* 1980;65(2):226-231

17. Freeman NC, Sheldon L, Jimenez M, Melnyk L, Pellizari ED, Berry M. Contribution of children's activities to lead contamination of food. *J Expo Anal Environ Epidemiol.* 2001;11(5):407-413

18. Jacobs DE, Clickner RP, Zhou JY, et al. The prevalence of lead-based paint hazards in U.S. housing. *Environ Health Perspect.* 2002;110(10):A599-A606

19. Farfel MR, Chisolm JJ. An evaluation of experimental practices for abatement of residential lead-based paint: Report on a pilot project. *Environ Res.* 1991;55(2):199-212

20. Centers for Disease Control and Prevention. Death of a child after ingestion of a metallic charm—Minnesota, 2006. *MMWR Morb Mortal Wkly Rep.* 2006;55(12):340-341

21. Lanphear BP, Hornung R, Khoury JC, et al. Low-level environmental lead exposure and children's intellectual function: an international pooled analysis. *Environ Health Perspect.* 2005;113(7):894-899

22. Chen A, Dietrich KN, Radcliffe J, Ware JH, Rogan WJ. IQ and blood lead from 2 to 7 years: are the effects in older children the residual from high blood lead in 2-year-olds? *Environ Health Perspect.* 2005;113(5):597-601

23. Centers for Disease Control and Prevention. *Screening Young Children for Lead Poisoning: Guidance for State and Local Public Health Officials.* Atlanta: CDC; 1997

24. Binns HJ, Campbell C, Brown MJ. Interpreting and managing blood lead levels of less than 10 µg/dL in children and reducing childhood exposure to lead: recommendations of the Centers for Disease Control and Prevention Advisory Committee on Childhood Lead Poisoning Prevention. *Pediatrics.* 2007;120(5):e1285-e1298

25. Centers for Disease Control and Prevention. Elevated blood lead levels in refugee children— New Hampshire, 2003–2004. *MMWR Morb Mortal Wkly Rep.* 2005;54(2):42-46

26. Schwartz J, Otto D. Lead and minor hearing impairment. *Arch Environ Health.* 1991;46(5): 300-305

27. Bhattacharya A, Shukla R, Bornschein RL, Dietrich KN, Keith R. Lead effects on postural balance of children. *Environ Health Perspect.* 1990;89:35-42

28. Sciarillo WG, Alexander G, Farrell KP. Lead exposure and child behavior. *Am J Public Health.* 1992;82(10):1356-1360

29. Needleman HL, Schell A, Bellinger D, Leviton A, Allred EN. The long-term effects of exposure to low doses of lead in childhood: an 11-year follow-up report. *N Engl J Med.* 1990;322(2):83-88

30. Needleman HL, Riess J, Tobin M, Biesecker G, Greenhouse J. Bone lead levels and delinquent behavior. *JAMA.* 1996;275(5):363-369

31. Rice D. Behavioral effects of lead: commonalities between experimental and epidemiologic data. *Environ Health Perspect.* 1996;104(Suppl):337-351

32. Markovac J, Goldstein GW. Picomolar concentrations of lead stimulate brain protein kinase C. *Nature.* 1988;334(6177):71-73

33. Cecil KM, Brubaker CJ, Adler CM, et al. Decreased brain volume in adults with childhood lead exposure. *PloS Med.* 2008;5:e112

34. Brubaker CJ, Schmithorst VJ, Haynes EN, et al. Altered myelination and axonal integrity in adults with childhood lead exposure: a diffusion tensor imaging study. *Neurotoxicology.* 2009;30(6):867-875

35. Yuan W, Holland S, Cecil KM, et al. The impact of early childhood lead exposure on brain organization: a functional magnetic resonance imaging study of language function. *Pediatrics.* 2006;118(3):971-977

36. McIntire MS, Wolf GL, Angle CR. Red cell lead and d-amino levulinic acid dehydratase. *Clin Toxicol.* 1973;6(2):183-188

37. Selevan SG, Rice D, Hogan KD, Euling SY, Pfahles-Hutchens A, Bethel J. Blood lead concentration and delayed puberty in girls. *N Engl J Med*. 2003;348(16):1527-1536

38. Centers for Disease Control and Prevention, Advisory Committee on Childhood Lead Poisoning Prevention. Recommendations for blood lead screening of young children enrolled in Medicaid: targeting a group at high risk. *MMWR Recomm Rep*. 2002;49(RR-14):1-13

39. Wengrovitz AM, Brown MJ. Recommendations for blood lead screening of Medicaid-eligible children aged 1–5 years: an updated approach to targeting a group at high risk. *MMWR Recomm Rep*. 2009;58(RR-9):1-11

40. Centers for Disease Control and Prevention. *Guidelines for the Identification and Management of Lead Exposure in Pregnant and Lactating Women*. Atlanta, GA: US Department of Health and Human Services, 2010. Available at: www.cdc.gov/nceh/lead/publications/LeadandPregnancy2010.pdf. Accessed March 22, 2011

41. Esteban E, Rubin CH, Jones RL, Noonan G. Hair and blood as substrates for screening children for lead poisoning. *Arch Environ Health*. 1999;54(6):436-440

42. Manton WI, Angle CR, Stanek K, Reese Y, Kuehnemann T. Acquisition and retention of lead by young children. *Environ Res*. 2000;82(1):60-80

43. Centers for Disease Control and Prevention. *Managing Elevated Blood Lead Levels Among Young Children: Recommendations from the Advisory Committee on Childhood Lead Poisoning Prevention*. Atlanta, GA: Centers for Disease Control and Prevention; 2002

44. Dietrich KN, Ware JH, Salganick M, et al. Effect of chelation therapy on the neuropsychological and behavioral development of lead-exposed children following school entry. *Pediatrics*. 2004;114(1):19-26

45. American Academy of Pediatrics, Committee on Drugs. Treatment guidelines for lead exposure in children. *Pediatrics*. 1995;96(1 Pt 1):155-160

46. American Academy of Pediatrics, Council on Environmental Health and Committee on Infectious Diseases. Drinking water from private wells and risks to children. *Pediatrics*. 2009;123(6):1599-1605

Chapter 32

Mercury

■ ■ ■ ■ ■ ■

Mercury (Hg) occurs in 3 forms: the metallic element (Hg^0, quicksilver or elemental mercury), inorganic salts (Hg^{1+}, or mercurous salts, and Hg^{2+}, or mercuric salts), and organic compounds (methylmercury, ethylmercury, and phenylmercury). Solubility, reactivity, biological effects, and toxicity vary among these forms. Mercury has been used for more than 3000 years in medicine and industry.

Naturally occurring mercury sources include cinnabar (ore) and fossil fuels, such as coal and petroleum. Environmental contamination has resulted from mining, smelting, and industrial discharges (principally by burning fossil fuels). Atmospheric mercury contributes to local and global contamination. Mercury in lakes and stream sediments can be converted by bacteria into organic mercury compounds (eg, methylmercury) that accumulate in the food chain and progressively increase in concentration as they ascend the food chain (ie, biomagnification). The result is that certain predator fish from oceans (eg, shark, tuna, swordfish) or freshwater (eg, bass, pike, trout, etc) may contain higher levels of mercury. Very high exposures to methylmercury in fish in the 1950s following industrial release of mercury into Minamata Bay, Japan, caused serious disturbances in fetal brain development among exposed pregnant women and thousands of cases of acute adult methylmercury toxicity, and an estimated 200 000 individuals had neurologic manifestations of chronic methylmercury exposure.[1] To reduce consumption of most highly contaminated fish species, states have issued advisories about consumption of locally caught fish, which may vary by fish species or body of water or be applied on a statewide basis. Recommendations on limiting intake of large ocean fish, such as tuna, swordfish, king mackerel, tilefish, and shark have been issued by the US Environmental Protection Agency (EPA) and Food and Drug Administration (FDA).

Methylmercury has also been used as a fungicide on seed grains. Consumption of mercury-treated seed grains caused widespread mercury poisoning among people in Iraq and China and has been responsible for neurologic disorders in wildlife.[2]

Elemental mercury has been used in sphygmomanometers, thermometers, and thermostat switches. Dental amalgams contain 40% to 50% mercury as well as silver and other metals. Fluorescent light bulbs, including tubes and compact bulbs, and disc ("button") batteries also contain mercury. Indiscriminate disposal of these items is a source of environmental mercury contamination when they are buried in landfills or burned in waste incinerators rather than recycled. Elemental mercury also is used in some folk remedies, such as those of Santeria, practiced by some groups of Hispanic Americans.[3,4]

ROUTES OF EXPOSURE

Elemental Mercury

Elemental mercury is a liquid at room temperature and readily volatilizes to a colorless and odorless vapor. When inhaled, elemental mercury vapor easily passes through pulmonary alveolar membranes and enters the blood, where it distributes primarily into red blood cells and is carried to all tissues of the body, including crossing the blood-brain barrier. Once in a cell, mercury is oxidized to Hg^{2+}, which hinders its excretion. Approximately 80% of inhaled mercury is absorbed in the body. In contrast, less than 0.1% of elemental mercury is absorbed from the gastrointestinal tract after ingestion, and only minimal absorption occurs with dermal exposure.[5]

Inorganic Mercury

Inorganic mercury salts are poorly absorbed after ingestion, although mercuric salts tend to be extremely caustic.

Organic Mercury

In general, organic mercury compounds are lipid soluble and are well absorbed from the gastrointestinal tract. Methylmercury is 95% absorbed after ingestion, contributing to concern about consumption of methylmercury-contaminated fish.[6] Methylmercury passes through the placenta, is concentrated in the fetus, and is transferred into human milk. This form of mercury also is well absorbed after inhalation. Phenylmercury is well absorbed after ingestion and dermal contact. In contrast to other organic mercury compounds, the carbon-mercury chemical bond of phenylmercury is relatively unstable, resulting in the release of elemental mercury that can be inhaled and absorbed across pulmonary membranes.

Ethylmercury is found in thimerosal (merthiolate) and has been used as an antiseptic and as a preservative for vaccines and other drug therapies. Thimerosal contains 49.6% mercury by weight. Until fall 1999, many vaccines had 12.5 to 25 μg of mercury in each dose. In 1999, recognizing the potential for increasing exposure as more vaccines were added to the routinely recommended immunization schedule for children, the American Academy of Pediatrics (AAP), along with the American Academy of Family Physicians, the Advisory Committee on Immunization Practices of the Centers for Disease Control and Prevention (CDC), and the US Public Health Service issued a joint recommendation that thimerosal be removed from vaccines as quickly as possible.[7,8] Since 2001, no new vaccine licensed by the FDA for use in children has contained thimerosal as a preservative. All vaccines routinely recommended for children younger than 6 years of age, except for influenza vaccine in multidose vials, have been free of thimerosal, or contain only trace amounts. Multidose vials of influenza vaccine contain thimerosal as a preservative, but single-dose units of influenza vaccine formulated for pediatric use are thimerosal free. Meningococcal conjugate vaccine, available as 2 different thimerosal-free products, is the preferred vaccine for children and adolescents. Multidose vials of a third meningococcal vaccine contain thimerosal.

SYSTEMS AFFECTED AND CLINICAL EFFECTS

Elemental Mercury

At high concentrations, mercury vapor inhalation produces an acute necrotizing bronchitis and pneumonitis, which can lead to death from respiratory failure.[9] Fatalities have resulted from heating elemental mercury in inadequately ventilated areas.[10]

Long-term exposure to mercury vapor primarily affects the central nervous system (CNS). Early nonspecific signs include insomnia, forgetfulness, loss of appetite, and mild tremor and may be misdiagnosed as psychiatric illness. Continued exposure leads to progressive tremor and erethism, characterized by red palms, emotional lability, hypertension, and visual and memory impairments.[11-16] Salivation, excessive sweating, and hemoconcentration are accompanying signs. Mercury also accumulates in kidney tissues. Renal toxicity includes proteinuria or nephrotic syndrome, alone or in addition to other signs of mercury exposure.[17,18] Isolated renal effects may be immunologic in origin.

Mercury exposure from dental amalgams has provoked concerns about subclinical or unusual neurologic effects. The federal governments of Norway, Finland, Denmark, and Sweden have enacted legislation requiring that dental patients receive informed consent information about the dental restorative material that will be used. In the United States, a few state governments have enacted informed consent legislation for dental patients receiving dental restorations.[19]Although dental amalgams are a source of mercury exposure and are associated with slightly higher urinary mercury excretion, there is no scientific evidence for any measurable clinical toxic effects other than rare hypersensitivity reactions.[20-25] Two randomized clinical trials failed to demonstrate neurobehavioral or neuropsychological differences between children exposed to dental amalgam and those who were not.[26-28]

Inorganic Mercury

Mercuric bichloride (Hg^{2+}) is well described by its common name, corrosive sublimate. Ingestions usually are inadvertent or with suicidal intent, and gastrointestinal tract ulceration or perforation and hemorrhage are rapidly produced, followed by circulatory collapse. Breakdown of intestinal mucosal barriers leads to extensive mercury absorption and distribution to the kidneys. Acute renal toxic effects include proximal tubular necrosis and anuria.

Acrodynia, or childhood mercury poisoning, was frequently reported in the 1940s among infants exposed to calomel teething powders containing mercurous chloride.[29,30] Cases also have been reported in infants exposed to phenylmercury used as a fungicidal diaper rinse[31] and in children exposed to phenylmercuric acetate from interior latex paint.[32] Children's individual susceptibility to develop acrodynia is poorly understood, but a maculopapular rash, swollen and painful extremities, peripheral neuropathy, hypertension, and renal tubular dysfunction develop in affected children.[33,34]

Organic Mercury

Organic mercury toxicity occurs with long-term exposure and affects the CNS. Signs progress from paresthesias to ataxia, followed by generalized weakness, visual and hearing impairment, tremor and muscle spasticity, and then coma and death. Organic mercury also is a potent teratogen, causing disruption of the normal patterns of neuronal migration and nerve cell histology in the developing brain. In the Minamata Bay disaster with contaminated fish and the Iraq epidemic with contaminated seed grain, mothers who were asymptomatic or showed mild toxic effects gave birth to severely affected infants. Typically, the infants seemed normal at birth, but psychomotor retardation, blindness, deafness, and seizures developed over time.[35]

Because the fetus and infant are more susceptible to the neurotoxic effects of methylmercury, investigators have looked for subclinical effects among children whose mothers' diets include large amounts of fish or marine mammals containing methylmercury and whose blood mercury concentrations are higher than those commonly seen in the United States. There are 3 such longitudinal studies—one in the Seychelles (islands in the Indian Ocean about 1000 miles off the east coast of Africa), one in the Faroe Islands (islands off the coast of Iceland), and the third from New Zealand. Approximately 900 Faroese children were evaluated at 7 and 14 years of age; higher maternal hair mercury concentrations were associated with deficits in motor, attention, and verbal test results, and these deficits did not change between the test occasions.[36] However, despite similar exposures, this pattern of deficits was not found among 643 children examined through 9 years of age in the Seychelles.[37] Data from all 3 studies were evaluated to estimate a dose-response relationship between maternal mercury and childhood IQ; for each increase by 1 part per million (ppm) in maternal hair mercury, child IQ loss was estimated at −0.18 IQ points (95% confidence interval, −0.378 to −0.009).[38] It is possible that results from these studies have limitations attributable to confounding, because seafoods are rich sources of omega-3 fatty acids, which have important beneficial effects on fetal neurodevelopment.[39] Further studies with appropriate biological markers, psychological assessments, and considerations of biologic variations in mercury metabolism may be necessary to clarify effects.[40,41]

The US EPA has reviewed methylmercury toxicity to determine a reference dose for mercury. A reference dose is a daily dosage of a chemical that is likely to be without risk of adverse effects when experienced over a lifetime; it is used to provide a basis for establishing safety standards and guidelines. The US EPA concluded that the reference dose for mercury, on the basis of development of neurobehavioral toxicity, should be established at 0.1 μg/kg per day to achieve a cord blood concentration of <5.8 μg mercury/L—a concentration below which no adverse effects are expected.[42] In the 1999-2002 National Health and Nutrition Examination Survey (NHANES, a series of surveys of the health and nutritional status of the United States population conducted by the CDC), an estimated 6% of US women had a blood total mercury concentration of ≥5.8 μg/L.[43] However, these data may not be representative of women who eat large amounts of fish, nor do they account for concentration of methylmercury in the fetus (a maternal blood mercury concentration of 3.5 μg/L would be expected to achieve a fetal blood mercury concentration of 5.8 μg/L).[44] Analysis of data from adult women gathered in the 1999-2004 National Health and Nutrition Examination Surveys identified 10.4% with a mercury concentration above 3.5 μg/L and 4.7% of women with mercury concentration above 5.8 μg/L. Risk of elevated mercury concentrations was highest among women living in the Northeast or who were of Asian descent or had higher income.[45]

Ethylmercury, although it may have similar toxicity to methylmercury, has been less well studied. A large number of medical/pharmaceutical products (eg, ear and eye drops, eye ointment, nasal sprays, and hemorrhoid relief ointment) may contain thimerosal as a preservative (see www.epa.gov/mercury for a list). Very high exposures to thimerosal-containing products have resulted in toxicity, including acrodynia, chronic mercury toxicity, renal failure, and neuropathy.[46-50] Merthiolate used to irrigate the external auditory canals in a child with tympanostomy tubes caused fatal mercury poisoning.[51]

There has been concern that organic mercury exposure from thimerosal-containing vaccines and other sources has played a role in the growing incidence of autism. However, a substantial number of scientific studies fail to support a causal relationship.[52-60]

DIAGNOSTIC METHODS

Diagnosis of mercury poisoning usually is made on the basis of history and physical examination. Urine and blood tests may demonstrate elevated mercury concentrations. Normal blood mercury concentrations, however, do not exclude mercury poisoning.

Elemental Mercury

Increased mercury vapor concentrations can be measured in exhaled air from people with dental amalgams, but the biological significance is uncertain. Also unclear is the significance of the slight increase in urinary mercury excretion detected after dental amalgams are placed.

Inorganic Mercury

Inorganic mercury exposure can be measured by urinary mercury determination, preferably using a 24-hour urine collection. Results greater than 10 to 20 µg/day are evidence of excessive exposure, and neurologic signs may be present at concentrations greater than 100 µg/L. However, the urinary mercury concentration does not necessarily correlate with chronicity or severity of toxic effects, especially if the mercury exposure has been intermittent or variable in intensity. Whole blood mercury can be measured, but concentrations tend to return to normal (<0.5–1.0 µg/L) within 1 to 2 days after the exposure to inorganic mercury ends.

Organic Mercury

Organic mercury compounds concentrate in red blood cells, so whole blood may be used to diagnose excessive exposure. In a 1999 to 2002 sample of the US population, the geometric mean blood mercury concentrations were 0.33 µg/L for children 1 to 5 years old and 0.92 µg/L for women 16 to 49 years old.[43] Blood mercury concentrations rarely exceed more than 1.5 µg/L in the unexposed population. Methylmercury also distributes into growing hair, thus providing a noninvasive means to estimate body burden and blood concentration over time in research studies. In the general population, the mercury concentration in hair is usually 1 part per million (1 µg/g) or less.[61] The ratio of hair mercury (µg/g) to blood mercury (µg/L) is approximately 0.25 in adults and varies with child age.[62] Although measuring hair mercury concentration is a well established method to quantify methylmercury exposure for research purposes, hair sampling for mercury is generally not useful in the clinical setting, particularly when performed by an outside source, such as a commercial laboratory. Typically, in this scenario, the rationale for measuring exposure is unknown, control for external contamination is usually not considered, and collection protocols are usually ad hoc.[63] There is no clinical cut point to establish toxicity on the basis of a child's hair mercury concentration. An elevated hair mercury concentration measured by an outside laboratory should, therefore, usually be followed up with a blood mercury measurement to establish current exposure levels.

TREATMENT

The most important and most effective treatment is to identify the mercury source and end the exposure. Mercury accumulates in blood and CNS and renal tissues and is very slowly eliminated. Chelating agents have been used to enhance mercury elimination, but whether chelation reduces toxic effects or speeds recovery in people who have been poisoned is unclear. Use of chelation agents (dimercaprol [BAL in oil], dimercaptosuccinic acid [DMSA, succimer], and 2,3-dimercaptopropane-1-sulfonate] DMPS, dimaval]) for severe to asymptomatic inorganic mercury poisoning has been reported.[14-16,64-69] There is no chelation agent approved by the FDA that is effective for methylmercury poisoning. Dimercaprol may increase the mercury concentration in the brain and should not be used in cases of methylmercury poisoning.[70] Succimer has been used for some severe organic mercury poisoning.[71] All mercury poisoning should be treated in consultation with a physician experienced in managing children with mercury poisoning. Children who have had mercury poisoning need periodic follow-up neurologic examinations and developmental assessments by a pediatrician and may need referral for further neurological and developmental evaluations.

Chelation for chronic mercury exposures to improve nervous system symptoms has been proposed by some as treatment of autism spectrum disorders. As noted in more detail in Chapter 46, monitored clinical trials are lacking, and chelation presents some serious dangers for children. Thus, chelation as a treatment for autism spectrum disorders is not indicated and may, in fact, be dangerous.[72]

PREVENTION OF EXPOSURE

Many mercury compounds are no longer sold in the United States. Electronic equipment has replaced many mercury-containing oral thermometers and sphygmomanometers in medical settings. Additionally, because the costs of abatement after a mercury spill (even a spill as seemingly trivial as a broken sphygmomanometer) can be very expensive, elimination of mercury has significant cost savings. Pediatricians who still have mercury-containing devices should safely eliminate their use, and families should be encouraged to do the same.[73]

Sources of mercury in school settings should also be catalogued and safely eliminated. Local programs for the safe disposal of mercury-containing devices may be available.

Organic mercury fungicides, including phenylmercury (once used in latex paints), are no longer licensed for commercial use. Newer enclosed methods for preparing mercury amalgams have reduced the likelihood of mercury spillage and exposure during dental amalgam preparation.

The amount of mercury in thermometers is small and usually insufficient to produce clinically significant exposure. If a mercury thermometer breaks, the bead of elemental mercury should be carefully rolled onto a sheet of paper and then put in a jar or an airtight container for appropriate disposal. Use of a vacuum cleaner should be avoided, because it causes elemental mercury to vaporize in the air, creating greater health risks.[74] If a thermometer spill occurs on carpet, the affected carpet area needs to be carefully removed and discarded. Specific instructions on mercury spills from broken thermometers are available (www.epa.gov/mercury). In the event of a larger elemental mercury spill, consultation with the local health department and a certified environmental cleaning company is advised.[75]

Compact fluorescent light bulbs and other fluorescent light bulbs contain small amounts of mercury. In the event of breakage, the room should be aired out, and forced air heating and air conditioning systems should be turned off for 15 minutes. Special instructions for cleaning broken debris and mercury from broken bulbs off hard surfaces and carpets or rugs are found on the EPA Web site (www.epa.gov/mercury). Clothing in contact with the broken bulb should be discarded, but clothes exposed to mercury vapor during cleanup can be washed. Local programs for the safe disposal of used fluorescent light bulbs are available in many areas (see www.epa.gov/mercury).

Most regulatory standards or advisories pertain to the workplace. Nonoccupational standards have been established by the EPA for drinking water (2 µg/L) and by the FDA for fish (1 part per million) and bottled drinking water (2 µg/L).

The FDA has set a regulatory limit for methylmercury in commercial fish of 1 part per million (1 µg/g).[76] In March 2001, the FDA issued an advisory to pregnant women, women of childbearing age, nursing mothers, and young children to avoid consumption of shark, king mackerel, swordfish, and tilefish. For other types of fish, including canned light tuna, the FDA has advised that consumption by children, pregnant women, and those who may become pregnant be kept below 12 oz per week. (Canned albacore and fresh tuna have approximately 3 times higher methylmercury concentration than does canned light tuna.) The risks of exposure to methylmercury from fish have to be balanced with the health benefits of eating fish. Fish are an important source of lean protein and contain unsaturated fatty acids (including omega-3 fatty acids) and other beneficial nutrients important to child development. For some populations, locally caught fish may be the only good alternative for a nutritious diet, but local advisories should be consulted, because fish from some lakes and streams have higher concentrations of contaminants than commercially available fish. Beneficial effects on child IQ from fish intake (>2 meals/week) during pregnancy must be weighed with negative effects from mercury in the fish.[77] If fish with lower mercury levels are available, then it is prudent to substitute these rather than eat fish that have methylmercury advisories. There are many types of commercial fish and shellfish with low methylmercury concentration, some of which are also high in omega-3 fatty acids (salmon, pollock, scallops), which are critical nutrients for the development of the fetal brain. Mercury content of many various commercial seafood varieties can be found on the FDA Web site (see Table 32.1 for a partial list).

Although the levels of mercury in commercial fish are regulated by the FDA, the federal government does not regulate the levels of mercury in fish caught for sport. Because of the potential for mercury contamination, states have issued advisories recommending public limits or the avoidance of consuming certain fish caught for sport from specific bodies of water. These include freshwater species, such as trout, walleye, pike, muskie, and bass, which may have levels of mercury that would result in substantial mercury intakes from a meal of fish. Current state fish consumption advisories can be found on the EPA Web site (http://www.epa.gov/OST/fish).

Vaporized mercury can contaminate home air when mercury spills occur (eg, broken thermometers or compact fluorescent light bulbs). In the event of a spill, the Agency for Toxic Substances and Disease Registry suggests that acceptable residential air mercury levels should not exceed 0.5 µg/cubic meter.[78]

Frequently Asked Questions

Q   *My child swallowed the mercury from an oral thermometer. What do I do?*
A   Elemental mercury in these thermometers is poorly absorbed from the gastrointestinal tract. No treatment is needed. (The fragments of broken glass are of greater concern.) Because mercury vapor can be absorbed, sporadic cases of acrodynia have resulted from children playing on a carpet contaminated by metallic mercury. Special care should be taken when cleaning up mercury spills from thermometers (see http://www.epa.gov/mercury); particularly, children and pregnant women should not be allowed to help, and windows and doors in the affected rooms should be opened to the outside and closed off from other rooms.

Q   *Should pregnant women or women planning pregnancy avoid eating fish?*
A   There is no known risk that outweighs the benefit of eating commercially caught fish. See www.epa.gov/mercury for handouts on how to get the

Table 32.1: Mercury Concentration in Selected Commercial Seafood*

SEAFOOD	MEAN MERCURY CONCENTRATION (ppm)
Highest Levels	
Tilefish (Gulf of Mexico)	1.450
Shark	0.988
Swordfish	0.976
King Mackerel	0.730
Moderate Levels	
Orange roughy	0.554
Grouper (all species)	0.465
Chilean Bass	0.386
Tuna (fresh/frozen)	0.383
Tuna (canned, albacore)	0.353
Lowest Levels	
Tuna (canned, light)	0.118
Trout, freshwater	0.072
Crab	0.060
Scallops	0.050
Catfish	0.049
Pollock	0.041
Salmon (fresh/frozen)	0.014
Tilapia	0.010
Clams	Nondetectable
Salmon (canned)	Nondetectable
Shrimp	Nondetectable

*Selected data from http://www.cfsan.fda.gov/~frf/sea-mehg.html. Other contaminants, such as PCBs
 (see Chapter 18), may alter the safety of eating particular fish.
ppm indicates parts per million.

positive health benefits from eating fish and shellfish while minimizing mercury exposure for women who may become pregnant, pregnant women, nursing mothers, and young children. Recommendations include:
— Avoid eating shark, king mackerel, tilefish, and swordfish
— Limit consumption of fish low in mercury to 12 oz/week. Albacore (white) tuna should be limited to no more than 6 oz/week.
— For fish that are caught from local waters, no more than 6 oz/week should be consumed and no other fish should be eaten that week. Check fish advisories for your state at www.epa.gov/OST/fish.

Q *Should my child have nonmercury fillings? or Should the mercury fillings be replaced?*
A Mercury amalgams are a durable material for filling dental caries. There is no scientific evidence that this commonly used dental material causes harm to a child, although mercury exposure may occur from the presence of dental amalgams. It is not necessary to replace amalgams just because of the mercury content; furthermore, the removal process may weaken the tooth.

Q *Someone spilled some mercury at my child's school. How should it be cleaned up?*
A It is necessary to enlist a specialist's help to clean up even small mercury spills in schools. The janitor should not vacuum it up, because this may spread the mercury aerosol. The local health department can provide the names of local environmental companies with expertise in mercury cleanup. School children should not play with the spilled mercury or take it home from the school.

Resources

State and local public health and environmental agencies
They may be of assistance if a mercury spill occurs, if clinically significant poisoning is suspected, or to evaluate possible environmental exposure sources.

US Environmental Protection Agency
Web site: www.epa.gov/mercury
This Web site provides a wide array of information on mercury, including a link to state fish advisories, a list of consumer products that contain mercury, handouts about fish consumption advisories for pregnant women and children, and household hazardous waste collection centers that accept mercury-containing equipment and used fluorescent light bulbs.

US Food and Drug Administration
Web site: www.cfsan.fda.gov/~frf/sea-mehg.html
This Web site provides information on mercury content in commercial fish.

Institute of Medicine

Seafood Choices: Balancing Benefits and Risks

Web site: www.iom.edu/Reports/2006/Seafood-Choices-Balancing-Benefits-and-Risks.aspx

World Health Organization

Children's Exposure to Mercury Compounds (2010)

Web site: www.who.int/ceh/publications/children_exposure/en/index.html

References

1. Ekino S, Susa M, Ninomiya T, Imamura K, Kitamura T. Minamata disease revisited: an update on the acute and chronic manifestations of methyl mercury poisoning. *J Neurol Sci.* 2007;262 (1-2):131-144

2. Clarkson TW, Magos L, Myers GJ. Human exposure to mercury: the three modern dilemmas. *J Trace Elem Exp Med.* 2003;16:321-343

3. Ozuah PO. Folk use of elemental mercury: a potential hazard for children? *J Natl Med Assoc.* 2001;93(9):320–322

4. Zayas LH, Ozuah PO. Mercury use in espiritismo: a survey of botanicas. *Am J Public Health.* 1996;86(1):111–112

5. Clarkson TW. The pharmacology of mercury compounds. *Annu Rev Pharmacol.* 1972;12: 375–406

6. US Environmental Protection Agency. Water quality criterion for the protection of human health: methyl mercury. Washington, DC: Office of Science and Technology, Office of Water, US Environmental Protection Agency; 2001. Publication No. EPA-823-R-01-001. Available at: http://www.waterboards.ca.gov/water_issues/programs/tmdl/records/region_1/2003/ref1799.pdf. Accessed March 28, 2011

7. American Academy of Pediatrics, Committee on Infectious Diseases, Committee on Environmental Health. Thimerosal in vaccines—an interim report to clinicians. *Pediatrics.* 1999;104(3 Pt 1):570–574

8. American Academy of Family Physicians, American Academy of Pediatrics, Advisory Committee on Immunization Practices, Public Health Service. Summary of the joint statement on thimerosal in vaccines. *MMWR Morb Mortal Wkly Rep.* 2000;49(27):622, 631

9. Jaffe KM, Shurtleff DB, Robertson WO. Survival after acute mercury vapor poisoning. *Am J Dis Child.* 1983;137(8):749–751

10. Solis MT, Yuen E, Cortez PS, Goebel PJ. Family poisoned by mercury vapor inhalation. *Am J Emerg Med.* 2000;18(5):599-602

11. Taueg C, Sanfilippo DJ, Rowens B, Szejda J, Hesse JL. Acute and chronic poisoning from residential exposures to elemental mercury—Michigan, 1989–1990. *J Toxicol Clin Toxicol.* 1992;30(1):63–67

12. Fawer RF, deRibaupierre Y, Guillemin MP, Berode M, Lob M. Measurement of hand tremor induced by industrial exposure to metallic mercury. *Br J Ind Med.* 1983;40(2):204–208

13. Smith PJ, Langolf GD, Goldberg J. Effect of occupational exposure to elemental mercury on short term memory. *Br J Ind Med.* 1983;40(4):413–419

14. Eyer F, Felgenhauer N, Pfab R, Drasch G, Zilker T. Neither DMPS nor DMSA is effective in quantitative elimination of elemental mercury after intentional IV injection. *Clin Toxicol (Phila).* 2006;44(4):395-397

15. Forman J, Moline J, Cernichiari E, et al. A cluster of pediatric metallic mercury exposure cases treated with meso-2,3-dimercaptosuccinic acid (DMSA). *Environ Health Perspect.* 2000;108:575-577

16. Michaeli-Yossef Y, Berkovitch M, Goldman M. Mercury intoxication in a 2-year-old girl: a diagnostic challenge for the physician. *Pediatr Nephrol.* 2007;22(6):903-906

17. Agner E, Jans H. Mercury poisoning and nephrotic syndrome in two young siblings. *Lancet.* 1978;2(8096):951

18. Tubbs RR, Gephardt GN, McMahon JT, et al. Membranous glomerulonephritis associated with industrial mercury exposure. Study of pathogenetic mechanisms. *Am J Clin Pathol.* 1982;77(4):409–413

19. Edlich RF, Greene JA, Cochran AA, et al. Need for informed consent for dentists who use mercury amalgam restorative material as well as technical considerations in removal of dental amalgam restorations. *J Environ Pathol Toxicol Oncol.* 2007;26(4):305-322

20. Clarkson TW, Friberg L, Hursh JB, Nylander M. The prediction of intake of mercury vapor from amalgams. In: Clarkson TW, Friberg L, Nordberg GF, Sager PR, eds. *Biological Monitoring of Toxic Metals.* New York, NY: Plenum Press; 1988:247–264

21. Eley BM. The future of dental amalgam: a review of the literature. Part 4: mercury exposure hazards and risk assessment. *Br Dent J.* 1997;182(10):373–381

22. Eley BM. The future of dental amalgam: a review of the literature. Part 6: possible harmful effects of mercury from dental amalgam. *Br Dent J.* 1997;182(10):455–459

23. Nur Ozdabak H, Karaoğlanoğlu S, Akgül N, Polat F, Seven N. The effects of amalgam restorations on plasma mercury levels and total antioxidant activity [published online September 13, 2008]. *Arch Oral Biol.* 2008;53(12):1101-1106

24. Brownawell AM, Berent S, Brent RL, et al. The potential adverse health effects of dental amalgam. *Toxicol Rev.* 2005;24(1):1-10

25. Mitchell RJ, Osborne PB, Haubenreich JE. Dental amalgam restorations: daily mercury dose and biocompatibility. *J Long Term Eff Med Implants.* 2005;15(6):709-721

26. DeRouen TA, Martin MD, Leroux BG, et al. Neurobehavioral effects of dental amalgam in children: a randomized clinical trial. *JAMA.* 2006;295(15):1784-1792

27. Bellinger DC, Trachtenberg F, Daniel D, Tavares MA, McKinlay S. A dose-effect analysis of children's exposure to dental amalgam and neuropsychological function: the New England Children's Amalgam Trial. *J Am Dent Assoc.* 2007;138(9):1210-1216

28. Bellinger DC, Caniel C, Trachtenberg F, Tavares M, McKinlay S. Dental amalgam restorations and children's neuropsychological function: the New England Children's Amalgam Trial. *Environ Health Perspect.* 2007;115(3):440-446

29. Cheek DB. Acrodynia. In: Kelley V, ed. *Brenneman's Practice of Pediatrics.* Vol I. New York, NY: Harper and Row Publishers; 1977;17D:1–12

30. Warkany J. Acrodynia—postmortem of a disease. *Am J Dis Child.* 1966;112(2):147–156

31. Gotelli CA, Astolfi E, Cox C, Cernichiari E, Clarkson TW. Early biochemical effects of an organic mercury fungicide on infants: "dose makes the poison." *Science.* 1985;227(4687): 638–640

32. Agocs MM, Etzel RA, Parrish RG, et al. Mercury exposure from interior latex paint. *N Engl J Med.* 1990;323(16):1096–1101

33. van der Linde AA, Lewiszong-Rutjens CA, Verrips A, Gerrits GP. A previously healthy 11-year-old girl with behavioural disturbances, desquamation of the skin and loss of teeth. *Eur J Pediatr.* 2009;168(4):509-511

34. Weinstein M, Bernstein S. Pink ladies: mercury poisoning in twin girls. *CMAJ.* 2003;168(2):201

35. Amin-Zaki L, Majeed MA, Elhassani SB, Clarkson TW, Greenwood MR, Doherty RA. Prenatal methylmercury poisoning. Clinical observations over five years. *Am J Dis Child.* 1979;133(2):172–177

36. Debes F, Budtz-Jørgensen E, Weihe P, White RF, Grandjean P. Impact of prenatal methylmercury exposure on neurobehavioral function at age 14 years. *Neuroxicol Teratol.* 2006;28(3):363-375

37. Myers GJ, Davidson PW, Cox C, et al. Prenatal methylmercury exposure from ocean fish consumption in the Seychelles child development study. *Lancet.* 2003;361(9370):1686-1692

38. Axelrad DA, Bellinger DC, Ryan LM, Woodruff TJ. Dose-response relationship of prenatal mercury exposure and IQ: an integrative analysis of epidemiologic data. *Environ Health Perspect.* 2007;115(4):609-615

39. Budtz-Jørgensen E, Grandjean P, Weihe P. Separation of risks and benefits of seafood intake. *Environ Health Perspect.* 2007;115(3):323-327

40. Spurgeon A. Prenatal methylmercury exposure and developmental outcomes: review of the evidence and discussion of future directions. *Environ Health Perspect.* 2006;114(2):307-312

41. Canuel R, de Grosbois SB, Atikessé L, et al. New evidence on variations of human body burden of methylmercury from fish consumption. *Environ Health Perspect.* 2006;114(2):302-306

42. National Academy of Sciences. *Methylmercury, Toxicological Effects of Methylmercury.* Washington, DC: National Academies Press; 2000

43. Jones, RL, Sinks T, Schober SE, Pickett M. Blood mercury levels in young children and childbearing-aged women—United Status, 1999-2002. *MMWR Morb Mortal Wkly Rep.* 2004;53(43):1018-1020

44. Stern AH, Smith AE. An assessment of the cord blood-maternal blood methylmercury ratio: implications for risk assessment. *Environ Health Perspect.* 2003;113(1):155-163

45. Mahaffey KR, Clickner RP, Jeffries RA. Adult women's blood mercury concentrations vary regionally in USA: association with patterns of fish consumption (NHANES 1999-2004) *Environ Health Perspect.* 2009;117(1):47-53

46. Axton JH. Six cases of poisoning after a parenteral organic mercurial compound (Merthiolate). *Postgrad Med J.* 1972;48(561):417–421

47. Fagan DG, Pritchard JS, Clarkson TW, Greenwood MR. Organ mercury levels in infants with omphaloceles treated with organic mercurial antiseptic. *Arch Dis Child.* 1977;52(12):962–964

48. Lowell JA, Burgess S, Shenoy S, Peters M, Howard TK. Mercury poisoning associated with hepatitis-B immunoglobulin. *Lancet.* 1996;347(8999):480

49. Matheson DS, Clarkson TW, Gelfand EW. Mercury toxicity (acrodynia) induced by long-term injection of gammaglobulin. *J Pediatr.* 1980;97(1):153–155

50. Pfab R, Muckter H, Roider G, Zilker T. Clinical course of severe poisoning with thiomersal. *J Toxicol Clin Toxicol.* 1996;34(4):453–460

51. Rohyans J, Walson PD, Wood GA, MacDonald WA. Mercury toxicity following Merthiolate ear irrigations. *J Pediatr.* 1984;104(2):311–313

52. Stratton K, Gable A, McCormick MC, eds. *Immunization Safety Review: Thiomersal-Containing Vaccines and Neurodevelopmental Disorders.* Washington, DC: National Academies Press; 2001

53. Thompson WW, Price C, Goodson, et al. Early thimerosal exposure and neuropsychological outcomes at 7 to 10 years. *N Engl J Med.* 2007;357(13):1281-1292

54. Parker SK, Schwartz B, Todd J, Pickering LK. Thimerosal-containing vaccines and autistic spectrum disorder: a critical review of published original data. *Pediatrics.* 2004;114(3):793-804

55. Stehr-Green P, Tull P, Stellfeld M, et al. Autism and thimerosal-containing vaccines: lack of consistent evidence for an association. *Am J Prev Med.* 2003;25(2):101-106

56. Madsen KM, Lauritsen MB, Pedersen CB, et al. Thimerosal and the occurrence of autism: negative ecological evidence from Danish population-based data. *Pediatrics* 2003;112(3 Pt 1):604-606

57. Hviid A, Stellfeld M, Wohlfahrt J, Melbye M. Association between thimerosal-containing vaccine and autism. *JAMA.* 2003;290(13):1763-1766

58. Heron J, Golding J. Thimerosal exposure in infants and developmental disorders: a prospective cohort study in the United Kingdom does not support a causal association. *Pediatrics.* 2004;114(3):577-583

59. Andrews N , Miller E, Grant A, et al. Thimerosal exposure in infants and developmental disorders: a retrospective cohort study in the United Kingdom does not support a causal association. *Pediatrics.* 2004;114(3):584-591

60. Price CS, Thompson WW, Goodson B, et al. Prenatal and infant exposure to thimerosal from vaccines and immunoglobulins and risk of autism. *Pediatrics.* 2010;126(4):656-664

61. McDowell MA, Dillon CF, Osterloh J, et al. Hair mercury levels in U.S. children and women of childbearing age: reference range data from NHANES 1999-2000. *Environ Health Perspect.* 2004;112(11):1165-1171

62. Budtz-Jørgensen E, Grandjean P, Jørgensen PJ, Weihe P, Keiding N. Association between mercury concentrations in blood and hair in methylmercury-exposed subjects at different ages. *Environ Res.* 2004;95(2):385-393

63. Nuttall KL. Interpreting hair mercury levels in individual patients. *Ann Clin Lab Sci.* 2006;36(3):248-261

64. Garza-Ocanas L, Torres-Alanis O, Pineyro-Lopez A. Urinary mercury in twelve cases of cutaneous mercurous chloride (calomel) exposure: effect of sodium 2,3-dimercaptopropane-1-sulfate (DMPS) therapy. *J Toxicol Clin Toxicol.* 1997;35(6):653–655

65. Hohage H, Otte B, Westermann G, et al. Elemental mercurial poisoning. *South Med J.* 1997;90(10):1033–1036

66. Gonzalez-Ramirez D, Zuniga-Charles M, Narro-Juarez A, et al. DMPS (2,3-dimercaptopropane-1-sulfonate, dimaval) decreases the body burden of mercury in humans exposed to mercurous chloride. *J Pharmacol Exp Ther.* 1998;287(1):8–12

67. Risher JF, Amler SN. Mercury exposure: evaluation and intervention: the inappropriate use of chelating agents in the diagnosis and treatment of putative mercury poisoning. *Neurotoxicology.* 2005;26(4):691-699

68. Tominack R, Weber J, Blume C, et al. Elemental mercury as an attractive nuisance: multiple exposures from a pilfered school supply with severe consequences. *Pediatr Emerg Care.* 2002;18(2):97-100

69. Torres AD, Rai AN, Hardiek ML. Mercury intoxication and arterial hypertension: report of two patients and review of the literature. *Pediatrics.* 2000;105(3):e34

70. Agency for Toxic Substances and Disease Registry. Mercury toxicity. *Am Fam Physician.* 1992;46(6):1731–1741

71. Bates BA. Mercury. In: Haddad LM, Shannon MW, Winchester JF, eds. *Clinical Management of Poisoning and Drug Overdose.* 3rd ed. Philadelphia, PA: WB Saunders; 1998:750–756

72. Myers SM; Johnson CP; American Academy of Pediatrics, Council on Children with Disabilities. Management of children with autism spectrum disorders. *Pediatrics.* 2007;120(5):1162-1182

73. Goldman LR; Shannon MW; American Academy of Pediatrics, Committee on Environmental Health. Technical report: mercury in the environment: implications for pediatricians. *Pediatrics.* 2001;108(1):197–205

74. Bonhomme C, Gladyszacak-Kholer J, Cadou A, Ilef D, Kadi Z. Mercury poisoning by vacuum-cleaner aerosol. *Lancet.* 1996;347(8994):115

75. Baughman T. Elemental mercury spills. *Environ Health Perspect.* 2006;114(2):147-152

76. US Environmental Protection Agency. *What You Need to Know About Mercury in Fish and Shellfish. 2004 EPA and FDA Advice For: Women Who Might Become Pregnant, Women Who are Pregnant, Nursing Mothers, Young Children.* Publication No. PA-823-R-04-005. Washington, DC: US Environmental Protection Agency; March 2004. Available at: www.cfsan.fda.gov/~dms/admehg3.html.

77. Oken E, Radesky JS, Wright RO, et al. Maternal fish intake during pregnancy, blood mercury levels, and child cognition at age 3 years in a US cohort. *Am J Epidemiol.* 2008;167(10):1171-1181

78. Agency for Toxic Substances and Disease Registry. *Preliminary Health Assessment, Olin Chemical Co, Charleston, TN.* Atlanta, GA: Agency for Toxic Substances and Disease Registry; 1988

Chapter 33

Nitrates and Nitrites in Water

■ ■ ■ ■ ■ ■

Nitrogen, an essential nutrient, is absorbed and incorporated by plants from nitrate or ammonium in soil. The use of nitrogen fertilizer for improved crop yields has generally increased in the United States and globally since the 1950s, peaking in the United States around 1990.[1] Nitrate contamination of water supplies is a potential environmental consequence of modern agricultural activity and increasing urbanization. Nitrate concentrations in shallow groundwater and some surface waters have increased as a result of use of nitrogen fertilizers, intensive livestock operations that produce large amounts of animal waste, substandard private septic systems, and municipal wastewater treatment discharges.[2] A recent US Geological Survey National Water Quality Assessment Program report documents elevated nitrate concentrations in 4 of 33 major aquifers sampled in rural and urban areas.[3] Poorly constructed shallow wells in rural areas are at greatest risk of nitrate contamination. In general, nitrite is not as prevalent in water supplies as nitrate, because nitrite is rapidly converted to nitrate, depending on aerobic and bacterial conditions.[4]

High nitrate concentrations in water can potentially have adverse effects on ecology and public health. Nitrate and other nutrients have been linked to blue-green algal blooms, which can produce toxic bacteria that can negatively affect wildlife and humans.[5,6] Methemoglobinemia in infants may result from ingestion of water contaminated with nitrate.[7] Two cases of methemoglobinemia, also known as "blue baby syndrome," were reported in 2000 by the Wisconsin Department of Health in infants fed formula reconstituted with water from private wells with nitrate-nitrogen (NO_3-N) concentrations of 22.9 and 27.4 mg/L.[8] There is great interindividual variability in risk of methemoglobinemia related to nitrate contamination of drinking water. In adults, genetic reductase deficiencies are potential risk factors. Infants younger than 6 months are at high risk, and those younger than 1 month are at highest risk. It has been suggested that coincident gastrointestinal tract infection may be a significant contribution to risk. Gastrointestinal tract infection, diarrhea, and/or vomiting can lead to methemoglobinemia in infants without exposure to high nitrate concentrations from drinking water or foods.[9]

NITRATE IN US WATER SUPPLIES

The trend for US water supplies has been a general increase in nitrate concentrations.[10] The US Environmental Protection Agency (EPA) drinking water standard (maximum contaminant level [MCL]) for public water supplies is 10 mg/L (10 parts per million [ppm]) for NO_3-N and 1 mg/L (1 part per million) for nitrite.[11] These maximum contaminant levels were set in response to concerns regarding methemoglobinemia in infants. EPA drinking water standards, however, do not apply to private wells, nor are these wells subject to federal regulations of the Navajo Nation (which has its own EPA). Wells are minimally regulated by states. Well owners are usually responsible for their own wells. Approximately 15% to 20% of US households obtain their water from private wells.

It was estimated that approximately 1.5 million people, including 22 500 infants, or 1.2% of those served by private wells, and 3 million people, including 43 500 infants, or 2.4% of those served by public community wells, were exposed to drinking water nitrate concentrations above the maximum contaminant level.[12] The 1994 Midwest Well Water Survey collected water samples from 5500 domestic wells located in 9 states. Of those samples, 13.4% exceeded the nitrate maximum contaminant level, with Kansas (24.6%) and Iowa (20.6%) having the highest proportion of samples with nitrate maximum contaminant level greater than 10 parts per million.[13] Proximity to heavy agricultural activity may exacerbate the situation. A North Carolina study (1998) sampled 1600 wells in 15 counties where intensive livestock facilities were located. Of the wells tested, 10.2% had nitrate greater than 10 parts per million.[14] Nitrates in well water are interpreted as an indication of surface contamination and, thus, are often markers of other contamination, typically of agricultural origin, including fecal coliform bacteria, pesticides, and other land applications.

ROUTE AND SOURCES OF EXPOSURE

Drinking water is the main source of nitrate for infants. In breastfed infants, there is no evidence of increased risk of methemoglobinemia from maternal ingestion of nitrate-contaminated water with NO_3-N concentrations as high as 100 parts per million, because these mothers do not produce milk with high nitrate concentrations.[15] It is uncertain whether transplacental transfer of nitrates occurs. Acquired methemoglobinemia has been linked to a variety of oxidizing agents, including topical benzocaine, silver nitrate burn therapy, laundry inks, and other agents.[16]

CLINICAL EFFECTS

Nitrate is rapidly absorbed from the proximal small intestine, and approximately 70% of ingested nitrate is found in urine within 24 hours. Ordinarily, most ingested nitrate is metabolized and excreted unless conditions favor reduction to nitrite. Although few recent data are available, approximately 2000 cases of acquired methemoglobinemia were reported in North America and Europe between 1945 and 1971.[10]

Although nitrate does not cause methemoglobinemia, it can be converted to nitrite by gut flora. In turn, nitrite converts ferrous iron (Fe^{+2}) in hemoglobin to ferric iron (Fe^{+3}), resulting in methemoglobin, which is incapable of carrying oxygen. Infants younger than 6 months who are fed formula reconstituted with well water containing nitrate are at the greatest risk of methemoglobinemia. The gastric pH of infants is higher than that of older children and adults, with resultant proliferation of lower intestinal bacteria that reduce ingested nitrate to more reactive nitrite.[7] The system responsible for reduction of induced methemoglobin to normal ferrous hemoglobin has only about half the activity in infants as in adults.[17] Infants younger than 6 months are particularly at risk of methemoglobinemia as a result of lesser amounts and activity of methemoglobin reductase, the enzyme that reduces ferric iron in methemoglobin back to ferrous iron, regenerating hemoglobin. Infants begin making adult levels of methemoglobin reductase at around 6 months of age.

Methemoglobinemia generally presents with few clinical signs other than cyanosis. Methemoglobin is dark brown and results in obvious cyanosis at concentrations as low as 3%. Symptoms are generally minimal until methemoglobin concentrations exceed 20%. Usually, cyanosis is manifest well before other symptoms appear unless exposure is intense. The mucous membranes of infants with methemoglobinemia-induced cyanosis tend to have a brownish cast. The brown discoloration increases with the concentration of methemoglobin, as do irritability, tachypnea, altered mental status, and complaints of headache in older children. In the absence of respiratory symptoms, history of cardiovascular disease, abnormal pulse, or abnormal oximetry, a diagnosis of methemoglobinemia should be considered in a child who becomes cyanotic and unresponsive to oxygen administration.[18]

TREATMENT OF METHEMOGLOBINEMIA

Health care professionals who suspect that a child has methemoglobinemia should consult with their local poison control center or a toxicologist to help guide management. An asymptomatic child with cyanosis who has a methemo-globin concentration of less than 20% usually requires no treatment other than identifying and eliminating the source of exposure. For methemoglobin concentrations above 30%, methylene blue (dosage 1 mg/kg, intravenously, over a period of several minutes) and 100% oxygen are therapeutic antidotes. Methylene blue acts as an electron carrier for the hexose monophosphate alternate pathway that reduces methemoglobin to hemoglobin. A rapid disappearance of cyanosis in response to methylene blue would be expected within 1 hour but might not occur if the patient has erythrocyte glucose-6-phosphate dehydrogenase (G6PD) or nicotinamide adenine dinucleotide phosphate diaphorase deficiency or if methemoglobinemia is attributable to the ingestion of compounds such as aniline or dapsone. More information on diagnosis and treatment can be found elsewhere.[16,17]

PREVENTION OF METHEMOGLOBINEMIA

Clinical treatment alone for methemoglobinemia is not sufficient. It is critical to identify and eliminate exogenous sources of exposure. Infants with gastro-intestinal infection, diarrhea, dehydration, and/or acidosis may be especially susceptible. Assessment of potential nitrate exposure includes asking about family residence, occupation, drinking water, foods ingested, and use of topical medications or folk remedies. Children may be exposed at child care or school or when visiting vacation homes or camps. Prenatal and newborn care for patients with private wells should include a recommendation for testing well water for nitrate contamination.[19] Water with elevated nitrate concentrations should not be ingested by infants younger than 1 year or used to prepare infant formula. Well waters with high nitrate concentrations typically have elevated concentrations of various pesticides and fecal coliform bacteria. Care must be taken when boiling water before mixing formula, because this may concentrate nitrate and other chemical contaminants. Boiling water for 1 minute generally is sufficient to kill microorganisms without overconcentrating nitrate and other chemical contaminants.[20] Effective in-home systems for nitrate removal include ion exchange resins and reverse-osmosis systems, which are available but expensive. Water testing for nitrate, pesticides, and fecal coliforms can be performed by any reference or public health laboratory using EPA-approved laboratory methods.

CHRONIC EFFECTS

Epidemiologic studies have reported increased risks associated with elevated concentrations of nitrate in drinking water for a variety of noncancer outcomes, including hyperthyroidism[21] and insulin-dependent diabetes.[22] Several studies have found associations between birth defects and high nitrate concentrations in water supplies.[22-25] Anecdotal reports of spontaneous abortions in Indiana

(1991–1993) describe a case study in which 3 women experienced a total of 6 spontaneous abortions; the women resided in proximity to each other and consumed drinking water from private wells containing high concentrations of NO_3-N (19–26 parts per million).[26]

Cancer risk during adulthood from exposure to nitrate in drinking water is another potential public health concern. Ingested nitrate is reduced endogenously to nitrite through bacterial reactions in the saliva, and nitrite can be converted to N-nitroso compounds via reaction with secondary amines (from common dietary sources or pesticides) in the stomach, intestine, and bladder.[27] N-nitroso compounds are known to induce cancer in a variety of organs in more than 40 animal species including higher primates. Epidemiologic studies on nitrate in drinking water and cancer risk have shown mixed results.[28] Some studies have demonstrated elevated risk of cancer of the esophagus, colon, nasopharynx, bladder, and prostate as well as non-Hodgkin lymphoma.[28,29] Ecologic studies of stomach cancer in Slovakia, Spain, and Hungary with historical measurements and exposure levels near or above the maximum contaminant level have found positive correlations with stomach cancer incidence or mortality.[30-32] In the Slovakian study, incidence of non-Hodgkin lymphoma and colon cancer were significantly elevated among men and women exposed to public water supplies with NO_3-N concentrations of 4.5 to 11.3 mg/L. Despite some uncertainty about nitrate contamination of water's contribution to cancer, the International Agency for Research on Cancer (IARC) reviewed the evidence in 2006 and determined that ingested nitrate or nitrite under conditions that result in endogenous nitrosation is probably carcinogenic to humans (Group 2A).[33]

Frequently Asked Questions

Q *Do commercial treatment systems sufficiently protect against nitrate contamination?*

A Water softeners and charcoal filters do not significantly reduce nitrate concentrations. Reverse–osmosis systems and ion exchange resins do remove nitrate but are expensive.

Q *Is low-grade nitrate contamination a risk for cancer?*

A We don't know for sure. Published studies of exposure to nitrate in drinking water and cancer risk are not all in agreement, but the International Agency for Research on Cancer has determined that ingesting nitrate probably increases the risk for cancer.

Q *Are the current maximum contaminant levels sufficiently strict to protect the population?*

A Most of the population is protected from methemoglobinemia or other potential adverse effects of nitrate at current maximum contaminant levels. The EPA's drinking water standards for nitrate (10 parts per million) and nitrite (1 part per million) are designed to protect the health even of people who are considered most susceptible. These standards, however, only apply to public water supplies.

Q *Should I have my well water tested? How often?*

A Indications for having a well tested would include having a new baby, recent damage to the well, or living in a neighborhood where there is known well water nitrate contamination. Individuals with private wells should have them tested for nitrates and coliform bacteria on a yearly basis. Risk factors for increased nitrate contamination include shallow well depth and regional nitrate contamination. Collect the sample during wet weather (late spring and early summer), when runoff and excess soil moisture carry contaminants into shallow groundwater sources or through defects in your well. Do not test during dry weather or when the ground is frozen.

Q *I have a young baby and will be staying in a vacation home for a couple of weeks. I don't know whether the well has been tested. Can I give my baby the well water?*

A The well water should be tested before being offered to an infant. If this is not possible, it may be safer and more convenient to use bottled water for the baby and others staying in the vacation home.

References

1. Brown LR, Renner M, Flavin C. *Vital Signs 1997: The Environmental Trends That Are Shaping Our Future.* New York, NY: WW Norton & Co; 1997
2. Nolan BT, Ruddy BC, Hitt KJ, Helsel DR. A national look at nitrate contamination of groundwater. *Water Conditioning and Purification.* 1998;40:76–79
3. US Geological Survey. *The Quality of Our Nation's Waters: Nutrients and Pesticides.* Reston, VA: US Department of the Interior, US Geological Survey; 1999. US Geological Survey Circular 1225
4. Mackerness CW, Keevil CW. Origin and significance of nitrite in water. In: Hill M, ed. *Nitrates and Nitrites in Food and Water.* Chichester, England: Ellis Horwood; 1991:77–92
5. Burgess C. A wave of momentum for toxic algae study. *Environ Health Perspect.* 2001;109(4):A160–A161
6. Carmichael WW, Azevedo SM, An JS, et al. Human fatalities from cyanobacteria: chemical and biological evidence for cyanotoxins. *Environ Health Perspect.* 2001;109(7):663–668
7. McKnight GM, Duncan CW, Leifert C, Golden MH. Dietary nitrate in man: friend or foe? *Br J Nutr.* 1999;81(5):349–358
8. Knobeloch L, Salna B, Hogan A, Postle J, Anderson H. Blue babies and nitrate-contaminated well water. *Environ Health Perspect.* 2000;108(7):675-678
9. Avery AA. Infantile methemoglobinemia: reexamining the role of drinking water nitrates. *Environ Health Perspect.* 1999;107(7):583-586
10. Reynolds KA. The prevalence of nitrate contamination in the United States. *Water Conditioning and Purification.* 2002;44(1). Available at: http://www.wcponline.com/column.cfm?T=T&ID=1330&AT=T. Accessed August 25, 2010
11. US Environmental Protection Agency. National Primary Drinking Water Regulations: Final Rule, 40. CFR Parts 141, 142, and 143. *Fed Regist.* 1991;56(20):3526–3597

12. US Environmental Protection Agency. *Another Look: National Pesticide Survey: Phase II Report.* Washington, DC: US Environmental Protection Agency; 1992

13. National Center for Environmental Health. *A Survey of the Quality of Water Drawn From Domestic Wells in Nine Midwest States.* Atlanta, GA: Centers for Disease Control and Prevention; 1995. Available at: http://www.cdc.gov/nceh/hsb/disaster/pdfs/A%20Survey%20 of%20the%20Quality%20ofWater%20Drawn%20from%20Domestic%20Wells%20in%20 Nine%20Midwest%20States.pdf. Accessed August 25, 2010

14. North Carolina Division of Public Health. *Contamination of Private Drinking Well Water by Nitrates.* Raleigh, NC: North Carolina Division of Public Health; 1998. Available at: http:// www.epi.state.nc.us/epi/mera/ilocontamination.html. Accessed August 25, 2010

15. Dusdieker LB, Stumbo PJ, Kross BC, Dungy CI. Does increased nitrate ingestion elevate nitrate levels in human milk? *Arch Pediatr Adolesc Med.* 1996;150(3):311–314

16. Wright RO, Lewander WJ, Woolf AD. Methemoglobinemia: etiology, pharmacology, and clinical management. *Ann Emerg Med.* 1999;34(5):646–656

17. Smith RP. Toxic responses of the blood. In: Amdur MO, Doull J, Klaassen CD, eds. *Casarett and Doull's Toxicology, The Basic Science of Poisons.* 4th ed. New York, NY: Pergamon Press; 1991:257–281

18. Agency for Toxic Substances and Disease Registry. *Case Studies in Environmental Medicine (CSEM). Nitrate/Nitrite Toxicity.* Available at: http://www.atsdr.cdc.gov/csem/nitrate/no3cover. html. Accessed June 11, 2011

19. Greer FR; Shannon M; American Academy of Pediatrics, Committee on Nutrition, Committee on Environmental Health. Clinical report: infant methemoglobinemia: the role of dietary nitrate in food and water. *Pediatrics.* 2005;116(3):784–786. Reaffirmed April 2009

20. American Academy of Pediatrics, Committee on Environmental Health and Committee on Infectious Diseases. Policy statement: drinking water from private wells and risks to children. *Pediatrics.* 2009;123(6):1599–1605

21. Seffner W. Natural water contents and endemic goiter—a review [article in German]. *Zentralbl Hyg Umweltmed.* 1995;196(5):381–398

22. Kostraba JN, Gay EC, Rewers M, Hamman RF. Nitrate levels in community drinking waters and risk of IDDM. An ecological analysis. *Diabetes Care.* 1992;15(11):1505–1508

23. Arbuckle TE, Sherman GJ, Corey PN, Waters D, Lo B. Water nitrates and CNS birth defects: a population-based case-control study. *Arch Environ Health.* 1988;43(2):162–167

24. Scragg RK, Dorsch MM, McMichael AJ, Baghurst PA. Birth defects and household water supply. Epidemiological studies in the Mount Gambier region of South Australia. *Med J Aust.* 1982;2(12):577–579

25. Croen LA, Todoroff K, Shaw GM. Maternal exposure to nitrate from drinking water and diet and risk of neural tube defects. *Am J Epidemiol.* 2001;153(4):325–331

26. Centers for Disease Control and Prevention. Spontaneous abortions possibly related to ingestion of nitrate-contaminated well water—LaGrange County, Indiana, 1991–1994. *MMWR Morb Mortal Wkly Rep.* 1996;45(26):569–572

27. Walker R. Nitrates, nitrites and N-nitroso compounds: a review of the occurrence in food and diet and the toxicological implications. *Food Addit Contam.* 1990;7(6):717–768

28. Cantor KP. Drinking water and cancer. *Cancer Causes Control.* 1997;8(3):292–308

29. Ward MH, deKok TM, Levallois P, et al. Workgroup Report: Drinking-Water Nitrate and Health—Recent Findings and Research Needs *Environ Health Perspect.* 2005;113(11): 1607–1614

30. Gulis G, Czompolyova M, Cerhan JR. An ecologic study of nitrate in municipal drinking water and cancer incidence in Trnava District, Slovakia. *Environ Res.* 2002;88(3):182–187

31. Morales-Suarez-Varela MM, Llopis-Gonzalez A, Tejerizo-Perez ML. Impact of nitrates in drinking water on cancer mortality in Valencia, Spain. *Eur J Epidemiol.* 1995;11(1):15–21

32. Sandor J, Kiss I, Farkas O, Ember I. Association between gastric cancer mortality and nitrate content of drinking water: ecological study on small area inequalities. *Eur J Epidemiol.* 2001;17(5):443–447

33. International Agency for Research on Cancer. *IARC Monographs on the Evaluation of Carcinogenic Risks to Humans.* Volume 94: Ingested Nitrates and Nitrites, and Cyanobacterial Peptide Toxins. Lyon, France: International Agency for Research on Cancer; 2006. Available at: http://monographs.iarc.fr/ENG/Monographs/vol94/mono94-1.pdf. Accessed August 25, 2010

Chapter 34

Noise

■ ■ ■ ■ ■ ■

Noise is undesirable sound. Sound is vibration in a medium, usually air, and has frequency (pitch), intensity (loudness), periodicity, and duration. The frequency of sound is measured in cycles per second and is expressed in hertz (Hz) (1 Hz = 60 cycles per second). People respond to frequencies ranging from 20 to 20 000 Hz but are most sensitive to sounds in the range of 500 to 3000 Hz, the band of frequencies that includes human speech.

The loudness of sound is measured in terms of pascals (Pa) or decibels (dB). The range of sound limits in human hearing is 0.00002 Pa (the weakest sound that a keen human adult ear can detect under quiet conditions) to 200 Pa (the pressure causing pain in the adult ear). The dB is a method of compressing this range by expressing the ratio of one sound energy level to another. The unit most commonly used is dB SPL, indicating that the ratio of sound pressure levels (SPL) is being used. Human speech is approximately 50 dB SPL.

The perceived loudness of sound varies with the frequency. For example, to match the perceived loudness of a 40 dB SPL 1000-Hz tone requires more than 80 dB SPL at 50 Hz and more than 60 dB SPL at 10 000 Hz. This 40 dB SPL equivalency curve is used to determine the measure of sound intensity, referred to as the decibel weighted by the A scale (dBA). Periodicity refers to either continuous sound or impulse sound. Duration is the total length of time of exposure to sound. Reviews of sound characteristics and hearing are available.[1,2]

Few studies have been performed to estimate children's exposure to noise. On the basis of available data, it is likely that children are routinely exposed to more noise than the 24-hour equivalent noise exposures (Leq24) of 70 dBA recommended as an upper limit by the US Environmental Protection Agency (EPA) in 1974.[3] A longitudinal study of hearing in suburban and rural Ohio children 6 to 18 years of age found that Leq24 varied from 77 to 84 dB, and exposures were higher in boys than in girls.[4]

ROUTES OF EXPOSURE

Sound waves enter the ear through the external auditory canal and vibrate the eardrum. This vibration, in turn, travels through the 3 ossicles of the middle ear (the malleus, incus, and stapes), where the stapes vibrates through the oval window, vibrating the fluid of the cochlea of the inner ear. Within the cochlea, the basilar membrane covers the organ of Corti, which is composed of hair cells. Each hair cell responds to a specific frequency of the vibration and converts this signal to a nerve impulse. The impulses, transmitted by auditory nerves, are interpreted as sound or noise by the brain. Loss of hearing originating in the external auditory canal, eardrum, ossicles, or middle ear is called conductive hearing loss and is usually treatable. Loss of hearing originating in the hair cells or sites within the central nervous system is called sensorineural hearing loss and is usually irreversible.

Although sound vibration also may be transmitted to the body directly through the skin, this is not discussed here.

CLINICAL EFFECTS

Noise affects hearing and results in several adverse physiological and psychological effects.[5,6] Susceptibility to noise-induced hearing loss is highly variable; although some individuals are able to tolerate high noise levels for prolonged periods, other people in the same conditions may lose some hearing.[7] Other variables, such as cardiovascular risks, including smoking, enhance the negative effects of noise on hearing thresholds.[8]

Noise exposure that causes trauma to the hair cells of the cochlea results in hearing loss. Prolonged exposure to sounds louder than 85 dBA is potentially injurious.[9] Continuous exposure to hazardous levels of noise tends to have its maximum effect in the high-frequency regions of the cochlea. Noise-induced hearing loss usually is most severe around 4000 Hz, with downward extension toward speech frequencies with prolonged exposure. This pattern of loss of frequency perception is true regardless of the frequency of the noise exposure. Impulse noise is more harmful than continuous noise because it bypasses the body's natural protective reaction to noise, the dampening of the ossicles mediated by the facial nerve.[10]

Exposure to loud noise may result in tinnitus and a temporary decrease in the sensitivity of hearing. This condition, called temporary noise-induced threshold shift (NITS), lasts for several hours, depending on the degree of exposure, and may become permanent depending on the severity and duration of noise exposure. The prevalence of noise-induced threshold shift in one or both ears among a national sample of children 6 to 19 years of age was 12.5% (or

5.2 million children affected).[11] Most children with noise-induced threshold shift had an early phase of noise-induced threshold shift in only 1 ear and involving only a single frequency. However, among children with noise-induced threshold shift, 4.9% had moderate to profound noise-induced threshold shift. Noise-induced threshold shift may be reversible; however, continued excessive noise exposure could lead to progression of noise-induced threshold shift to include other frequencies and to increase severity and irreversibility. Farm youth may have a particularly high frequency of hearing loss and noise-induced threshold shift.[12] The average sound level at a music festival was 95 dBA, and 36% of surveyed attendees reported tinnitus after listening to the music.[13]

The consequences of these measured episodes of noise-induced threshold shift may be enormous if they progress to a persistent minimal sensorineural hearing loss. In school-aged children, minimal sensorineural hearing loss has been associated with poor school performance and social and emotional dysfunction.[14]

Little evidence is available to suggest that the organs of hearing are more sensitive to noise-induced hearing loss in children than in adults. Infants, however, cannot remove themselves from noxious noise; therefore, infants may be at higher risk of prolonged exposure to noise and its consequences.

Children are at increased risk of increased exposure to noise related to their behaviors. Children can damage hearing through play with firecrackers and cap pistols,[15] which can produce noise levels of 134 dBA[16] (see Table 34.1). Teenagers may not realize that they are susceptible to the adverse effects of excessive noise and that the results of such exposure can be permanent. Approximately 60% of teenagers and young adults exposed to sounds >87 dBA did not consider the noise to be too loud.[17] College student listeners of portable music devices typically use a medium to loud volume of 71.6 to 87.7 dB SPL,[18] which, for most, would not be hazardous to hearing. However, those listening at a very loud setting (approximately 97.8 dB) may be affected.[18]

Evidence that exposure to excessive noise during pregnancy may result in high-frequency hearing loss in newborn infants is inconclusive.[19,20] Neonates may be especially sensitive to sound. Newborn physiologic response to noise has prompted the development of permissible noise criteria to be applied to newly constructed or renovated hospital nurseries.[21] Noise levels often exceed those recommended.[22,23] Incorporation of individualized environmental care (including reduction of noise) to the management of preterm infants decreases their time on a ventilator and oxygen.[24,25] Strategies have been suggested to decrease sound in neonatal care units.[26]

Although children with autism have been reported to have atypical reactions to sounds, including difficulty filtering out background noise, and hypo- or hyperreactivity to sound, several studies have failed to confirm substantial differences in hearing between children with and without autism.[27,28]

Physiological Effects of Noise

Noise causes a stress response. For people, the hypothalamic-pituitary-adrenal axis is sensitive to noise as low as 65 dBA, resulting in a 53% increase in plasma 17-OH-corticosteroid concentrations.[29] Increased excretion of adrenaline and noradrenaline has been demonstrated in humans exposed to noise at 90 dBA for 30 minutes.[30]

Noise contributes to sleep deprivation.[31,32] Noise levels at 40 to 45 dBA result in a 10% to 20% increase in awakening or arousal changes on electroencephalograms (EEGs). Noise levels at 50 dBA result in a 25% probability of arousal features on EEGs.[33]

Noise has undesirable cardiovascular effects. Exposure to noise levels greater than 70 dBA causes increases in vasoconstriction, heart rate, and blood pressure.

A stress response consisting of acute terror and panic was described in children in Labrador, Canada, and Germany on exposure to sonic booms.[34] Biochemical evidence of the stress response (elevated urinary cortisol concentrations) was found. Most studies of children at schools with high levels of aircraft or traffic noise did not find effects on physiologic markers of stress but demonstrated negative effects on difficult cognitive tests or reading comprehension.[35]

Psychological Effects of Noise

Exposure to moderate levels of noise can cause psychological stress.[36] Annoyance, including feelings of bother, interference with activity, and symptoms such as headache, tiredness, and irritability are common psychological reactions to noise. The degree of annoyance is related to the nature of the sound and individual tolerance. Intense noise can cause personality changes and a reduced ability to cope. Sudden, unexpected noise can cause a startle reaction, which may provoke physiological stress responses.

Work performance can be affected by noise. At low levels, it can improve the performance of simple tasks. However, noise may impair intellectual function and performance of complex tasks. Ambient noise may negatively affect the understanding of speech in the classroom. Guidelines on classroom noise that consider child age and vulnerable conditions have been proposed.[37] For those with normal speech processing, maximum classroom ambient noise is recommended to be 40 dBA for children 12 years and older, 39 dBA for children 10 to 11 years of age, 34.5 dBA for children 8 to 9 years of age, and 28.5 dBA for children 6 to 7 years of age. Vulnerable groups—those suspected of delayed speech processing in noise—need quieter environments (21.5 dBA at 6 to 7 years of age).

DIAGNOSIS OF NOISE-INDUCED HEARING LOSS

Parental concern about a child's hearing, speech, or language delay indicates a need for further evaluation.[38] The typical finding in noise-induced hearing loss is a dip in hearing threshold around 4000 Hz on an audiogram. Physicians in facilities that are unable to provide pure tone audiograms should refer their patients for evaluation. Audiologic evaluation, including pure tone audiometry, should be performed to determine whether there is hearing loss (induced by noise or resulting from other causes) in children who have no evidence of acute or serous otitis media but have a history of:

- Excessive environmental noise exposure, such as prolonged exposure to cap pistols or "boom boxes"
- Poor school performance
- Short attention span
- Complaining of ringing in the ears, a feeling of fullness in the ears, muffling of hearing, or difficulty in understanding speech
- Speech delay

The American Academy of Pediatrics recommends hearing screening for all newborn infants and periodic screening for every child through adolescence.[39,40]

TREATMENT OF CLINICAL SYMPTOMS

Although noise-induced threshold shifts may be temporary, there is no known treatment to reverse noise-induced hearing loss. Children with such loss should have appropriate audiology evaluations and be fitted with personal amplification devices, as necessary. To quantify hearing, 0 dB is an arbitrary zero defined as the faintest sound that a young sensitive human ear can hear. Because the decibel scale is logarithmic, every 3 dB increase represents a doubling of sound intensity. A 10 dB increase represents a ten-fold increase in sound intensity and will be perceived as twice as loud. An 80 dB sound is 10 times more intense than a 70 dB sound but is only perceived as being twice as loud. Categories of hearing loss (HL) include: 20 to 40 dB HL, mild hearing loss; 41 to 60 dB HL, moderate hearing loss; 61 to 90 dB HL, severe hearing loss; greater than 90 dB HL, profound hearing loss. Pediatricians should counsel children and teenagers who have hearing loss as well as their parent, about ways to preserve existing hearing and prevent additional hearing loss.

PREVENTION OF EXPOSURE

Pediatricians should discuss noise exposure during routine health supervision visits. To reduce noise exposure, parents, children, and adolescents should be advised to:

- Avoid loud noises, especially loud impulse noise, whenever possible.
- Avoid toys that make loud noise, especially cap pistols. If a toy seems too loud for a parent, then it likely is too loud for the child. A parent may put tape over the speakers or remove the batteries of toys already owned that are too loud.[41]

Table 34.1: Average Peak Sound Levels for Selected Toys	
TOY	PEAK NOISE LEVEL (dBA)
Music box	79
Toy mobile phone	85
Sit-on fire truck	87
Laser pistol	87
Musical telephone	89
Robot soldier	94
Pull turtle	95
Police machine gun	110
Cap gun fired without caps	114
Cap gun fired with caps	134

*Adapted from the National Institute of Public Health Denmark.[16]
dBA indicates decibels weighted by the A scale.

(There currently is no regulation on the amount of noise toys can make. Voluntary noise standards are enforced by the Consumer Product Safety Commission, at their discretion.)

- Avoid the use of firecrackers to protect hearing and to avoid other injury.
- Reduce the volume on televisions, computers, radios, and personal music devices (iPods, etc).
- Turn off televisions, computers, and radios when not in use.
- Use headphones and earbuds with caution. The volume level of the radio or personal digital player should be low enough so that normal conversation can still be heard.
- Use earplugs if attending a loud event (such as a rock concert or dance event). If the level of noise is perceived as uncomfortable or painful, it is prudent to leave the event.
- When flying or riding in a train, consider using noise-canceling headphones. These headphones cover the entire outer ear and work by picking up ambient noise outside the headphones and then emitting a counter frequency that cancels out the incoming noise.
- Create a "stimulus haven," the quietest room in the house for play and interactions.[42]

See Table 34.2 for common exposures to noise. Aircraft noise varies by position in the airplane, with high levels (90 dBA) in the back of the cabin during takeoff and average noise levels at 78 to 84 dBA over the duration of the flight.[43]

Table 34.2: Decibel Ranges and Effects of Common Sounds

EXAMPLE	SOUND PRESSURE (dBA)	EFFECT FROM EXPOSURE
Breathing	0–10	Threshold of hearing
Whisper, rustling leaves	20	Very quiet
Quiet rural area at night	30	
Library, soft background music	40	
Quiet suburb (daytime), conversation in living room	50	Quiet
Conversation in restaurant or average office, background music, chirping bird	60	Intrusive
Freeway traffic at 15 m, vacuum cleaner, noisy office or party, TV audio	70	Annoying
Garbage disposal, clothes washer, average factory, freight train at 15 m, food blender, dishwasher, arcade games	80	Possible hearing damage
Busy urban street, diesel truck	90	Hearing damage
Power lawn mower, iPod or other MP3 player, motorcycle at 8 m, outboard motor, farm tractor, printing plant, jack hammer, garbage truck, jet takeoff (305 m away), subway	100	
Automobile horn at 1 m, boom box stereo held close to ear, steel mill, riveting	110	
Front row at live rock music concert, siren, chain saw, stereo in cars, thunderclap, textile loom, jet takeoff (161 m away)	120	Human pain threshold
Earphones at maximum level, armored personnel carrier, jet takeoff (100 m away)	130	
Aircraft carrier deck	140	
Toy cap pistol, firecracker, jet takeoff (25 m away)	150	Eardrum rupture

dBA indicates decibels weighted by the A scale; m, meters.

When noise reduction is not possible, hearing protectors need to be worn, such as during occupational exposures, use of power lawn mowers, recreational exposures such as loud concerts, and other situational noise exposures. There are 2 types of hearing protectors—earplugs or earmuffs. Earplugs should fit properly; a slight tug required to remove them indicates correct fit. They are available in most drug stores. Earplugs should be checked while chewing, because jaw motion may loosen them. Earmuffs are the most effective type of ear protector and are available at most hardware stores. They have cups lined with sound-absorbing material that are held against the head with a spring band or oil-filled ring that provides a tight seal.

Unfortunately, environmental noise often cannot be controlled, which makes noise reduction or hearing protection difficult. Government regulations are needed to protect parents, children, and adolescents from these noises. If the workplace time-weighted average noise level exceeds 85 dBA, the employer must offer a hearing conservation program. Hearing protection must be provided and worn by all workers with 8 hours of exposure to 90 dBA, 4 hours at 95 dBA, and 2 hours at 100 dBA, with no exposure allowed to continuous noise above 115 dBA or impulse noise above 140 dBA. In nonoccupational settings, environmental noise is expressed as a day-night average sound level (DNL). For the protection of public health, the EPA proposed a DNL of 55 dB during waking hours and 45 dB during sleeping hours in neighborhoods, and 45 dB in daytime and 35 dB at night in hospitals. In 1972, Congress passed the Noise Control Act, giving the EPA a mandate to regulate environmental noise. The EPA's Office of Noise Abatement of Control was established at that time but was closed in 1982. State and local governments now have the primary responsibility of responding to many noise pollution matters.

During an emergency situation, it is to be expected that noise will occur when alarms, sirens, or other systems are activated automatically. When appropriate, caregivers and children can be taught to evacuate or to move away from the area near the noise. When this is not possible (because of a lockdown or other situation in which it is not safe to move away from the noise), pediatricians can work with child care, school, hospital, or other local facility administrators to ensure that the facility's emergency or disaster plan includes information on what to do to turn down the volume of the alarms or turn off the alarms as appropriate. Training for children and caregivers on what each alarm or siren signals is also important and should be addressed.

Frequently Asked Questions

Q *We live near an airport and the jets fly directly over our house as they take off and land. Will this be harmful to my newborn baby?*

A If the noise is causing discomfort to the parents' ears, it may be causing pain to the infant. The infant should be observed for sleep disturbances and response to the noise. The Federal Aviation Administration program on Airport Noise Compatibility Planning may be contacted for assessment of noise and possible mitigation. The local state programs listing participating airports can be found at http://www.faa.gov. Noise has physical and psychological effects on adults as well as children. To promote health and well-being for all family members, parents can consider moving to a quieter setting, if such a move is feasible.

Q *Are there unique hazards to the use of earbuds or headphones? How loud is too loud?*

A There are several reports of hearing loss secondary to the use of personal audio players using either headphones or earbuds. Although the data on damage are not conclusive, children and adolescents should be educated about the potential danger of loud music, whether heard at concerts, dances, and other social events or through earbuds or headphones. The personal digital audio player should be set at approximately 60% of maximum (maximum volume is about 100-110 dBA), and listening should be limited to 60 minutes daily. The user should be able to hear conversations going on around him or her while listening to the music. Earbuds generally have tighter seals with the ear canal than do headphones, so sound transfer may be more efficient with earbuds. Ringing or a feeling of fullness in the ear definitely means the music was too loud.

Resources

US Environmental Protection Agency, Office of Air and Radiation
Web site: www.epa.gov/air/noise.html

World Health Organization Regional Office for Europe
Night Noise Guidelines for Europe. Geneva, Switzerland: World Health Organization; 2009. www.euro.who.int/__data/assets/pdf_file/0017/43316/E92845.pdf

References

1. Philbin MK, Graven SN, Robertson A. The influence of auditory experience on the fetus, newborn, and preterm infant: report of the sound study group of the national resource center: the physical and developmental environment of the high risk infant. *J Perinatol.* 2000;20(8 Suppl):S1–S142

2. Nave CR. Hyperphysics: Sound and Hearing. Available at: http://hyperphysics.phy-astr.gsu.edu/hbase/HFrame.html. Accessed March 28, 2011

3. DeJoy DM. Environmental noise and children: a review of recent findings. *J Aud Res.* 1983;23(3):181–194

4. Roche AF, Chumleawc RM, Siervogel RM. *Longitudinal Study of Human Hearing, Its Relationship to Noise and Other Factors. III. Results From the First 5 Years.* Washington, DC: US Environmental Protection Agency/Aerospace Medical Research Lab; 1982. Report No. AFAMRL-TR-82-68

5. Daniel E. Noise and hearing loss: a review. *J Sch Health.* 2007;77(5):225-231

6. Evans GW. Child development and the physical environment. *Annu Rev Psychol.* 2006;57: 423-451

7. Henderson D, Hamernik RP. Biologic bases of noise-induced hearing loss. *Occup Med.* 1995;10(3):513–534

8. Agrawal Y, Platz EA, Niparko JK. Risk factors for hearing loss in US adults: data from the National Health and Nutrition Examination Survey, 1999 to 2002. *Otol Neurotol.* 2009;30(2):139-145

9. Prince MM, Stayner LT, Smith RJ, Gilbert SJ. A re-examination of risk estimates from the NIOSH Occupational Noise and Hearing Survey (ONHS). *J Acoust Soc Am.* 1997;101:950–963

10. Jackler RK, Schindler DN. Occupational hearing loss. In: LaDou J, ed. *Occupational Medicine.* Norwalk, CT: Appleton and Lange; 1990:95–105

11. Niskar AS, Kieszak SM, Holmes AE, Esteban E, Rubin C, Brody DJ. Estimated prevalence of noise-induced hearing threshold shifts among children 6–19 years of age: the Third National Health and Nutrition Examination Survey, 1988–1994, United States. *Pediatrics.* 2001;108(1):40–43

12. Renick KM, Crawford JM, Wilkins JR. Hearing loss among Ohio farm youth: a comparison to a national sample. *Am J Ind Med.* 2009;52(3):233-239

13. Mercier V, Luy D, Hohmann BW. The sound exposure of the audience at a music festival. *Noise Health.* 2003;5(19):51-58

14. Bess FH, Dodd-Murphy J, Parker RA. Children with minimal sensorineural hearing loss: prevalence, educational performance, and functional status. *Ear Hear.* 1998;19(5):339–354

15. Segal S, Eviatar E, Lapinsky J, Shlamkovitch N, Kessler A. Inner ear damage in children due to noise exposure from toy cap pistols and firecrackers: a retrospective review of 53 cases. *Noise Health.* 2003;5(18):13-18

16. National Institute of Public Health Denmark. *Health Effects of Noise on Children and Perception of the Risk of Noise.* Bistrup ML, ed. Copenhagen, Denmark: National Institute of Public Health Denmark; 2001:29

17. Mercier V, Hohmann B. Is electronically amplified music too loud? What do young people think? *Noise Health.* 2002;4(16):47-55

18. Torre P. Young adults' use and output level settings of personal music systems. *Ear Hear.* 2008;29(5):791-799

19. American Academy of Pediatrics, Committee on Environmental Health. Noise: a hazard for the fetus and newborn. *Pediatrics.* 1997;100(4):724–727

20. Rocha EB, Frasson de Azevedo M, Ximenes Filho JA. Study of the hearing in children born from pregnant women exposed to occupational noise: assessment by distortion product otoacoustic emissions. *Rev Bras Otorrinolaringol.* 2007;73(3):359-369

21. Philbin MK, Robertson A, Hall JW III. Recommended permissible noise criteria for occupied, newly constructed or renovated hospital nurseries. The Sound Study Group of the National Resource Center. *J Perinatol.* 1999;19(8 Pt 1):559-563

22. Darcy AE, Hancock LE, Ware EJ. A descriptive study of noise in the neonatal intensive care unit. Ambient levels and perceptions of contributing factors. *Adv Neonatal Care.* 2008;8(3): 165-175

23. Lasky RE, Williams AL. Noise and light exposures for extremely low birth weight newborns during their stay in the neonatal intensive care unit. *Pediatrics*. 2009;123(2):540-546

24. Als H, Lawhon G, Brown E, et al. Individualized behavioral and environmental care for the very low birth weight preterm infant at high risk for bronchopulmonary dysplasia: neonatal intensive care unit and developmental outcome. *Pediatrics*. 1986;78(6):1123–1132

25. Buehler DM, Als H, Duffy FH, McAnulty GB, Liederman J. Effectiveness of individualized developmental care for low-risk preterm infants: behavioral and electrophysiologic evidence. *Pediatrics*. 1995;96(5 Pt 1):923–932

26. Philbin KM. Planning the acoustic environment of a neonatal intensive care unit. *Clin Perinatol*. 2004;31(2):331–352

27. Tharpe AM, Bess FH, Sladen DP, Schissel H, Couch S, Schery T. Auditory characteristics of children with autism. *Ear Hear*. 2006;27(4):430-441

28. Gravel JS, Dunn M, Lee WW, Ellis MA. Peripheral audition of children on the autistic spectrum. *Ear Hear*. 2006;27(3):299–312

29. Henkin RI, Knigge KM. Effect of sound on hypothalamic pituitary-adrenal axis. *Am J Physiol*. 1963;204:701–704

30. Frankenhaeuser M, Lundberg U. Immediate and delayed effects of noise on performance and arousal. *Biol Psychol*. 1974;2(2):127–133

31. Falk SA, Woods NF. Hospital noise—levels and potential health hazards. *N Engl J Med*. 1973;289(15):774–781

32. Cureton-Lane RA, Fontaine DK. Sleep in the pediatric ICU: an empirical investigation. *Am J Crit Care*. 1997;6(1):56-63

33. Thiessen GJ. Disturbance of sleep by noise. *J Acoust Soc Am*. 1978;64(1):216–222

34. Rosenberg J. Jets over Labrador and Quebec: noise effects on human health. *Can Med Assoc J*. 1991;144(7):869–875

35. Clark C, Martin R, van Kempen E, et al. Exposure–effect relations between aircraft and road traffic noise exposure at school and reading comprehension: The RANCH Project. *Am J Epidemiol*. 2006;163(1):27-37

36. Morrison WE, Haas EC, Shaffner DH, Garrett ES, Fackler JC. Noise, stress, and annoyance in a pediatric intensive care unit. *Crit Care Med*. 2003;31(1):113-119

37. Picard M, Bradley JS. Revisiting speech interference in classrooms. *Audiology*. 2001;40(5):221-244

38. American Academy of Pediatrics, Committee on Practice and Ambulatory Medicine and Section on Otolaryngology and Bronchoesophagology. Hearing assessment in infants and children: recommendations beyond neonatal screening. *Pediatrics*. 2003;111(2):436-440

39. Hagan JF, Shaw JS, Duncan PM, eds. *Bright Futures: Guidelines for Health Supervision of Infants, Children, and Adolescents*. 3rd ed. Elk Grove Village, IL: American Academy of Pediatrics; 2008

40. American Academy of Pediatrics, Joint Committee on Infant Hearing. Year 2007 position statement: principles and guidelines for early hearing detection and intervention programs. *Pediatrics*. 2007;120(4):898-921

41. Hear-it AISBL. Noisy toys are not for delicate ears. Available at: http://www.hear-it.org/page.dsp?area=898. Accessed April 22, 2011

42. Wachs TD. Nature of relations between the physical and social microenvironment of the two-year-old child. *Early Dev Parenting*. 1993;2:81–87

43. Torsten Lindgren T, Wieslander G, Nordquist T, Dammström, BG, Norbäck D. Hearing status among cabin crew in a Swedish commercial airline company. *Int Arch Occup Environ Health*. 2009;82(7):887–892

Chapter 35

Persistent Organic Pollutants — DDT, PCBs, PCDFs, and Dioxins

■ ■ ■ ■ ■ ■ ■

The term "persistent organic pollutants" (POPs) generally refers to compounds with one or more aromatic rings, with bromine or chlorine substituting for some of the hydrogens. These compounds degrade slowly or incompletely and, thus, remain in the environment for long periods. POPs are fat soluble and, thus, not excreted in urine and have low vapor pressure and, thus, are not excreted through the lungs. Consequently, when they are released into the environment in large quantities, they concentrate up food chains and appear in the tissues of higher-order predators, including human beings. The archetype is dichlorodiphenyltrichloroethane (DDT), an organochlorine pesticide. It was banned from manufacture in 1972 after 4 decades of extensive global use. This decision was based on, among other things, its widespread appearance in human tissue and its effects on wildlife, especially reproduction in pelagic birds (birds that live in the open sea rather than in coastal or inland waters).[1] A recent, more specific use of the term persistent organic pollutants comes from the Stockholm Convention (http://chm.pops.int/default.aspx), an international agreement adopted in 2001, which aims to protect human health and the environment by eliminating and reducing the worldwide production, use, and emission of persistent organic pollutants. The Stockholm Convention initially targeted global elimination of the "dirty dozen," 12 widespread, toxic agents broadly believed to have sufficient toxicity to outweigh any benefit from continued use. In 2009, 9 additional chemicals named as persistent organic pollutants were listed by the Stockholm Convention. Many of these "living chemicals" are still produced and in use.

In this chapter, 4 of the "dirty dozen" are discussed—DDT and its derivatives, polychlorinated biphenyls (PCBs), dibenzofurans, and polychlorinated dibenzodioxins (PCDDs), especially 2,3,7,8 tetrachlorodibenzodioxin (TCDD). Chlordane, heptachlor, and hexachlorobenzene are discussed in Chapter 15. The others—aldrin, dieldrin, endrin, mirex, and toxaphene—are no longer used in the United States, and clinical questions about them seldom arise. Besides the "dirty dozen," other persistent agents of concern include polybrominated biphenyls (PBBs; see Chapter 28) and polybrominated diphenyl ethers (PBDEs; see Chapter 36).

PCBs are compounds with 2 linked phenyl rings and variable degrees of chlorination. They are clear, nonvolatile, hydrophobic oils. Approximately 1.5 million metric tons were produced starting in the 1930s. They were banned in the United States and northern Europe in the late 1970s. Much of what was made is still somewhere in the environment. PCBs were used primarily in the electrical industry as insulators and dielectrics, especially for applications in which a fire hazard was present, such as in heavy transformers. During the 1960s, analytical chemists interested in DDT residues in the tissues of pelagic birds began identifying background peaks in their chromatograms as PCBs. Since then, numerous studies throughout the world have shown detectable levels of PCBs in human tissue and human milk; except for DDT and its analogues, PCBs are the most dispersed of the halogenated hydrocarbon pollutant chemicals,[2] although the polybrominated diphenyl ethers may be catching up.[3]

Polychlorinated dibenzofurans are partially oxidized PCBs. They were not made intentionally but appear as contaminants in PCBs that have undergone high temperature applications or have been in fires or explosions. Polychlorinated dibenzodioxins, commonly referred to as dioxins, also are contaminants. These compounds were formed during the manufacture of hexachlorophene, pentachlorophenol, and the phenoxyacid herbicides 2,4,5 trichloro-phenoxyacetic acid (a component of Agent Orange, used as a defoliant during the Vietnam War) and silvex, under what would now be considered poorly controlled conditions. They also are formed, albeit at very low yield, during paper bleaching and waste incineration. One dioxin congener, tetrachlorodibenzo-p-dioxin (TCDD), may be the most toxic synthetic chemical known.[4]

ROUTES AND SOURCES OF EXPOSURE

Children may be exposed through ingestion, inhalation, and dermal exposure. The source of exposure for most people to all of these compounds is contaminated food. Because the chemicals are not well metabolized or excreted, even very small daily doses accumulate to measurable amounts over years. The most concentrated source is sport fish from contaminated waters. Persistent organic pollutant residues bioconcentrate in fish, a food that is high on the food chain and commonly consumed by people. Bioconcentration also increases exposure for native people of the Arctic, who eat blubber of sea mammals, themselves fish eaters.[5] In certain areas of the Arctic, dietary intakes exceed established national and international guidelines.[6] In areas where PCB contamination has been a problem, state and local health departments have issued advisories that recommend limiting the consumption of contaminated fish. The major dietary source for young children is human milk, from which they absorb and store these chemicals (see Chapter 15).

Predictable occupational exposure to these compounds is now rare and would be most likely for those involved in the cleanup of hazardous waste sites or repair work for electrical utilities. Heavy electrical equipment produced decades ago still is in service, and transformers may leak or become damaged during fires or explosions, thus exposing workers and the environment to PCBs or polychlorinated dibenzofurans (PCDFs). Substantial quantities of PCBs still are present in older industrial facilities other than electric utilities, such as railroads. Modern herbicides are not contaminated with polychlorinated dibenzodioxins, and although there is exposure from waste incineration and paper bleaching, the amounts are very small. DDT is or was used as an indoor spray to control malaria in several countries, mostly in sub-Saharan Africa. Workers who do the spraying and residents of the sprayed houses have high exposures, and these workers may become immigrants to the United States. There should be no occupational exposure to DDT in the United States, but there is some suspicion that DDT is still used internationally in agriculture and, thus, those who handle imported food or fiber might be exposed. Immigrants to the United States may also have been exposed in their country of origin.

SYSTEMS AFFECTED AND CLINICAL EFFECTS

At the population level, exposure to commonly encountered levels of PCBs is associated with lower developmental/IQ test scores, including lower psychomotor scores from the newborn period through 2 years of age,[7] defects in short-term memory in 7-month-olds[8] and 4-year-olds,[9] and lowered IQs in 42-month-olds[10,11] and 11-year-olds.[12] Prenatal exposure to PCBs from the mother's body burden, rather than exposure through human milk, seems to account for most but not all[11] of the findings. There also may be subclinical effects on thyroid function in the newborn infant, but this has been an inconsistent finding[13] (see Chapter 28).

DDT, mostly as DDE (dichlordiphenyldichloroethylene, a degradation product of DDT), has been studied in several cohorts, with most showing some effects on developmental test scores in young children.[14] Results from a Catalonian[15] birth cohort showed that prenatal exposure to p,p'-DDE was associated with a delay in mental and psychomotor development at 13 months of age; a study in mostly migrant women in California showed similar developmental delays but in association with DDT, the parent compound.[16] Long-term breastfeeding was found to be beneficial to neurodevelopment in both studies, despite exposure to these chemicals through human milk. See Table 35.1 for a list of reported signs and symptoms by age at occurrence.

Exposure to DDE has been associated with preterm birth.[24] Although estrogen-like effects have been observed in some studies, it is not clear whether this results in a shorter duration of lactation[25-28] (see Chapter 15).

Table 35.1: Reported Signs and Symptoms by Age at Occurrence from PCBs, PCDFs, PCDDs, TCDD, and DDT/DDE

PRENATAL EXPOSURE TO LOW LEVELS OF PCBs

■ Newborns	Decrease in birth weight[17]
■ Infants	Motor delay detectable from birth to 2 years[18]
■ 7-month-olds	Defects in visual recognition memory[8]
■ 42-month-olds	Lower IQ (may be some contribution from postnatal exposure)[10]
■ 4-year-olds	Defects in short-term memory[9]
■ 11-year-olds	Delays in cognitive development[12]

PRENATAL EXPOSURE TO HIGH LEVELS OF PCBs/PCDFs (ASIAN POISONINGS)

■ Newborns	Low birth weight, conjunctivitis, natal teeth, pigmentation[19]
■ Infant through school age	Delays on all cognitive domains tested; behavior disorders; growth retardation; abnormal development of hair, nails, and teeth; pigmentation; increased risk of bronchitis[20]
■ Puberty	Small penis size but normal development in boys; growth delay but normal development in girls[21]

DIRECT INGESTION OF HIGH DOSES OF PCBs/PCDFs

■ Any age	Chloracne, keratoses, and pigmentation; mixed peripheral neuropathy; gastritis[22]

DERMAL EXPOSURE TO HIGH LEVELS OF TCDD

■ Children	Probably higher absorbed dose for a given exposure than adults, chloracne, liver function test abnormalities[23]

EXPOSURE TO LOW LEVELS OF DDT/DDE

■ Children	Delays in psychomotor test scores in preschool children[14]

DDT indicates dichlorodiphenyltrichloroethane; DDE, dichlordiphenyldichloroethylene; PCBs, polychlorinated biphenyls; PCDFs, polychlorinated dibenzofurans; PCDDs, polychlorinated dibenzodioxins; TCDD, 2,3,7,8-tetra-chlorobenzo-p-dioxin.

Two mass poisonings occurred in Asia in which cooking oil was inadvertently mixed with PCBs that were heat-degraded and, thus, heavily contaminated with polychlorinated dibenzofurans. In 1968, an epidemic of acne among residents of Kyushu province in Japan was traced to the use of such cooking oil. Approximately 2000 people were eventually given the diagnosis of Yusho (oil disease).[29] Among 13 women who were pregnant around the time of exposure, one of the children was stillborn and was deeply and diffusely pigmented (a "cola-colored" baby). Some of the live-born children were small, hyperbilirubinemic, and pigmented and had conjunctival swelling with dilation of the sebaceous glands of the eyelid. Follow-up of the children up to 9 years later showed apathy, lethargy, and soft neurologic signs. The growth deficit apparent at birth resolved by approximately 4 years of age. An extraordinarily similar outbreak occurred in Taiwan in 1979.[30] In Taiwan, 117 children who were born during or after the food contamination in 1979 and, thus, exposed to their mothers' body burden of PCBs and polychlorinated dibenzofurans were examined in 1985[24] and have been followed since. They have a variety of ectodermal defects, such as excess pigmentation, carious teeth, poor nail formation, and short stature. They have persistent behavioral abnormalities[31] and cognitive impairment, on the average about 5 to 8 IQ points. Furthermore, the delay is as severe in children born up to 6 years after exposure as it is in those born in 1979.[32]

A chemical plant explosion in Seveso, Italy, in 1975 released kilogram quantities of TCDD. The highest recorded serum concentrations of TCDD in humans occurred in children in the most heavily exposed areas in this incident.[33] Children in the area near the explosion had chloracne, most pronounced on areas unprotected by clothing,[34] and some had abnormal liver function tests.[23] Further follow-up of men exposed as infants or adolescents showed alterations in sperm production and sex hormones.[35] In Vietnam, spraying with Agent Orange during the Vietnam War has left a legacy of TCDD contamination still detectable in human milk.[36] There are anecdotal reports of toxicity in children, but no systematic study has been reported. The offspring of male Vietnam veterans who may have had exposure from Agent Orange show no clear excess of malformations[37]; no data are available on the offspring of female veterans. Studies assessing the carcinogenic potential of PCBs in animals and humans have shown inconsistent results.[38] TCDD, however, is a highly potent carcinogen and is categorized as a known human carcinogen by the International Agency for Research on Cancer.[39]

A single study in the United States demonstrated an association between prenatal exposure to DDE and taller, heavier boys at age 14 years.[40] This finding was not confirmed in another prospective study of 304 adolescent boys.[41]

DIAGNOSTIC METHODS

Although many laboratories can measure DDT/DDE and PCBs, there are no quality assurance programs or reference values available, and no laboratory is licensed to measure these chemicals for diagnostic or therapeutic use. Thus, any measurement would have to be regarded as research and would be interpretable only within a research project. The polychlorinated dibenzofurans and polychlorinated dibenzodioxins are much more difficult to measure, and no clinical interpretation is available if the measurement is performed. Because any of these compounds can appear in human milk, it occasionally seems useful to measure them in a clinical setting. However, any reasonably sensitive method will detect DDE and PCBs in most samples of human milk. Thus far, all expert bodies that have considered this topic recommend breastfeeding and do not recommend testing of human milk. More information is included in Chapter 15.

TREATMENT

No regimen is known to lower body burden of these compounds. In Asia, treatments that have been tried include cholestyramine, sauna bathing, and fasting, none of which were effective. Breastfeeding does lower the levels, by approximately 20% for each 6 months of lactation. Theoretically, this would increase the risk to the child, but so far the morbidity attributable to exposure to these compounds has come from prenatal exposure to maternal body burden rather than from exposure through human milk (see Chapter 15).

REGULATION

DDT was banned in the United States in 1972. PCBs are banned from new production throughout the world. Any waste substance, commonly waste oils, with more than 50 parts per million (ppm) of PCBs must be handled as a hazardous substance and disposed of as hazardous waste. PCBs are unavoidable contaminants of foods, so they have "temporary tolerances," which are levels that, if found in a food in commerce, result in a requirement from the US Food and Drug Administration that the food be removed from the market. For infant and junior foods, the tolerance is 1.5 parts per million fat basis for PCBs; for fish, it is 5 parts per million fat basis. There are no tolerances for polychlorinated dibenzofurans or polychlorinated dibenzodioxins.

The Food and Agriculture Organization and the World Health Organization (WHO) publish "allowable daily intakes." For PCBs, the allowable daily intake is 6 µg/kg per day, which is about the median for a fully breastfed 5-kg infant. There are no allowable daily intakes for polychlorinated dibenzofurans or polychlorinated dibenzodioxins. There is a "tolerable daily intake" (reflecting greater uncertainty in the data) of 4 picograms (pg)/kg per day of toxic equivalents of TCDD. Similarly, there is a tolerable daily intake for total DDT of 0.01 mg/ kg day. Although intake by breastfed children might commonly exceed this level, the WHO explicitly advised there be no change in the organization's policy to recommend breastfeeding despite the presence of the pollutant chemicals.[42,43]

The concept of "toxic equivalency" arises out of the dilemma faced by those who regulate these compounds. Exposure to a single compound of this class is unusual; rather, most human exposure is to mixtures of dozens or more of these compounds. Many PCBs, polychlorinated dibenzofurans, and dioxins other than TCDD have a spectrum of toxic effects similar to that of TCDD, but the doses at which they produce those effects vary over orders of magnitude, with TCDD being the most potent. Much, if not all, of the toxicity of TCDD is thought to begin when it binds to the aryl hydrocarbon hydroxylase (Ah) receptor. This receptor is structurally similar to steroid hormone receptors but has no known endogenous ligand. It is distributed widely in mammalian tissue and may have evolved as part of a detoxification pathway. There are assays available that measure Ah receptor binding; thus, a given compound can be compared to TCDD in terms of its abilities to bind to the receptor. The ratio of receptor binding can be used as a conversion factor to estimate the toxicity of a compound relative to TCDD; multiplying the amount of the compound times its conversion factor yields a "toxic equivalent" (TEQ) amount of TCDD. The conversion factors are thus called "toxic equivalency factors." They can be calculated for any compound that binds to the Ah receptor. The "toxic equivalent" amount for a mixture can be estimated by adding the "toxic equivalent" amounts for the individual compounds present. The 1998 revision of the tolerable daily intake for TCDD was the first time that it was expressed in "toxic equivalents," rather than as an amount of TCDD per se. This makes biological sense, because the typical diet contains more "toxic equivalents" from compounds other than TCDD, especially PCBs, than from TCDD itself; thus, it makes little sense to consider only part of a mixture of compounds with similar toxicity. On the other hand, there are other forms of toxicity that some of these compounds possess, such as neurotoxicity, that are not related to Ah receptor binding and, thus, will not be captured by the "toxic equivalent" approach. Nonetheless, using "toxic equivalents" to think about the problem of mixtures of compounds with relatively similar toxicity seems like a step in the right direction, recognizing that the toxicology of mixtures in general is not well understood and a great deal of work will be necessary before it is understood. There is a good discussion of the use of toxic equivalency in the documents supporting the 1998 tolerable daily intake recommendation for TCDD.[44]

ALTERNATIVES

PCBs have been replaced mostly by mineral oils. Polychlorinated dibenzodioxins and polychlorinated dibenzofurans were never made deliberately, and no product is now contaminated at the levels seen during the 1960s. DDT has been supplanted for all agricultural uses by other pesticides or improved agricultural practice. For malaria control, it can probably be replaced by bed nets and other means of controlling vectors.

Frequently Asked Questions

Q   *Should I be concerned about dioxins in coffee filters, diapers, tampons, etc?*

A   Paper products usually are bleached by using chlorine bleaches. The reaction between the chlorine and the lignins in the wood fiber produces many complex chlorinated organic compounds, among them TCDD. The amounts are minuscule, and avoiding products that have been bleached using chlorine is unlikely to produce a discernable health benefit. Unbleached products or products bleached using oxygen are sometimes available and can be substituted. They should be free of such residues.

Q   *How do I know whether fish or other foods have PCBs or dioxins in them?*

A   The food supply has trace amounts of all of these compounds. Commercial foods are regulated, so they should not have more than minimal amounts. Among unregulated foods, the most likely source of higher exposure is sport fish. States in which these compounds have been a problem, such as those around the Great Lakes, have advisories concerning the consumption of noncommercial fish, and these should be available from the state health department.

Q   *If PCBs were banned in the 1970s and are no longer produced, why are they still a problem?*

A   PCBs and compounds like them were used and dispersed at a time when their persistence seemed to be desirable and the consequences of that persistence unappreciated. PCBs and DDT break down either very slowly or not at all in the environment. Parts of the Great Lakes and the Hudson River still have sludge heavily contaminated by PCBs that were probably made in the 1960s. Compounds with this degree of persistence are no longer used for applications that allow such pollution to occur, but the amounts in the environment when the ban occurred were sufficient to produce contaminated sediment for subsequent decades, with no clear end in sight.

Resources

US Environmental Protection Agency (EPA)
Web site: www.epa.gov/OST/fish
This site lists EPA guidelines for states for the development of fish advisories for PCBs and other persistent contaminants.

World Health Organization (WHO)
Persistent Organic Pollutants: Impact on Child Health (2010).
www.who.int/ceh/publications/persistent_organic_pollutant/en/index.html

References

1. Rogan WJ, Chen AM. Health risks and benefits of bis(4-chlorophenyl)-1,1,1-trichloroethane (DDT). *Lancet*. 2005;366(9487):763-773
2. International Programme on Chemical Safety. *Polychlorinated Biphenyls and Terphenyls. Environmental Health Criteria 140*. Geneva, Switzerland: World Health Organization; 1993
3. Noren K, Meironyte D. Certain organochlorine and organobromine contaminants in Swedish human milk in perspective of past 20-30 years. *Chemosphere*. 2000;40(9-11):1111-1123
4. Baarschers W. *Eco-Facts and Eco-Fiction: Understanding the Environmental Debate*. London, England: Routledge; 1996
5. Dewailly E, Ryan JJ, Laliberte C, et al. Exposure of remote maritime populations to coplanar PCBs. *Environ Health Perspect*. 1994;102(Suppl 1):205-209
6. Zung A, Glaser T, Kerem Z, Zadik Z. Breast development in the first 2 years of life: an association with soy-based infant formulas. *J Pediatr Gastroenterol Nutr*. 2008;46(2):191-195
7. Gladen BC, Rogan WJ. Effects of perinatal polychlorinated biphenyls and dichlorodiphenyl dichloroethene on later development. *J Pediatr*. 1991;119(1 Pt 1):58-63
8. Jacobson SW, Fein GG, Jacobson JL, Schwartz PM, Dowler JK. The effect of intrauterine PCB exposure on visual recognition memory. *Child Dev*. 1985;56(4):853-860
9. Jacobson JL, Jacobson SW, Humphrey HE. Effects of *in utero* exposure to polychlorinated biphenyls and related contaminants on cognitive functioning in young children. *J Pediatr*. 1990;116(1):38-45
10. Patandin S, Lanting CI, Mulder PGH, Boersma ER, Sauer CP, Weisglas-Kuperus N. Effects of environmental exposure to polychlorinated biphenyls and dioxins on cognitive abilities in Dutch children at 42 months of age. *J Pediatr*. 1999;134(1):33-41
11. Walkowiak J, Wiener JA, Heinzow B, et al. Environmental exposure to polychlorinated biphenyls and quality of the home environment: effects on psychodevelopment in early childhood. *Lancet*. 2001;358(9293):1602-1607
12. Jacobson JL, Jacobson SW. Intellectual impairment in children exposed to polychlorinated biphenyls *in utero*. *N Engl J Med*. 1996;335(11):783-789
13. Brouwer A, Longnecker M, Birnbaum L, et al. Characterization of potential endocrine-related health effects at low-dose levels of exposure to PCBs. *Environ Health Perspect*. 1999;107 (Suppl 4):639-649
14. Rosas LG, Eskenazi B. Pesticides and child neurodevelopment. *Curr Opin Pediatr*. 2008;20(2): 191-197
15. Ribas-Fito N, Julvez J, Torrent M, Grimalt JO, Sunyer J. Beneficial effects of breastfeeding on cognition regardless of DDT concentrations at birth. *Am J Epidemiol*. 2007;166(10):1198-1202

16. Adeoya-Osiguwa SA, Markoulaki S, Pocock V, Milligan SR, Fraser LR. 17 beta-Estradiol and environmental estrogens significantly affect mammalian sperm function. *Hum Reprod.* 2003;18(1):100-107

17. Fein GG, Jacobson JL, Jacobson SW, Schwartz PM, Dowler JK. Prenatal exposure to polychlorinated biphenyls: effects on birth size and gestational age. *J Pediatr.* 1984;105(2): 315-320

18. Gladen BC, Rogan WJ, Hardy P, Thullen J, Tingelstad J, Tully M. Development after exposure to polychlorinated biphenyls and dichlorodiphenyl dichloroethene transplacentally and through human milk. *J Pediatr.* 1988;113(6):991-995

19. Miller RW. Congenital PCB poisoning: a reevaluation. *Environ Health Perspect.* 1985;60: 211-214

20. Rogan WJ, Gladen BC, Hung KL, et al. Congenital poisoning by polychlorinated biphenyls and their contaminants in Taiwan. *Science.* 1988;241(4863):334-336

21. Guo YL, Lai TJ, Ju SH, Chen YC, Hsu CC. Sexual developments and biological findings in Yucheng children. In: Fiedler H, Frank H, Hutzinger O, Parzefall W, Riss A, Safe S, eds. *Organohalogen Compounds.* 14th ed. Vienna, Austria: Federal Environmental Agency; 1993:235-238

22. Kuratsune M, Yoshimura T, Matsuzaka J, Yamaguchi A. Epidemiologic study on Yusho, a poisoning caused by ingestion of rice oil contaminated with a commercial brand of polychlorinated biphenyls. *Environ Health Perspect.* 1972;1:119-128

23. Mocarelli P, Marocchi A, Brambilla P, Gerthoux PM, Young DS, Mantel N. Clinical laboratory manifestations of exposure to dioxin in children. A six-year study of the effects of an environmental disaster near Seveso, Italy. *JAMA.* 1986;256(19):2687-2695

24. Longnecker MP, Klebanoff M, Zhou H, Brock J. Association between maternal serum concentration of the DDT metabolite DDE and preterm and small-for-gestational-age babies at birth. *Lancet.* 2001;358(9276):110-114

25. Gladen BC, Rogan WJ. DDE and shortened duration of lactation in a Northern Mexican town. *Am J Public Health.* 1995;85(4):504-508

26. Karmaus W, Davis S, Fussman C, Brooks K. Maternal concentration of dichlordiphenyl dichloroethylene (DDE) and initiation and duration of breast feeding. *Paediatr Perinat Epidemiol.* 2005;19(5):388-398

27. McGuiness B, Vena JE, Buck GM, et al. The effects of DDE on the duration of lactation among women in the New York State Angler Cohort. *Epidemiology.* 1999;10:359

28. Cupul-Uicab LA, Gladen BC, Hernandez-Avila M, Weber JP, Longnecker MP. DDE, a degradation product of DDT, and duration of lactation in a highly exposed area of Mexico. *Environ Health Perspect.* 2008;116(2):179-183

29. Harada M. Intrauterine poisoning: Clinical and epidemiological studies and significance of the problem. *Bull Inst Const Med Kumamoto Univ.* 1976;25(Suppl):1-66

30. Hsu S, Ma C, Hsu SK, Wu S, Hsu NH, Yeh C. Discovery and epidemiology of PCB poisoning in Taiwan. *Am J Ind Med.* 1984;5(1-2):71-79

31. Chen Y-CJ, Yu M-LM, Rogan WJ, Gladen BC, Hsu CC. A six-year follow-up of behavior and activity disorders in the Taiwan Yu-Cheng children. *Am J Public Health.* 1994;84(3):415-421

32. Lai TJ, Liu X, Guo YL, et al. A cohort study of behavioral problems and intelligence in children with high prenatal polychlorinated biphenyl exposure. *Arch Gen Psychiatry.* 2002;59(1061):1066

33. Mocarelli P, Needham LL, Morocchi A, et al. Serum concentrations of 2,3,7,8-tetrachlorodibenzo-p-dioxin and test results from selected residents of Seveso, Italy. *J Toxicol Environ Health.* 1991;32(4):357-366

34. Caramaschi F, del-Corno G, Favaretti C, Giambelluca SE, Montesarchio E, Fara GM. Chloracne following environmental contamination by TCDD in Seveso, Italy. *Int J Epidemiol.* 1981;10(2):135-143

35. Mocarelli P, Gerthoux PM, Patterson DG, et al. Dioxin exposure, from infancy through puberty, produces endocrine disruption and affects human semen quality. *Environ Health Perspect.* 2008;116(1):70-77

36. Schecter A, Dai LC, Thuy LT, et al. Agent Orange and the Vietnamese: the persistence of elevated dioxin levels in human tissues. *Am J Public Health.* 1995;85(4):516-522

37. Erickson JD, Mulinare J, McClain PW. Vietnam veterans' risks for fathering babies with birth defects. *JAMA.* 1984;252(7):903-012

38. Cogliano VJ. Assessing the cancer risk from environmental PCBs. *Environ Health Perspect.* 1998;106(6):317-323

39. International Agency for Research on Cancer. *Polychlorinated Dibenzo-para-dioxins and Polychlorinated dibenzofurans.* Lyon, France: International Agency for Research on Cancer; 1997

40. Gladen BC, Ragan NB, Rogan WJ. Pubertal growth and development and prenatal and lactational exposure to polychlorinated biphenyls and dichlorodiphenyl dichloroethene. *J Pediatr.* 2000;136(4):490-496

41. Gladen BC, Klebanoff M, Hediger ML, et al. Prenatal DDT exposure in relation to anthropometric and pubertal measures in adolescent males. *Environ Health Perspect.* 2004;112(17): 1761-1767

42. Pronczuk J, Moy G, Vallenas C. Breast milk: an optimal food. *Environ Health Perspect.* 2004;112(13):A722-A723

43. World Health Organization. *Persistent Organic Pollutants: Impact on Child Health.* Geneva, Switzerland, World Health Organization; 2010. Available at: http://www.who.int/ceh/ publications/persistent_organic_pollutant/en/index.html. Accessed June 11, 2011

44. van den Berg M, van Birgelen APJM, Birnbaum L, et al. Consultation on assessment of the health risk of dioxins; re-evaluation of the tolerable daily intake (TDI): executive summary. *Food Addit Contam.* 2000;17:223-240

Chapter 36

Persistent Toxic Substances

■ ■ ■ ■ ■ ■

The term "persistent toxic substances" (PTSs) is synonymous with persistent bioaccumulative toxic substances (PBTs). Persistent toxic substances overlap with another category of environmental toxicants, the persistent organic pollutants (POPs [see Chapter 35]), generally categorized as a group of 12 specific halogenated chemicals (aldrin, chlordane, dichlorodiphenyltrichloroethane [DDT], dieldrin, endrin, heptachlor, hexachlorobenzene, mirex, polychlorinated biphenyls [PCBs], dioxins, dibenzofurans, and toxaphene). Persistent toxic substances include toxicants with the following features: (1) they degrade slowly or not at all over time or through exposure to sunlight, water, or other mechanisms; (2) they have potential for long-distance transport by air or water with settling in remote regions of the globe; (3) they have long elimination half-lives, leading to bioaccumulatation in humans and other living creatures; and (4) they are known to have or strongly suspected of having human toxicity. These chemicals include a broad range of substances (Table 36.1), such as organic compounds (eg, pentachlorophenol, polyaromatic hydrocarbons), metals (eg, lead, mercury), pesticides (eg, lindane), and halogenated compounds. The number of substances labeled as persistent toxic substances continues to grow, corresponding to their use in the manufacture of consumer products.

Because of their environmental persistence, spread, and bioaccumulation, exposure to these chemicals is a concern, especially for fetuses, nursing infants, and children.

Among persistent toxic substances, the halogenated compounds have received the greatest attention. Chlorinated chemicals have the longest history of concern, not only because of their health effects but because of their effect on diminishing stratospheric ozone (the "ozone layer"), the protective blanket that absorbs

Table 36.1: Common Persistent Toxic Substances*	
	COMMON SOURCES
ORGANIC MOLECULES	
Methyl tertiary butyl ether (MTBE)	Gasoline additive
Alkylphenols	Clothing treatment solutions
Endosulfan	Insecticide
Phthalates	Plastics
METALS AND ORGANOMETALS	
Lead and tetraethyl lead	Paint, gasoline additive
Mercury and organomercury	Air, food
Cadmium	Tobacco smoke
Organotin compounds	Marine paint, outdoor air
Methylcyclopentadienyl manganese tricarbonyl (MMT)	Gasoline additive
HALOGENATED COMPOUNDS	
Perfluoroalkyl chemicals	Teflon, Scotchguard, nonstick materials
Polybrominated diphenyl ethers	Fire retardants, food, water, indoor air, dust
Perchlorates	Food, water
Lindane	Insecticide (lice, scabies)
Pentachlorophenol	Wood preservative
Atrazine	Herbicide

The term persistent toxic substances includes the class of compounds known as persistent organic pollutants (POPs). The 12 original persistent organic pollutants, all of which are chlorinated compounds, consist of aldrin, chlordane, dichlorodiphenyltrichloroethane (DDT), dieldrin, endrin, heptachlor, hexachlorobenzene, mirex, polychlorinated biphenyls, dioxins, dibenzofurans, and toxaphene.

significant amounts of the sun's harmful ultraviolet radiation. This environmental damage, coupled with suspected toxicity of halogenated compounds, led to the removal of chlorofluorocarbons (CFCs) from refrigerators, air conditioners, spray cans, and multiple-dose inhalers. However, chemicals made with the halides chlorine (Cl^-), bromine (Br^-), and fluorine (Fl^-) remain prevalent.

This chapter reviews three widely used persistent toxic substances—polybrominated diphenyl ethers, perchlorates, and perfluoroalkyl compounds.[1] These substances serve as examples to illustrate some of the issues relevant to other such pollutants.

POLYBROMINATED DIPHENYL ETHERS

The polybrominated diphenyl ethers (PBDEs) are a family of chemicals (also known as brominated flame retardants [BFRs]) used primarily as fire retardants. Structurally related to PCBs, the polybrominated diphenyl ethers have a base structure of 2 phenyl rings linked by an oxygen atom. Polybrominated diphenyl ethers additionally have attached bromide atoms that vary in number (from 4 to 10) and position to form more than 200 distinct chemicals.[2] Each polybrominated diphenyl ether variant is referred to as a congener. There are three types of commercial products, c-pentabrominated diphenyl ether (c-pentaBDE), c-octabrominated diphenyl ether (c-octaBDE), and c-decabrominated diphenyl ether (c-decaBDE); each contains a mixture of congeners.

The development and use of polybrominated diphenyl ethers has been hailed as an industrial advance, responsible for a marked reduction in the morbidity and mortality from fires in homes and businesses. Over the last 2 decades, fire retardants containing polybrominated diphenyl ethers have saved lives, prevented harm, and reduced the economic consequences of fire.[2] At the same time, their increasing use has led to greater environmental contamination. As high-production chemicals, polybrominated diphenyl ethers are manufactured in amounts exceeding 67 000 metric tons annually. More than 50% of the global use of polybrominated diphenyl ethers is in the United States.

With their potent fire-retardant effects, polybrominated diphenyl ethers have become ubiquitous in consumer products. They are found in building materials, furniture, motor vehicles, paints, plastics, foams, furniture, mattresses, and clothing. Consumer products typically have concentrations of 5% to 30% by weight.[2] They also are used extensively in children's clothing as a result of legislation requiring such clothes to retard flames. Polybrominated diphenyl ethers are similar to other persistent toxic substances, because they have significant environmental persistence with elimination half-lives as long as 2 years (although some have elimination half-lives as short as 15 days).[3] They differ from many other persistent toxic substances, because they are primarily used indoors (in consumer products) rather than outdoors.[3] Polybrominated diphenyl ethers also differ from other persistent toxic substances in the method by which they are disposed. Unlike many consumer products, which must be recycled and/or managed as toxic waste because of their harmful constituents, products containing polybrominated diphenyl ethers are discarded, leading to uncontrolled discharge into the environment.[4] Concentrations of polybrominated diphenyl ethers are rising in wildlife, including invertebrates, fish, birds, and marine mammals.[5] Concentrations in humans also have been rising rapidly over the last few decades, particularly in the Americas.[3] Women who have recently emigrated to the United States from rural Mexico have lower concentrations of polybrominated diphenyl ethers in their blood,[6] consistent with greater use of these chemicals in the United States as well as its presence in modern interior environments. Concentrations in the blood of US adults are 10 to 100 times higher than those found in Europe and Japan.[7]

Polybrominated diphenyl ethers are also found extensively in food. Canned sardines and other fish have the highest concentrations, followed by meat and dairy products.[4] On the basis of typical food consumption patterns, meat accounts for the highest single food source of polybrominated diphenyl ethers in children and adults. Intake from food is estimated at 2 to 5 nanograms (ng)/kg daily for children and 1 ng/kg daily in adults.

Polybrominated diphenyl ethers accumulate in human milk, leading to significant concentrations.[8] Human milk concentrations in US women are as much as 75 times higher than concentrations in European women.[4,9] Human milk contains an average of 1056 picograms (pg)/g wet weight of polybrominated diphenyl ethers.[4] As a result, the highest exposure in humans occurs in nursing infants, who ingest an average 307 ng/kg of body weight daily, versus 1 ng/kg daily for adults (Fig 36.1). This corresponds with average concentrations of 24 to 114 parts per billion (ppb) of polybrominated diphenyl ethers in children's blood, a concentration considerably higher than blood concentrations in adults. In contrast to PCBs and other persistent organic pollutants, concentrations of polybrominated diphenyl ethers decrease with age.

Food intake does not entirely account for the concentrations of polybrominated diphenyl ethers found in children and adults.[4] People also are exposed from the ingestion of water and from inhalation. In a study of a single family, concentrations of polybrominated diphenyl ethers were higher in September than December. They were also higher in the children than they were in the adults.[3] The primary source of exposure was thought to be house dust. The lower concentration found in adults was attributed to a lower degree of exposure to dust and to the specific type of polybrominated diphenyl ether measured, since some of these chemicals have very short elimination half-lives. According to current estimates, house dust accounts for up to 80% of total exposure to polybrominated diphenyl ethers in toddlers, compared with 14% for adults. Exposure to dust can lead to as much as a 100-fold higher concentration in toddlers.[3]

Exposure to polybrominated diphenyl ethers is potentially toxic to the reproductive and neurologic systems. Polybrominated diphenyl ethers also appear to act as primary endocrine disrupters, affecting the estrogen and thyroid axes. According to the US Environmental Protection Agency (EPA), polybrominated diphenyl ethers are significantly neurotoxic in experimental animals, producing

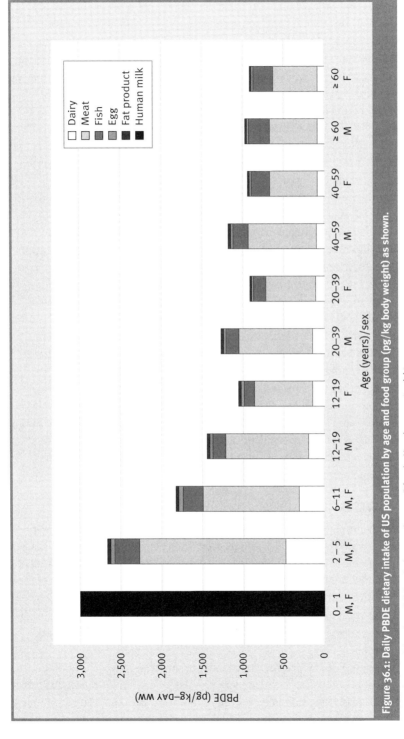

Figure 36.1: Daily PBDE dietary intake of US population by age and food group (pg/kg body weight) as shown.

PBDE indicates polybrominated diphenyl ether; pg, picogram; F, female; M, male; ww, wet weight.
Reprinted with permission from Schecter et al.[3]

hyperactivity and other changes in behavior.[10] In animal models, toxicity is similar to that of the PCBs, including endocrine disruption, reproductive and developmental toxicity, and central nervous system effects.[2,4] Effects on the hypothalamic-pituitary-thyroid axis have received the most attention.[6] Exposed animals have reduced circulating thyroid hormone concentrations[2,6]; this appears to be a central nervous system effect attributable to disturbances of thyroid hormone signaling at multiple levels of the hypothalamic-pituitary-thyroid axis. This has led to theories that polybrominated diphenyl ethers can alter neurogenesis in the fetus and newborn infant.[6] One study reported inverse associations between polybrominated diphenyl ethers measured in cord blood and measures of neurodevelopment through 6 years of age.[11] Adverse reproductive effects can be produced in laboratory animals at exposures to concentrations less than 302 ng/g lipid weight, a concentration reached by 5% of US women.[7]

On the basis of growing concerns, legislative and regulatory actions have been passed to reduce human exposure. The EPA has set a reference dose (a scientific estimate of a daily exposure level that is not expected to cause adverse health effects in humans) for polybrominated diphenyl ethers of 7 μg/kg/day. The European Union has mandated the phase-out of certain polybrominated diphenyl ethers. In August 2003, the State of California outlawed the sale of penta- and octabrominated diphenyl ether and products containing them as of January 2008. However, decabrominated diphenyl ether and other congeners remain in high production and use.[4]

Reducing exposures is possible by limiting sources in homes. Because many consumer products, such as pillows and mattresses, must have flame retardant treatment to comply with regulations, it may be difficult to minimize exposure without changes in current regulations. Risks and benefits of using any alternative flame-retardant products must be weighed and compared with using polybrominated diphenyl ethers.

PERCHLORATES

Perchlorates are salts that carry the perchlorate (ClO_4^-) ion. Perchlorates were used until the mid 20th century as a treatment for hyperthyroidism.[12,13] Because they are potent oxidizers, perchlorates are commonly used in many industries. Ammonium perchlorate is used in the production of solid rocket fuel, propellants, explosives, automobile airbags, pyrotechnic compounds (eg, fireworks), and blasting equipment.[14] A small amount of perchlorate is also formed naturally. Natural sources and use by industry have led to widespread environmental contamination.[15]

In the United States, perchlorate contamination of water wells and other drinking water sources has become more prevalent. Perchlorate concentrations greater than 4 parts per billion have been found in the drinking water consumed by more than 11 million people in 35 states.[12] In these water sources, concentrations of perchlorate range from 4 to 420 µg/L.[13] People are also exposed through food. Perchlorates found in cow milk were traced back to animals grazing on crops irrigated with perchlorate-contaminated water. Perchlorates have been found in fruits, vegetables, and grains.[14,15] Human exposure is substantial as a result of this contamination of food and water. Perchlorate is found in human milk at an average concentration of 0.5 µg/L.

The main health concern resulting from exposure is possible inhibition of thyroid function, an effect that appears to occur predominantly by competitive inhibition of iodide transport that reduces the amount of iodide available for hormone production.[12] In experimental animals, exposure to perchlorates produces abnormal central nervous system development[14]; neuroanatomic disturbances in the hippocampus, in the absence of overt neurotoxicity, have been observed.[14] These effects may be of relevance to human neurodevelopment. Children with congenital hypothyroidism develop mental retardation if the hypothyroidism is not detected promptly and treated. Without treatment, children born with even mild subclinical deficiencies of thyroid function have reduced intelligence, a high incidence of attention-deficit/hyperactivity disorder (ADHD), and visuospatial difficulties.[14,16] Most serious sequelae attributable to perchlorate exposures may be in the first trimester of pregnancy, when the fetus is dependent on the maternal supply of iodine and thyroid hormones, and during exclusive breastfeeding because of the presumed action of perchlorate to decrease iodide uptake into milk.[17] Because perchlorates accumulate in human milk, there is concern about breastfed infants because they rely completely on human milk for iodine.[14] Data also suggest that there are genetic influences on thyroid hormone synthesis, indicating that certain population subgroups are more susceptible to the effects of environmental goitrogens (substances that suppress thyroid function), such as perchlorate.[17]

Although studies in animals link perchlorate exposure prenatally and postnatally with adverse health outcomes, human epidemiologic studies associating exposure with adverse effects in children show inconsistent results. In a 2005 review, the National Academy of Sciences (NAS) noted a lack of firm evidence to show that perchlorates produced important human toxicity.[18] On the basis of their review, however, the National Academy of Sciences recommended a reference dose for perchlorate in human milk of 0.0007 mg/kg/day (or 0.7 µg/kg/day).[18] Other scientists have suggested that this dose is not low enough to protect health.[19] In 2006, scientists from the Centers for Disease Control and Prevention (CDC) described a strong association between perchlorate concentrations in US women and their circulating thyroid hormone concentrations.[15] In that study, perchlorate was a significant negative predictor of thyroxine (T_4) concentrations in adults. According to current theories, the goitrogenic effects of perchlorates alone may be low. In the context of exposure to other environmental goitrogens such as thiocyanate (found in tobacco smoke) and nitrates (found in well water), however, perchlorate exposure may lead to a significant effect on the thyroid axis. In this combined effect theory, the discrete effect of perchlorates might be missed in epidemiologic investigations. Among environmental goitrogens, perchlorate is estimated to be 10 times more potent than thiocyanate and 300 times more potent than nitrate at inhibiting iodide uptake by the thyroid.[17] A recent study in infants revealed that higher urinary concentrations of perchlorate were associated with higher urinary concentrations of thyroid-stimulating hormone (TSH) in infants who had lower urinary iodide.[20]

The EPA established an official reference dose of 0.7 μg/kg/day of perchlorate, consistent with the recommended reference dose included in the National Academy of Sciences report.[21] The EPA has not established a national regulation for perchlorate in drinking water, and the permissible or recommended amounts in public water supplies differ by state or do not exist; private wells are not regulated. Consultation with the local health department about perchlorate regulations and its presence in public water or well water may be advisable in certain areas, such as the desert west, where there is arid soil and dry conditions, or anywhere if the question arises. In addition, mothers and children, in general, and lactating women, in particular, need adequate iodine, either through the use of iodized salt or as part of a supplement, because inadequate iodine increases susceptibility to any perchlorate-induced effect on the thyroid.

POLYFLUOROALKYL CHEMICALS

The polyfluoroalkyl chemicals (PFCs) are a family of fluorinated compounds used heavily in industry and in consumer products. Perfluorooctanoic acid (PFOA) and perfluorooctane sulfonate (PFOS) are the most prominent members of this group. The widespread use of polyfluoroalkyl chemicals has led to substantial human exposure.[1] For example, perfluorooctanoic acid is found in consumer products such as carpeting, microwave popcorn bags, fire-resistant foams, all-weather clothing, paint, upholstery, household cleansers, and Teflon.[1] Since its creation in the 1970s, Teflon has become one of the most widely used chemicals in the world, having revolutionized the cooking industry by creating a nonstick surface on pans. Polyfluoroalkyl chemicals have been widely used in the manufacture of stain-resistant carpets; common products include Stainmaster and Scotchguard.

Widespread use of perfluorooctanoic acid, perfluorooctane sulfonate, and other polyfluoroalkyl chemicals has resulted in environmental contamination with evidence of extensive exposure in wildlife and humans.[1] Human exposure to perfluorooctanoic acid occurs primarily from food and water consumption, inhalation of outdoor air, and inhalation or ingestion of household dust. Microwave popcorn bags, which contain a layer of polyfluoroalkyl chemicals to prevent sticking, are a significant source of perfluorooctanoic acid, containing 6 to 290 parts per million (ppm).[22] Small amounts of polyfluoroalkyl chemicals are also emitted into the environment when new nonstick cookware is used.[23] Perfluorooctanoic acid and other polyfluoroalkyl chemicals can also enter the food chain in feed animals and crops.

Human exposure to perfluorooctanoic acid is extensive; it can be measured in the blood of most Americans.[1] Data from the 2003–2004 National Health and Nutrition Examination Survey (NHANES) identified polyfluoroalkyl chemicals in more than 98% of Americans 12 years and older; the mean serum concentration of perfluorooctanoic acid was 3.5 parts per billion. Concentrations of perfluorooctane sulfonate were higher in males than in females. Individuals with occupational exposure to polyfluoroalkyl chemicals have serum concentrations ranging from 200 to 2500 parts per million.[24] Perfluorooctanoic acid, perfluorooctane sulfonate, and other polyfluoroalkyl chemicals cross the placenta.

Exposure of the fetus and child to polyfluoroalkyl chemicals raises concerns about neurotoxicity and potential mutagenicity. Children have been shown to have higher concentrations of perfluorooctanoic acid and perfluorooctane sulfonate than adults.[25] In experimental animals and humans, polyfluoroalkyl chemicals are associated with reduced fetal growth.[25] A study in Japan demonstrated that in utero exposure to relatively low levels of perflurooctanesulfonate was negatively correlated with birth weight.[26] Perfluorooctanoic acid has been associated with a broad range of birth defects and an increased risk of cancer.[1] The Scientific Advisory Board of the EPA has recommended that perfluorooctanoic acid be considered a likely human carcinogen.[27] Perfluorooctanoic acid has been implicated in other toxicities, including endocrine disruption.[28] Higher concentrations of perfluorooctanoic acid and perfluorooctane sulfonate have been associated with thyroid disease.[29] Several human epidemiologic studies have not found significant health effects associated with polyfluoroalkyl chemicals. A study of pregnant women exposed to perfluorooctanoic acid/perfluorooctane sulfonate did not find adverse neuromuscular or neurologic effects.[25]

Although there are no federal standards for exposure to perfluorooctanoic acid, limits of exposure have been suggested. The EPA has recently set a provisional health advisory level of 0.4 parts per billion in drinking water.

The extent of environmental contamination by perfluorooctanoic acid and perfluorooctane sulfonate, along with persistent concerns about their health effects, has led to an accelerated phase-out. In 2006, the major manufacturers of perfluorooctanoic acid arrived at an agreement with the EPA to eliminate perfluorooctanoic acid from consumer products by 2015; 95% of this reduction was to occur by 2010.[30] Cross-sectional data suggest that concentrations of perfluorooctanoic acid and perfluorooctane sulfonate in humans are falling as a result of this phaseout.[1]

Prevention of children's exposure to perfluorooctanoic acid, perfluorooctane sulfonate, and related polyfluoroalkyl chemicals begins with advocacy to remove these products from food containers, particularly coated boxes and microwave popcorn bags. Until these products are completely removed from sale in the United States, new nonstick cookware should be used in well-ventilated environments until it "ages" sufficiently to have minimal emission when heated.

References

1. Calafat A, Wong L, Kuklenyik Z, Reidy J, Needham L. Polyfluoroalkyl chemicals in the U.S. population: data from the National Health and Nutrition Examination Survey (NHANES) 2003-2004 and comparisons with NHANES 1999-2000. *Environ Health Perspect.* 2007;115(11):1596-602

2. Birnbaum LS, Staskal DF. Brominated flame retardants: cause for concern? *Environ Health Perspect.* 2004;112(1):9-17

3. Schecter A, Papke O, Harris TR, et al. Polybrominated diphenyl ether (PBDE) levels in an expanded market basket survey of U.S. food and estimated PBDE dietary intake by age and sex. *Environ Health Perspect.* 2006;114(10):1515-1520. doi:10.1289/ehp.9121

4. Athanasiadou M, Cuadra SN, Marsh G, Bergman A, Jakobsson K. Polybrominated diphenyl ethers (PBDEs) and bioaccumulative hydroxylated PBDE metabolites in young humans from Managua, Nicaragua. *Environ Health Perspect.* 2008;116(3):400-408

5. Lema SC, Dickey JT, Schultz IR, Swanson P. Dietary exposure to 2,2',4,4'-tetrabromodiphenyl ether (PBDE-47) alters thyroid status and thyroid hormone-regulated gene transcription in the pituitary and brain. *Environ Health Perspect.* 2008;116(12):1694-1699

6. Bradman A, Fenster L, Sjodin A, Jones RS, Patterson DG Jr, Eskenazi B. Polybrominated diphenyl ether levels in the blood of pregnant women living in an agricultural community in California. *Environ Health Perspect.* 2007;115(1):71-74

7. Fischer D, Hooper K, Athanasiadou M, Athanassiadis I, Bergman A. Children show highest levels of polybrominated diphenyl ethers in a California family of four: a case study. *Environ Health Perspect.* 2006;114(10):1581-1584

8. Lind Y, Darnerud P, Atuma S, et al. Polybrominated diphenyl ethers in breast milk from Uppsala County, Sweden. *Env Res.* 2003;93(2):186-194

9. Lunder S, Jacob A. *Fire Retardants in Toddlers and Their Mothers.* Washington, DC: Environmental Working Group; 2008

10. Anonymous. Developmental exposure to low-dose PBDE-99: effects on male fertility and neurobehavior in rat offspring. *Environ Health Perspect.* 2005;113(2):149-154

11. Herbstman JB, Sjodin A, Jurzon M, et al. Prenatal exposure to PBDEs and neurodevelopment. *Environ Health Perspect.* 2010;118(5):712–719

12. Buffler PA, Kelsh MA, Lau EC, et al. Thyroid function and perchlorate in drinking water: an evaluation among California newborns, 1998. *Environ Health Perspect.* 2006;114(5):798-804

13. Godley AF, Stanbury JB. Preliminary experience in the treatment of hyperthyroidism with potassium perchlorate. *J Clin Endocrinol Metab.* 1954;14(1):70-78

14. Gilbert ME, Sui L. Developmental exposure to perchlorate alters synaptic transmission in hippocampus of the adult rat. *Environ Health Perspect.* 2008;116(6):752-760

15. Blount BC, Pirkle JL, Osterloh JD, Valentin-Blasini L, Caldwell KL. Urinary perchlorate and thyroid hormone levels in adolescent and adult men and women living in the United States. *Environ Health Perspect.* 2006;114(12):1865-1871

16. Haddow J, Palomaki G, Allan W, et al. Maternal thyroid deficiency during pregnancy and subsequent neuropsychological development of the child. *New Engl J Med.* 1999;341(8):549-555

17. Scinicariello F, Murray HE, Smith L, Wilbur S, Fowler BA. Genetic factors that might lead to different responses in individuals exposed to perchlorate. *Environ Health Perspect.* 2005;113(11):1479-1484

18. National Research Council, Committee to Assess the Health Implications of Perchlorate Ingestion. *Health Implications of Perchlorate Ingestion.* Washington, DC: National Research Council; 2005

19. Ginsberg G, Rice D. The NAS perchlorate review: questions remain about the perchlorate RfD. *Environ Health Perspect.* 2005;113(9):1117-1119

20. Cao Y, Blount BC, Valentin-Blasini L, Bernbaum JC, Phillips T, Rogan WJ. Goitrogenic anions, thyrotropin, and thyroid hormone in infants. *Environ Health Perspect.* 2010;118(9): 1332-1337

21. US Environmental Protection Agency, Federal Facilities Restoration and Reuse Office. Perchlorate. Available at: http://www.epa.gov/fedfac/documents/perchlorate.htm. Accessed March 29, 2011

22. Begley T, White K, Honigfort P, Twaroski M, Neches R, Walker R. Perfluorochemicals: potential sources of and migration from food packaging. *Food Addit Contam.* 2005;22(1):23-31

23. Sinclair E, Kim S, Akinleye H, Kannan K. Quantitation of gas-phase perfluoroalkyl surfactants and fluorotelomer alcohols released from nonstick cookware and microwave popcorn bags. *Environ Sci Technol.* 2007;41(4):1180-1185

24. Olsen G, Mair D, Church T, et al. Decline in perfluorooctanesulfonate and other polyfluoroalkyl chemicals in American Red Cross adult blood donors, 2000-2006. *Environ Sci Technol.* 2008;42(13):4989-4995

25. Fei C, McLaughlin JK, Lipworth L, Olsen J. Prenatal exposure to perfluorooctanoate (PFOA) and perfluorooctanesulfonate (PFOS) and maternally reported developmental milestones in infancy. *Environ Health Perspect.* 2008;116(10):1391-1395

26. Washino N, Saijo Y, Sasaki S, et al. Correlations between prenatal exposure to perfluorinated chemicals and reduced fetal growth. *Environ Health Perspect.* 2009;117(4):660-667

27. US Environmental Protection Agency. Perfluorooctanoic Acid (PFOA) and Fluorinated Telomers: Risk Assessment. Available at: http://www.epa.gov/opptintr/pfoa/pubs/pfoarisk.html. Accessed March 29, 2011

28. Jensen AA, Leffers H. Emerging endocrine disruptors: perfluoroalkylated substances. *Int J Androl.* 2008;31(2):161-169

29. Melzer D, Rice N, Depledge MH, Henley WH, Galloway TA. Association between serum perfluorooctanoic acid (PFOA) and thyroid disease in the U.S. National Health and Nutrition Examination Survey. *Environ Health Perspect.* 2010;118(5):686–692

30. Dooley EE. The Beat. PFOA to be eliminated. *Environ Health Perspect.* 2006;114(4):A217

Chapter 37

Pesticides

■ ■ ■ ■ ■ ■

As defined by the US Environmental Protection Agency (EPA), a pesticide is a substance or mixture of substances intended for preventing, destroying, repelling, or mitigating any pest. Pests include insects; mice and other animals; unwanted plants, such as weeds; fungi; or microorganisms, including bacteria and viruses. In addition to insecticides, the term "pesticide" also applies to herbicides, fungicides, and other substances used to control pests. Pesticides are ubiquitous in the environment.

The mechanism by which some pesticides kill pests includes cytotoxic or neurotoxic effects that can also harm or kill human beings. The EPA estimates that in the year 2000, 74% of households were using 1 or more pesticides in the home or immediate environment.[1] Recent efforts by the EPA to reduce residential usage of products most commonly associated with acute poisonings has been associated with more than a 40% reduction in incidence of serious pesticide poisonings from 1995 to 2004.[2]

Pesticides have numerous beneficial effects. When used appropriately for control of insects and rodents, pesticides can assist in the prevention or the spread of disease. Pesticides can have a positive effect on crop yields. These compounds, however, also can be toxic to adults and children. Because pesticides are present in food, homes, schools, and parks, children are frequently exposed. Children at increased risk of pesticide exposure include those whose parents are farmers or farm workers, pesticide applicators, or landscapers or children who live adjacent to agricultural areas.[3,4] Children and teenagers may work or play near their parents in the fields, where they may be exposed to pesticides. People who work with pesticides may use these agricultural-strength chemicals at home.[4] Inappropriate applications may increase exposure and cause illness and death.

Food Quality Protection Act (FQPA) of 1996

Actions generated by the Food Quality Protection Act, modifying the Federal Insecticide, Fungicide and Rodenticide Act and the Federal Food, Drug, and Cosmetic Act:

- Established a single health-based standard for all pesticides in food.
- Benefits, in general, cannot override the health-based standard.
- Prenatal and postnatal effects are to be considered.
- In the absence of data confirming the safety to infants and children, because of their special sensitivities and exposures, an additional uncertainty factor of up to 10 times is required to be added to safety values.
- Aggregate risk, the sum of all exposures to the chemical, must be considered in establishing safe levels.
- Cumulative risk, the sum of all exposures to chemicals with similar mechanisms of action, must be considered in establishing safe levels.
- Endocrine disrupters are to be included in the evaluation of safety.
- All existing pesticide registrations are to be reviewed by 2006.
- Expedited review is possible for safer pesticides.
- Risks are to be determined for 1-year and lifetime exposure.

In response to concerns about children's exposure to pesticides via food, Congress passed the Food Quality Protection Act of 1996 (Pub L No. 104-170).[5] This law was unique in that it explicitly required that the EPA ensure a "reasonable certainty that no harm will result in infants and children" from exposure to pesticides and that the effects of chemicals that have the same mechanism of action be considered cumulatively. Additional information regarding chronic exposure to small amounts of pesticides from food is included in Chapter 18.

This chapter focuses on acute and chronic effects of pesticides and prevention measures.

INSECTICIDES

The major classes of insecticides are organophosphates, carbamates, pyrethrum and synthetic pyrethroids, organochlorines, and boric acid and borates.

Organophosphates

Organophosphate pesticides are a major category of insecticides used in the United States and are responsible for most acute pesticide poisonings. Effective in 2000 and in 2003, respectively, 2 of the most toxic organophosphate pesticides—chlorpyrifos and diazinon—were banned for household use. A few household uses of organophosphate pesticides remain, including in flea collars (tetrachlorvinphos), in pest strips (dichlorvos), and for head lice and general use (malathion). Malathion is still widely used as a home and garden insecticide. Organophosphate pesticides are widely used in agriculture, where they sometimes drift into nearby communities, and they are commonly detected as residues on food. In addition, many people may still have these products stored in their homes. Therefore, the clinician should remain alert to these risks.

N-Methyl Carbamates

N-methyl carbamates are similar to organophosphates. The most toxic carbamate is aldicarb, which is used on food crops. Carbaryl and propoxur are available for a variety of household uses, and propoxur is used in some types of flea collars, which can leave an insecticidal residue on pet fur. Carbaryl is a widely used garden insecticide, with 2 to 4 million pounds applied for household use in 2001. These chemicals are moderately toxic, and propoxur is considered by the EPA to be a probable human carcinogen.[6]

Pyrethrum and Synthetic Pyrethroids

Pyrethrum, an extract of dried chrysanthemum flowers, refers to a composite of 6 insecticidal ingredients known as pyrethrins. Natural pyrethrins are used mainly for indoor bug bombs and aerosols because of their instability in light and heat. Antilice shampoos, such as A200 and Rid, contain pyrethrins. Pyrethroids, synthetic chemicals based on the structure and biological activity of pyrethrum, are modified to increase their stability. The pyrethroids are classified as type I or type II (or cyano-pyrethroids); type II pyrethroids generally are more toxic than the type I pyrethroids. Pyrethroids are used in agriculture, gardening, and homes for control of structural pests (eg, termites), for flea control, and against lice and scabies (as permethrin [eg, Elimite]). Permethrin (Permanone, Duranon) is marketed as a spray for tents and clothing and is sold in pesticide-impregnated outdoor clothing.[7,8] Pyrethrum and pyrethroids rapidly penetrate insects and paralyze them. As residential uses of organophosphate pesticides have become more restricted since 2000, pyrethrin and pyrethroids have taken their place. The incidence of poison center calls and visits to health care facilities related to organophosphates have steadily declined from 2000 to 2005, while those related to pyrethrum and pyrethroid pesticides have correspondingly increased.[9]

Organochlorines

Halogenated hydrocarbons were developed in the 1940s for use as insecticides, fungicides, and herbicides. Organochlorines are lipid soluble, have low molecular weight, and persist in the environment. Dichlorodiphenyltrichloroethane (DDT), chlordane, and other organochlorines were enormously successful because of their efficacy and low acute toxicity. Production of DDT and most other organochlorine compounds was banned in the United States in the 1970s because of concern about their persistence, bioaccumulation in the food chain, effects on wildlife, and possible long-term carcinogenicity. Organochlorines continue to be used in developing countries, including those exporting food to the United States. Lindane (Kwell) continues to be prescribed for lice and scabies, although safer preparations are available. Lindane poses a serious risk of poisoning if accidentally ingested or misused topically. According to the Food and Drug Administration, lindane is to be used only in patients who have failed to respond to adequate doses of other approved agents and with caution in those weighing less than 110 lb.[10] As of January 2002, the state of California no longer allowed the sale of pharmaceutical lindane.[11] A survey of California pediatricians indicated that the ban did not cause significant problems, and at the same time, it has nearly eliminated poisonings from lindane in California.[12] The ban has eliminated discharge of water contaminated with lindane into waterways by water-treatment facilities.

Boric Acid and Borates

Boric acid commonly is available as a pellet or powder for household insect control. Boric acid and borates generally are considered to be among the less toxic chemicals used for insect control and increasingly are used instead of organophosphate pesticides in settings where children may be present. Although less toxic, this class of compounds was used extensively in the 1950s and 1960s, with reports of significant toxicity, especially when ingested.[13,14] Poison control centers increasingly are receiving reports of ingestions of boric acid pellets or powders by children younger than 6 years.[15]

FLEA-CONTROL PRODUCTS

Children may come into direct contact with pesticides through use of household products. Some products that are readily available to consumers have significant toxicity and should be avoided when possible; others have been associated with little or no toxicity. Flea-control products are widely used in the United States. Two-thirds of US households contain a pet, and the market for flea control products is more than $1 billion per year. Because children frequently are in close contact with their pets and may sleep with their pets, exposure to these products is of significant concern.

Flea collars legally may contain highly toxic organophosphate or N-methyl carbamate products, such as tetrachlorvinphos and propoxur. These collars are designed to slowly release pesticides onto the fur of the pet, where residues are bioavailable to children through direct contact.[16] Many of the pet shampoos, dips, and sprays contain permethrin. Although the toxicity of permethrin is less than that of some other insecticides, it has been identified as a likely human carcinogen by the EPA.[17] Less toxic choices are imidacloprid (Advantage) or fipronil (Frontline) products, although these have some neurotoxicity and can be transferred to a child's hand when petting an animal. These newer agents are discussed individually in this chapter. Selamectin (Revolution), a botanical insecticide/antiparasitic, is a derivative of avermectin, another botanical insecticide. It is not considered to have significant health hazards, but it is a relatively new product for which fewer data are available compared with older alternatives.

Preferred approaches to flea control include regular flea combing and bathing of pets, regular vacuuming of carpets, and washing of pet's bedding in hot water. If necessary, a systemic flea-control preparation, such as lufenuron (Program), or an insect-growth regulator, such as S-methoprene, fenoxycarb, or pyriproxyfen (Nylar), are the least toxic alternatives.

Neonicotinoids

Neonicotinoids may be used as flea control for pet animals. These insecticides are becoming more widely used in the agricultural setting. There are several in this class, including acetamiprid, thiacloprid, and imidacloprid, the latter of which is the most commonly used active ingredient in this class. They work as agonists to nicotinic acetylcholine receptors (nAChRs), but their uniqueness lies in their highly selective affinity for insect nAChRs, compared with those of mammals. In addition, they are water soluble, which decreases their ability to cross the mammalian blood-brain barrier.[18,19]

Fipronil

This is the most common example of another relatively newer class of insecticides known as N-phenylpyrazoles. Fipronil is also widely used on pet animals for flea control as well as lawn treatments, agricultural crops, and in bait stations for ant and roach control. These agents inhibit gamma-aminobutyric acid (GABA) channels, leading to hyperexcitability of the cell. Although this mechanism of action is similar to organochlorines, the N-phenylpyrazoles are selective for $GABA_A$ channels, whereas organochlorines inhibit $GABA_A$ and $GABA_C$ channels.[20]

OTHER PESTICIDES

Herbicides

Herbicides are pesticides that kill unwanted plants in agriculture, in homes, on lawns, in gardens, in parks, on school grounds, and along roadways where children walk, play, and ride bicycles. Herbicides are used by approximately 14 million households annually.

Glyphosate (Roundup, Rodeo)

Glyphosate is a broad-spectrum herbicide used to kill unwanted plants in agriculture and landscapes. It is the second most common household pesticide in the United States, with 5 to 8 million pounds applied in 2001, according to national estimates.

Bipyridyls

The bipyridyls paraquat and diquat are nonselective herbicides. Paraquat is acutely toxic and is a restricted use pesticide unavailable to home-owners. Diquat is available for household use as a general purpose weed killer.

Chlorophenoxy Herbicides

These include 2,4-dichlorophenoxy-acetic acid (2,4-D). 2,4-D is the most common household pesticide used in the United States, with between 8 and 11 million pounds per year applied to lawns, parks, and athletic fields. The mixture of 2,4-D and the now-banned chlorophenoxy herbicide 2,4,5-trichlorophenoxy-acetic acid was known as Agent Orange. This mixture was used heavily in South Vietnam and Cambodia for defoliation by the US Armed Forces. The mixture was contaminated with 2,3,7,8-tetrachlorodibenzo-p-dioxin, a known human carcinogen and developmental toxicant.

Fungicides

Fungicides include substituted benzenes, thiocarbamates, ethylene bisdithiocarbamates, copper, organotin, cadmium compounds, elemental sulfur, and miscellaneous compounds such as captan, benomyl, and vinclozolin. Organomercury compounds have been banned in the United States because of their extreme toxicity. Fungicides are used to protect grains and perishable produce from mold. These chemicals also are used as seed treatments, on ornamental plants, and in soil. Some fungicides are available in stores for use on garden plants. Fungicides most commonly are applied as a wettable powder or in granular form, and are generally poorly absorbed in these forms via dermal or respiratory routes.

Wood Preservatives

Wood preservatives include pentachlorophenol and chromated copper arsenate (CCA). These preservatives were banned from materials other than wood by the EPA in 1987. Pentachlorophenol is used as a wood preservative for utility poles, cross arms, and fence posts and is a known carcinogen. Chromated copper arsenate was used in pressure-treated wood commonly used to construct decks, porches, and playground equipment but was banned for residential use in 2004 (see Chapter 9). Older outdoor wood structures may still contain arsenic, which can get on children's hands.

Rodenticides

Rodenticides commonly used in US homes are anticoagulants or cholecalciferol. Anticoagulants interfere with the activation of vitamin K-dependent factors (II, VII, IX, X). Examples include warfarins, the 10-fold more potent indanediones, and superwarfarins (eg, brodifacoum), approximately 100 times more potent than the warfarins. Cholecalciferol (vitamin D) is poisonous to rodents at high doses. In 2008, the EPA removed the more potent superwarfarins from products available to consumers and required retail products to be in the form of child resistant bait stations rather than loose pellets. Yellow phosphorus, strychnine, and arsenic rodenticides no longer are registered but may be in use from existing stored supplies.

Insect Repellents

N,N-diethyl-meta-toluamide (also known as N,N-diethyl-3-methyl-benzamide)—DEET—is the active ingredient in many insect repellent products. DEET is used to repel insects, such as mosquitoes, that may transmit viral encephalitis (eg, West Nile virus) or malaria and ticks that may carry Lyme disease. Marketed in the United States since 1956 and used by about one third of the US population each year, DEET is available in many commercial products as an aerosol, liquid, lotion, or stick and in impregnated materials such as wristbands. Some sunscreen formulations also include DEET as a convenient multipurpose product. Commercial products registered for direct application to human skin contain from 4% to 99.9% DEET. Concentrations above 30% provide no increase in protection. Using separate DEET and sunscreen products at the same time is an acceptable practice. However, the use of combination products is not recommended, because the sunscreen needs to be reapplied after exertion or swimming, whereas the mosquito repellent generally does not need to be reapplied, and the risk of toxicity increases with reapplication.

Alternatives to DEET include Picaridin (1-methylpropyl 2-[2-hydroxyethyl]-1-piperidinecarboxylate, also known as KBR 3023) and oil of lemon eucalyptus. Picaridin and DEET have similar effectiveness at comparable concentrations. Estimated protection time varies depending on the study and type of mosquito being tested, but the range for both has been between 3 and 7 hours in most studies.[21] Oil of lemon eucalyptus (*p*-menthane-3,8-diol) is close behind DEET and Picaridin, followed by 2% soybean oil; all other substances are less effective than these.[21]

Products containing citronella, sold as insect repellents, are not as effective as DEET and, therefore, are not recommended when concern exists about arthropodborne disease. Pure oil of eucalyptus (eg, essential oil) has not been tested for safety and effectiveness and should not be used.[7]

Inert Ingredients

Although there are approximately 900 pesticides registered for use in the United States, these chemicals are sold in more than 20 000 different products. Each product contains one or more active ingredients (the 1 or 2 that actually kill the pest) and a mixture of other ingredients—sometimes called "inerts." A typical pesticide formulation may contain less than 2% active ingredients and more than 98% inert ingredients. These other ingredients function as dispersants, carriers, solvents, synergists, or ingredients that help the pesticide adhere to surfaces and resist rapid degradation. Despite the term "inert," these ingredients may be toxic. For example, xylene (an inert ingredient in some pyrethroid formulations) is a central nervous system depressant and reproductive toxicant. Other inert ingredients may be respiratory or dermal irritants or sensitizers or may even have potential chronic effects, such as potential carcinogenicity or reproductive toxicity. Synergists (chemicals that inhibit the detoxification process in insects), such as piperonyl butoxide and sulfoxide, are generally of low toxicity.

Inert ingredients are not subject to the same level of scrutiny as the active ingredients and may be untested for toxicity. Active ingredients must be listed on the product label, whereas it is very difficult to obtain any information about the other ingredients in a pesticide product. If a patient experiences an adverse effect from exposure to a pesticide, it is important to realize that the offending chemical may be one of the other ingredients that are not listed on the label. A clinician treating a patient who was exposed to a specific product can legally obtain information about other ingredients directly from the manufacturer by calling the phone number on the product label.

SOURCES OF EXPOSURE

Children in the United States are almost universally exposed to pesticides; home and garden pesticide use may result in increased levels of exposure in both urban and rural settings.[22]

Prenatal and early childhood exposures may be especially significant because of the susceptibility of developing organ systems as well as behavioral, physiological, and dietary characteristics of children. Metabolites of organophosphate pesticides were shown to be present in the meconium of all of the 20 newborn infants tested in a study in New York City.[23] This is indicative of ubiquitous exposure to these chemicals, even in utero.

The Centers for Disease Control and Prevention (CDC) conducts regular national biomonitoring surveys to test for residues of pesticides in adults and in children older than 6 years. The Fourth National Report on Human Exposure to Environmental Chemicals, published in 2009, reported on 45 pesticides and pesticide metabolites in blood or urine of the noninstitutionalized US population.[24] Twenty six pesticides were detected in the majority of children tested.

In general, the organochlorine insecticides were found at higher concentrations in adults, although children younger than 12 years were not sampled for organochlorines. Pesticides found at notably higher concentrations in children as compared with adults included the organophosphate insecticides and the fungicide/disinfectant ortho-phenylphenol. The CDC study did not provide information on whether the concentrations found in humans are toxic, but it does provide a comparison range for current exposures to certain pesticides in the general population, including children.

ROUTES OF EXPOSURE

Children may be exposed to pesticides through inhalation, ingestion, and dermal absorption.

Inhalation

Pesticides applied as dusts, mists, sprays, or gases may reach the mucous membranes or the alveoli, where they are absorbed into the bloodstream. Where suburban neighborhoods are interspersed with agricultural lands, chemicals from aerial spraying or fumigation may drift into residential areas.

Inhalation of the noninsecticide group of pesticides is usually relatively minor, because their volatility is low and, with the exception of the chlorophenoxy herbicides, they are rarely distributed by aerial spraying. Fungicides may be inhaled during the process of application, but once applied they are subject to limited inhalation.

Ingestion

Ingestion of pesticides may result in acute poisoning. Pesticides stored in food containers (eg, soft drink bottles) pose a special hazard for children. An EPA survey reported that nearly half of US households with a child younger than 5 years had a pesticide stored within the reach of children.[25]

The major problem with ingestion of pesticides is from foods that have been treated with them, especially those grown in home gardens. Infants and children may be exposed through their diets to trace amounts of pesticides applied to food crops (see Chapter 18). People also may be exposed to low levels of organochlorines by eating crops grown in contaminated soil and eating fish from contaminated waters. Pesticides are found in some water supplies: a 1999 EPA survey found that 10.7% of community water system wells contained one or more pesticides that were not removed by standard water treatment technologies (see Chapter 17).[26]

In addition, young children consume measurable amounts of soil, and children with pica can consume up to 100 g/day of soil that may contain persistent organic pesticides as well as heavy metals, such as arsenic.

Table 37.1: Number of Calls to Poison Control Centers About Pediatric Pesticide Poisonings, 2006[27]		
PESTICIDE	AGE <6 YEARS	AGE 6–19 YEARS
Anticoagulant rodenticides	11 592	360
Pyrethroids	5468	1801
Insect repellents	6738	1625
Organophosphates	1096	429
Borates/boric acid	3447	131
Glyphosate	1133	321
Carbamates	1062	235
Naphthalene	1042	106

Wood treated with chromated copper arsenate is a potential source of childhood exposure to arsenic. Arsenic is leached from the wood with aging and can accumulate on the wood surface or the soil under playground equipment and decks made with treated wood. Young children are at particular risk of exposure from hand-to-mouth activity.

Accidental ingestion may occur with any of these compounds, especially with the rodenticides. Whether by ingestion or inhalation, children frequently have serious exposures to pesticides, as indicated by calls to poison control centers (see Table 37.1).

Dermal Absorption

Many pesticides are readily absorbed through the skin. The potential for dermal exposures in children is high because of their relatively large body surface area and extensive contact with lawns, gardens, and floors by crawling and playing on the ground. Lindane (Kwell, for topical scabies and lice treatment) and DEET are absorbed through the skin. Dermal exposure to herbicides and fungicides generally results in skin irritation and rarely in systemic effects.

SYSTEMS AFFECTED AND CLINICAL EFFECTS

Parental and Prenatal Exposures

Effects that have been associated with parental or prenatal pesticide exposures include intrauterine growth restriction and prematurity,[28] birth defects,[29] fetal death,[30] and spontaneous abortion.[31] More research is needed to further clarify whether these associations are causal.

ACUTE EFFECTS

Organophosphates

Organophosphates phosphorylate the active site of the enzyme acetylcholinesterase at the nerve ending, irreversibly inhibiting this enzyme. The signs and symptoms of acute organophosphate poisoning result from the accumulation of acetylcholine at cholinergic receptors (muscarinic effects) as well as at voluntary muscles (including the diaphragm) and autonomic ganglia (nicotinic effects). Accumulation of acetylcholine in the brain causes sensory and behavioral disturbances, impaired coordination, depressed cognition, and coma (see Table 37.2).

Organophosphates are rapidly distributed throughout the body after inhalation or ingestion. Symptoms usually develop within 4 hours of exposure but may be delayed up to 12 hours with dermal exposure. Initial symptoms may include headache, dizziness, miosis, nausea, abdominal pain, and diarrhea; anxiety and restlessness may be prominent. With progressive worsening, muscle twitching, weakness, bradycardia, hypersecretion (sweating, salivation, rhinorrhea, bronchorrhea), and profuse diarrhea may develop. Central nervous system effects include headache, blurred vision, anxiety, confusion, emotional lability, ataxia, toxic psychosis, vertigo, convulsions, and coma. Cranial nerve palsies have been noted.[32]

More severe intoxications result in sympathetic and nicotinic manifestations with muscle weakness and fasciculations including twitching (particularly in eyelids), tachycardia, muscle cramps, hypertension, and sweating. Finally, paralysis of respiratory and skeletal muscles and convulsions may develop. Children are more likely than adults to have central nervous system signs such as coma and seizures.

N-Methyl Carbamates

Carbamates act similarly to organophosphates in binding acetylcholinesterase, but the bonds are more readily reversible. The clinical symptoms produced are not easily differentiated from those of organophosphate poisoning. Although acetylcholinesterase may be low in organophosphate poisoning, it usually is normal in carbamate poisoning.[32] Carbamates may be highly toxic, although the effects of exposure are more short lived, with some cases abating within 6 to 8 hours.

Pyrethrum and Synthetic Pyrethroids

Pyrethrum and synthetic pyrethroids are absorbed from the gastrointestinal and respiratory tracts but only very slightly through the skin. Because pyrethrins are metabolized very rapidly by the liver and most metabolites are promptly excreted by the kidneys, they have low toxicity when ingested.[32] Most problematic are allergic reactions, which have occurred in the form of contact dermatitis,

Table 37.2: Acute Effects of Common Pesticide Classes[32]

PESTICIDE CATEGORY	EXAMPLES	MECHANISM OF EFFECTS, ACUTE SYMPTOMS	DIAGNOSIS AND TREATMENT
Organophosphates	Chlorpyrifos, diazinon, tetrachlorvinphos, methyl parathion, azinphos-methyl, naled, malathion, acephate	Irreversible acetylcholinesterase inhibition; nausea, vomiting, hypersecretion, bronchoconstriction, headache	Cholinesterase levels; supportive care, atropine, pralidoxime
N-methyl carbamates	Carbaryl, aldicarb, propoxur	Reversible acetylcholinesterase inhibition; nausea, vomiting, hypersecretion, bronchoconstriction, headache	Cholinesterase levels; supportive care, atropine
Pyrethrins	Pyrethrum	Allergic reactions; anaphylaxis, tremor, ataxia at high doses	No diagnostic test; treat allergic reactions with antihistamines or steroids, as needed
Pyrethroids —Type I	Allethrin, permethrin, tetramethrin	Tremors, ataxia, irritability, enhanced startle response	No diagnostic test; decontamination, supportive care, symptomatic treatment
—Type II	Deltamethrin, cypermethrin, fenvalerate	Choreoathetosis, salivation, seizures	Skin contact may cause highly unpleasant, temporary paresthesias, best treated with vitamin E oil preparations
Organochlorines	Lindane, endosulfan, dicofol	GABA blockade; uncoordination, tremors, sensory disturbances, dizziness, seizures	Detectable in blood; decontamination, supportive care, cholestyramine to clear enterohepatic recirculation

Table 37.2: Acute Effects of Common Pesticide Classes[32], *continued*

PESTICIDE CATEGORY	CHEMICAL EXAMPLES	MECHANISM OF EFFECTS, ACUTE SYMPTOMS	DIAGNOSIS AND TREATMENT
Chlorophenoxy compounds	2,4-Dichloro-phenoxyacetic acid (2,4-D)	Acidosis, neuropathy, myopathy, nausea and vomiting, myalgia, headache, myotonia, fever	Detectable in urine; decontamination, forced alkaline dieresis
Bipyridyl compounds	Paraquat, diquat	Free radical formation; pulmonary edema, acute tubular necrosis, hepatocellular toxicity	Urine dithionite test (colorimetric); decontamination, do NOT administer oxygen, aggressive hydration, hemoperfusion
Anticoagulant rodenticides	Warfarin, brodifacoum, diphencoumarin, diphacinone, pindone	Vitamin K antagonism; hemorrhage	Elevated PT; vitamin K administration

GABA indicates gamma-aminobutyric acid; PT, prothrombin time.

anaphylaxis, or asthma. Paresthesias (described as stinging, burning, or itching) may occur when liquid or volatile compounds contact the skin; these rarely last more than 24 hours.[32] Absorption of extraordinarily high doses rarely may cause incoordination, dizziness, headaches, nausea, and diarrhea. A fatal asthma attack in a child attributed to shampooing her dog with a flea-control shampoo containing pyrethrin has been described.[33]

Organochlorines

The toxic action of organochlorines is primarily on the nervous system. By interfering with the flux of cations across nerve cell membranes, organochlorines produce abnormal nerve function and irritability, which may result in seizures. Disturbances of sensation, coordination, and mental function are characteristic. Lindane poisoning presents with nausea, vomiting, and central nervous system stimulation or generalized seizures.

Boric Acid and Borates

Boric dust is irritating to the skin, upper airways, and lower respiratory tract. Ingestion of borates can result in severe gastroenteritis, headache, lethargy, and an intensely erythematous skin rash similar in appearance to staphylococcal scalded skin syndrome.[34] Metabolic acidosis may be observed, and shock can occur in severe cases.

Neonicotinoids

Although dermal exposure has been documented, most symptomatic cases of poisoning have resulted from ingestion. Most reports have been individual case reports, but there are now 2 series reported—1 retrospective and 1 prospective.[18,19] Nonspecific symptoms include nausea, vomiting, dizziness, and diaphoresis. Ulcerative lesions in the gastrointestinal tract may occur, particularly when accompanied by the solvent N-methyl-2-pyrrolidone (NMP). Other, more serious effects include aspiration pneumonia, respiratory failure, coma, and arrthymia.[18,19]

Fipronil

Most reports of human poisoning to date have documented self-limiting symptoms, including nausea, vomiting, and aphthous ulcers. In severe cases, mental status changes and seizures may occur. For the most part, these are also self-limiting and have not required long-term treatment beyond supportive care.[35]

Herbicides

Glyphosate

At usual exposure levels, glyphosate has a low level of acute toxicity. Ingestions of three quarters of a cup or more (usually as a suicide attempt) have been fatal.[36] Symptoms include abdominal pain, vomiting, pulmonary edema, kidney damage, and renal failure. More commonly, lower levels cause skin and eye irritation. The surfactant polyethoxylated tallowamine, added to improve product application, is more toxic than the active ingredient glyphosate. The 2 mixed together (Roundup) may show a synergistic increase in toxicity.

Bipyridyls (Paraquat and Diquat)

Acute bipyridyl toxicity is thought to involve the production of free radical oxygen and, secondarily, interference with nicotinamide adenine dinucleotide phosphate and nicotinamide adenine dinucleotide phosphate (reduced form). Paraquat and diquat are corrosive to the tissues they contact directly. Initially, local effects of paraquat result in caustic burns to the skin or mucosa. This is followed by a period of multisystem injury with pulmonary edema and damage to the liver, kidney, myocardium, and skeletal muscle. Two to 14 days following exposure, progressive pulmonary failure occurs as a result of irreversible alveolar fibrosis. Diquat is less damaging to the skin and does not concentrate in the lungs. Intense nausea, vomiting, and diarrhea may be followed by hypertension, dehydration, renal failure, and shock. Death has occurred after ingestion of as little as 10 mL of a 20% concentration of paraquat in an adult and is common in ingestions exceeding 40 mg/kg. Sufficient amounts of paraquat may be absorbed dermally to produce systemic toxicity and death.

Chlorophenoxy Herbicides

Chlorophenoxy herbicides primarily are irritants, causing cough, nausea, and emesis. Few cases of large ingestions have been reported. Symptoms include coma, miosis, fever, hypertension, muscle rigidity, and tachycardia. Pulmonary edema, respiratory failure, and rhabdomyolysis may occur.[32,37]

Fungicides

Because a large variety of compounds are used in fungicides, the systems affected and clinical effects vary with each compound. Fungicides rarely are associated with acute poisonings in children because of their low toxicity, poor absorption, and use patterns. However, many of these chemicals are serious respiratory and skin irritants, some are associated with allergic sensitization, and some are linked to chronic effects such as endocrine disruption.[38] Common responses to acute fungicide exposure include rashes, mucous membrane irritation, and respiratory symptoms.

Rodenticides

Anticoagulants

Anticoagulants may produce bleeding and are the number one cause of pesticide-related calls to poison control centers for children younger than 6 years. However, data reported by the American Association of Poison Control Centers show no fatalities after anticoagulant ingestion.[39,40]

Insect Repellents

Occasionally, people who use DEET experience adverse reactions, generally consisting of temporary irritation to the skin and eyes. A portion of dermally applied DEET is absorbed systemically.[41] Increased absorption of DEET has been reported in a mouse model when combined with sunscreen use.[42] In 1961, a case of encephalitis linked to DEET was reported.[43] Since that time, additional reports of adverse reactions included rashes, fevers, seizures, and death (mostly in children).[44,45] The major features of each of these cases have been reviewed.[46] Despite broad usage in the United States for many decades with serious problems reported rarely, the relationship between exposure to DEET and reported neurologic symptoms is of concern. Most of the cases of toxicity involved the use of DEET concentration from 10% to 50% and were related to overdose and misuse. Clinicians evaluating children with unexplained encephalopathy or seizures should consider the possibility of exposure to DEET.[8,47] Picaridin was introduced in the United States in 2005 but has been in use in Europe and Australia since 1998. Although the experience is less extensive than with DEET, no serious toxicity has been reported. No evidence of dermal, organ, or reproductive toxicity or carcinogenicity from Picaridin has been demonstrated in animals.[48]

SUBCLINICAL EFFECTS

A statistical simulation by a committee of the National Academy of Sciences suggested that for some pesticides, the reference dose (the dose of a non-cancer-causing toxicant at which no health effects are likely) may be exceeded by thousands of children daily. Some children may display mild symptoms of inattention and gastrointestinal, or flulike, symptoms related to dietary pesticides.[49] Multiple exposures from a variety of sources (ie, food, yard, school) may be cumulative.

CHRONIC SYSTEMIC EFFECTS

Many organochlorine pesticides are linked to chronic health effects such as developmental abnormalities in animals,[50] cancer, and endocrine disruption. Exposures to pesticides and herbicides during the first year of life have been associated with an increased risk of developing asthma by 5 years of age.[51]

CHRONIC NEUROTOXIC EFFECTS

Chronic neurobehavioral or neurologic effects have been reported in a small proportion of organophosphate poisonings in adults. Symptoms reported to persist for months or years include headaches, visual difficulties, problems with memory and concentration, confusion, unusual fatigue, irritability, and depression. In serious poisonings with some organophosphates in adults, there have been reports of organophosphate-induced delayed polyneuropathy associated with paralysis in the legs, sensory disturbances, and weaknesses. In one well-documented case, an infant with hypertonia was diagnosed and treated for cerebral palsy prior to the discovery that she was suffering from chronic poisoning by an organophosphate pesticide. Her house had been sprayed by uncertified applicators prior to her birth and continued to have excessive levels of chemical 9 months later.[52]

Delayed or chronic neurotoxicity may be associated with pesticide exposure during central nervous system development. Although there is plasticity inherent in the development of the nervous system in the infant and child, toxic exposures during the brain growth spurt may exert subtle, permanent effects on the structure and function of the brain. Exposure to neurotoxicants during early life may result in abnormal behavioral traits, such as hyperactivity, decreased attention span, and neurocognitive deficits. Recently, maternal body burden of dichlordiphenyl-dichloroethylene (DDE, a degradation product of DDT) has been associated with impaired neurodevelopmental outcomes in children 6 to 24 months of age.[53] Prenatal exposure to chlorpyrifos (an organophosphate) has been associated with delays on the Psychomotor Development Index and Mental Development Index, attention problems, attention-deficit/hyperactivity disorder (ADHD), and pervasive developmental disorder at 3 years of age (as identified by the Child Behavioral Checklist).[54] Other studies have found similar associations between prenatal organophosphate exposure and developmental delays.[55]

Animal studies have demonstrated periods of vulnerability to neurotoxicants during early life. Single, relatively modest doses of organophosphate, pyrethroid, or organochlorine pesticides during the brain growth spurt in rodents lead to permanent changes in muscarinic receptor levels in the brain and behavioral changes into adulthood.[56,57] These findings are supported by evidence that acetylcholinesterase may play a direct role in axonal outgrowth and neuronal differentiation.[58] The widely used organophosphate pesticides chlorpyrifos and diazinon are suspected neuroteratogens and now have been banned by the EPA for residential use. Adult rats exposed only as neonates to permethrin show alterations in dopaminergic activity in the striatum (a part of the basal ganglia) and in behavior.[59] These findings support the hypothesis that early life exposures to pesticides increase risk for Parkinson disease and other neurologic diseases related to aging.[60]

CARCINOGENIC EFFECTS

Several organophosphates are probable (ie, dichlorvos) or possible (ie, malathion, tetrachlorvinphos) human carcinogens.[61] Permethrin is classified by the EPA as a likely human carcinogen. A variety of fungicides are also suspected carcinogens. Epidemiologic studies have found associations between certain childhood cancers (eg, all brain cancers, non-Hodgkin lymphoma, and leukemia) and pesticide exposure.[62-64] A large review of 30 epidemiologic studies supported a possible role for pesticides in childhood leukemia.[65] Most, but not all, of the studies reported elevated risks among children whose parents were occupationally exposed to pesticides or who used pesticides in the home or garden.[66] Several studies have linked home use of pesticides with childhood brain tumors.[67] Particular behaviors associated with an increased chance of developing brain tumors included using sprays or foggers to dispense flea or tick treatments, flea collars, home pesticide bombs, fumigation for termites, pest strips, and lindane shampoo.

ENDOCRINE DISRUPTION

In the mid-1990s, evidence emerged that numerous chemicals in the environment can mimic hormones in laboratory animals, wildlife, and humans. Over the past decade, much research has focused on these so-called "endocrine disrupters." Many of the organochlorine insecticides have been discovered to exert some of their toxic effects through an endocrine mechanism. For example, DDT is estrogenic, and its metabolite DDE is antiandrogenic. Babies with cryptorchidism or hypospadias had a more than 2.5-fold increased risk of having detectable levels of DDT, DDE, lindane, and several other organochlorine pesticides in their blood.[68] Some pesticides, including DDE and hexachlorobenzene, have been shown to suppress thyroid hormone levels in neonates.[69] The widely used herbicide, atrazine, has been found to be an aromatase agonist, thereby stimulating the endogenous conversion of androgens to estrogen.[70] This pesticide has been linked to intersex abnormalities in amphibian populations living near agricultural fields. Some studies have linked atrazine to mammary tumors in rats.[71] Even low-level exposures to hormonally active agents may pose a risk to the health of infants and children, because subtle alterations of hormone function during critical periods of neurologic and sexual development may have long-term effects. Endocrine disruption is discussed in greater detail in Chapter 28.

DIAGNOSTIC METHODS

The history of exposure is of particular importance. In a review of 190 acute pesticide poisonings, laboratory tests were not often found to be diagnostically helpful.[72] In addition, symptoms of pesticide exposure are likely to be nonspecific. In the case of organophosphate or N-methyl carbamate poisoning, measurement of plasma pseudocholinesterase or red blood cell acetylcholinesterase concentrations are generally rapidly available and may be helpful in confirming a diagnosis. However, because of population variability, these tests are neither sensitive nor specific and must be considered in the context of the clinical situation.

Urine metabolites of some pesticides (organophosphates, chlorophenoxy herbicides, pyrethroids) are measurable, but these tests are available only through specialty laboratories and should only be ordered in unusual circumstances. Organochlorine pesticides and their metabolites are measurable in blood. Population surveys have shown widespread low-level residues in the general population. The Centers for Disease Control and Prevention's National Biomonitoring Study measures 45 pesticides and metabolites and has generated current reference ranges by age group, sex, and ethnicity.[24] The Centers for Disease Control and Prevention survey includes only children older than 6 years. Testing for pesticides should be reserved for unusual circumstances, and the results should be interpreted with caution. The mainstay for the diagnosis of pesticide poisoning is maintenance of a high index of suspicion and a careful exposure history.

TREATMENT

When a poisoning has occurred, the label of the chemical should be obtained whenever possible. Many pesticides have confusingly similar names. Many different active ingredients are sold using the same trade names. Therefore, it is important to ascertain the exact ingredients for any product of concern. The EPA-mandated label contains concise information on specific treatment guidelines, symptoms, and signs and a toll-free telephone number for manufacturer assistance. In an agricultural exposure, the country cooperative extension service agent can provide valuable knowledge of the local crops, chemical usage patterns, and modes of application.

Regional poison control centers can help with patient evaluation and management and have a medical toxicologist available for consultation. The National Pesticide Telecommunications Network can help answer questions about pesticide identification, toxicology, acute and chronic symptoms, and treatment (see Resources).

Serious poisonings should be managed with guidance from a medical toxicologist and/or a regional poison control center. Immediate decontamination is important. If there is an ingestion, gastric decontamination may be indicated. If the exposure is dermal, clothing should be removed and the patient should be washed with soap and water. Caregivers should avoid exposure to the chemical. Latex examination gloves are insufficient personal protective equipment, as many pesticides readily penetrate these gloves. Grossly contaminated patients may need to be decontaminated outside with rescuers using chemical protective gear. Care should be taken to identify other children or adults who may have had similar exposure and need evaluation and treatment. Eliminating a source of contamination may prevent future exposures.[37]

Insecticides

Organophosphates

The patient should be decontaminated. Patients who are asymptomatic or only have minor symptoms should be closely observed. Individuals with muscarinic signs and symptoms of organophosphate poisoning are treated with atropine—very large doses may be required to reverse muscarinic symptoms. The most common life-threatening problem is respiratory arrest from bronchorrhea and diaphragmatic paralysis. The most reliable end-point of adequate atropinization is control of bronchorrhea (drying of the secretions and clear lungs). Tachycardia before administration of atropine is not a contraindication to administration, because early in the acute poisoning, stimulation of autonomic ganglionic nicotinic receptors can activate the sympathetic pathway resulting in transient tachycardia. Eventually stimulation of cardiac muscarinic receptors predominates, resulting in bradycardia.

Pralidoxime (2-PAM, Protopam) breaks the bond in the acetylcholinesterase-phosphate complex and should be used as an antidote for most clinically significant organophosphate poisonings. Pralidoxime affects nicotinic and muscarinic effects of organophosphates. The bond in the acetylcholinesterase-phosphate complex takes up to 24 hours to become an irreversible bond that pralidoxime cannot break. Thus, it is important to administer pralidoxime early to prevent irreversible bonding and to preserve diaphragmatic function and prevent intubation. The neuromuscular junction is a nicotinic receptor and is unresponsive to atropine. If a blood sample for cholinesterase activity will be obtained, this should be done before administering pralidoxime, because pralidoxime quickly reactivates the enzyme. The decision to use pralidoxime should not await blood test results but is based on the clinical picture of the patient.

N-Methyl Carbamates

Treatment with atropine for carbamate poisoning is the same as for organophosphates. Pralidoxime therapy generally is unnecessary, and in some cases, severe reactions and sudden death have occurred with its use.[73] In mixed poisonings involving organophosphates and carbamates or unidentified agents, cautious use of pralidoxime should be considered.

Pyrethrum and Synthetic Pyrethroids

There is no specific antidote. Treatment is primarily supportive. In extremely large ingestions, intubation and lavage may be advised. Dermal paresthesias should be treated with topical application of vitamin E oil preparations. Seizures, if they occur, may be controlled with lorazepam. Allergic reactions should be treated as such, with follow-up intervention to prevent rechallenge with the allergen. It is important to distinguish poisoning from pyrethrum and synthetic pyrethroids from organophosphate poisoning, because some clinical features of synthetic pyrethroid poisoning can mimic organophosphate poisoning and unnecessary treatment with pralidoxime and atropine can be avoided.

Organochlorines

There is no specific antidote. Treatment is supportive with use of anticonvulsants for seizures and general supportive measures. Epinephrine is not advised for poisoning from organochlorines because of increased myocardial susceptibility to catecholamines and life-threatening dysrhythmias.

Boric Acid and Borates

Skin, eye, and gastrointestinal tract decontamination are the principal treatments. Aggressive hydration, treatment of metabolic acidosis, and oxygenation can be critical to supportive care.

Neonicotinoids

Treatment is primarily supportive. Although these agents also affect the cholinesterase receptor, they do not require the use of oximes nor the routine use of atropine. However, in certain circumstances, some patients who presented with severe muscarinic symptoms were successfully treated with atropine.[19]

Fipronil

There is no specific antidote. Treatment is primarily supportive. Treatment for seizures, if any occur, should be the same as in other insecticide poisoning.

Herbicides

Glyphosate

There is no specific antidote. Treatment is supportive.

Bipyridyl Herbicides (Paraquat and Diquat)

Hemoperfusion has been shown to be ineffective in reducing mortality. In paraquat poisoning, supplemental oxygen may increase lung damage and should be avoided if possible. Renal status should be closely monitored, particularly with diquat, because dialysis may be required.

Chlorophenoxy Herbicides

There is no specific antidote. The patient should be monitored for seizures and signs of multiple organ dysfunction (eg, gastrointestinal tract irritation or liver, kidney, and muscle damage). Alkalinization of the urine may enhance clearance.

Fungicides

Treatment for fungicide poisoning is guided by the specific compound ingested. Generally, decontamination and supportive care are the mainstays of treatment.

Rodenticides

Anticoagulants

Consulting with a poison control center can assist in determining the significance of the ingestion. In general, for one-time minor ingestions of warfarin-related or superwarfarin-related rodenticides in children younger than 6 years, no hospital visits, decontamination, or prothrombin time determinations are needed. The child should be observed at home, and parents should be advised to notify a physician if bleeding or bruising occurs. More severe poisonings require monitoring of prothrombin time at 24 and 48 hours following ingestion. Vitamin K preparations (such as phytonadione or AquaMEPHYTON) are appropriate for treatment of poisoning with the warfarins or superwarfarins. In several cases of poisoning with superwarfarins, treatment may need to continue for as long as 3 to 4 months.

Insect Repellents

There is no specific antidote. Treatment for poisoning from DEET is supportive.

PREVENTION: REDUCTION OF PESTICIDE-RELATED RISKS

With the exception of poison baits, as little as 1% of pesticides applied indoors reach the targeted pest. The rest may contaminate surfaces and air in the treated building. Outdoor pesticides may fall on nontargeted organisms, plants, animals, and outdoor furniture and play areas. In addition, material from the outdoor environment can be tracked indoors and add to exposure from dust, floors, and carpets.[74] They may contaminate groundwater, rivers, or wells.

Biomagnification of long-lasting compounds may result in exposure to animals (including humans) at the top of the food chain at concentrations tens of thousands of times greater than those at the bottom of the food chain.

Exposure assessment and counseling about safe practices should be a part of the health maintenance visit, especially for the children of farm workers, pesticide applicators, and others who work with pesticides. Safety precautions to safeguard the family's health should be stressed.

INTEGRATED PEST MANAGEMENT

Integrated pest management (IPM) is an increasingly useful approach to minimizing pesticide use while providing long-term pest control. It integrates chemical and nonchemical methods to provide the least toxic alternative for pest control. Integrated pest management uses regular monitoring to determine if and when treatments are needed. Management tactics include physical (eg, barriers, caulking), mechanical (eg, vacuuming up white flies), agricultural (eg, choosing plants well suited to the site), biological (eg, using predators, pathogens such as *Bacillus thurigiensis*, and naturally occurring bacteria that kill insects), and educational (eg, cleaning up roach- and ant-attracting foods in the kitchen). Treatments are not based on a predetermined schedule but rather on monitoring to indicate when the pest will cause unacceptable economic, medical, or aesthetic damage. Treatments are chosen and timed to be most effective and least hazardous to nontargeted organisms and the general environment. Integrated pest management programs have been successfully adopted by personal homes, school systems, cities and counties (for parks and roadways), gardens, and farms across the United States and often have resulted in substantial cost savings. The national PTA passed a resolution to work toward pesticide-free schools.[76,77]

Studies have demonstrated integrated pest management to be superior to conventional pest control methods. When implemented during pregnancy, integrated pest management was shown to reduce maternal and fetal exposure to pesticides.[78] In public housing units, integrated pest management methods have been documented to be both effective pest control and cost-effective.

Encourage Families to Avoid the Following Unsafe Pesticide Practices*

- Do not enter a field that has been posted with a sign indicating pesticide treatment. Treated fields should not be entered by anyone until pesticide dust has settled, plants are dry from spray, or the worker is wearing protective clothing.

- Do not use water in drainage ditches or any irrigation system for drinking, washing food or clothing, swimming, or fishing.

- Do not carry lunch or drinks into a treated field.

- Do not put pesticides in unmarked containers or food or drink jars.

- Never take pesticide containers home for use around the house. They are unsafe.

- Do not burn pesticide bags for fuel; they can give off poisonous fumes.

- Do not use pesticides from work around the house.

Encourage Families to Use Safe Pesticide Practices

- Wash work clothes separately from other laundry.

- Wash work clothes with detergent and hot water before wearing them again.

- Wash hands and arms after putting clothing into washing machine.

- Change clothing and wash with soap and water before picking up or playing with your children.

- Store pesticides in an area that children cannot access.

- Cover children's skin if they are with you at work.

- Keep the children and their toys and playthings indoors when there is nearby aerial spraying or spraying that may drift near the house.

- Children and teenagers should avoid work that involves mixing or spraying pesticides.

*Adapted from INFO Letter: Environmental and Occupational Health Briefs.[75]

Simple Steps That May Reduce the Need for Pesticides

1. Grow plant varieties that grow well in the area. A county extension agent or nursery personnel may have advice.
2. Time the watering and fertilizing of the plants according to their needs.
3. Follow recommendations given for mowing grass and pruning plants.
4. Decide what degree of damage from weeds, insects, and diseases can be tolerated, and do not take control measures unless that degree is exceeded.
5. Consider nonchemical options first when controls are needed. For example, determine whether weeds can be removed by hoeing or pulling.

Frequently Asked Questions

Q I am having pest problems in my lawn and garden. Should I get regular preventive applications by a professional service?

A Regular lawn treatment exposes people to pesticides unnecessarily. It also may kill insects that are beneficial in controlling the pest population, thereby requiring the use of more chemicals. Weed killers, especially combination products that include a fertilizer and an herbicide, are generally an unnecessary risk because they are used only for cosmetic purposes but leave a residue on the lawn that can be tracked into the home and may pose a long-term risk to children. If a professional lawn service is used, its personnel should (1) regularly monitor the lawn for pests and treat the lawn only when pests exist, (2) offer alternatives to the standard treatment, (3) give advance warning (including to neighbors) before applying any pesticides (this allows time to cover outdoor furniture and remove toys and pet food dishes), (4) be trained and certified, (5) give advance notification of the types of chemicals to be used and information on their effects on health, and (6) avoid applications under adverse weather conditions (eg, high winds).

Q Is an insect repellent containing DEET safe for use on my children?

A Products containing DEET are the most effective mosquito repellents currently available.[79] DEET is also an effective repellent for a variety of other insect pests, including ticks. DEET should be used in areas where there is concern about illness from insect bites. It also can be used when insects are likely to be a nuisance, such as at barbecues or at the beach. Although it generally is used without any problems, there have been rare reports of adverse effects. Usually, these problems have occurred with inappropriate use. No definitive studies exist in the scientific literature about what concentration of DEET is safe for children. Alternatives to DEET include Picaridin (1-methylpropyl 2-(2-hydroxyethyl)-1-piperidinecarbox-ylate, also known as KBR 3023) and oil of lemon eucalyptus. Picaridin and DEET have similar effectiveness at comparable concentrations.

The concentration of DEET in products may range from less than 10% to 100%. The efficacy of DEET plateaus at a concentration of 30%, the maximum concentration currently recommended for infants and children. The major difference in the efficacy of products relates to their duration of action. Products with concentrations around 10% are effective for periods of approximately 2 hours. As the concentration of DEET increases, the duration of activity increases; for example, a concentration of about 24% has recently been shown to provide an average of 5 hours of protection.

The safety of DEET does not seem to relate to differences in these concentrations. Thus, products with a concentration of 30% appear to be as

---

Precautions When Using Insect Repellants

1. Read and carefully follow all directions before using the product. Do not allow children to handle the product. When using on children, apply to your own hands first and then put it on the child. Do not apply to children's hands.

2. Wear long sleeves and pants when possible and apply repellent to clothing—a long-sleeved shirt with snug collar and cuffs is best. The shirt should be tucked in at the waist. Socks should be tucked over pants, hiking shoes, or boots.

3. Use just enough repellent to cover exposed skin and/or clothing. Heavy application and saturation generally are unnecessary for effectiveness. Do not use repellents underneath clothing.

4. Do not apply to eyes or mouth, and apply sparingly around ears. When using sprays, do not spray directly on face—spray on hands first and then apply to face.

5. Do not apply repellents over cuts, wounds, or irritated skin.

6. Wash treated skin with soap and water when returning indoors. Wash treated clothing.

7. Avoid using sprays in enclosed areas. Do not use repellents near food.

8. If a child develops a rash or other apparent allergic reaction from an insect repellent, stop using the repellent, wash it off with mild soap and water and call a pediatrician or a local poison control center for further guidance.

safe as products with a concentration of 10% when used according to the directions on the product labels. A prudent approach would be to select the lowest concentration effective for the amount of time spent outdoors. It is generally agreed that DEET should not be applied more than once a day.

Some properties of infant and toddler skin may differ from those of adult skin until children are at least 2 years of age.[47] Because studies suggest the possibility that young skin may have greater permeability to chemicals, DEET should be applied sparingly and only when needed, weighing the risks of exposure to vectorborne illness to the possible risks of absorption. No data are available to show infants and children's blood levels following DEET application.

DEET should not be used in a product that combines the repellent with a sunscreen. Sunscreens are often applied repeatedly because they can be washed away through swimming and sweating. DEET is not water soluble and will last up to 8 hours. Repeated application may increase the potential toxic effects of DEET. Sunscreens and insect repellants may be used together as individual products applied separately as indicated.

Q *We have rodents in and around our home. How can we safely get rid of them?*

A Most pesticides for controlling rats (rodenticides) available for home use today are the anticoagulants warfarin or superwarfarin (coumarins) or indanediones. They kill the rodents by causing internal bleeding. These anticoagulants also can cause bleeding in children if ingested and, therefore, must be used carefully. Each year, more than 10 000 children are exposed to these products, making anticoagulant baits one of the most common pesticide ingestions in children younger than 6 years. Fortunately, the amounts usually eaten by young children rarely cause serious injury. Poisoning can be avoided by following the product label and using common sense. In 2008, the EPA took further measures aimed at decreasing the number of significant pediatric ingestions of rodenticides. "Consumer sized" products may no longer contain brodifacoum, difethialone, bromadiolone, or difenacoum (the second-generation anticoagulants). Use of tamper-resistant bait stations with solid bait will reduce children's access to these products, and therefore, sales to consumers will only be allowed in this form in the future. Because rodenticides have a long shelf-life, the older consumer products may remain in use for some time to come. If it is suspected that a child may have ingested a product containing anticoagulants, a physician or poison control center or the emergency department of the nearest hospital should be contacted immediately. Alternatives to rodenticides include careful sealing of cracks and crevices, cleaning up brush and debris from outdoor areas where rats may hide, and careful sanitation to leave no food scraps for rodents to eat. Mechanical traps can be effective for controlling a minor rodent problem.

These can include snap traps or glue traps. The latter are less likely to cause injuries to small children who might come into contact with the traps.

Q *What is the best way to treat a roach problem?*

A Hygiene measures are key. Cockroaches are found where there is water and food. Eating should be discouraged in areas other than the kitchen. All foodstuffs should be stored in closed containers. Water sources should be eliminated by caulking cracks around faucets and pipe fittings. Cracks and crevices where cockroaches can enter the home should be sealed.

A prudent approach is to minimize exposure to sprays whenever possible. Individual bait stations are recommended. If possible, baiting should be done outside the home as well. Boric acid, formulated for use as a pesticide, is comparatively less toxic than cholinesterase inhibitors and pyrethroids, and can be used in cracks and crevices in areas inaccessible to children.

If these measures are not successful, the family should consult a professional exterminator. If professional extermination is to be done, be certain

---

Measures That May Reduce the Danger of Exposure to Rodenticides

1. Place all rodenticides out of the reach of children and nontarget animals in tamper-proof bait boxes. Outdoors, place bait inside the entrance of a burrow and then collapse the entrance over the bait.

2. Securely lock or fasten shut the lids of all bait boxes.

3. Use a solid bait and place in the baffle-protected lockable feeding chamber, never in the runway of the box.

4. Always use sanitation measures in conjunction with pesticides to limit rodent access to food and hiding places. Work with neighbors to secure the neighborhood. If baiting alone is used without sanitation measures, the rodent population will rebound each time the baiting stops. Measures include using rat-proof garbage cans and food storage precautions (including keeping food in the refrigerator), and frequently raking up garden waste (including fallen fruit).

5. Modify the habitat by rodent-proofing buildings and changing landscaping to eliminate hiding places.

6. Continue to monitor periodically to ensure that rodents are not recolonizing.

that it is a licensed firm and find out what insecticide will be used and its possible toxic effects. Before using any insecticide in the home, all food, dishes, cooking utensils, children's toys, and clothing should be removed or protected from contamination. After application of the insecticide, young children and pregnant women should stay out of the area for as long as possible. The room should be aired well by cross ventilation for 4 to 8 hours before people and pets return. Crawling babies should not be allowed in the area until it has been well vacuumed or mopped and the residents can be certain that the pesticide was not applied in an area where the infant can reach. For example, if the pesticide is applied to the wall, a crawling infant could hold onto the wall or wipe his hands and sustain a significant exposure.

Families should avoid using over-the-counter bug sprays and bug bombs. *The Cockroach Control Manual,* an excellent resource, is available from the University of Nebraska. It includes complete information on an integrated pest management approach including "least toxic methods." It is available for purchase or free download at http://pested.unl.edu/cocktoc.htm.

Q   *What is the best way to control fleas on a dog or cat?*

A   There are a wide variety of flea-control products. The safest approach to flea control is to avoid pesticide products altogether. This can be done by bathing the pet with a regular pet shampoo at least every other week, and simultaneously washing the pet's bedding in hot water with a regular laundry detergent. Vacuuming rugs at least weekly is also very important. If your pet is scratching, then carefully comb its fur with a fine-toothed flea comb to look for "flea dirt" and adult fleas. Flea dirt is a red-brown particulate that appears rusty red if pressed onto paper. It represents the blood-filled feces from the fleas. If regular bathing, vacuuming, laundry, and flea combing is not sufficient to control fleas, then the best option is an oral agent such as lufenuron (Program, Sentinel). The flea products to avoid include flea collars (which generally contain tetrachlorvinphos or propoxur) and permethrin shampoos.

Q   *My house is overrun with ants. Should I get an exterminator to spray?*

A   Spraying for ants is generally ineffective. Ants are relatively easy to control using the principles of integrated pest management (IPM). First, it is important to discover how the ants are getting in to the house. Once the entry point is identified, it can be sealed off. If it's not possible to seal, then ant bait could be placed in that location, as long as it is out of reach of children. It is also important to discover where the ants are going and to remove all food sources by sealing food items in containers or zip lock bags. The ant trail should be wiped clean with dish soap and water to remove the scent that the ants are following. This set of actions will cause the ant problem to completely resolve within a few days. If a professional pest control company is needed, look for one that is certified by Green Shield, which maintains standards for integrated pest management pest control (www.greenshield certified.org).

Resources

Extoxnet
Web site: http://ace.ace.orst.edu/info/extoxnet
A cooperative effort among the University of California at Davis, Oregon State University, Michigan State University, and Cornell University that provides updated pesticide information in understandable terms. It includes toxicology briefs and information on carcinogenicity, testing, and exposure assessment.

National Center for Environmental Assessment Publications and Information
Phone: 513-489-8190
Offers free fact sheets on lawn care, pesticide labels, and pesticide safety.

National Pesticide Telecommunications Network
Phone for health professionals: 800-858-7377; phone for general public: 800-858-7378
Web site: http://npic.orst.edu/index.html
A toll-free EPA and Oregon State University-sponsored information service.

Organophosphate Pesticides and Child Health: A Primer for Health Care Providers.
Online CME course: http://depts.washington.edu/opchild/

Texas Agricultural Extension Service, Physician's Guide to Pesticide Poisoning
Web site: www-aes.tamu.edu/doug/med/pgpp.htm

Toxnet
Web site: http://toxnet.nlm.nih.gov
A cluster of databases on toxicology, hazardous chemicals, and related areas.

University of Nebraska Cooperative Extension, Signs and Symptoms of Pesticide Poisoning
Web site: www.ianr.unl.edu/pubs/pesticides/ec2505.htm

US Environmental Protection Agency

Web site: www.epa.gov

- *Recognition and Management of Pesticide Poisonings.* 5th ed. Available at: www.epa.gov/oppfead1/safety/healthcare/handbook/handbook.htm (available in English and Spanish)
- EPA online resources in case of suspected pesticide poisoning: www.epa.gov/oppfead1/safety/incaseof.htm
- EPA pamphlets
  - *Citizen's Guide to Pest Control and Pesticide Safety*
  - *Pest Control in the School Environment*
  - *Healthy Lawn, Healthy Environment*

References

1. Kiely T, Donaldson D, Grube AH. *Pesticide Industry Sales and Usage: 2000 and 2001 Market Estimates.* US Environmental Protection Agency, Office of Pesticide Programs; Washington, DC: US Environmental Protection Agency; 2004. Available at: http://www.epa.gov/oppbead1/pestsales/01pestsales/market_estimates2001.pdf. Accessed October 12, 2010

2. Blondell JM. Decline in pesticide poisonings in the United States from 1995 to 2004 *Clin Toxicol.* 2007;45(5):589–592

3. Lu C, Fenske RA, Simcox NJ, Kalman D. Pesticide exposure of children in an agricultural community: evidence of household proximity to farmland and take home exposure pathways. *Environ Res.* 2000;84(3):290–302

4. Fenske RA, Kissel JC, Lu C, et al. Biologically based pesticide dose estimates for children in an agricultural community. *Environ Health Perspect.* 2000;108(6):515–520

5. Food Quality Protection Act of 1996. Pub L No 104-170, 110 Stat 1489

6. Reregistration Eligibility Decision Fact Sheet. R.E.D. Facts. Propoxur. 1997. Available at http: www.epa.gov/oppsrrd1/REDs/factsheets/2555fact.pdf. Accessed October 12, 2010

7. Centers for Disease Control and Prevention. Updated information regarding mosquito repellents May 8, 2008. Available at: http://www.cdc.gov/ncidod/dvbid/westnile/resources/uprepinfo.pdf. Accessed October 12, 2010

8. Brown M, Hebert AA. Insect repellents: an overview. *J Am Acad Dermatol.* 1997;36(2 Pt 1): 243–249

9. Power LE, Sudakin DL. Pyrethrin and pyrethroid exposures in the United States: a longitudinal analysis of incidents reported to poison centers. *J Med Toxicol.* 2007;3(3):94-99

10. Food and Drug Administration. FDA Public Health Advisory: Safety of Topical Lindane Products for the Treatment of Scabies and Lice. Rockville, MD: Food and Drug Administration; 2009. Available at: http://www.fda.gov/Drugs/DrugSafety/PostmarketDrugSafetyInformationforPatientsandProviders/ucm110845.htm. Accessed October 12, 2010

11. California Health and Safety Code. State of California Assembly Bill 2318, §111246 (2000)

12. Humphreys EH, Janssen S, Heil A, Hiatt P, Solomon G, Miller MD. Outcomes of the California ban on pharmaceutical lindane: clinical and ecologic impacts. *Environ Health Perspect.* 2008;116(3):297-302

13. Goldbloom RB, Goldbloom A. Boric acid poisoning: report of four cases and a review of 109 cases from the world literature. *J Pediatr.* 1953;43(6):631–643

14. Wong LC, Heimbach MD, Truscott DR, Duncan BD. Boric acid poisoning: report of 11 cases. *Can Med Assoc J.* 1964;90:1018–1023

15. Litovitz TL, Klein-Schwartz W, White S, et al. 1999 annual report of the American Association of Poison Control Centers Toxic Exposure Surveillance System. *Am J Emerg Med.* 2000;18(5):517–574

16. Davis MK, Boone JS, Moran JE, Tyler JW, Chambers JE. Assessing intermittent pesticide exposure from flea control collars containing the organophosphorus insecticide tetrachlorvinphos. *J Expo Sci Environ Epidemiol.* 2008;18(6)564-570. doi:10.1038/sj.jes.7500647

17. US Environmental Protection Agency. Permethrin Facts. Reregistration Eligibility Decision (RED) Fact Sheet. 2006. Available at: http://www.epa.gov/oppsrrd1/REDs/factsheets/ permethrin_fs.htm. Accessed October 12, 2010

18. Mohamed F, Gawarammana I, Robertson TA, Roberts MS, et al. Acute human self-poisoning with imidacloprid compound: a neonicotinoids insecticide. *PloS One. 2009;4(4):e5127*

19. Phua DH, Lin CC, Wu ML, et al. Neonicotinoid insecticides: an emerging cause of acute pesticide poisoning. *Clin Toxicol.* 2009;47:336-341

20. Ratra GS, Casida JE. GABA receptor subunit composition relative to insecticide potency and selectivity. *Toxicol Lett.* 2001;122(3):215-222

21. Fradin MS, Day JF. Comparative efficacy of insect repellents against mosquito bites. *N Engl J Med.* 2002;347(1):13–18

22. Lu C, Knutson DE, Fisker-Andersen J, Fenske RA. Biological monitoring survey of organophosphorus pesticide exposure among pre-school children in the Seattle metropolitan area. *Environ Health Perspect.* 2001;109(3):299–303

23. Whyatt RM, Barr DB. Measurement of organophosphate metabolites in postpartum meconium as a potential biomarker of prenatal exposure: a validation study. *Environ Health Perspect.* 2001;109(4):417–420

24. Centers for Disease Control and Prevention. *Fourth National Report on Human Exposure to Environmental Chemicals.* Atlanta, GA: Centers for Disease Control and Prevention; 2009. Available at: http://www.cdc.gov/exposurereport. Accessed June 11, 2011

25. Whitmore RW, Kelly JE, Reading PL. *National Home and Garden Pesticide Survey: Final Report, Volume 1.* Research Triangle Park, NC: Research Triangle Institute; 1992. Publication RTI/5100/17-01F

26. US Environmental Protection Agency, Office of Water. *A Review of Contaminant Occurrence in Public Water Systems.* Washington, DC: US Environmental Protection Agency; 1999. EPA Publication 816-R-99-006

27. Bronstein AC, Spyker DA, Cantilena LR Jr, Green J, Rumack BH, Heard SE. 2006 Annual Report of the American Association of Poison Control Centers' National Poison Data System (NPDS). *Clin Toxicol (Phila).* 2007;45(8):815-917

28. Longnecker MP, Klebanoff MA, Zhou H, Brock JW. Association between maternal serum concentration of the DDT metabolite DDE and preterm and small-for-gestational-age babies at birth. *Lancet.* 2001;358(9276):110–114

29. Garry VF, Schreinemachers D, Harkins ME, Griffith J. Pesticide appliers, biocides, and birth defects in rural Minnesota. *Environ Health Perspect.* 1996;104(4):394–399

30. Bell EM, Hertz-Picciotto I, Beaumont JJ. A case-control study of pesticides and fetal death due to congenital anomalies. *Epidemiology.* 2001;12(2):148–156

31. Arbuckle TE, Lin Z, Mery LS. An exploratory analysis of the effect of pesticide exposure on the risk of spontaneous abortion in an Ontario farm population. *Environ Health Perspect.* 2001;109(8):851–857

32. Reigart JR, Roberts JR. *Recognition and Management of Pesticide Poisonings.* 5th ed. Washington, DC: US Environmental Protection Agency; 1999

33. Wagner SL. Fatal asthma in a child after use of an animal shampoo containing pyrethrin. *West J Med.* 2000;173(2):86–87

34. Tangermann RH, Etzel RA, Mortimer L, Penner GD, Paschal DG. An outbreak of a food-related illness resembling boric acid poisoning. *Arch Environ Contam Toxicol.* 1992;23(1): 142–144

35. Mohamed F, Senarathna L, Percy A, et al. Acute human self-poisoning with the N-phenylpyrazole insecticide fipronil—a GABA$_A$-gated chloride channel blocker. *J Toxicol Clin Toxicol.* 2004;42(7):955-963

36. Talbot AR, Shiaw MH, Huang JS, et al. Acute poisoning with a glyphosate-surfactant herbicide (Roundup): a review of 93 cases. *Hum Exp Toxicol.* 1991;10:1–8

37. American Academy of Pediatrics, Committee on Injury and Poison Prevention. *Handbook of Common Poisonings in Children.* Rodgers GC Jr, ed. 3rd ed. Elk Grove Village, IL: American Academy of Pediatrics; 1994

38. Kelce WR, Monosson E, Gamcsik MP, Laws SC, Gray LE Jr. Environmental hormone disruptors: evidence that vinclozolin developmental toxicity is mediated by antiandrogenic metabolites. *Toxicol Appl Pharmacol.* 1994;126(2):276–285

39. Litovitz T, Manoguerra A. Comparison of pediatric poisoning hazards: an analysis of 3.8 million exposure incidents. A report from the American Association of Poison Control Centers. *Pediatrics.* 1992;89(6 Pt 1):999–1006

40. Litovitz TL, Klein-Schwartz W, Dyer KS, Shannon M, Lee S, Powers M. 1997 annual report of the American Association of Poison Control Centers Toxic Exposure Surveillance System. *Am J Emerg Med.* 1998;16(5):443–497

41. Selim S, Hartnagel RE Jr, Osimitz TG, Gabriel KL, Schoenig GP. Absorption, metabolism, and excretion of N,N-diethyl-m-toluamide following dermal application to human volunteers. *Fundam Appl Toxicol.* 1995;25(1):95–100

42. Ross EA, Savage KA, Utley LJ, Tebbett IR. Insect repellent interactions: sunscreens enhance DEET (N,N-diethyl-m-toluamide) absorption. *Drug Metab Dispos.* 2004;32(8):783-785

43. Gryboski J, Weinstein D, Ordway N. Toxic encephalopathy apparently related to the use of an insect repellent. *N Engl J Med.* 1961;264:289–291

44. Centers for Disease Control and Prevention. Seizures temporally associat-ed with use of DEET insect repellent—New York and Connecticut. *MMWR Morb Mortal Wkly Rep.* 1989;38(39):678–680

45. Veltri JC, Osimitz TG, Bradford DC, Page BC. Retrospective analysis of calls to poison control centers resulting from exposure to the insect repellent N,N-diethyl-m-toluamide (DEET) from 1985–1989. *J Toxicol Clin Toxicol.* 1994;32(1):1–16

46. Roberts JR, Reigart JR. Insect repellents: does anything beat DEET? *Pediatr Ann.* 2004;33(7):443-453

47. Giusti F, Martella A, Bertoni L, Seidenari S. Skin barrier, hydration, Ph of skin of infants under two years of age. *Pediatr Dermatol.* 2001;18(2):93-96

48. Abramowicz M. Picaridin—a new insect repellent. *Med Lett Drugs Ther.* 2005;47(1210):46-47

49. National Research Council. *Pesticides in the Diets of Infants and Children.* Washington, DC: National Academies Press; 1993

50. Vonier PM, Crain DA, McLachlan JA, Guillette LJ Jr, Arnold SF. Interaction of environmental chemicals with the estrogen and progesterone receptors from the oviduct of the American alligator. *Environ Health Perspect.* 1996;104(12):1318–1322

51. Salam MT, Li YF, Langholz B, Gilliland FD. Early life environmental risk factors for asthma: findings from the Children's Health Study. *Environ Health Perspect.* 2004;112(6):760-765

52. Wagner SL, Orwick DL. Chronic organophosphate exposure associated with transient hypertonia in an infant. *Pediatrics.* 1994;94(1):94–97

53. Fenster L, Eskenazi B, Anderson M, Bradman A, Hubbard A, Barr DB. In utero exposure to DDT and performance on the Brazelton neonatal behavioral assessment scale. *NeuroToxicology.* 2007;28(3):471–477

54. Rauh VA, Garfinkel R, Perera FP, et al. Impact of prenatal chlorpyrifos exposure on neurodevelopment in the first 3 years of life among inner-city children. *Pediatrics.* 2006;118(6):e1845-e1859

55. Eskenazi, Rosas LG, Marks AR, et al. Pesticide toxicity and the developing brain. *Basic Clin Pharmacol Toxicol.* 2008;102(2):228–236

56. Ahlbom J, Fredriksson A, Eriksson P. Exposure to an organophosphate (DFP) during a defined period in neonatal life induces permanent changes in brain muscarinic receptors and behaviour in adult mice. *Brain Res.* 1995;677(1):13–19

57. Ahlbom J, Fredriksson A, Eriksson P. Neonatal exposure to a type-I pyrethroid (bioallethrin) induces dose-response changes in brain muscarinic receptors and behaviour in neonatal and adult mice. *Brain Res.* 1994;645(1-2):318–324

58. Brimijoin S, Koenigsberger C. Cholinesterases in neural development: new findings and toxicologic implications. *Environ Health Perspect.* 1999;107(Suppl 1):59–64

59. Nasuti C, Gabbianelli R, Falcioni ML, Di Stefano A, Sozio P, Cantalamessa F. Dopaminergic system modulation, behavioral changes, and oxidative stress after neonatal administration of pyrethroids. *Toxicology.* 2007;229(3):194-205

60. Logroscino G. The role of early life environmental risk factors in Parkinson disease: what is the evidence? *Environ Health Perspect.* 2005;113(9):1234-1238

61. US Environmental Protection Agency, Office of Pesticide Programs. List of Chemicals Evaluated for Carcinogenic Potential. Washington, DC: US Environmental Protection Agency; 2000. Available at: http://www.epa.gov/pesticides/carlist. Accessed October 12, 2010

62. Kristensen P, Andersen A, Irgens LM, Bye AS, Sundheim L. Cancer in offspring of parents engaged in agricultural activities in Norway: incidence and risk factors in the farm environment. *Int J Cancer.* 1996;65(1):39–50

63. Alexander FE, Patheal SL, Biondi A, et al. Transplacental chemical exposure and risk of infant leukemia with MLL gene fusion. *Cancer Res.* 2001;61(6):2542–2546

64. Buckley JD, Meadows AT, Kadin ME, LeBeau MM, Siegel S, Robinson LL. Pesticide exposures in children with non-Hodgkin lymphoma. *Cancer.* 2000;89(11):2315–2321

65. Infante-Rivard C, Weichenthal S. Pesticides and childhood cancer: an update of Zahm and Ward's 1998 review. *J Toxicol Environ Health Part B.* 2007;10:81-99

66. Zahm SH, Ward MH. Pesticides and childhood cancer. *Environ Health Perspect.* 1998;106(Suppl 3):893–908

67. Davis JR, Brownson RC, Garcia R, Bentz BJ, Turner A. Family pesticide use and childhood brain cancer. *Arch Environ Contam Toxicol.* 1993;24(1):87–92

68. Fernandez MF, Olmos B, Granada A, et al. Human exposure to endocrine-disrupting chemicals and prenatal risk factors for cryptorchidism and hypospadias: a nested case-control study. *Environ Health Perspect.* 2007;115(Suppl 1):8-14

69. Maervoet J, Vermeir G, Covaci A, et al. Association of thyroid hormone concentrations with levels of organochlorine compounds in cord blood of neonates. *Environ Health Perspect.* 2007;115(12):1780-1786

70. Fan W, Yanase T, Morinaga H, et al. Atrazine-induced aromatase expression is SF-1 dependent: implications for endocrine disruption in wildlife and reproductive cancers in humans. *Environ Health Perspect.* 2007;115(5):720-727

71. Cooper RL, Laws SC, Das PC, et al. Atrazine and reproductive function: mode and mechanism of action studies. *Birth Defects Res B Dev Reprod Toxicol.* 2007;80(2):98-112

72. Lessenger JE, Estock MD, Younglove T. An analysis of 190 cases of suspected pesticide illness. *J Am Board Fam Pract.* 1995;8(4):278–282

73. Kurtz PH. Pralidoxime in the treatment of carbamate intoxication. *Am J Emerg Med.* 1990;8(1): 68–70

74. Nishioka MG, Lewis RG, Brinkman MC, Burkholder HM, Hines CE, Menkedick JR. Distribution of 2,4-D in air and on surfaces inside residences after lawn applications: comparing exposure estimates from various media for young children. *Environ Health Perspect.* 2001;109(11):1185–1191

75. INFO Letter: Environmental and Occupational Health Briefs. Vol. 9, No. 4. Piscataway, NJ: Environmental and Health Risk Communications Division; 1996

76. Child Proofing our Communities Campaign. *Poisoned Schools: Invisible Threats, Visible Actions.* Falls Church, VA: Center for Health, Environment, and Justice; 2001

77. Rose RI. Pesticides and public health: integrated methods of mosquito management. *Emerg Infect Dis.* 2001;7(1):17–23

78. Williams MK, Barr DB, Camann DE, et al. An intervention to reduce residential insecticide exposure during pregnancy among an inner-city cohort. *Environ Health Perspect.* 2006;114(11):1684-1689

79. Fradin MS, Day JF. Comparative efficacy of insect repellents against mosquito bites. *N Engl J Med.* 2002;347(1):13–18

Chapter 38

Plasticizers

■ ■ ■ ■ ■ ■

INTRODUCTION

Plastics are made up of 2 types of components. The main components are polymers, or resins, that make up the bulk of the plastic material. Examples include polyvinyl chloride (PVC), polycarbonate (PC), high-density polyethylene (HDPE) and polypropylene (PP). The second components are additives. Additives are small but important parts of the overall plastic composition. Additives give plastics useful properties, such as color, fire resistance, strength, or flexibility. To a large extent, it is additives that give plastics most of their functions.

"Plasticizer" is a term used to describe some of the additives added to polymers or resins to give them more flexibility (eg, phthalates), or to make them more rigid (eg, bisphenol A [BPA]). This chapter focuses on some of the most commonly used and well studied additives that have known or potential links to human health, particularly in children.

PHTHALATES

Phthalates are a class of commonly used plasticizers.[1] In particular, dioctyl phthalate (DOP) is extensively used as a plasticizer for polyvinyl chloride. Factors such as flexibility and wide availability make phthalates optimal chemicals for industrial use. Phthalates migrate to the surface of plastics and can then evaporate or leach into the surrounding environment. Because of their widespread use, phthalates have become some of the most abundant industrial pollutants in the environment.[2] Many phthalates, including dioctyl phthalate, are classified as toxic chemicals by the US Environmental Protection Agency

Table 38.1: Sources of Phthalate Exposure

PHTHALATE PARENT COMPOUND	POTENTIAL SOURCES OF EXPOSURE
Di(2-ethylhexyl) phthalate (DEHP)	Polyvinyl chloride-containing medical tubing, blood storage bags, medical devices, food contamination, food packaging, indoor air, plastic toys, wall coverings, tablecloths, floor tiles, furniture upholstery, shower curtains, garden hoses, swimming pool liners, rainwear, baby pants, dolls, some toys, shoes, automobile upholstery and tops, packaging film and sheets, sheathing for wire and cable
Diethyl phthalate (DEP)	Cosmetics, nail polish, deodorant, perfumes/cologne, lotions, after shave, pharmaceuticals/herbal products, insecticide
Di-isononyl phthalate (DINP)	Children's toys
Dibutyl phthalate (DBP)	Nail polish, makeup, after shave, perfumes, coatings on pharmaceuticals/herbal products, chemiluminescent glow sticks
Di-n-octyl phthalate (DnOP)	Children's toys
Di-n-butyl phthalate (DnBP)	Medicines, cosmetics, cellulose acetate plastics, latex adhesives, nail polish and other cosmetic products, plasticizers in cellulose plastics, solvent for certain dyes
Butyl benzyl phthalate (BBP)	Vinyl flooring, adhesives, sealants, food packaging, furniture upholstery, vinyl tile, carpet tiles, artificial leather, adhesives
Dimethyl phthalate (DMP)	Insecticides, indoor air, adhesives, hairstyling products, shampoo, after shave

(EPA)'s Toxic Release Inventory. Low-molecular weight phthalates, such as diethyl phthalate (DEP) and dibutyl phthalate (DBP), are commonly used as components of fragrance and color stabilizers in cosmetics and personal care products. They are found in lotions, after shave, perfumes, nail polish, and other products used on a daily basis. High-molecular weight phthalates include di(2-ethylhexyl) phthalate (DEHP) and benzyl butyl phthalate (BBP). Di(2-ethylhexyl) phthalate is used in polyvinyl chloride products, flexible plastics, and intravenous (IV) tubing.

ROUTES OF EXPOSURE

Phthalates leach out of products easily and can, therefore, be inhaled, ingested, or dermally absorbed or enter the bloodstream directly through the IV route. Children are exposed to phthalates through multiple sources and routes of exposure (see Table 38.1). Phthalates leach out from these products at higher concentrations when they are heated.

Table 38.2: Selected Review of Effects of Phthalates on Children's Health

HEALTH OUTCOME STUDIED	REFERENCE	STUDY TYPE AND PATIENT GROUP	RESULTS	WEAKNESSES OF STUDY
Endocrine/ Reproductive	10	Retrospective cohort, 19 adolescents (ages 14-16) who underwent ECMO in NICU	1. 18 adolescents were growing and developing normally relative to population estimates 2. All serum tests/hormone concentrations were within the normal range relative to pubertal maturation stage	1. Do not know what true phthalate exposures were (may not have used phthalate-containing medical tubing) 2. No internal biomarkers of phthalate concentrations 3. Small sample size
	3	Prospective cohort, 85 mother/infant pairs (2-36 months)	1. Found a relationship between increased maternal phthalate concentration in third trimester of pregnancy and decreased anogenital distance in infants	1. Only one pregnancy measurement in 3rd trimester (as opposed to first trimester, when genital development occurs) 2. Small sample size
	4	Prospective cohort, 130 mother/infant pairs (3 months of age)	1. Found positive correlations between MEP, MBP concentrations in human milk and serum hormone binding globulin 2. Did not find a relationship between phthalate concentrations and incidence of cryptorchidism	1. Do not know infant postnatal phthalate internal dose; this could be related to outcomes studied 2. Measurements may have included some contribution from diester contamination
Immune/ Inflammatory	11	Retrospective cohort study, 84 infants	1. Found a 1-week decrease in gestational age at delivery in infants with detectable concentrations of MEHP in cord blood as compared with infants with nondetectable MEHP concentrations in cord blood	1. Plausible hypothesis? 2. Do not know true fetal exposures 3. Potentially poor analytic methods 4. Small sample size and retrospective design

continued on page 552

continued from page 551

Table 38.2: Selected Review of Effects of Phthalates on Children's Health, *continued*

HEALTH OUTCOME STUDIED	REFERENCE	STUDY TYPE AND PATIENT GROUP	RESULTS	WEAKNESSES OF STUDY
Immune/ Inflammatory, *continued*	5	Case/control, 198 children with persistent allergy/ asthma cases/202 child controls	1. Found higher concentrations of BBP in indoor dust of cases compared with controls 2. BBP in indoor dust associated with allergies/ eczema symptoms in dose-response fashion 3. DEHP in indoor dust associated asthma in dose-response fashion	1. No internal biomarkers of phthalate concentrations 2. Cross-sectional nature of study does not help elucidate pathophysiology for development of symptoms (ie, do phthalates exacerbate atopic status or cause atopic status to develop?)
	8	Prospective cohort, 404 mothers	1. Found positive association between (how much change in) low-molecular weight phthalate exposure in third trimester of pregnancy and 0.97 day longer gestation and increased head circumference	1. Unclear whether single urine phthalate measurement during third trimester reflects exposure during entire pregnancy 2. Results may be attributable to residual confounding of other anthropometric factors
	12	Prospective cohort, 283 mothers	1. Found that women in second or third trimester of pregnancy at the 75th percentile for DEHP exposures had a 2-day longer gestation as compared with women at the 25th percentile 2. Log-unit increases in MEHP and MEOHP exposure in women within second and third trimester of pregnancy associated with increased odds of Cesarean delivery, delivery 41 weeks or later	1. Unclear clinical significance of 2-day increased gestational period 2. Unclear whether single urine phthalate measurement reflects exposure during entire pregnancy

Table 38.2: Selected Review of Effects of Phthalates on Children's Health, *continued*

HEALTH OUTCOME STUDIED	REFERENCE	STUDY TYPE AND PATIENT GROUP	RESULTS	WEAKNESSES OF STUDY
Immune/ Inflammatory, *continued*	7	Prospective cohort, 295 mother/neonate pairs	1. Found an inverse relationship between the sum of high-molecular weight phthalates in third trimester of pregnancy and orientation on Brazelton Neonatal Behavioral Assessment Scale, and Quality of Alertness in girls 2. Found a positive relationship between the sum of low-molecular weight phthalates in third trimester of pregnancy and improved motor performance scores on Brazelton Neonatal Behavioral Assessment Scale	1. Unclear whether single urine phthalate measurement during third trimester reflects exposure during entire pregnancy 2. Only 1 measure of neonatal behavior within 5 days of birth – unclear how this may predict future behaviors

ECMO indicates extracorporeal membrane oxygenation; NICU, neonatal intensive care unit; MEP, monoethyl phthalate; MBP, monobutyl phthalate; MEHP, mono-2-ethylhexyl phthalate; BBP, benzyl butyl phthalate; DEHP, di(2-ethylhexyl) phthalate; MEHP, mono(2-ethylhexyl) phthalate; MEOHP, mono-(2-ethyl-5-oxohexyl) phthalate.

SYSTEMS AFFECTED AND CLINICAL EFFECTS

Phthalates are known as "endocrine-disrupting chemicals" and affect the endocrine system through multiple mechanisms of action (see Chapter 28). Di(2-ethylhexyl) phthalate and dibutyl phthalate are the most toxic to the reproductive system. Studies in animals have found antiandrogenic effects in fetal and early postnatal development leading to male reproductive tract abnormalities, including undescended testes, hypospadias, and decreased fertility. These studies are, however, difficult to assess given the ubiquity of phthalates in animal feed, cages, and other products (Table 38.1). The most sensitive time period for phthalate exposure and effects in humans is thought to be during weeks 10 to 13 of gestation, a period of extensive reproductive system development. In male infants, increased maternal urinary concentrations of di(2-ethylhexyl) phthalate metabolite during the mother's third trimester of pregnancy (which may or may not be a surrogate for first trimester exposure) were associated with decreased anogenital distance (a sensitive measure of fetal androgen exposure).[3] In addition, increased phthalate exposure through human milk has been associated with changes in luteinizing hormone, free testosterone, and sex-hormone binding globulin in male infants.[4] Phthalate exposure has also been associated with changes in thyroid hormone concentrations in adults, but no studies that examined fetal or childhood exposures and thyroid outcomes have been published.

More recently, exposures to di(2-ethylhexyl) phthalate and butyl benzyl phthalate have been associated with changes in inflammatory and immunologic function. In a cross-sectional study, butyl benzyl phthalate in indoor dust was associated with an increased risk of allergic rhinitis and eczema among school-aged children, and di-2-ethylhexl phthalate in dust was associated with an increased risk of asthmatic symptoms.[5] It is hypothesized that mono(2-ethylhexyl) phthalate (MEHP, a hydrolytic product of di[2-ethylhexyl] phthalate) induces proinflammatory prostaglandins and thromboxanes in the lungs, leading to increased respiratory symptoms. Laboratory studies in mice show that phthalate exposure exerts an adjuvant effect with a coallergen (ovalbumin), leading to increased atopic-like skin lesions.[6] Exposure to phthalates was implicated in potential nervous system inflammation in a study in which prenatal phthalate exposure was associated with changes in Brazelton scores in newborn infants.[7] Epidemiologic studies have found prenatal phthalate exposure to be associated with both an increase[8] and decrease in gestational age.[9] One proposed mechanism is via perturbation of prostaglandin or other inflammatory mechanisms, leading to uterine contractions.

Scientific panels, advocacy groups, and industry groups have analyzed the literature on di(2-ethylhexyl) phthalate and di-isononyl phthalate (DINP) and have come to different conclusions about safety. The controversy exists because risk to humans must be extrapolated from animal data that demonstrate differences in toxicity depending on the species, route of exposure, and age at exposure and because of persistent uncertainties in human exposure data. It is important to note that effects in animals are usually demonstrated at high doses, well above exposures encountered in the general human population.

PREVENTION

Phthalates are ubiquitous in the environment, and childhood exposures are widespread. Pediatricians can inform families about how to avoid exposure and identify alternatives to phthalate-containing products. It is important to know sources of exposure (Table 38.1), potential health effects (Table 38.2), and how to avoid phthalate exposures, including avoiding heating up plastics and using safe alternatives (Table 38.3). For example, pediatricians may suggest that parents avoid plastics with recycling code No. 3 (polyvinyl chloride or vinyl may contain phthalates). It is difficult to know whether a specific product contains phthalates, because labeling is not required by federal law. In August 2008, the federal government enacted the Consumer Product Safety Act, which creates a permanent ban on di-2-ethylhexl phthalate, dibutyl phthalate, and butyl benzyl phthalate in toys for children younger than 12 years and all child-care items for children 3 years and younger. It also created an interim ban on 3 additional phthalates (di-isononyl phthalate, di-isodecyl phthalate [DIDP], and di-*n*-octyl phthalate [DnOP]) until more research is conducted about potential adverse health outcomes. Several state-based policies are being developed. In general, it may be prudent to avoid exposure to phthalates when possible until the scientific basis of safety or harm from low level exposure is more clearly established.

BISPHENOL A

Bisphenol A is a chemical produced in large quantities, primarily to impart rigidity in the production of polycarbonate plastics and epoxy resins. Polycarbonate plastics have applications including use in some food and drink packaging (eg, water and infant bottles), compact discs, impact-resistant safety equipment, and medical devices. Epoxy resins are used as lacquers to coat metal products, such as food cans, bottle tops, and water supply pipes. Some dental sealants and composites may also contribute to bisphenol A exposure.

Human exposure to bisphenol A is widespread. Since 1999, more than a dozen studies using different analytical techniques have measured free, unconjugated bisphenol A in human serum at concentrations ranging from 0.2 to 20 ng/mL.[13] The relatively high concentrations of bisphenol A in the sera of pregnant women, umbilical cord blood, and fetal plasma indicate that bisphenol A crosses the placenta. The 2003-2004 Third National Health and Nutrition Examination Survey (NHANES III) conducted by the Centers

Table 38.3: Tips on How to Avoid Exposures to Phthalates and Bisphenol A

- Look at the recycling code on the bottom of products to find the plastic type.
- Avoid plastics with recycling code No. 3 (phthalates), No. 6 (styrenes), and No. 7 (bisphenol A) unless plastics labeled No. 7 are labeled as "biobased" or "greenware," meaning that they are made from corn and do not use bisphenol A.
- Plastic codes No. 1, 2, 4, and 5 are considered safer alternatives.
- Do not microwave food or beverages (including infant formula) in plastic.
- Do not microwave or heat plastic cling wraps.
- Avoid placing plastics in the dishwasher.
- Use alternatives, such as glass, when possible.
- Buy phthalate-free toys or those approved by the European Union.

for Disease Control and Prevention (CDC) found detectable concentrations of bisphenol A in 93% of 2517 urine samples from a representative sample of people in the United States 6 years and older.[14]

SYSTEMS AFFECTED AND CLINICAL EFFECTS

Assays are available to measure the *in vitro* estrogenic activity of possible endocrine disrupters, including bisphenol A.[15] Assays to determine the *in vivo* estrogenicity of bisphenol A have demonstrated that estrogen receptor binding is very weak, compared with the natural estrogen 17 β-estradiol. When prepubescent CD-1 mice were treated with doses of bisphenol A ranging from 0.1 to 100 mg/kg of body weight, estrogenic responses, including increased uterine wet weight, luminal epithelial height, and increased expression of the estrogen-inducible protein lactoferrin were observed.[16] There is also some evidence that bisphenol A binds to thyroid hormone receptor, acting as a thyroid hormone antagonist by preventing the binding of T_3. One study found that the affinity of bisphenol A for this receptor was several fold lower than its affinity for the estrogen receptors.[17]

Few human epidemiologic data exist to connect bisphenol A exposure in children to health effects. Limited cross-sectional data from adult studies link exposure to bisphenol A with reduced sexual function,[18] including ovarian dysfunction[19]; higher rates of diabetes[20] and heart disease[21]; and other potential consequences.[22] Some studies in animals report effects in fetuses and newborn infants exposed to bisphenol A.[23] One small study in pregnant women[24] linked prenatal exposure to bisphenol A with behavioral changes in children.

PREVENTION

Guidance is available about reducing exposures to bisphenol A in infants and children (Table 38.3).

Frequently Asked Questions

Q *Why is there controversy over bisphenol A?*
A Studies have shown effects on endocrine functions in animals exposed to bisphenol A. The controversy arises because there are few studies showing harmful effects in infants or children. There is concern, however, that children are rapidly growing and developing and may, therefore, be especially susceptible to chemicals such as bisphenol A. Additional research studies and reviews by the US Food and Drug Administration may be able to determine what level of exposure to bisphenol A might cause similar effects in humans.

Q *What precautionary measures can parents take to reduce babies' exposure to bisphenol A?*
A Avoid clear plastic bottles or containers with the recycling No. 7 and the letters "PC" (indicating "polycarbonate") imprinted on them—many of these contain bisphenol A. Alternatives include polyethylene or polypropylene that should not contain bisphenol A. Glass is also an alternative but can be hazardous if dropped or broken. Because heat may cause the release of bisphenol A from plastic, it is prudent to consider the following:
    — Do not boil polycarbonate bottles;
    — Do not microwave polycarbonate bottles; and
    — Do not wash polycarbonate bottles in the dishwasher.

Q *Should I stop using canned liquid formula?*
A The lining of cans may contain bisphenol A, so avoiding canned formula is one way to reduce exposure. If you are considering switching from liquid to powdered formula, note that the mixing procedures may differ, so pay special attention when preparing formula from powder.
    — If your baby is on a special formula to address a medical condition, you should not switch to another formula, as the known risks would outweigh any potential risks posed by bisphenol A.
    — Risks associated with giving your baby homemade condensed milk formulas or soy or goat milk are far greater than the potential effects of bisphenol A.

Q *Will breastfeeding reduce my baby's exposure to bisphenol A?*
A Although low concentrations of bisphenol A have been detected in human milk, breastfeeding a baby is one way to reduce exposure to bisphenol A that leaches from plastic bottles or formula can linings. The American Academy of Pediatrics recommends exclusive breastfeeding for a minimum of 4 months

but preferably for 6 months. Breastfeeding should be continued, with the addition of complementary foods, at least through the first 12 months of age and thereafter as long as mutually desired by mother and infant.

Q *Is anything being done to advocate for safety testing of chemicals before they are put on the market? It seems as though we are always finding possible and actual hazards of new chemicals, but not until after they have been released into the environment.*

A The American Academy of Pediatrics and other organizations, strongly advocate for protecting children, pregnant women, and the general population from the hazards of chemicals before the chemicals are marketed.[25]

Resources For Providers And Patients

US Food and Drug Administration
Subcommittee Report on Bisphenol A (17-page summary)
www.fda.gov/ohrms/dockets/ac/08/briefing/2008-4386b1-05.pdf

National Institute of Environmental Health Sciences (NIEHS) fact sheet:
www.niehs.nih.gov/health/docs/bpa-factsheet.pdf

Pediatric Environmental Health Specialty Units (PEHSUs)
Health Care Provider Fact Sheet (English)
www.aoec.org/PEHSU/documents/physician_bpa_final.pdf

Health Care Provider (Spanish)
www.aoec.org/PEHSU/documents/physician_bpa_spanish_final.pdf

Patient Fact Sheet (English)
www.aoec.org/PEHSU/documents/patient_bpa_final.pdf

Patient Fact Sheet (Spanish)
www.aoec.org/PEHSU/documents/patient_bpa_spanish_final.pdf

References

1. Shea KM; American Academy of Pediatrics, Committee on Environmental Health. Pediatric exposure and potential toxicity of phthalate plasticizers. *Pediatrics*. 2003;111(6 Pt 1):1467–1474
2. Phthalates activate estrogen receptors. *Sci News*. 1995;148(3):47
3. Swan SH, Main KM, Liu F, et al. Decrease in anogenital distance among male infants with prenatal phthalate exposure. *Environ Health Perspect*. 2005;113(8):1056–1061
4. Main KM, Mortensen GK, Kaleva MM, et al. Human breast milk contamination with phthalates and alterations of endogenous reproductive hormones in infants three months of age. *Environ Health Perspect*. 2006;114(2):270–276
5. Bornehag CG, Sundell J, Weschler CJ, et al. The association between asthma and allergic symptoms in children and phthalates in house dust: a nested case-control study. *Environ Health Perspect*. 2004;112(14):1393–1397

6. Hill SS, Shaw BR, Wu AH. Plasticizers, antioxidants, and other contaminants found in air delivered by PVC tubing used in respiratory therapy. *Biomed Chromatogr.* 2003;17(4):250–262

7. Engel SM, Zhu C, Berkowitz GS, et al. Prenatal phthalate exposure and performance on the Neonatal Behavioral Assessment Scale in a multiethnic birth cohort. *Neurotoxicology.* 2009;30(4):522–528

8. Wolff MS, Engel SM, Berkowitz GS, et al. Prenatal phenol and phthalate exposures and birth outcomes. *Environ Health Perspect.* 2008;116(8):1092-1097

9. Whyatt RM, et al. Prenatal di(2-ethylhexyl)phthalate exposure and length of gestation among an inner-city cohort. *Pediatrics.* 2009;124(6):e1213-e1220

10. Rais-Bahrami K, Nunez S, Revenis ME, Luban NL, Short BL. Follow-up study of adolescents exposed to di(2-ethylhexyl) phthalate (DEHP) as neonates on extracorporeal membrane oxygenation (ECMO) support. *Environ Health Perspect.* 2004;112(13):1339-1340

11. Latini G, De Felice C, Presta G, et al. In utero exposure to di-(2-ethylhexyl)phthalate and duration of human pregnancy. *Environ Health Perspect.* 2003;111(14):1783-1785

12. Adibi JJ, Hauser R, Williams PL, Whyatt RM, Calafat AM, Nelson H, Herrick R, Swan SH. Maternal urinary metabolites of Di-(2-Ethylhexyl) phthalate in relation to the timing of labor in a US multicenter pregnancy cohort study. *Am J Epidemiol.* 2009;15;169(8):1015-1024

13. Vandenberg LN, Hauser R, Marcus M, Olea N, Welshons WV. Human exposure to bisphenol A (BPA). *Reprod Toxicol.* 2007;24(2):139–177

14. Calafat AM, Ye X, Wong LY, Reidy JA, Needham JL. Exposure of the U.S. population to bisphenol A and 4-tertiary-octylphenol: 2003–2004. *Environ Health Perspect.* 2008;116(1):39–44

15. Soto AM, Maffini MV, Schaeberle CM, Sonnenschein C. Strengths and weaknesses of in vitro assays for estrogenic and androgenic activity. *Best Pract Res Clin Endocrinol Metab.* 2006;20(1):15–33

16. Markey CM, Michaelson CL, Veson EC, Sonnenschein C, Soto AM. The mouse uterotrophic assay: a re-evaluation of its validity in assessing the estrogenicity of bisphenol A. *Environ Health Perspect.* 2001;109(1):55–60

17. Moriyama K, Tagami T, Akamizu T, et al. Thyroid hormone action is disrupted by bisphenol A as an antagonist. *J Clin Endocrinol Metab.* 2002;87(11):5185–5190

18. Vandenberg LN, Maffini MV, Sonnenschein C, Rubin BS, Soto AM. Bisphenol-A and the great divide: a review of controversies in the field of endocrine disruption. *Endocr Rev.* 2009;30:75-95

19. Takeuchi T, Tsutsumi O, Ikezuki Y, Takai Y, Taketani Y. Positive relationship between androgen and the endocrine disruptor, bisphenol A, in normal women and women with ovarian dysfunction *Endocr J.* 2004;51(2):165–169

20. Lang IA, Galloway TS, Scarlett A, et al. Association of urinary bisphenol A concentration with medical disorders and laboratory abnormalities in adults. *JAMA.* 2008;300(11):1303-1310

21. Melzer D, Rice NE, Lewis C, Henley WE, Galloway TS. Association of urinary bisphenol A concentration with heart disease: evidence from NHANES 2003/06. *PLoS One.* 2010;5(1):e8673

22. Lakind JS, Naiman DQ. Daily intake of bisphenol A and potential sources of exposure: 2005–2006 National Health and Nutrition Examination Survey. *J Exp Sci Env Epidemiol.* 2011;21(3):272-279

23. The National Toxicologic Program. Available at: http://cerhr.niehs.nih.gov/evals/bisphenol/bisphenol.pdf. Accessed March 30, 2011

24. Braun JM, Yolton K, Dietrich KN, et al. Prenatal bisphenol A exposure and early childhood behavior. *Environ Health Perspect.* 2009;117(12):1945-1952

25. American Academy of Pediatrics, Council on Environmental Health. Policy statement: chemical-management policy: prioritizing children's health. *Pediatrics.* 2011;127(5):983-990

Chapter 39

Radon

■ ■ ■ ■ ■ ■

Radon is a colorless, odorless, inert radioactive gas released during the natural decay of thorium and uranium, which are common, naturally occurring elements found in varying amounts in rock and soil.[1-3] Radon-222 decays into radioactive elements, including polonium, bismuth, and lead. These decay products are often termed "daughters" or "progeny." Some of these radioactive progeny, such as polonium-218 and polonium-214, emit alpha particles that can cause tissue damage. Radon is classified as a Class A human carcinogen by the US Environmental Protection Agency (EPA),[2] meaning that it is known to cause cancer in humans. Radon in air is measured in picocuries per liter (pCi/L); a picocurie is 1 trillionth of a curie. The curie is a standard measure for the intensity of radioactivity contained in a sample of radioactive material.

SOURCES AND ROUTES OF EXPOSURE

Radon accounts for approximately 55% of the total background radiation.[4] In the outdoors, radon is diluted and poses minimal risk. Higher levels may be found indoors or in areas with poor ventilation. Radon gas in the soil can enter homes and other buildings through cracks in concrete floors and walls, floor drains, construction joints, and tiny cracks or pores in hollow-block walls.[2]

Inhalation of radon gas is the major route of exposure. The EPA estimates that nearly 1 in 15 homes has elevated radon levels.[2] Different parts of the country have varying levels of radon in the ground. The EPA or state radon offices can provide information on which areas have higher levels. The amount of radon within an individual home and between neighboring homes can be variable because of differences in ventilation, construction, and design. The most important component of radon dose comes from its short-lived decay products.[5,6] Radon itself is an inert gas with a half-life of about 4 days, and almost all of the gas that is inhaled will be exhaled. However, because the decay products are isotopes of solid elements, they may attach to molecules of water and other atmospheric gases. These decay products are then deposited on the surface of the respiratory tract and, because of their short half-lives (less than 30 minutes), will decay there. This may result in local tissue damage.

Radon is soluble in water but it is also highly volatile and, thus, mostly removed from public water supplies.[7] Its concentration in water can vary widely, however, depending on geographic location and water source. Ingestion as a route of exposure may be important if high radon concentrations are present in drinking water.[5,6] Estimates of the length of time that ingested radon may stay in the stomach are based on studies of water and food gastrointestinal tract transit times. The most significant organ to receive a radon dose through ingestion seems to be the stomach wall.[7] After passing from the stomach to the small intestine, any remaining radon is transferred to the blood and rapidly removed from the body. It is possible for radon gas to be released from water during showering. In most instances, radon entering the home through water is a small source of risk.

SYSTEMS AFFECTED AND CLINICAL EFFECTS

Lung Cancer

Underground miners were noted to have increased rates of lung cancer nearly a century ago.[1] A large number of independent epidemiologic studies of thousands of miners around the world carried out over more than 50 years have shown increased lung cancer rates in underground miners, even after controlling for other exposures, such as smoking, asbestos, silica, diesel fumes, arsenic, chromium, nickel, and ore dust.[8-11] Laboratory studies of animals support this finding. Mice exposed to radon have increased rates of lung cancer, pulmonary fibrosis, and emphysema and a shortened lifespan.[8]

Several challenges exist in converting cancer risk estimates in individuals occupationally exposed to radon to individuals with only residential exposures. Underground miners are exposed to radon at much higher levels than are nonminers and may have other risk factors for cancer or lung disease. However, several epidemiologic studies have suggested that there is an increased risk of lung cancer from residential radon exposure.[12-16] Consensus meetings of the US EPA, National Research Council, and World Health Organization (WHO) have concluded that radon is a human carcinogen that contributes to a large number of lung cancer deaths each year.[1-3] Radon is estimated to cause approximately 21 000 lung cancer deaths in the United States each year.[2] Smoking greatly increases the risk of lung cancer at a given level of radon exposure. For instance, at a radon level of 4 pCi/L of air, the percentage of people estimated to

Table 39.1: Lifetime Risk of Lung Cancer Death (per Person) from Radon Exposure in Homes[17,a]			
RADON LEVEL (pCi/L)[b]	NEVER SMOKERS	CURRENT SMOKERS	GENERAL POPULATION[c]
20	36 out of 1000	26 out of 100	11 out of 100
10	18 out of 1000	15 out of 100	56 out of 1000
8	15 out of 1000	12 out of 100	45 out of 1000
4	73 out of 10 000	62 out of 1000	23 out of 1000
2	37 out of 10 000	32 out of 1000	12 out of 1000
1.25	23 out of 10 000	20 out of 1000	73 out of 10 000
0.4	73 out of 100 000	64 out of 10 000	23 out of 10 000

[a] Estimates are subject to uncertainties as discussed in Chapter VII of *EPA's Assessment of Risks from Radon in Homes.*[17]
[b] Assumes constant lifetime exposure in homes at these levels.
[c] Includes smokers and nonsmokers.

develop lung cancer with lifetime exposure is 6.2% for smokers, a rate nearly 9 times higher than the percentage of 0.7% for nonsmokers.[17] Table 39.1 illustrates risks for smokers and nonsmokers at different levels of lifetime radon exposure.

Radon represents a significant preventable cause of lung cancer. The public health impact of the 21 000 US deaths attributable to radon in 2003 can be compared with deaths in 2001 from drunk driving (17 400), falls in the home (8000), drowning (3900), and home fires (2800).[2]

Stomach Cancer

Higher rates of stomach cancer were noted in atomic bomb survivors[18] and in miners exposed to radon.[19] However, the study of miners did not find trends in mortality related to dose. There are very few studies of cancer and ingestion of water containing radon. One ecologic study reported a positive correlation between stomach cancer and radon levels as reported by county in Pennsylvania.[20] Ecologic studies look at groups and area-wide exposure data but cannot make links at an individual level. A case-cohort study in Finland did not find an association between stomach cancer and exposure to radon or other radionuclides.[21]

Leukemia

The effects of radon exposure in childhood are not well understood. It is possible that radon exposure could increase leukemia risk, because bone marrow is vulnerable to the effects of ionizing radiation. Most studies to date have focused on residential radon exposure and childhood leukemia. Eleven of 12 descriptive (ecologic) studies suggest that there could be increased risk of childhood cancer associated with radon exposure (reviewed in Evrard et al[22] and Raaschou-Nielsen[23]). In some of these studies, the effect of radon exposure was higher for acute myelogenous leukemia than for acute lymphocytic leukemia. However, the 7 case-control studies conducted to date have shown inconsistent results; some found an association between residential radon and childhood leukemia, but others did not (reviewed in Evrard et al[22] and Raaschou-Nielsen[23]).

Overall, the literature suggests that there may be an association between leukemia and residential radon exposure. However, larger, prospective studies are required to more thoroughly understand these risks.

DIAGNOSTIC METHODS AND MEASUREMENT OF EXPOSURE

The EPA recommends that all homes be tested for radon; additional details can be found on the EPA's Web site and in the publication *A Citizen's Guide to Radon*.[2] There are 2 general ways to test homes for radon: short-term testing and long-term testing. Testing should usually be performed in the basement or on the first floor, because radon levels are usually higher than on upper floors. Short-term testing is generally carried out for between 2 and 90 days. Several types of detectors used for short-term testing can give good results, but because radon levels can vary daily, they do not give a good year-round estimate. The most common form of detector is charcoal based. In a blinded study that tested commercially available short-term radon detectors, it was noted that increased humidity and temporal fluctuations in radon concentrations could have a negative influence on the accuracy and precision of some short-term detectors.[24] Long-term tests remain in the home for more than 90 days and are more likely to give a better estimate of year-round average of radon levels in the home. Anyone can perform these tests without professional help. Test kits are generally reliable, inexpensive, and readily available through state radon offices or directly from commercial vendors. The test kit is sent back to the company in a prepaid mailer for analysis, and processing time is measured in days.

PREVENTION OF EXPOSURE

The US EPA, WHO, and other groups have strongly recommended initiatives to reduce indoor exposure to radon.[2,3] Some municipalities require new homes to be constructed in a radon-resistant manner, that radon testing be conducted whenever a home is sold, and that radon testing be performed in all schools. When levels of radon higher than 4 pCi/L are found, repairs should be made to reduce the level. Remediation should be considered at levels between 2 and 4 pCi/L. It is often difficult to reduce radon levels that are below 2 pCi/L. The average indoor air radon level is estimated at about 1.3 pCi/L.

In general, radon exposure can be reduced by increasing ventilation and by reducing the influx of radon in the home. These repairs are not expensive and can usually be completed for about the same cost as other common home repairs. Key components of radon remediation include:

- Adjusting existing central ventilation systems
- Sealing cracks in the foundation
- Creating negative pressure under the basement floor with the installation of a radon sub-slab soil suction system
- Prohibiting the use of building materials containing excessive radium

More detailed information about home radon abatement measures is available from the EPA (http://www.epa.gov/iaq/radon).

Most importantly, pediatricians should advise families about the hazards of radon exposure and that testing and remediation are easy and affordable. They should also point out that cigarette smoking dramatically magnifies the radon-induced risk of lung cancer.

Frequently Asked Questions

Q *Should I test for radon in my home?*
A The EPA recommends that all homes be checked. An inexpensive home-testing kit can be obtained from home improvement stores, the National Safety Council, and from some local or state radon programs. The sample obtained should be sent to a certified laboratory for analysis. Mitigation measures should be taken if the level of radon exceeds 4 pCi/L and considered for levels between 2 and 4 pCi/L. Further information can be obtained from the Resources section of this chapter.

Q *What are the health effects from exposure to radon?*
A There are no immediate medical problems related to radon exposure. However, radon in indoor air is estimated to cause about 21 000 lung cancer deaths in the United States each year. Some studies suggest an increased risk of childhood leukemia with radon exposure. There is no evidence that respiratory diseases, such as asthma, are caused by radon exposure.

Q *What about radon in schools?*
A Children spend a third or more of their weekdays in schools, making radon in schools a potential concern. The EPA recommends that all schools be tested for radon. Radon problems in schools are often remedied by adjusting settings of central ventilation systems. The other approaches listed above can also be applied. More detailed information is available at www.epa.gov/iaq/schools/environmental.html.

Resources

US Environmental Protection Agency (EPA)
Web site: www.epa.gov/radon/pubs
This Web site has links to several EPA publications, information on home testing and remediation, and geographical maps of radon exposure.
US EPA Radon Hotline: 800-767-7236

State and Regional Indoor Environments Contact Information
Web site: www.epa.gov/iaq/whereyoulive.html

The International Radon Project
Web site: www.who.int/ionizing_radiation/env/radon/en/index.html
A World Health Organization Initiative to reduce lung cancer risk around the world.

References

1. National Research Council, Committee on Health Risks of Exposure to Radon. *The Health Effects of Exposure to Indoor Radon: BEIR VI.* Washington, DC: National Academies Press; 1998. Executive summary available at: http://epa.gov/radon/beirvi.html. Accessed August 25, 2010

2. US Environmental Protection Agency. *A Citizen's Guide to Radon: The Guide to Protecting Yourself and Your Family From Radon.* Washington, DC: US Environmental Protection Agency; 2009. Publication No. US EPA 402-K-07-009. Available at: http://www.epa.gov/radon/pdfs/citizensguide.pdf. Accessed August 25, 2010

3. World Health Organization. *WHO Handbook on Indoor Radon: A Public Health Perspective.* Geneva, Switzerland: World Health Organization; 2009. Available at: http://www.nrsb.org/pdf/WHO%20Radon%20Handbook. Accessed August 25, 2010

4. National Research Council, Committee to Assess Health Risks from Exposure to Low Levels of Ionizing Radiation. *Health Risks from Exposure to Low Levels of Ionizing Radiation: BEIR VII Phase 2.* Washington, DC: National Academies Press; 2006

5. Kendall GM, Smith TJ. Doses to organs and tissues from radon and its decay products. *J Radiol Prot.* 2002;22(4):389-406

6. Kendall GM, Smith TJ. Doses from radon and its decay products to children. *J Radiol Prot.* 2005;25(3):241-256

7. Khursheed A. Doses to systemic tissues from radon gas. *Radiat Prot Dosimetry.* 2000;88(2):171-181

8. US Environmental Protection Agency. *A Physician's Guide - Radon.* US Environmental Protection Agency; 1999. Publication No. US EPA 402-K-93-008

9. Lubin JH, Boice JD Jr, Edling C, et al. Lung cancer in radon-exposed miners and estimation of risk from indoor exposure. *J Natl Cancer Inst.* 1995;87(11):817-827

10. Vacquier B, Caer S, Rogel A, et al. Mortality risk in the French cohort of uranium miners: extended follow-up 1946-1999. *Occup Environ Med.* 2008;65(9):597-604

11. Samet JM, Eradze GR. Radon and lung cancer risk: taking stock at the millenium. *Environ Health Perspect.* 2000;108(Suppl 4):635-641

12. Darby S, Hill D, Deo H, et al. Residential radon and lung cancer—detailed results of a collaborative analysis of individual data on 7148 persons with lung cancer and 14,208 persons without lung cancer from 13 epidemiologic studies in Europe. *Scand J Work Environ Health.* 2006;32(Suppl 1):1-83

13. Field RW. A review of residential radon case-control epidemiologic studies performed in the United States. *Rev Environ Health.* 2001;16(3):151-167

14. Lubin JH, Boice JD Jr. Lung cancer risk from residential radon: meta-analysis of eight epidemiologic studies. *J Natl Cancer Inst.* 1997;89(1):49-57

15. Neuberger JS, Gesell TF. Residential radon exposure and lung cancer: risk in nonsmokers. *Health Phys.* 2002;83(1):1-18

16. Pavia M, Bianco A, Pileggi C, Angelillo IF. Meta-analysis of residential exposure to radon gas and lung cancer. *Bull World Health Organ.* 2003;81(10):732-738

17. US Environmental Protection Agency. *Report: EPA's Assessment of Risks from Radon in Homes.* Washington, DC: US Environmental Protection Agency; 2003. Publication No. US EPA 402-R-03-003

18. Preston DL, Shimizu Y, Pierce DA, Suyama A, Mabuchi K. Studies of mortality of atomic bomb survivors. Report 13: Solid cancer and noncancer disease mortality: 1950-1997. *Radiat Res.* 2003;160(4):381-407

19. Darby SC, Radford EP, Whitley E. Radon exposure and cancers other than lung cancer in Swedish iron miners. *Environ Health Perspect.* 1995;103(Suppl 2):45-47

20. Kjellberg S, Wiseman JS. The relationship of radon to gastrointestinal malignancies. *Am Surg.* 1995;61(9):822-825

21. Auvinen A, Salonen L, Pekkanen J, Pukkala E, Ilus T, Kurttio P. Radon and other natural radionuclides in drinking water and risk of stomach cancer: a case-cohort study in Finland. *Int J Cancer.* 2005;114(1):109-113

22. Evrard AS, Hemon D, Billon S, et al. Ecological association between indoor radon concentration and childhood leukaemia incidence in France, 1990-1998. *Eur J Cancer Prev.* 2005;14(2):147-157

23. Raaschou-Nielsen O. Indoor radon and childhood leukaemia. *Radiat Prot Dosimetry.* 2008;132(2):175-181

24. Sun S, Budd G, McLemore S, Field RW. Blind testing of commercially available short-term radon detectors. *Health Phys.* 2008;94(6):548-557

Chapter 40

Tobacco Use and Secondhand Tobacco Smoke Exposure

■ ■ ■ ■ ■ ■

Tobacco use and secondhand tobacco smoke (SHS) exposure are uniquely linked in the pediatric setting. The most significant source of secondhand smoke exposure of children is smoking by an adult living with the child.[1] Most tobacco use begins before age 18 years,[2] influenced by exposure to tobacco use by parents or peers, glamorous depictions in movies and other media, advertising that targets children and adolescents, and other environmental, social, and cultural factors.[2,3] The connection between children and tobacco use is so strong that the Commissioner of the US Food and Drug Administration declared smoking a "pediatric disease" in 1995.[4]

Secondhand smoke is a dynamic mixture of exhaled smoke and smoke released from the smoldering end of cigarettes, cigars, and pipes. It contains more than 4000 chemical compounds, many of which are poisons.[5] Cigarette smoking is the most important factor determining the level of particulate matter in the indoor air, and concentrations of particulates less than 2.5 micrometers (a size that reaches the lower airways) can be 2 to 3 times higher in homes with smokers than in homes without smokers.[6] In 1992, the US Environmental Protection Agency (EPA) declared that secondhand smoke is a group A carcinogen, indicating that secondhand smoke causes cancer in people.[7]

Although the prevalence of tobacco use and exposure to secondhand smoke has declined significantly, 20.6% of US adults still used tobacco in 2009.[8] During 2007–2008, approximately 88 million nonsmokers 3 years or older in the United States were exposed to secondhand smoke. Of these, 32 million were 3 to 19 years of age, reflecting the higher prevalence of exposure among children and youths. For children 3 to 11 years of age, 53.6% were exposed to secondhand smoke.[9] These numbers are much higher outside the United States, in countries in which tobacco use is more prevalent and people may be less aware of the dangers of exposure.[10] Using data from 192 countries, the World Health Organization estimated the burden of disease worldwide from exposure to secondhand smoke to be approximately 1% of total mortality and 0.7% of total worldwide burden of disease in disability-adjusted life years (DALYs).[11]

ROUTES AND SOURCES OF EXPOSURE

The primary route of exposure is through inhalation, although some exposure may occur through contact with particles that settle on surfaces and then are ingested through the gastrointestinal tract.[12]

Most children exposed to secondhand smoke are exposed in their own homes, and because many young children spend a large proportion of their time indoors with their families,[1] their exposure may be significant. Because the components of smoke remain in the space long after the source of smoke is extinguished, exposure can occur even after the smoker has left. Settings in which children may be exposed include child care settings; the homes of relatives and friends; smoking areas of restaurants, bars, and airports; and motor vehicles. Adolescents may be exposed in their workplaces.

MECHANISMS OF EFFECT

Secondhand smoke contains more than 50 carcinogens, including polycyclic aromatic hydrocarbons, N-nitrosamines, aromatic amines, aldehydes, and other organic (eg, benzene) and inorganic (eg, heavy metals, polonium^{210}) compounds.[13] Although the mechanisms of carcinogenesis have not been determined for all of these chemicals, tobacco-specific carcinogens have been measured in the urine of nonsmokers, including children, exposed to second-hand smoke.[14]

Several mechanisms by which exposure to secondhand smoke causes injury to the respiratory tract have been described. Prenatal exposure to nicotine causes changes in synthesis of airway tissues. These changes may be attributable to effects on nicotinic acetylcholine receptors that are abundant in the developing lung. Postnatal exposure induces bronchial hyperreactivity, which may be attributable to increases in neuroendocrine cells in the lungs that synthesize and release bronchoconstrictors. Other mechanisms include altered neural control of the airway, causing bronchoconstriction, mucus secretion, and microvascular leakage. Increased concentrations of serum immunoglobulin E (IgE) and poor immune cell function have been described in exposed children. These altered immune responses may contribute to the increased incidence of wheezing, asthma, impaired macrophage function, altered mucociliary clearance, enhanced bacterial adherence, and disruption of the respiratory epithelium. Changes in nitric oxide production contribute to bronchial hyperreactivity.[13]

Infants exposed to secondhand smoke have an increased risk of sudden infant death syndrome (SIDS). Although the mechanism resulting in the increased risk has not been completely described, several studies have demonstrated deficient cardiorespiratory control, probably resulting from nicotine's effects on the nicotinic receptors in the peripheral and central nervous systems. Some of the effects on nervous system function may be attributable to changes that occur during fetal development resulting from maternal smoking or exposure to secondhand smoke.[13]

Changes in the cardiovascular system associated with exposure to secondhand smoke include inflammatory responses, vasodilatation, platelet activation, lower high-density lipoprotein (HDL) levels, impaired oxygen delivery, formation of free radicals, and changes in heart rate.[13]

CLINICAL EFFECTS

In adult nonsmokers, the effects of exposure to secondhand smoke include increased risk of some cancers, heart disease, reproductive, and respiratory effects.[5,7,13] There is increasing evidence of other adverse health effects.

The adverse health effects of exposing children to secondhand smoke are well established, and many researchers suggest that children are more susceptible to the these health effects than are adults.[13] Short-term effects are primarily respiratory and include increased incidence and severity of upper and lower respiratory infections, otitis media with effusion, SIDS, and asthma exacerbations.[5] Each year in the United States, an additional 430 deaths from SIDS; 24 500 infants born with low birth weight; 71 900 preterm births; 202 300 episodes of asthma; and 790 000 visits for otitis media can be attributed to exposure to secondhand smoke.[5]

A growing body of evidence indicates that long-term exposure during childhood, especially early childhood, results in decreased lung function, increased incidence of asthma (including asthma in adulthood), and increased incidence of cancers.[13,15] Several authors have demonstrated a gene-environment association for these and other illnesses associated with exposure to secondhand smoke.[5,16,17] Children exposed to secondhand smoke are more likely to develop dental caries[18] and have respiratory complications when undergoing general anesthesia.[19] Among children 4 to 16 years of age, exposure is significantly associated with 6 or more days of school absence in the past year.[20] Children living in households with smokers are at greater risk of injury and death from fires.[21] For children younger than 10 years, playing with cigarette lighters or matches causes approximately 100 000 fires and 300 to 400 child deaths each year.[22]

The effects of exposure to secondhand smoke on cognition and behavior are under investigation,[23-26] but most studies are limited, because they do not include many variables that affect behavior and cognition.

SCREENING METHODS

Screening for children's exposure to secondhand smoke in the clinical setting is typically done by questioning the child or accompanying adult. Groner et al[27] used hair nicotine levels to validate a series of 3 questions ([1] Does the mother smoke?; [2] Do others smoke?; and [3] Do others smoke inside?) and developed a decision tree with probabilities for use in the clinical setting. No other validation studies of questions used in the clinical setting have been performed. School-based studies include a Turkish study that compared parental report of "smoking in the same room" as the child to urine cotinine concentrations (sensitivity 39%, specificity 80%)[28]; and a study of German and Dutch children that compared parental report of smoking in the living room with ambient levels of nicotine (sensitivities 61% to 78%, specificities 81% to 96%).[29] A study of parents and youth 13 to 17 years of age compared telephone interview responses to salivary cotinine; sensitivity and specificity of the youths' responses to the question about smoking by a parent were 43% and 93%, respectively. When the responses of parent and youth agreed, sensitivity and specificity were 85% and 90%, respectively.[30]

PREVENTION OF EXPOSURE

Secondhand smoke permeates any environment in which tobacco is smoked. Ott et al[31] demonstrated this effect in a 2-bedroom house in which a single cigar was smoked. The door between the room in which the cigar was smoked (the kitchen) and the adjacent living room was opened 3 inches; the door from the living room to the bedroom in which the measurement was taken was closed. No bedroom windows were open, to reduce air exchange in the bedroom. Approximately 30 minutes after the cigar was lit, carbon monoxide levels rose in the bedroom.

Counseling Parents to Maintain Smoke-Free Homes and Other Environments

If a parent is not able or not willing to quit smoking, an intermediate method that reduces (but does not eliminate) exposure to secondhand smoke is to establish and enforce smoke-free rules. Smoking should not be allowed within any structure attached to the home or within range of open windows or doors or in any vehicle used to transport children. Because components of secondhand smoke persist in the environment for days after the source of smoke is gone,[12] smoke-free rules should be enforced even when children are absent.

Counseling Parents to Quit Smoking

Quitting smoking may be the most effective way for a parent to eliminate a child's exposure to secondhand smoke. Pediatricians are in a good position to provide tobacco use cessation counseling to parents. Because many parents lack health insurance and access to primary health care for themselves, pediatricians may be the only physicians some parents visit on a regular basis, serving as the primary source of health information for the family.[32,33] Just as pediatricians counsel parents about diet and safety, it is appropriate for pediatricians to counsel parents about ways to reduce children's exposure to secondhand smoke. The US Public Health Service Guideline, *Treating Tobacco Use and Dependence*, recommends that clinicians "…ask parents about tobacco use and offer them cessation advice and assistance."[34] Many "teachable moments" occur when a child has a medical condition exacerbated by exposure to secondhand smoke, such as asthma or recurrent otitis media.[35]

Despite the similarity between counseling about smoking and counseling about other parental behaviors that affect children, many pediatricians express concerns about their role in counseling parents about tobacco use cessation. One concern is a fear of alienating the parent by asking the parent to change behavior. A survey of parents, however, found that more than 50% agreed that it is the pediatrician's job to advise parents to quit smoking; 52% of current smokers surveyed responded they would welcome advice to quit.[36] In a study of parents of children hospitalized for an illness that could be exacerbated by exposure to secondhand smoke, all parents who smoked and participated in the study believed that pediatricians should offer parents the chance to participate in a smoking-cessation program.[37] Other barriers to counseling parents about smoking cessation reported by pediatricians include time, lack of training, and lack of reimbursement.[34]

Counseling parents to eliminate exposure of children to secondhand smoke is effective in increasing parents' interest in tobacco use cessation, making quit attempts, and the success of those attempts.[38,39] Counseling parents about the adverse effects of exposure and ways to eliminate exposure is associated with reduced exposure of children.[40]

The Process of Quitting

At baseline, without counseling or any other intervention, approximately 4% to 8% of tobacco users quit each year.[34] Success increases with each quit attempt, and interventions such as advice to quit, counseling, and pharmacotherapies increase the likelihood of success for each attempt.[34] Approximately 10% of all smokers who receive counseling from a physician stop smoking.[34] Although this rate may not seem significant within the context of an individual practice, it reflects a tremendous public health impact at a population level. If there were a

10% rate of cessation in patients in all physician practices in the United States, 2 million smokers would quit each year.[34] Over time, advice from physicians also may influence family members to quit using tobacco entirely, reduce the numbers of cigarettes they smoke, or change the venue of smoking (ie, from indoors to outdoors).

Treating Adult Tobacco Use and Dependence

The US Public Health Service updated its clinical practice guideline on tobacco use cessation counseling in 2008.[34] In addition to comprehensively reviewing the efficacy of tobacco use cessation strategies, the guideline strongly recommends that all health care professionals routinely assess tobacco use status at every medical visit, regardless of the reason for the visit. Health care professionals are urged to provide counseling at each visit and assess the eligibility of their patients for pharmacotherapies.[34] Table 40.1 gives further information on counseling.

Billing for Counseling Parents About Smoking Cessation

Unfortunately, there is currently no reimbursement or *Current Procedural Terminology* (CPT) code for counseling parents about tobacco use cessation. Coding for diagnosis and treatment is an important step that will help to develop the evidence supporting the benefits of tobacco dependence treatment in the pediatric setting. Two diagnosis codes may be particularly useful: 989.84 (toxic effects of tobacco) and V15.89 (other specified personal history presenting hazards to health [list exposure to secondhand smoke as the hazard]).[41] Similarly, naming exposure to secondhand smoke as a factor in insurance claims, death certificates, and other documents may aid in assessing the impact of secondhand smoke on health and the need for reimbursement for treatment of exposure to secondhand smoke.

Despite barriers, counseling parents effectively in the context of a busy practice is possible, because the intervention can be very brief. The simple statement, "you should quit smoking," when delivered by a member of the health care team, increases quit attempts and the success of quit attempts.[34] Following up on the advice with additional counseling or referral to community-based cessation programs, including the 1-800-Quit Now "Quitline" (a free counseling delivered over the phone) are important next steps. Because the consequences of second-hand smoke exposure are so great and the effects of even brief intervention are so powerful, a busy pediatrician can and should deliver tobacco use cessation counseling to patients and their families.

Strategies for Adolescents

Most tobacco use begins in the teenage years, and prevention of the initiation of tobacco use—including "experimentation"—is an important goal for

Table 40.1: Strategies for Counseling Parents and Caregivers in Tobacco Use Cessation[34]

The **"Five A's"** tobacco use cessation approach includes the following components:

1. *Ask* about tobacco use at every opportunity, and assess status with specific attention to the user's motivation and barriers to change.

2. *Advise* the tobacco user to quit.

3. *Assess* by determining the tobacco user's readiness to quit within the next 2 to 4 weeks.

4. *Assist* the tobacco user with the change.

5. *Arrange* follow-up.

Although these steps are fairly brief, concern is frequently expressed about the limited time available for cessation counseling during a child's visit. Even brief advice from pediatricians, however, may have a positive impact on reducing parental tobacco use and relapse rates.

An alternative to the 5 A's is "Ask, Advise, and Refer":

Ask about tobacco use at every opportunity.

Advise the tobacco user to quit and make the child's environment smoke and tobacco free. Consider prescribing pharmacotherapies whenever appropriate.

Refer the tobacco user or family member to 1-800-QUIT NOW or other cessation resource.

Pharmacotherapies

Nicotine is highly addictive, and pharmacotherapy plays an important role in cessation. Unfortunately, many people do not use pharmacotherapies correctly, including using medications for too short a period. Pediatricians should understand the correct use of pharmacotherapies and barriers to their use, even if they do not prescribe them for family members of patients. Many resources are available, including the American Academy of Family Physicians' prescribing guide, found at: http://www.aafp.org/online/etc/medialib/ aafp_org/documents/clinical/pub_health/askact/prescribguidelines.Par.0001.File.tmp/ PrescribGdln.pdf.

pediatricians. It is important to discuss the role of the media in tobacco use initiation and maintenance. Advertisements for tobacco products, including chewing tobacco, cigars, and snuff, are pervasive in the United States,[34] despite the 1998 ban on youth-targeted tobacco advertisements.[42] More subtle advertising to youth is delivered by depicting tobacco use in movies and other media; multiple studies have shown that when children and adolescents view smoking in movies, they are more likely to accept and initiate tobacco use.[3]

Early identification of the adolescent at risk of tobacco use is important. The US Surgeon General has identified 4 categories of risk factors for adolescent tobacco use.[43]

- *Personal*—belief that use of tobacco will make the teenager fit better into the social scene
- *Behavioral*—lack of strong educational goals, lack of attachment to school and social clubs
- *Socioeconomic*—low socioeconomic status
- *Environmental*—tobacco use by peers and/or parents, exposure to tobacco products and advertisements

The effectiveness of physicians' counseling of teenagers who use tobacco is less well established than it is with adults. The US Public Health Service guideline recommends using the same counseling strategies with teenagers that have been shown to be effective with adults but with advice tailored to teenagers. Messages can focus on the short-term effects of smoking, such as cost, bad breath, smelly clothes, decreased physical performance, and social unacceptability. It may be useful to raise teenagers' awareness of attempts by tobacco companies to "hook" them on tobacco through seductive advertising campaigns. Discussing the effects of exposure to secondhand smoke with children and teenagers also may be useful in reducing their exposure and increasing the rate at which their parents quit.[34]

Nicotine-replacement medications have been shown to be safe in adolescents, but there is insufficient evidence of effectiveness of pharmacotherapies for tobacco dependence treatment of adolescents. They are, therefore, not recommended as components of pediatric tobacco intervention by the US Public Health Service.[43] The 2009 US Food and Drug Administration warning regarding bupropion and varenicline are of particular interest to pediatricians.[44] This warning noted that depressed mood, agitation, changes in behavior, suicidal ideation, and suicide had been reported in patients attempting to quit tobacco use while using bupropion or varenicline.

Some pediatricians may consider using pharmacotherapy products for certain adolescent smokers. When doing so, pediatricians should determine how many cigarettes are smoked on a typical day, the degree of dependence (assessed using a standard scale, such as the Hooked on Nicotine Checklist [HONC]; see Table 40.2), any contraindications to or concerns about using pharmacotherapy, body weight, and the teenager's intent to quit. Confidentiality can be an issue, especially when pharmacotherapies are prescribed for teenagers. Because most insurance companies do not cover cessation counseling, and some do not reimburse for cessation pharmacotherapies, cost can be a concern.[34] Table 40.3 identifies steps to help teenagers stop using tobacco.

The American Academy of Pediatrics addressed tobacco use and exposure to secondhand smoke in the policy statement, "Tobacco Use: A Pediatric Disease,"[46] and 2 technical reports, "Secondhand and Prenatal Tobacco Smoke Exposure"[47] and "Tobacco as a Substance of Abuse."[43] Readers are referred to these sources for a more complete discussion of adolescents and tobacco use.

Table 40.2: The Hooked on Nicotine Checklist (HONC)[45]

QUESTION	NO	YES
Have you ever tried to quit, but couldn't?	☐	☐
Do you smoke now because it is really hard to quit?	☐	☐
Have you ever felt like you were addicted to tobacco?	☐	☐
Do you ever have strong cravings to smoke?	☐	☐
Have you ever felt like you really needed a cigarette?	☐	☐
Is it hard to keep from smoking in places where you are not supposed to?	☐	☐
When you haven't used tobacco for a while … **OR When you tried to stop smoking …**		
Did you find it hard to concentrate because you couldn't smoke?	☐	☐
Did you feel more irritable because you couldn't smoke?	☐	☐
Did you feel a strong need or urge to smoke?	☐	☐
Did you feel nervous, restless or anxious because you couldn't smoke?	☐	☐

SCORING

The Hooked on Nicotine Checklist is scored by counting the number of YES responses.

Dichotomous Yes/No Scoring: The Hooked on Nicotine Checklist can be used as an indicator of diminished autonomy.

Individuals who score a zero on the Hooked on Nicotine Checklist by answering NO to all 10 questions enjoy full autonomy over their use of tobacco. Because each symptom measured by the Hooked on Nicotine Checklist has face validity as an indicator of diminished autonomy, a smoker has lost full autonomy if any symptom is endorsed. In schools and clinics, smokers who have scores above zero can be told that they are already hooked. Many youths become hooked before they even consider themselves to be smokers, because they don't smoke every day. Research indicates that dichotomous scoring is helpful when the Hooked on Nicotine Checklist is used to predict the trajectory of smoking.

Continuous Scoring: The Hooked on Nicotine Checklist can be used to measure the severity of diminished autonomy. The number of symptoms a person endorses serves as a measure of the extent to which autonomy has been lost. Some researchers prefer to provide multiple response options for questionnaire items (eg, *never, sometimes, most of the time, always*). In certain situations, this can improve the statistical properties of a survey. When this has been done with the Hooked on Nicotine Checklist, its performance was not improved. Having more response options complicates the scoring, because the total score does not coincide with the number of individual symptoms. Therefore, we recommend the Yes/No response format. Researchers who wish to measure frequency or severity of symptoms may do so by adding to the yes/no format additional questions about any item endorsed by a smoker. Here is an example:

Have you ever felt like you were addicted to tobacco? A smoker who checked "yes" would then respond to:
— How often have you felt addicted? *Rarely, Occasionally, Often, Very Often*
— On a scale from 1 (*hardly at all*) to 10 (*extremely*), how addicted have you felt?

Table 40.3: Steps to Help Teenagers Stop Using Tobacco

1. Ask teenagers to consider that most adults who smoke started when they were teenagers, and wish that they had quit as teenagers. Mention that tobacco companies actively solicit teenagers to try smoking.

2. Ask teenagers to make a list of reasons why someone might want to quit. Then talk about any that might apply to them.

3. Point out that the longer it is that a person smokes, the harder it is to quit.

4. Ask teenagers who are not willing to discontinue use to promise that they will not increase the amount that they smoke.

5. Ask teenagers who say that tobacco is not a problem for them, "At what point would tobacco become a problem for you?"

6. Ask teenagers who say that they are not addicted to enter into a verbal contract with you to avoid tobacco for a month. Follow up by telephone.

7. Once the teenager has made a commitment to stop, the pediatrician's task is to encourage and educate. Suggest that teenagers who are determined to give up tobacco do the following:

   — Consider the logical arguments in favor of cessation, including health hazards.
   — Learn about ways to quit.
   — Think about how and why they use tobacco.
   — Develop a plan to cope with (or avoid) situations where the urge to use is great.
   — Make the commitment.
   — Get the help they need (eg, pharmacotherapies, cessation clinics, quitting partners).
   — Decide on a cessation plan and stay with it.
   — Anticipate and prepare for occasional urges to smoke long after discontinuing use.

Strategies for Preadolescents

It is important for pediatricians to begin disseminating a "don't start smoking" message as early as possible and to engage parents, even those who smoke, during this stage. One powerful message that can be delivered by a parent who uses tobacco is that "quitting is hard, and I wish I had never started." Teenagers whose parents use tobacco are more likely to use tobacco themselves. The process of initiation is rapid and can occur within moments of the first inhalation.[43]

REDUCING TOBACCO USE INITIATION

Effective techniques to reduce initiation of tobacco use include (1) increasing the unit price for tobacco products; (2) mass media education campaigns (when combined with other interventions); and (3) community mobilization to restrict minors' access to tobacco products (when combined with other interventions).

Interventions directed at retailers of tobacco products, including laws and education of retailers or the community, have not been shown to be effective.[48] Strategies to reduce tobacco use initiation should be part of a larger, state- or nationwide program of tobacco control. Successful programs are described in *Best Practices for Comprehensive Tobacco Control Programs*[49] and include:

1. State and community interventions that support, implement, and unite organizations, systems, and networks that encourage and support tobacco-free behavior choices.
2. Health communication interventions that deliver messages supporting tobacco-free behavior choices through many venues and to many groups.
3. Cessation interventions based in, but not limited to, the health care system, to ensure that all patients are screened for tobacco use, receive brief cessation interventions, and are offered more intensive services and cessation medications.
4. Surveillance and evaluation of tobacco-related attitudes, behaviors, and health outcomes at regular intervals.
5. Administration and management that provides funding for the skilled staff, effective managers, and strong leaders needed to implement these programs.

THE PEDIATRICIAN'S OFFICE AND TOBACCO USE

Reinforcing the antitobacco message is important, and the office setting and office staff can play important roles in delivering these messages (Table 40.4).[34] One of the most important steps a practice can take is to screen all patients and families for tobacco use and exposure to secondhand smoke. A systematic screening procedure can be as simple as adding "tobacco use or exposure to secondhand smoke" to the vital signs collected at every visit. The information should be recorded in a standard place on the patient's chart. When developing or updating electronic health records (EHRs), pediatricians should make sure that the EHR section on vital signs has the capability to reflect active smoking or exposure to secondhand smoke. Making sure that cessation materials are readily available, including the 1-800-Quit Now phone number, is another important step (see Table 40.4).

Frequently Asked Questions From Parents

Q   If I smoke, can I breastfeed?

A   Breastfeeding is best for infants, whether or not you use tobacco. However, for the same reasons we highly recommend that pregnant women do not use tobacco, breastfeeding mothers should not use tobacco, because nicotine and other toxicants are transferred through human milk to the infant. Another reason not to use tobacco is that infants of women who smoke are weaned at an earlier age. If you do continue to use tobacco, never breastfeed while

Table 40.4: Office Interventions

1. Set an example.
Pediatricians should be role models and should not use tobacco. Clinical buildings and associated grounds should be tobacco free, have signs stating so, and have enforcement plans. Subscribe to magazines that do not carry tobacco advertisements or advertisements written by tobacco manufacturers.

2. Systematically assess parents' tobacco use status and children's exposure to secondhand smoke.
Systematic strategies for identifying tobacco users, such as stickers on the medical chart or a vital sign form that includes tobacco use status, should be implemented. The goal is to prompt any staff member who has contact with patients or parents who use tobacco to provide information about cessation and smoke-free homes. It is important to ask about the tobacco use status of parents and household members In the context of a child's health assessment. The issue of tobacco use by parents or household members should be entered into the problem list and addressed at each visit.

3. Involve several staff members in providing information about smoking cessation.
Educating additional office staff (eg, a nurse or health educator) in tobacco use cessation counseling can extend the physician's efforts and provide effective support.

4. Serve as an "agenda setter."
The pediatrician may serve as a catalyst for a parent to quit using tobacco. The pediatrician may initiate the process and then provide referrals to specialists in and resources for cessation and maintenance of a tobacco-free lifestyle.

5. Provide patient education materials.
Materials can be obtained free or at low cost from many organizations (see Resources) and on the Internet.

6. Use local resources. Local resources are available in most areas.
Physician referrals should include a specific agency or program, telephone number, and description of what to expect. Self-help materials are available from many agencies. The makers of tobacco use cessation pharmacotherapies offer self-help programs as adjuncts to their products.

Adapted from Fiore et al.[34]

smoking, because a high concentration of smoke will be in close proximity to your infant.

Q *When visitors come to my home, they ask if they can smoke in another room. What should I tell them?*

A Children's homes should be completely smoke-free. Even if smokers smoke in a separate room, smoke-filled air is spread throughout the home, exposing everyone in the house to secondhand smoke. Visitors to your home should honor your request not to smoke. If they cannot do this, insist that they smoke outside, away from open doors and windows. Keep in mind that residual smoke on their clothing and their belongings may release toxins into your home.

Q *I can't stop smoking right now. How can I reduce my child's exposure to secondhand smoke?*

A Because your child will be exposed to secondhand smoke if you smoke in any part of your home, be sure that you only smoke outside the house, and never smoke in your car or any vehicle in which a child rides. Choose a smoke-free child care setting, and avoid taking your child to places where smoking is permitted, such as bars or restaurants (even if there is a separate smoking area), airport smoking lounges, etc.

Q *Is there good evidence that exposure to secondhand smoke is linked to the development of asthma in young children?*

A Yes, there is sufficient evidence showing a strong association between exposure to secondhand smoke and the development of asthma or wheezing in young children.

Q *We live in my parent's home. They smoke in their bedroom. How can I ask them to smoke outside of their own home?*

A There are a couple of things you can do. If you feel comfortable (and safe) telling them about how harmful secondhand smoke is to your child, you can say that the pediatrician asked if they would make their home smoke free. Or, if you prefer, your pediatrician can write a note to them asking them to make their home smoke free. Making their home smoke free may have the added benefits of reducing the number of cigarettes they smoke and encouraging them to take the next step towards quitting.

Q *I've tried to quit using the gum and the patch before. They didn't work. Why should I try them now?*

A Each time you make a quit attempt, you learn more about the quitting process and what works (or does not work) to help you quit. Most people make several quit attempts before they succeed. I recommend you call 1-800-QUIT NOW and talk to a counselor who will help you plan your next quit attempt. The service is free, and it really works.

Q *I've heard that the new medicine, varenicline, is really helpful. What do you know about it?*

A Varenicline has been effective in helping many smokers quit, but there also are concerns about its safety in some users. It is a good idea to discuss the benefits and risks of using this medication with your doctor or nurse practitioner. Another good source for information is 1-800-QUIT NOW.

Q *We do not smoke but we live in a large apartment building and we smell smoke through the walls. Is this a problem, and if so, what can we do about it?*

A A recent study showed that children in apartments had higher mean cotinine levels than did children in detached houses.[50] Potential causes for this result could be seepage through walls or shared ventilation systems. You should consider working for a smoking ban in your apartment building. Smoking bans in multiunit housing may reduce children's exposure to tobacco smoke.[51]

Frequently Asked Questions From Clinicians

Q *Parents have been asking me about thirdhand smoke. What is that?*

A "Thirdhand" smoke is residual tobacco smoke that remains after a cigarette is extinguished. Research indicates an association between smoking in the home and persistently high levels of tobacco pollutants even after active smoking has ceased, meaning that children can still be exposed. Toxins include particulate matter that deposits in a layer onto surfaces and in loose household dust, and volatile toxic compounds that "off gas" into the air over days, weeks, and months.[50] All homes should be smoke free.

Q *How do I counsel anyone in the context of a busy practice?*

A Even the briefest of statements, such as, "You should quit smoking," have been shown to effectively increase the number and success of quit attempts. Most pediatricians already make these or similar statements to parents when treating a child with asthma or other respiratory illness. Referring the patient or parent to 1-800-QUIT NOW or another cessation resource adds only a few minutes and can make the message much more effective.

Q *How can a pediatrician be expected to counsel when counseling is not covered by most insurance plans?*

A Unfortunately, many insurance companies do not reimburse for preventive services counseling. Because the consequences of secondhand smoke exposure to children and families are so great, and the time needed to deliver a brief "stop using tobacco" message is short, many pediatricians find the time to provide this important service.

Resources

Agency for Health Care Research and Quality
Phone: 800-358-9295
Web site: www.ahrq.gov

American Academy of Pediatrics, Richmond Center of Excellence
Phone: 847-434-4264
Web site: www.aap.org/richmondcenter

American Cancer Society
Phone: 800-ACS-2345
Web site: www.cancer.org

American Lung Association, Environmental Health
Phone: 800-LUNG-USA or 800-548-8252 or 202-785-3355
Web site: www.lungusa.org
Freedom From Smoking: www.ffsonline.org

Asthma and Allergy Foundation of America
Phone: 800-7-ASTHMA or 800-727-8462 or 202-466-7643
Web site: www.aafa.org

CEASE, Clinical Effort Against Secondhand Smoke Exposure
Web site: www.ceasetobacco.org

Centers for Disease Control and Prevention, Office on Smoking and Health
Phone: 800-CDC-INFO or 800-232-4636 or 770-488-5701
Web site: www.cdc.gov/tobacco

National Cancer Institute
Phone: 800-4-CANCER or 800-422-6237
Web site: www.nci.nih.gov

Nicotine Anonymous
Phone: 415-750-0328
Web site: www.nicotine-anonymous.org

Smoke Free Homes
Phone: 202-476-4746
Web site: www.kidslivesmokefree.org

US Environmental Protection Agency, Indoor Air Quality Publications
Phone: 800-490-9198
Web site: www.epa.gov/iaq/pubs

US Environmental Protection Agency, Smoke-free Homes and Cars Program
Phone: 866-SMOKE-FREE or 866-766-5337
Web site: www.epa.gov/smokefree

References

1. Schwab M, McDermott A, Spengler J. Using longitudinal data to understand children's activity patterns in an exposure context: data from the Kanawha County Health Study. *Environ Int.* 1992;18:173-189
2. Centers for Disease Control and Prevention. *Preventing Tobacco Use Among Young People: A Report of the Surgeon General.* Atlanta, GA: US Department of Health and Human Services, Public Health Service, Centers for Disease Control and Prevention, National Center for Chronic Disease Prevention and Health Promotion, Office on Smoking and Health; 1994

3. Wellman RJ, Sugarman DB, DiFranza JR, Winickoff JP. The extent to which tobacco marketing and tobacco use in films contribute to children's use of tobacco: a meta-analysis. *Arch Pediatr Adolesc Med.* 2006;160(12):1285-1296

4. FDA head calls smoking a "pediatric disease." *Columbia University Record.* March 24, 1995

5. California Environmental Protection Agency. *Proposed Identification of Environmental Tobacco Smoke as a Toxic Air Contaminant.* Sacramento, CA: Air Resources Board, Office of Environmental Health Hazard Assessment, California Environmental Protection Agency; 2005

6. Spengler JD, Dockery DW, Turner WA, Wolfson JM, Ferris BG Jr. Long term measurements of respirable sulfates and particles inside and outside homes. *Atmosph Environ.* 1981;15(1):23-30

7. US Environmental Protection Agency. *Respiratory Health Effects of Passive Smoking: Lung Cancer and Other Disorders.* Washington, DC: US Environmental Protection Agency, Office of Research and Development, Office of Air and Radiation; 1992

8. Centers for Disease Control and Prevention. Vital signs: current cigarette smoking among adults aged ≥18 years—United States, 2009. *MMWR Morb Mortal Wkly Rep.* 2010;59(35):1135-1140

9. Centers for Disease Control and Prevention. Vital signs: nonsmokers' exposure to secondhand smoke—United States, 1999–2008. *MMWR Morb Mortal Wkly Rep.* 2010;59(35):1141-1146

10. The GTSS Collaborative Group. A cross country comparison of exposure to secondhand smoke among youth. *Tob Control.* 2006;15(Suppl 2):ii4-ii19

11. Oberg M Jaakkola MS Woodward A, Peruga A, Pruss-Usten A. Worldwide burden of disease from exposure to second-hand smoke: a retrospective analysis of data from 192 countries. *Lancet.* 2011;377(9760):139-146

12. Matt GE, Quintana PJ, Hovell MF, et al. Households contaminated by environmental tobacco smoke: sources of infant exposures. *Tob Control.* 2004;13(1):29-37

13. US Department of Health and Human Services. *The Health Consequences of Involuntary Exposure to Tobacco Smoke: A Report of the Surgeon General.* Atlanta, GA: US Department of Health and Human Services, Centers for Disease Control and Prevention, Coordinating Center for Health Promotion, National Center for Chronic Disease Prevention and Health Promotion, Office on Smoking and Health; 2006

14. Hecht SS, Ye M, Carmella SG, et al. Metabolites of a tobacco-specific lung carcinogen in the urine of elementary school-aged children. *Cancer Epidemiol Biomarkers Prev.* 2001;10(11): 1109-1116

15. Chuang SC, Gallo V, Michaud D, et al. Exposure to environmental tobacco smoke in childhood and incidence of cancer in adulthood in never smokers in the European Prospective Investigation into Cancer and Nutrition. *Cancer Causes Control.* 2011;22(3):487-494

16. Palmer CN, Doney AS, Lee SP, et al. Glutathione S-transferase M1 and P1 genotype, passive smoking, and peak expiratory flow in asthma. *Pediatrics.* 2006;118(2):710-716

17. Wang C, Salam MT, Islam T, Wenten M, Gauderman WJ, Gilliland FD. Effects of in utero and childhood tobacco smoke exposure and {beta}2-adrenergic receptor genotype on childhood asthma and wheezing. *Pediatrics.* 2008;122(1):e107-114

18. Aligne CA, Moss ME, Auinger P, Weitzman M. Association of pediatric dental caries with passive smoking. *JAMA.* 2003;289(10):1258-1264

19. Drongowski RA, Lee D, Reynolds PI, et al. Increased respiratory symptoms following surgery in children exposed to environmental tobacco smoke. *Paediatr Anaesth.* 2003;13(4):304-310

20. Mannino DM, Moorman JE, Kingsley B, Rose D, Repace J. Health effects related to environmental tobacco smoke exposure in children in the United States: data from the Third National Health and Nutrition Examination Survey. *Arch Pediatr Adolesc Med.* 2001;155(1): 36-41

21. Leistikow BN, Martin DC, Milano CE. Fire injuries, disasters, and costs from cigarettes and cigarette lights: a global overview. *Prev Med.* 2000;31(2 Pt 1):91-99

22. Leistikow BN, Martin DC, Jacobs J, Rocke DM, Noderer K. Smoking as a risk factor for accident death: a meta-analysis of cohort studies. *Accid Anal Prev.* 2000;32(3):397-405

23. Yolton K, Khoury J, Hornung R, Dietrich K, Succop P, Lanphear B. Environmental tobacco smoke exposure and child behaviors. *J Dev Behav Pediatr.* 2008;29(6):450-457

24. Julvez J, Ribas-Fitó N, Torrent M, Forns M, Garcia-Esteban R, Sunyer J. Maternal smoking habits and cognitive development of children at age 4 years in a population-based birth cohort. *Int J Epidemiol.* 2007;36(4):825-832

25. Fagnano M, Conn KM, Halterman JS. Environmental tobacco smoke and behaviors of inner-city children with asthma. *Ambul Pediatr.* 2008;8(5):288-293

26. Rückinger S, Rzehak P, Chen C-M, et al. Prenatal and postnatal tobacco exposure and behavioral problems in 10-year-old children: results from the GINI-plus prospective birth cohort study. *Environ Health Perspect.* 2010;118(1):150-154

27. Groner JA, Hoshaw-Woodard S, Koren G, Klein J, Castile R. Screening for children's exposure to environmental tobacco smoke in a pediatric primary care setting. *Arch Pediatr Adolesc Med.* 2005;159(5):450-455

28. Boyaci H, Etiler N, Duman C, Basyigit I, Pala A. Environmental tobacco smoke exposure in school children: parent report and urine cotinine measures. *Pediatr Int.* 2006;48(4):382-389

29. Gehring U, Leaderer BP, Heinrich J, et al. Comparison of parental reports of smoking and residential air nicotine concentrations in children. *Occup Environ Med.* 2006;63(11):766-772

30. Lee DJ, Arheart KL, Trapido E, Soza-Vento R, Rodriguez R. Accuracy of parental and youth reporting of secondhand smoke exposure: the Florida youth cohort study. *Addict Behav.* 2005;30(8):1555-1562

31. Ott WR, Klepeis NE, Switzer P. Analytical solutions to compartmental indoor air quality models with application to environmental tobacco smoke concentrations measured in a house. *J Air Waste Manag Assoc.* 2003;53(8):918-936

32. Devoe JE, Baez A, Angier H, Krois L, Edlund C, Carney PA. Insurance + access not equal to health care: typology of barriers to health care access for low-income families. *Ann Fam Med.* 2007;5(6):511-518

33. Weissman JS, Zaslavsky AM, Wolf RE, Ayanian JZ. State Medicaid coverage and access to care for low-income adults. *J Health Care Poor Underserved.* 2008;19(1):307-319

34. Fiore M, Jaen C, Baker T, et al. *Treating Tobacco Use and Dependence: 2008 Update. Clinical Practice Guideline.* Rockville, MD: US Department of Health and Human Services, Public Health Service; 2008

35. McBride CM, Emmons KM, Lipkus IM. Understanding the potential of teachable moments: the case of smoking cessation. *Health Educ Res.* 2003;18(2):156-170

36. Frankowski BL, Weaver SO, Secker-Walker RH. Advising parents to stop smoking: pediatricians' and parents' attitudes. *Pediatrics.* 1993;91(2):296-300

37. Winickoff JP, Hibberd PL, Case B, Sinha P, Rigotti NA. Child hospitalization: an opportunity for parental smoking intervention. *Am J Prev Med.* 2001;21(3):218-220

38. Winickoff JP, Buckley VJ, Palfrey JS, Perrin JM, Rigotti NA. Intervention with parental smokers in an outpatient pediatric clinic using counseling and nicotine replacement. *Pediatrics.* 2003;112(5):1127-1133

39. Winickoff JP, Hillis VJ, Palfrey JS, Perrin JM, Rigotti NA. A smoking cessation intervention for parents of children who are hospitalized for respiratory illness: the stop tobacco outreach program. *Pediatrics.* 2003;111(1):140-145

40. Sharif I, Oruwariye T, Waldman G, Ozuah PO. Smoking cessation counseling by pediatricians in an inner-city setting. *J Natl Med Assoc.* 2002;94(9):841-845

41. American Academy of Pediatrics. Coding Corner. What diagnosis code should I use for parental smoke exposure? *AAP News.* 2003;23(1):31

42. National Association of Attorneys General. Master Settlement Agreement. *Settlement Documents.* Washington, DC: National Association of Attorneys General; 1998. Available at: http://www.naag.org/settlement_docs.php. Accessed March 31, 2011

43. Sims TH; American Academy of Pediatrics, Committee on Substance Abuse. Technical report—tobacco as a substance of abuse. *Pediatrics.* 2009;124(5):e1045-e1053

44. US Food and Drug Administration. Information for Healthcare Professionals: Varenicline (marketed as Chantix) and Bupropion (marketed as Zyban, Wellbutrin, and generics). Available at: http://www.fda.gov/Drugs/DrugSafety/PostmarketDrugSafetyInformationfor Patient sand Providers/DrugSafetyInformationforHealthcareProfessionals/ucm169986.htm. Accessed March 31, 2011

45. DiFranza JR, Savageau JA, Fletcher K, Ockene JK, Rigotti NA, McNeill AD, Coleman M, Wood C. Measuring the loss of autonomy over nicotine use in adolescents: The Development and Assessment of Nicotine Dependence in Youths (DANDY) Study. *Arch Pediatr Adolesc Med.* 2002;156(4):397-403

46. American Academy of Pediatrics, Committee on Environmental Health, Committee on Substance Abuse, Committee on Adolescence, Committee on Native American Child Health. Policy statement—tobacco use: a pediatric disease. *Pediatrics.* 2009;124(5):1474-1487

47. Best D; American Academy of Pediatrics, Committee on Environmental Health, Committee on Native American Child Health, Committee on Adolescence. Technical report—secondhand and prenatal tobacco smoke exposure. *Pediatrics.* 2009;124(5):e1017-1044

48. Centers for Disease Control and Prevention. *The Community Guide. Tobacco Use.* Atlanta, GA: The Community Guide, Epidemiology Analysis Program Office, Office of Surveillance, Epidemiology, and Laboratory Services, Centers for Disease Control and Prevention; 2003. Available at: http://www.thecommunityguide.org/tobacco/default.htm. Accessed March 31, 2011

49. Centers for Disease Control and Prevention. *Best Practices for Comprehensive Tobacco Control Programs—2007.* Atlanta, GA: US Department of Health and Human Services, Centers for Disease Control and Prevention, National Center for Chronic Disease Prevention and Health Promotion, Office on Smoking and Health; 2007. Available at: http://www.cdc.gov/tobacco/stateandcommunity/best_practices/pdfs/2007/bestpractices_complete.pdf. Accessed June 19, 2011

50. Wilson KM, Klein JD, Blumkin AK, Gottlieb M, Winickoff JP. Tobacco-smoke exposure in children who live in multiunit housing. *Pediatrics.* 2011;127(1):85-92

51. Kline RL. Smoke knows no boundaries: legal strategies for environmental tobacco smoke incursions into the home within multi-unit residential dwellings. *Tob Control.* 2000;9(2):201-205

52. Winickoff JP, Friebely J, Tanski SE, et al. Beliefs about the health effects of "thirdhand" smoke and home smoking bans. *Pediatrics.* 2009;123(1):e74-e79

Chapter 41

Ultraviolet Radiation

■ ■ ■ ■ ■ ■

The sun sustains life on earth. The sun is needed for photosynthesis, provides warmth, drives biological rhythms, and promotes feelings of well-being. Sunlight is needed for vitamin D production in skin. Despite beneficial effects, exposure to the ultraviolet (UV) component of the sunlight spectrum results in adverse effects on human health.

The sun emits electromagnetic radiation ranging from short-wavelength high-energy X-rays to long-wavelength lower energy radio waves. Ultraviolet radiation (UVR, "above violet") waves range from 200 to 400 nanometers (nm). UVR waves are longer than X-rays and shorter than visible light (400–700 nm) and infrared radiation (>700 nm, "below red" or "heat"). UVR is divided into UVA (320–400 nm, further subdivided into UVA2 [320–340] and UVA1 [340–400]), also called black (invisible) light; UVB (290–320 nm); and UVC (<290 nm). UVC rays possess the highest energy but are completely absorbed by stratospheric ozone; no UVC reaches the earth's surface. Thus, UVB, UVA, visible light, and infrared waves have the greatest biological significance.

Solar radiation that reaches the earth's surface comprises about 95% UVA and 5% UVB.[1] Most UVB is absorbed by stratospheric ozone, but no UVA is absorbed.[2] The ozone layer does not have uniform thickness; ozone concentration tends to increase toward the poles but is thinning in some areas.[2] Ozone depletion has a significant effect on the amount of UVB reaching the earth.[3]

UVB is more intense during the summer than during the winter, at midday compared with early morning or late afternoon, in places closer to the equator than in temperate zones, and at high altitudes compared with sea level. Sand, snow, concrete, and water can reflect up to 85% of sunlight, resulting in greater exposure.[4] Water is not a good photoprotectant, because UVR can penetrate to a depth of 60 cm, resulting in a significant exposure. In contrast to the variability of UVB, UVA is relatively constant throughout the day and the year.

UVR can be produced by manmade lamps (such as sunlamps) and tools (such as welding tools), but the sun is the primary source of UVR for most people.[5] UVR has been used for decades to treat skin diseases, especially psoriasis.[1]

ROUTE OF EXPOSURE

Individuals are exposed to UVR through direct contact to the skin and eyes while they are outdoors in the sunlight or when they are exposed to artificial sources of UVR emitted by sunlamps and sunbeds.

SYSTEMS AFFECTED

The skin, eyes, and immune system are affected.

CLINICAL EFFECTS

Effects on Skin

The skin is the organ most exposed to environmental UVR.

Erythema and Sunburn

Erythema and sunburn are acute reactions to excessive amounts of UVR. Exposure to UVR causes vasodilatation and an increase in the volume of blood in the dermis, resulting in erythema. The minimal erythema (or erythemal) dose depends on factors such as skin type and thickness, the amount of melanin in the epidermis and the capacity of the epidermis to produce melanin after sun exposure, and the intensity of the radiation. A classification system of 6 sun-reactive skin classifications was developed, taking into account an individual's expected sunburn and suntan tendency (Table 41.1).

The ability of UVR to produce erythema depends on the radiation wavelength expressed as the erythema "action spectrum." For erythema and sunburn, the action spectrum is mainly in the UVB range.[6]

Tanning

Tanning is a protective response to sun exposure.[7] Immediate tanning (or immediate pigment darkening) is the result of oxidation of existing melanin after exposure to visible light and UVA. Immediate pigment darkening becomes visible within several minutes and usually fades within 1 to 2 hours. Delayed tanning occurs when new melanin is formed as a result of UVB exposure. Delayed tanning becomes apparent 2 to 3 days after exposure, peaks at 7 to 10 days, and may persist for weeks or months. According to recent evidence, the tanning response means that DNA damage has occurred in skin.[8]

Table 41.1: Fitzpatrick Classification of Sun-Reactive Skin Types

SKIN TYPE	HISTORY OF SUNBURNING OR TANNING
I	Always burns easily, never tans
II	Always burns easily, tans minimally
III	Burns moderately, tans gradually and uniformly (light brown)
IV	Burns minimally, always tans well (moderate brown)
V	Rarely burns, tans profusely (dark brown)
VI	Never burns, deeply pigmented (black)

Phototoxicity and Photoallergy

Chemical photosensitivity refers to an adverse cutaneous reaction that occurs when certain chemicals or drugs are applied topically or taken systemically at the same time that a person is exposed to UVR or visible radiation. *Phototoxicity* is a form of chemical photosensitivity that does not depend on an immunologic response, because the reaction can occur on the person's first exposure to the offending agent. Most phototoxic agents are activated in the UVA range (320–400 nm). Drugs associated with phototoxic reactions include those commonly used by adolescents, such as nonsteroidal anti-inflammatory drugs (NSAIDs); tetracyclines and tretinoin; other medications, such as phenothiazines, psoralens, sulfonamides, and thiazides; and para-amino benzoic acid (PABA) esters.[9] *Photoallergy* is an acquired altered reactivity of the skin that depends on antigen-antibody or cell-mediated hypersensitivity.[9] Photoallergic reactions involve an immunologic response to a chemical or drug that is altered by UVR. PABA-containing sunscreens, fragrances, sulfonamides, and phenothiazines are associated with photoallergic reactions.[9]

People who take medications or use topical agents that are sensitizing should avoid all sun exposure, if possible, and completely avoid all UVA from artificial sources. The consequences of exposure can be uncomfortable, serious, or life threatening.

Phytophotodermatitis is a skin eruption resulting from the interaction of sunlight and photosensitizing compounds. The most common phototoxic compounds are the furocoumarins (psoralens) contained in a wide variety of plants, such as limes, lemons, and celery.

Up to 80% of patients with systemic lupus erythematosus have photosensitivity. The threshold UV dose triggering cutaneous or systemic reactions is much lower than that for sunburn. Many patients are not aware of the association of flares with UVR exposure, because the latency period between exposure and skin eruptions can range from several days to 3 weeks.[10]

Skin Aging (Photoaging)

Chronic unprotected exposure to UVR weakens the skin's elasticity, resulting in sagging cheeks, deeper facial wrinkles, and skin discoloration later in life. Photo-aged skin is characterized by alterations of cellular components and of the extracellular matrix.

Nonmelanoma Skin Cancer

Nonmelanoma skin cancer (NMSC) includes basal cell carcinoma and squamous cell carcinoma. In the US adult population, nonmelanoma skin cancer is by far the most common malignant neoplasm, with more than 2 million cases every year. The number of cases of nonmelanoma skin cancer in the United States is not precisely known, because physicians are not required to report these to cancer registries. Nonmelanoma skin cancer is rarely fatal unless left untreated; nevertheless, the American Cancer Society estimated that 2000 people die of nonmelanoma skin cancer per year.[11]

In general, nonmelanoma skin cancer occurs in maximally sun-exposed areas of fair-skinned people and is uncommon in black people and other people with increased natural pigmentation. Nonmelanoma skin cancer is more common in people older than 50 years, with the incidence in this age group rapidly increasing. The incidence of nonmelanoma skin cancer is also increasing in young adults.[12] Sun exposure is the main environmental cause of nonmelanoma skin cancer. Cumulative exposure over long periods, resulting in photodamage, is considered important in pathogenesis of squamous cell carcinoma.

Nonmelanoma skin cancer is extremely rare in children in the absence of predisposing conditions.

Melanoma

Melanoma is primarily a disease of the skin. Primary extracutaneous sites include the eye, mucous membranes, gastrointestinal tract, genitourinary tract, leptomeninges, and lymph nodes. Ninety-five percent of melanomas occur in the skin.[13]

Although much less common than nonmelanoma skin cancer, cutaneous malignant melanoma (hereafter referred to as "melanoma") is a serious public health issue. In the United States, melanoma is the fifth most common cancer in men and the sixth most common in women.[14] The incidence of melanoma is rising rapidly in the United States. In 1935, the lifetime risk for a person in the United States developing invasive melanoma was 1 in 1500. In 2007, this risk was 1 in 63 for invasive melanomas and 1 in 33 if in situ melanomas were included. Worldwide, melanoma is increasing faster than any other malignancy.[15] Melanoma accounts for less than 5% of skin cancer cases but causes the majority of skin cancer deaths. The American Cancer Society estimated that 68 130 melanomas would be diagnosed in 2009; approximately 8700 people were estimated to die of the disease.[16] Overall, the lifetime risk of getting melanoma is approximately 1 in 50 for white people, 1 in 200 for Hispanic people, and 1 in 1000 for black people.[16] Although melanoma has an excellent prognosis if detected in the early stages, melanoma that has metastasized has a grave prognosis. Thus, efforts have been directed toward prevention and early detection.

The reason for the increase in the incidence of melanoma is complex and incompletely understood but is likely to be related to changing patterns of dress favoring more skin exposure, a decrease in the earth's protective stratospheric ozone layer because of the widespread use of chlorofluorocarbons, more opportunities for leisure activities, and increased exposure to artificial sources of UVR for tanning purposes.

Melanoma is more likely to occur in males. Increasing age is a risk factor for melanoma, with most melanomas occurring in people older than 50 years. Family history also increases risk: a person's risk of developing melanoma increases if there are one or more first-degree relatives with melanoma. People at highest risk have light skin and eyes and sunburn easily. Melanoma also occurs in teenagers and young adults. It is the second most common cancer of women in their 20s and the third most common cancer of men in their 20s.[17] Melanoma incidence is increasing in young women 15 to 39 years of age.[18]

Although it is rare, melanoma occurs in children. Ferrari et al reviewed a 25-year experience with 33 Italian children with melanoma who were 14 years or younger at presentation. The children's lesions were not typical of melanoma lesions in adults.[19] Melanoma lesions in adults generally follow the "ABCDE's": they are **a**symmetric; with irregular **b**orders; variegated **c**olor; **d**iameter larger than 6 mm, the size of a pencil eraser; and changing or **e**volving. In the Ferrari series, however, many lesions in children were amelanotic (pink, pink-white, or red) and tended to be raised and to have regular borders. The key to diagnosis in these children was the recognition that the melanoma lesions were unlike any other lesions on the child.[19]

Evidence That UVR Causes Skin Cancer

In 1992, the International Agency for Research on Cancer (a part of the World Health Organization) reviewed the evidence for the carcinogenicity of solar radiation. They concluded that "There is sufficient evidence in humans for the carcinogenicity of solar radiation. Solar radiation causes cutaneous malignant melanoma and non-melanocytic skin cancer."[1] Since that time, further evidence has strengthened the link between sunlight exposure and skin cancer.

Epidemiologic evidence

1. *Latitude or estimated ambient solar UVR.* The rates of basal cell carcinoma and squamous cell carcinoma increase with increasing ambient solar UVR. There is a direct relationship between the incidence of nonmelanoma skin cancer and latitude, with higher rates found closer to the equator (where the amount of sunlight is greater).[15] The relationship of melanoma with latitude is not as clear cut as that for nonmelanoma skin cancer.[15]

2. *Race and pigmentation.* Basal cell carcinoma and squamous cell carcinoma occur primarily in white people. Incidence and mortality rates of melanoma are highest for white people.[20] There is, in general, an inverse relationship between skin cancer incidence and skin pigmentation of people in various countries in the world. Superficial epidermal melanin decreases the transmission of UVR. This may protect keratinocytes and melanocytes from sunlight-induced changes that lead to their malignant transformation.[7]

3. *History of sun exposure.* The pattern of sun exposure is important in the etiology of basal cell carcinoma, squamous cell carcinoma, and melanoma. Personal sun exposure is usually characterized by (1) total sun exposure over time; (2) occupational exposure (signifying a more chronic exposure); and (3) nonoccupational or recreational exposure (signifying intermittent exposure).[21] Squamous cell carcinoma is significantly associated with estimated total sun exposure and with occupational exposure. Chronic exposure to UVB is now considered as the main environmental cause of squamous cell carcinoma. Squamous cell carcinoma appears to be most straightforwardly related to the total sun exposure: these tumors occur on skin areas that are most regularly exposed (face, neck, and hands), and the risk rises with the lifelong accumulated dose of UVR.[22] Basal cell carcinoma and melanoma are significantly associated with intermittent sun exposure (ie, sunburning), but squamous cell carcinoma does not show this relationship. Melanoma is more strongly associated with intermittent sun exposures than is basal cell carcinoma.[21]

4. *Childhood sun exposure.* Childhood and adolescence are often considered to contain "critical periods of vulnerability" when people are especially susceptible to effects of toxic exposures. It has been estimated that approximately 25% of lifetime sun exposure occurs before 18 years of age.[23] Sun exposure and blistering sunburns during youth may be more intense than later in life because of child and adolescent behavior patterns. Sunlight exposure during childhood and adolescence is generally considered to confer increased risk of melanoma compared with exposure at older ages[24]; some conclude, however, that excessive UV exposure later in life may be as important a risk for melanoma as UV exposure earlier in life.[25]

   There is biological plausibility to support the heightened susceptibility of young melanocytes. Peak melanocytic activity occurs in early life, as demonstrated by the steady acquisition of nevi during childhood and adolescence. Freckling is also prominent at these ages; freckles in children often appear abruptly after high-dose sun exposure and are thought to represent clones of mutated melanocytes. The presence of freckles is associated with an increased risk of melanoma.[7] Young melanocytes may be especially vulnerable to the adverse effects of solar radiation. Sunlight may have both early and late effects on the development of melanoma (akin to cancer "initiation," "promotion," and "progression,"), and the biological effectiveness of sunlight in initiating melanoma is greatest during the period of peak melanocytic activity. Populations exposed to high sunlight levels in childhood will have more people with more initiated melanocytes than populations who experienced lower sunlight levels. This "melanoma potential" is retained when people move to a different environment.[24]

5. *Nevi.* Acute sun exposure is implicated in the development of nevi in children. The number of nevi increases with age,[26] nevi occur with more frequency on sun-exposed areas, and the number of nevi on exposed areas increases with the total cumulative sun exposure during childhood and adolescence.[27] Children with light skin who tend to burn rather than tan have more nevi at all ages, and children who have more severe sunburns have more nevi.[26]

There is a relationship between the number and type of melanocytic nevi and the development of melanoma. The presence of congenital melanocytic nevi (CMN [pigment cell malformations formed during gestation and visible at or shortly after birth]) also increases risk. In a review of 14 case series with adequate follow-up periods, investigators found an overall risk of melanoma arising in congenital melanocytic nevi of 0.7%; this was lower than expected. Melanoma risk was strongly dependent on the size of the congenital melanocytic nevi and was highest in garment nevi (defined as congenital nevi with hair growth situated on the trunk measuring >40 cm in largest diameter or expected to reach this size in adulthood).[28]

Dysplastic melanocytic nevi, which may represent a reaction to solar injury, are considered precursor lesions that increase melanoma risk.[29] The familial dysplastic nevus syndrome has the following features: (1) a distinctive appearance of abnormal melanocytic nevi; (2) unique histologic features of the nevi; (3) autosomal dominant pattern of inheritance; and (4) hypermutability of fibroblasts and lymphoblasts. Fibroblasts and lymphoblasts from patients with this syndrome are abnormally sensitive to UVR damage, and people with this syndrome are at markedly higher risk of developing melanoma.[30] Certain families with germline mutations in CDKN2A, CDK4, and other genes are at increased risk of developing dysplastic nevi and melanoma.[31]

6. *Exposure to artificial sources of UVR.* Exposure to sunbeds and sunlamps also is associated with increased risk of developing basal cell carcinoma, squamous cell carcinoma, and melanoma.

Biological evidence

Biological evidence also suggests that sunlight exposure is important in the pathogenesis of melanoma. Studies in opossums suggest that portions of the UVA spectrum may play a role in the pathogenesis of melanoma.[32] Portions of the UVA and UVB spectra promote the development of carcinomas in mice.[33] Melanoma has been induced in human foreskins grafted onto immunologically tolerant animals exposed to UVR.[34] Melanomas frequently are found in people with xeroderma pigmentosum and related disorders in which there is a genetically determined defect in the repair of DNA damaged by UVR and a high risk of nonmelanoma skin cancer.

Cellular studies

UVB exposure damages DNA, resulting in UVR-induced lesions, primarily cyclobutane pyrimidine dimers and pyrimidine (6-4) pyrimidone photoproducts.[7] The incomplete repair of DNA damage results in mutations.[7] UVA causes oxidative damage to DNA that is potentially mutagenic.[7]

Effects on the Eye

In adults, more than 99% of UVR is absorbed by the anterior structure of the eye, although some of it reaches the retina.[35] Acute exposure to UVR can result in photokeratitis.[36] Gazing directly into the sun (as can occur during an eclipse) can cause focal burns to the retina (solar retinopathy).[37] Chronic exposure to solar UVB is associated with an increased risk of cataracts.[38] Melanoma of the uveal tract, the most common primary intraocular malignant neoplasm in adults, is associated with light skin color, blond hair, and blue eyes.

Effects on the Immune System

UVR exposure is thought to have 2 effects: skin cancer induction and immune suppression, which is increasingly recognized as important in the development of skin cancer.[39] Experiments in mice chronically exposed to UVR show that tumors induced by UVR are highly antigenic and are recognized and rejected by animals with normal immune systems. The tumors grow progressively, however, when transplanted into mice, whose immune systems are compromised.[39] UVR exposure induces "systemic" immune suppression so that exposure on one body site suppresses the immune response when the antigen is introduced at a distant site that was not irradiated.[39]

Skin cancers are common in people exposed to immunosuppressive agents. In people with renal transplants, lifelong immunosuppressive treatment needed for adequate graft function leads to a reduction of immunosurveillance and an increased risk of various cancers, including nonmelanoma skin cancer. People who have had renal transplants also have an increased incidence of melanoma.[40] Because ongoing immunosurveillance is lacking, skin cancers in people who have received organ transplants are likely to behave aggressively with higher rates of local recurrence and a greater tendency to be invasive and metastatic.[41]

ARTIFICIAL SOURCES OF UVR

Sunlamps and sunbeds are the main sources of artificial UVR used for deliberate purposes. The "tanning industry" has grown quickly, with $5 billion of annual revenue, up from $1 billion in 1992.[42] Twenty-eight million visits are made to the 50 000 tanning facilities in the United States each year.[39] Artificial tanning is a common practice among teenagers, especially girls.[43,44]

Tanning beds primarily emit UVA radiation, although a small amount (<5%) is in the UVB range.[45] In terms of biological activity, the intensity of UVA radiation produced by large, powerful tanning units may be 10 to 15 times higher than that of the midday sun. Frequent indoor tanners may receive an annual UVA dose that is 1.2 to 4.7 times more than that received from sun exposure.[42] The intensity of tanning bed exposure is a new phenomenon and is not found in nature.

Artificial UVR exposure has been repeatedly shown to induce erythema and sunburn. Erythema or burning effects were reported by 18% to 55% of users of indoor tanning equipment in Europe and North America.[45] Even though UVB is much more potent than UVA in causing sunburn, high fluxes of UVA can cause erythema in individuals sensitive to sunlight. In people who tan easily, exposure to tanning appliances will lead first to immediate pigment darkening. A more permanent tan will occur with accumulated exposure, depending on individual tanning ability and the amount of UVB present in the light spectrum of the tanning lamps. Immediate pigment darkening has no photoprotective effect against UVR-induced erythema or sunburn.

Other frequently-reported effects of artificial tanning include skin dryness, pruritus, nausea, photodrug reactions, disease exacerbation (eg, systemic lupus erythematosus), and disease induction (eg, polymorphous light eruption). Long-term health effects include skin aging, effects on the eyes (eg, cataract formation), and carcinogenesis. A case-control study demonstrated a significant association between using any tanning device and the incidence of squamous cell carcinoma and basal cell carcinoma.[46] In 2006, the International Agency for Research on Cancer published an updated analysis of studies of the carcinogenicity of artificial UVR with regard to melanoma, squamous cell carcinoma, and basal cell carcinoma.[45] Any previous use of sunbeds was positively associated with melanoma (summary relative risk, 1.15; 95% confidence interval

[CI], 1.00–1.31), although there was no consistent evidence of a dose-response relationship. First exposure to tanning beds before age 35 significantly increased the risk of melanoma on the basis of 7 studies (summary relative risk, 1.75; 95% CI, 1.35–2.26). The summary relative risk of 3 studies of squamous cell carcinoma showed an increased risk. Studies did not support an association for basal cell carcinoma. The evidence did not support a protective effect of the use of tanning beds against damage to the skin from subsequent sun exposure.

In July 2009, the International Agency for Research on Cancer elevated UVR from tanning beds to a group 1 carcinogen, meaning "carcinogenic to humans." The group 1 designation places tanning beds in the same category as plutonium, tobacco, and asbestos.[47]

Because of mounting evidence about the carcinogenicity of artificial UVR, support for regulations to limit teenagers' access to tanning facilities has been widespread.[45] Currently (as of April 2011), more than 60% of states regulate tanning facilities for minors.[48] Some states completely ban salon access to children younger than 14 years, and other states ban access to those younger than 15 or 16 years. Some states require written parental consent or written consent with the parent present at the facility or a doctor's prescription. However, tanning legislation is often not enforced.[49]

There is some evidence that indoor tanning may be addictive in certain individuals.[50]

TREATMENT

Pediatricians will rarely encounter patients with nonmelanoma skin cancer or melanoma. Patients at high risk, including children with xeroderma pigmentosum and related disorders and those with a large number of nevi and a family history of melanoma, should be followed in collaboration with a dermatologist. Sunburns should be treated with cool compresses and analgesics. Instruction about preventing future sunburns should be given at the time of the burn.

PREVENTION OF EXPOSURE

Pediatricians have an important role in educating families about preventing skin cancer, beginning in infancy, and later when developmental stages result in new patterns of sun exposure (eg, when the child begins to walk, before starting school, and before entering adolescence). All parents and children should receive advice about protection from UVR. Not all children sunburn easily, but people of all skin types can experience skin cancer, skin aging, and sun-related damage to the immune system. Children who should receive special attention include those with xeroderma pigmentosum (who must avoid all UVR) and those with familial dysplastic nevus syndrome, with excessive numbers of nevi, or with first degree family members with melanoma. Children showing signs of excessive sun exposure (eg, freckles and/or nevi) also should receive special instruction. Performing a careful skin examination as part of a complete physical examination seems prudent and affords an opportunity to provide specific counseling.

Preteens and teenagers may need special reinforcement, because they often are susceptible to societal notions of beauty and health. Teen counseling should include a recommendation not to patronize tanning salons for any reason, including the desire for a "prevacation" or "preprom" tan.

Leading organizations (the American Cancer Society,[51] Centers for Disease Control and Prevention [CDC],[52] Healthy People,[53] National Council on Skin Cancer Prevention[54]) have recommended UVR-protective behaviors that include:

1. Do not burn. Avoid sun tanning and tanning beds.
2. Wear protective clothing and hats.
3. Seek shade.
4. Use extra caution near water, snow, and sand.
5. Apply sunscreen.
6. Wear sunglasses.

Avoiding Exposure

Because children and adolescents continue to experience high rates of sunburning,[55] advice about avoiding sunburning may be given during routine visits and at other times, such as when the child is noted to have a tan or presents with a sunburn.

Infants younger than 6 months should be kept out of direct sunlight. They should be dressed in cool, comfortable clothing and wear hats with brims. Whenever feasible, children's activities may be planned to limit peak-intensity midday sun (10 AM–4 PM). Advice should be framed in the context of promoting outdoor play, other physical activity, and visiting parks, zoos, and other natural environments.

Clothing and Hats

Clothes offer the simplest and often most practical means of sun protection. Protective factors in clothing include style, weave, and chemical enhancement. Clothes that cover more of the body provide more protection; sun-protective styles cover to the neck, elbows, and knees. A tighter weave lets in less sunlight than a looser weave. Darker clothes generally offer more protection. Treating fabrics with chemical absorbers or washing them with optical brighteners (dyes that absorb light in the ultraviolet and violet region of the electromagnetic spectrum and re-emit light in the blue region) increases UVR protectiveness.

The ultraviolet protection factor (UPF) measures a fabric's ability to block UVR from passing through the fabric and reaching the skin. The UPF is classified from 15 to 50+; 15 to 24 is rated as "Good," 25 to 39 is rated "Very Good," and 40 to 50+ is rated "Excellent" UV protection. The UPF of fabrics can be altered by shrinking, stretching, and wetness. Shrinking increases the UPF; stretching decreases the UPF. If cotton fabrics get wet, the UPF decreases. The US Federal Trade Commission monitors advertising claims about sun-protective clothing.[56]

Hats provide variable protection for head and neck, depending on the brim width, material, and weave. A wide-brimmed hat (3 inches) provides an SPF of 7 for the nose, 3 for the cheek, 5 for the neck, and 2 for the chin. Medium-brimmed hats (1–3 inches) provide an SPF of 3 for nose, 2 for the cheek and neck, and none for the chin. A narrow-brimmed hat provides an SPF of 1.5 for the nose but little protection for the chin and neck.[4]

Shade

Seeking shade is somewhat useful, but people can still sunburn, because light is scattered and reflected. A fair-skinned person sitting under a tree can burn in less than an hour. Shade provides relief from heat, possibly providing a false sense of security about UVR protection. Clouds decrease UVR intensity but not to the same extent that they decrease heat intensity, which also may result in overexposure.[4]

Window Glass

Standard clear window glass window glass absorbs wavelengths below 320 nm (UVB). UVA, visible light, and infrared radiation are transmitted through standard clear window glass.[57]

Sunscreen

Sunscreen is the method of sun protection most commonly used. Sunscreens reduce the intensity of UVR affecting the epidermis, thus preventing erythema and sunburn. Formulating, testing, and labeling of sunscreen products are regulated by the US Food and Drug Administration (FDA). Most FDA-approved sunscreen agents are organic chemicals that absorb various wavelengths of UVR, primarily in the UVB range; others are effective in the UVA range. Some agents are not photostable in the UVA range and degrade with sun exposure. Combinations of chemicals are needed to provide broad-spectrum protection and increase photostability.[58] The 2 FDA-approved physical sunscreens, zinc oxide and titanium dioxide, do not selectively absorb UVR but reflect and scatter all light. They are useful for patients with photosensitivity and other disorders who require protection from full-spectrum UVR. Because physical sunscreens are usually white or tinted after application, they may be cosmetically unacceptable. Some newer formulations are less visible on the skin but may be less effective.[58]

The sun protection factor (SPF) is a grading system developed to quantify the degree of protection from erythema provided by using a sunscreen. SPF pertains only to UVB; the higher the SPF, the greater the protection. For example, a person who would normally experience a sunburn in 10 minutes can be protected up to about 150 minutes (10 x 15) with an SPF-15 sunscreen. Sunscreens with an SPF of 15 or more theoretically filter more than 92% (1/15th) of the UVB responsible for erythema; sunscreens with an SPF of 30 filter out approximately 97% (1/30th) of the UVB. In actual use, the SPF often is substantially lower than expected, because the amount used is less than half the recommended amount.[59] An SPF of 15 should be adequate in most cases. For most users, proper application and reapplication are more important factors than using a product with a higher SPF. Products with a higher SPF have been recommended for some people, including those who have had skin cancer.[60]

The FDA has approved 17 sunscreen chemicals for use in the United States. Several more are available in the European Union. Four chemicals effective in the UVA range have been approved for use in the United States. In May 1999, the FDA published its final rule for over-the-counter sunscreen products that protect against UVB. Regulations concerning UVA were delayed until reliable testing methods could be developed. In June 2011, the FDA issued new rules regarding labeling of sunscreen products. Previous rules dealt almost exclusively with protection against UVB only. The 2011 FDA rule established a standard broad-spectrum test procedure to measure UVA radiation protection in relation to UVB radiation protection. Sunscreen products that pass the broad-spectrum test are allowed to be labeled as "Broad Spectrum," indicating protection against UVB and UVA. For "Broad Spectrum" sunscreens, the SPF also indicates the overall amount of protection provided. For Broad Spectrum sunscreens with SPF values of 15 or higher, FDA allows manufacturers to claim that these formulations help protect against not only sunburn but also skin cancer and early skin aging when used as directed with other sun-protection measures. These sun-protection measures include limiting time in the sun and wearing protective clothing. For sunscreen products labeled with SPF values but not as "Broad Spectrum," FDA states that the SPF value indicates the amount of protection against sunburn only. The new rule also states that manufacturers cannot label sunscreens as "waterproof" or "sweatproof" or identify their products as "sunblock," because these claims overstate effectiveness. Sunscreens cannot claim to provide sun protection for more than 2 hours without reapplication or to provide protection immediately after application (eg, "instant protection") without submitting data to support these claims and obtaining FDA approval. Water resistance claims on the front label must indicate whether the product remains effective for 40 minutes or 80 minutes while swimming or sweating, based on standard testing. Sunscreens that are not water resistant must include a direction instructing consumers to use a water-resistant sunscreen if swimming or sweating. All sunscreens must include standard "Drug Facts" information on the back and/or side of the container. These rules were not scheduled to take effect for 1 year (2 years for smaller sunscreen manufacturers), although consumers may start seeing labeling changes earlier.[61] Another rule currently proposed by the FDA would limit the maximum SPF value on sunscreen labels to "50+" because the FDA states that there are not sufficient data to show that products with SPF values higher than 50 provide greater protection for users than products with SPF values of 50.[62]

Regular use of a broad-spectrum sunscreen preparation has been shown to prevent solar (actinic) keratoses, lesions that may evolve to become squamous cell carcinoma.[63,64] One randomized clinical trial showed that regular sunscreen use compared with no regular sunscreen use decreased the incidence of squamous cell carcinoma.[65] In contrast, the role of sunscreen in preventing melanoma and basal cell carcinoma has not been fully elucidated. Some research has shown that sunscreen users have a higher risk of melanoma and basal cell carcinoma and more nevi.[66] These observations have led to concern that people who use sunscreens spend more time in the sun because they do not sunburn.[67] Two reviews, however, did not support the association between sunscreen use and an increased risk of melanoma.[68,69] Recently published results of a randomized trial of regular sunscreen use for a 5-year period appeared to reduce the incidence of new primary melanomas for up to 10 years after trial cessation.[70] The American Cancer Society, the American Academy of Dermatology, and many other organizations recommend sunscreen use as part of an overall program of reducing UVR exposure.

Sunscreens may be systemically absorbed. In 1 study, sunscreen products were studied in vitro to assess the extent of absorption following application to excised human skin. Half of the products were marketed specifically for children. Of the 5 chemical sunscreen ingredients present in the products, only oxybenzone (benzophenone-3 or BP-3) penetrated skin.[71] In another report, CDC researchers examined more than 2500 urine samples collected during 2003–2004 for oxybenzone. The samples selected were representative of the US population 6 years and older as part of the National Health and Nutrition Examination Survey (NHANES), an ongoing survey that assesses the health and nutritional status of the US civilian population. The analysis found oxybenzone in 97% of the samples,[72] suggesting widespread exposure of the population. Females and non-Hispanic white people had the highest concentrations regardless of age. Data are not available for children younger than 6 years. Sunscreen ingredients have been found in human milk.[73]

Studies in rats have shown alterations in liver, kidney, and reproductive organs in rats given oral or transepidermal doses of oxybenzone.[74] A study of 6 UVB and UVA commonly used sunscreens was conducted to determine estrogenicity in vivo and in vitro. Five of the 6 sunscreen ingredients (BP-3, homosalate, 4-methyl-benzylidene camphor [4-MBC], octyl methoxycin-namate [OMC], and octyl-dimethly-PABA) increased cell proliferation in breast cancer cells, and the sixth ingredient, butyl-methoxydibenzoylmethane (avoben-zone), was inactive. In the in vivo analysis, rats fed the sunscreen ingredients OMC, 4-MBC, and BP-3 showed dose-dependent increases in uterine weight. Epidermal application of one of the products (4-MBC) also increased uterine weight.[75] Researchers investigating human prenatal exposures to phthalate and phenol metabolites and their relationship to birth weight found that higher maternal concentrations of BP-3 were associated with a decrease in birth weight in girls but a greater birth weight in boys.[76]

Sunscreen products containing zinc and titanium oxides are increasingly manufactured using nanotechnology—the design and manipulation of materials on atomic and molecular scales. Nanoscale particles are measured in nanome-ters (nm), or billionths of a meter. Using nanoscale particles renders products containing zinc and titanium oxides nearly transparent, increasing cosmetic acceptability. Concerns have been raised, however, about the dearth of safety information available about nanoscale ingredients, including to skin that is damaged by sunburn. There are no data available about the effects of these products on infants and children. Advocacy groups have called on the FDA to require more testing and increased regulatory oversight.

Sunscreens should be used when a child might sunburn. There is no benefit in burning, and it should be avoided. Using sunscreen is recommended to decrease the known risks of sun exposure and sunburning, both of which increase the risk of developing skin cancer

The issue of whether sunscreen is safe for infants younger than 6 months is controversial. There are concerns that skin in infants younger than 6 months may have different absorptive characteristics and that biological systems that metabolize and excrete drugs may not be fully developed.[77] This is of particular concern for preterm infants, in whom the stratum corneum of the epidermis is thinner and a less effective barrier than that of full-term newborn infants and adults. Toxicity in infants and children from absorption of sunscreen ingredients, however, has not been reported. On the basis of available evidence, it is reason-able to tell parents what is known about the safety of sunscreens in infants younger than 6 months and to emphasize the importance of avoiding high-risk exposure. In situations in which the infant's skin is not protected adequately by clothing, it may be reasonable to apply sunscreen to small areas, such as the face and the backs of the hands.

Preparations that contain a combination of sunscreen with the insecticide N-N-diethyl-m-toluamide (DEET) should not be used, because they may result in overexposure to DEET (see Chapter 37).

The Ultraviolet (UV) Index

The UV index was developed in 1994 by the National Weather Service in consultation with the US Environmental Protection Agency (EPA) and the CDC. The UV index predicts the intensity of UV light for the following day on the basis of the sun's position, cloud movements, altitude, ozone data, and other factors. It is conservatively calculated on the basis of effects on skin types that burn easily. Higher numbers predict more intense UV light during midday of the following day: 0-2 = minimal; 3-4 = low; 5-6 = moderate; 7-9 = high; and 10+ = very high, with greater recommended avoidance behaviors as the UV index increases (eg, avoiding outdoor exposures from 10 am to 4 pm if UV index is 7 or higher). The index is available online for thousands of cities at http://www.weather.com. It is printed in the weather section of many daily newspapers and reported through weather reports of local radio, television, and weather stations.

Sunglasses

Sunglasses protect against sun glare and harmful radiation. The first sunglass standard was published in Australia in 1971; standards were subsequently adopted in Europe and the United States. The latest US sunglass standard was published in 2001 by the American National Standards Institute. This standard is voluntary and is not followed by all manufacturers.[57]

Major US visual health organizations recommend that sunglasses absorb 97% to 100%[78] or 99% to 100%[36] of the full UV spectrum (up to 400 nm). Expensive sunglasses do not necessarily provide better UVR protection. Purchasing sunglasses that meet standards for a safe level of UVR should be the goal. Wearing a hat with a brim can greatly reduce the UVR exposure to the eyes and surrounding skin. It is recommended that people wear sunglasses outdoors when working, driving, participating in sports, taking a walk, or running errands.[79] Sunglasses for infants and children are available.

VITAMIN D

Sun exposure and vitamin D concentrations are intricately intertwined. Humans get vitamin D from exposure to sun, from dietary sources (such as fortified milk and oily fish), and from vitamin supplements. Vitamin D synthesis in skin depends on skin type. An individual who burns easily after a first moderate UVR exposure will rapidly achieve maximal vitamin D synthesis. In contrast, dark-skinned individuals will have relatively limited vitamin D synthesis, because UVR will be absorbed by melanin rather than other cellular targets.[80] Because excess previtamin D_3 or vitamin D_3 is destroyed by sunlight, exposure to sunlight does not cause vitamin D intoxication.[81] The action spectrum that induces cutaneous vitamin D_3 synthesis is in the UVB range.[82]

Vitamin D is essential for normal growth and skeletal development. The actions of vitamin D that extend beyond bone mineral metabolism are increasingly becoming understood.[83] Many children, adolescents, and adults have insufficient or deficient levels of vitamin D.[83] Vitamin D is available through foods, supplements, and incidental sun exposure. Because current intake levels of vitamin D by children and adolescents may not prevent vitamin D deficiency, the AAP recommends that breastfed infants (as well as infants who consume less than 1000 mL of infant formula per day, older children, and teenagers) should receive daily supplementation with 400 IU of vitamin D.[84] The Institute of Medicine and others have recommended that children older than 1 year receive a daily supplement of 600 IU of vitamin D; infants younger than 1 year should receive 400 IU daily.[85,86] Additional vitamin D supplementation and laboratory evaluations of vitamin D status may be needed for some children in some areas. Overexposure to UVR from sunlight and exposure to UVR from artificial sources increase the risk of skin cancer, photoaging, and other adverse effects and should be avoided.

CHALLENGES

Pediatricians alone cannot change social concepts in which a suntan is equated with health and beauty. School programs and public education campaigns must continue to address this issue.

Several challenges to successful skin cancer prevention efforts have been identified.[87] First, sun-protection messages to avoid or limit time during peak sun hours may conflict with messages to promote physical activity. This potential conflict may be resolved by following the example of Australia, the country with the world's highest incidence of melanoma, to "Slip, Slop, Slap"—slip on a shirt, slop on some sunscreen, and slap on a hat. This message is consistent with conducting outdoor physical activity in a sun-protective manner. Next, there is controversy about how much sun exposure is needed for vitamin D synthesis, possibly resulting in excessive exposure to sun and deliberate exposure to artificial UVR. Third, it has been reported that skin cancer risk behaviors cluster with other risky behaviors, such as smoking and risky drinking. A greater understanding of these behaviors may help with interventions in high-risk groups. Lastly, the increasingly profitable tanning industry benefits from unrestrained selling of UVR. These challenges suggest that it is uncertain whether primary prevention efforts to reduce skin cancer through UVR protection will be successful.

Frequently Asked Questions

Q *Why is a baby at special risk from sunburn?*

A A baby's skin is thinner than an adult's and burns more easily. Even dark-skinned babies may be sunburned. Babies cannot tell you if they are too hot or beginning to burn and cannot get out of the sun without an adult's help. Babies also need an adult to dress them properly and to apply sunscreen.

Q *What can I do to protect my child?*

A Babies younger than 6 months should be kept out of direct sunlight because of the risk of heat stroke. They should be moved under a tree, umbrella, or stroller canopy, although on reflective surfaces, an umbrella or canopy may reduce UVR exposure by only 50%.

To avoid sunburn, infants and children may be dressed in cool, comfortable clothing, such as shirts and pants made of cotton, and should wear hats. Swimwear and other garments made of materials with high UPF ratings are available in stores and through the Internet. Sunscreen should be applied to the parts of the skin that will be exposed to the sun. Parents should apply sunscreen liberally and rub it in well before going outdoors, covering all exposed areas, especially the child's face, nose, ears, feet and hands, and the backs of the knees. Sunscreen should be used even on cloudy days, because the sun's rays can penetrate through the clouds. When choosing a sunscreen, parents should look for the words "broad-spectrum" on the label, meaning that the sunscreen will screen out most of the UVB and UVA rays. An SPF of 15 should be adequate in most cases. It is important to reapply after sweating or swimming. It is also important to remember that using sunscreen is only one part of a total program of sun protection. Sunscreens should be used to prevent burning and not as a reason to stay in the sun longer. Sunscreen may be applied to infants who are younger than 6 months to small areas of skin uncovered by clothing and hats.

Q *What factors in clothing can offer protection against sunburn?*

A Some fabrics have a UPF rating showing how much sun protection they offer. Even if a fabric does not have a UPF rating, it may offer excellent sun protection. Some fabrics, such as polyester crepe, bleached cotton, and viscose, are quite transparent to UVR and should be avoided in the sun. Other fibers, such as unbleached cotton, can absorb UVR. High-luster polyesters and even thin, satiny silk can be highly protective, because they reflect radiation. A fabric's weave also is important; in general, the tighter the weave or knit, the higher the protection offered. To assess protection, parents can hold the material up to a window or lamp and see how much light gets through. Darker clothes also generally offer more protection. Virtually all garments lose about a third of their sun-protective ability when wet.

Q *I'm concerned that using sunscreen on my child when she goes outside will lead to a low vitamin D level. Is this true?*

A Vitamin D helps the body to absorb calcium and so is needed for bone health in infants, children, teens and adults. The other actions of vitamin D are being studied by researchers. Although vitamin D is generated when the skin is exposed to direct sunlight, exposing the skin to the sun's ultraviolet rays raises the risk of developing skin cancer. Fortunately, vitamin D is available from certain foods (such as dairy products, salmon, and sardines) and vitamin supplements. Infants and children should, therefore, be protected from sun exposure with clothing, hats, and sunscreen. To ensure that infants and young children are protected from rickets (a bone disease that occurs when vitamin D levels are very low), the American Academy of Pediatrics recommends that all breastfed infants (as well as infants consuming less than 1000 mL of infant formula per day) receive daily supplementation with 400 International Units (IU) of vitamin D.[84]

The American Academy of Pediatrics recommends that older children and teenagers also receive 400 IU of vitamin D per day.[84] The Institute of Medicine and others recommend 600 IU of vitamin D per day for these age groups.[85,86]

Deliberate sun exposure or using tanning salons as a way to increase vitamin D levels, or for other reasons, raises skin cancer risk and should be avoided.

Q *I've heard that some sunscreen ingredients are absorbed into the body and aren't safe. What should I do?*

A Scientific research shows that some sunscreen chemicals are absorbed by people. Studies in laboratory animals show that some chemical sunscreen ingredients have hormone-like effects. There is concern that the vitamin A derivatives retinol and retinyl palmitate, added to many sunscreens, may raise cancer risk. The physical sunscreens titanium dioxide and zinc oxide are increasingly manufactured through nanotechnology, a new method that uses tiny particles. It is possible that these particles may be absorbed into the body; there are no research studies in children about this technology.

These concerns must be weighed against the known risks of sun exposure and sunburning. Keeping these pros and cons in mind, it is reasonable to use sunscreen with the goals of preventing sunburning and possibly decreasing the risk of certain skin cancers. Sunscreen use should be part of a total program of limiting sun exposure.

It may be prudent to avoid using products containing oxybenzone, a chemical with known hormone-like effects, especially on children.[83,88]

Q *Are tanning salons safe?*

A People who use sunlamps or go to tanning salons are exposed primarily to
UVA. The tan that occurs represents a protective response to the harmful
rays of the sun. Skin damage occurs whether a tan comes from the sun
itself or from artificial light from a tanning salon. Tanning in the tanning
salon raises the risk of developing skin cancer. Tanning salons are not safe
and should not be used by teenagers or others. The American Academy
of Pediatrics, the World Health Organization, the American Academy of
Dermatology, and the American Medical Association have urged states to
pass legislation that prohibits minors younger than 18 years from accessing
tanning salons.[83,88]

Q *Is using a spray tan safe?*

A "Spray tans," also known as "sunless" or "self-tanning" products, are
sometimes used by people to substitute for going outside or visiting a
tanning salon. Sunless tanners use dihydroxyacetone (DHA), a chemical
that reacts with amino acids in the stratum corneum (the top layer of skin)
to form brown-black compounds, melanoidins, which deposit in skin. DHA
is a mutagen that induces DNA strand breaks in certain strains of bacteria; it has not been shown to be carcinogenic in animal studies.[89] DHA is
the only color additive approved by the US FDA for use as a tanning agent.
DHA-containing tanning preparations may be applied to the consumer's
bare skin by misters at sunless tanning booths. Bronzers are water-soluble
dyes that temporarily stain the skin. Bronzers are easily removed with soap
and water.

   DHA-induced tans become apparent within 1 hour; maximal darkening occurs within 8 to 24 hours. Most users report that color disappears over
5 to 7 days. Because neither DHA nor melanoidins afford any significant
UVR protection, consumers must be advised that sunburn and sun damage
may occur unless they use sunscreen and other sun protection methods.
Consumers must also be warned that any sunless products containing added
sunscreen provide UVR protection during a few hours after application
and that additional sun protection must be used during the duration of the
artificial tan.

   Potential spray tan users may also be advised that it is probably healthier
to "love the skin you're in" rather than seeking a darker look.

Q *How do I choose sunglasses for my child?*

A There are no government regulations on the amount of UVR that sunglasses
must block. Sunglasses are regulated as medical devices by the FDA and may
be labeled as UV protective if they meet certain standards. Parents should
look for a label that states that the lenses block at least 99% of UVA and 99%
of UVB rays.

Protection is provided by a chemical coating applied to the lenses. Lens color has nothing to do with UV protection. Ski goggles and contact lenses with UV protection also are recommended.

It is never too early for a child, even an infant, to wear sunglasses. Larger lenses, well-fitted and close to the surface of the eye, provide the best protection.

Resources

American Academy of Pediatrics

Web site: www.aap.org
The AAP provides a patient education brochure titled "Fun in the Sun."

American Cancer Society

Web site: www.cancer.org

Centers for Disease Control and Prevention's Choose Your Cover Campaign

www.cdc.gov/ChooseYourCover

National Council on Skin Cancer Prevention

Web site: www.skincancerprevention.org
The council comprises organizations (including the AAP) whose staffs have experience, expertise, and knowledge in skin cancer prevention and education.

Skin Cancer Foundation

Web site: www.skincancer.org
The foundation is dedicated to nationwide public and professional education programs aimed at increasing public awareness, sun protection and sun safety, skin self-examination, children's education, melanoma understanding, and continuing medical education.

US Environmental Protection Agency SunWise Program

Web site: www.epa.gov/sunwise1/publications.html

World Health Organization (WHO)

Web site: www.who.int/en
Ultraviolet Radiation and Human Health:
www.who.int/mediacentre/factsheets/fs305/en/index.html
Sunbeds, tanning, and UV exposure:
www.who.int/mediacentre/factsheets/fs287/en/index.html

References

1. International Agency for Research on Cancer. *IARC Monographs on the Evaluation of Carcinogenic Risks to Humans. Volume 55. Solar and Ultraviolet Radiation. Summary of Data Reported and Evaluation.* Lyon, France: World Health Organization; 1997. Available at: http://monographs.iarc.fr/ENG/Monographs/vol55/volume55.pdf. Accessed April 3, 2011

2. Sparling B. *Basic Chemistry of Ozone Depletion.* Moffet Field, CA: NASA Advanced Supercomputing. Available at: http://www.nas.nasa.gov/About/Education/Ozone/chemistry. html. Accessed April 3, 2011

3. Kullavanijaya P, Lim HW. Photoprotection. *J Am Acad Dermatol.* 2005;52(6):937-958

4. Gilchrest BA. Actinic injury. *Annu Rev Med.* 1990;41:199–210

5. World Meteorological Organization. WMO UV Radiation Site. What is UV? Available at: http://uv.colorado.edu/what.html. Accessed April 3, 2011

6. Diffey BL. Ultraviolet radiation and human health. *Clin Dermatol.* 1998;16(1):83–89

7. Gilchrest BA, Eller MS, Geller AC, Yaar M. The pathogenesis of melanoma induced by ultraviolet radiation. *N Engl J Med.* 1999;340(17):1341–1348

8. Woo DK, Eide MJ. Tanning beds, skin cancer, and vitamin D: an examination of the scientific evidence and public health implications. *Dermatol Ther.* 2010;23(1):61-71

9. Weston WL, Lane AT, Morelli JG. Drug eruptions. In: *Color Textbook of Pediatric Dermatology.* St Louis, MO; Mosby; 2002:287-297

10. Obermoser G, Zelger B. Triple need for photoprotection in lupus erythematosus. *Lupus.* 2008;17(6):525–527

11. American Cancer Society. How Many People Get Basal and Squamous Cell Skin Cancers? http://www.cancer.org/Cancer/SkinCancer-BasalandSquamousCell/OverviewGuide/skin-cancer-basal-and-squamous-cell-overview-key-statistics. Accessed April 3, 2011

12. Christenson LJ, Borrowman TA, Vachon CM, et al. Incidence of basal cell and squamous cell carcinomas in a population younger than 40 years. *JAMA.* 2005;294(6):681-690

13. Markovic SN, Erickson LA, Rao RD, et al. Malignant melanoma in the 21st century, part 1: epidemiology, risk factors, screening, prevention, and diagnosis. *Mayo Clin Proc.* 2007;82(3): 364-380

14. Jemal A, Siegel R, Ward E, et al. Cancer statistics, 2009. *CA Cancer J Clin.* 2009;59(4):225-249

15. Rigel DS. Cutaneous ultraviolet exposure and its relationship to the development of skin cancer. *J Am Acad Dermatol.* 2008;58(5 Suppl 2):S129–S132

16. American Cancer Society. *How Many People Get Melanoma?* Available at: http://www.cancer. org/Cancer/SkinCancer-Melanoma/OverviewGuide/melanoma-skin-cancer-overview-key-statistics. Accessed April 3, 2011

17. Wu X, Groves FD, McLaughlin CC, Jemal A, Martin J, Chen VS. Cancer incidence patterns among adolescents and young adults in the United States. *Cancer Causes Control.* 2005;16(3):309–320

18. Purdue MP, Beane Freeman LE, Anderson WF, Tucker MA. Recent trends in incidence of cutaneous melanoma among us Caucasian young adults. *J Invest Dermatol.* 2008;128(12): 2906-2908

19. Ferrari A, Bono A, Baldi M, et al. Does melanoma behave differently in younger children than in adults? A retrospective study of 33 cases of childhood melanoma from a single institution. *Pediatrics.* 2005;115(3):649-654

20. Surveillance Epidemiology and End Results (SEER). Cancer Stat Fact Sheets. Melanoma of the Skin. Available at: http://www.seer.cancer.gov/statfacts/html/melan.html. Accessed April 3, 2011

21. Armstrong BK, Kricker A. The epidemiology of UV induced skin cancer. *J Photochem Photobiol B*. 2001;63(1-3):8-18

22. de Gruijl FR, van Kranen HJ, Mullenders LH. UV-induced DNA damage, repair, mutations and oncogenic pathways in skin cancer. *J Photochem Photobiol B*. 2001;63(1-3):19–27

23. Godar DE, Wengraitis SP, Shreffler J, Sliney DH. UV doses of Americans. *Photochem Photobiol*. 2001;73(6):621-629

24. Whiteman DC, Whiteman CA, Green AC. Childhood sun exposure as a risk factor for melanoma: a systematic review of epidemiologic studies. *Cancer Causes Control*. 2001;12(1): 69–82

25. Pfahlberg A, Kolmel K-F, Gefeller O. Timing of excessive ultraviolet radiation and melanoma: epidemiology does not support the existence of a critical period of high susceptibility to solar ultraviolet radiation-induced melanoma. *Br J Dermatol*. 2001;144(3):471–475

26. Gallagher RP, McLean DI, Yang CP, et al. Suntan, sunburn, and pigmentation factors and the frequency of acquired melanocytic nevi in children. Similarities to melanoma: the Vancouver Mole Study. *Arch Dermatol*. 1990;126(6):770–776

27. Holman CD, Armstrong BK. Pigmentary traits, ethnic origin, benign nevi, and family history as risk factors for cutaneous malignant melanoma. *J Natl Cancer Inst*. 1984;72(2):257–266

28. Krengel S, Hauschild A, Schafer T. Melanoma risk in congenital melanocytic naevi: a systematic review. *B J Dermatol*. 2006;155(1):1–8

29. Naeyaert JM, Brochez L. Dysplastic nevi. *N Engl J Med*. 2003;349(23):2233-2240

30. Clark WH Jr. The dysplastic nevus syndrome. *Arch Dermatol*. 1988;124(8):1207–1210

31. Tucker MA, Fraser MC, Goldstein AM, et al. A natural history of melanomas and dysplastic nevi: an atlas of lesions in melanoma-prone families. *Cancer*. 2002;94(12):3192–3209

32. Ley RD. Ultraviolet radiation A-induced precursors of cutaneous melanoma in Monodelphis domestica. *Cancer Res*. 1997;57(17):3682–3684

33. De Gruijl FR, Sterenborg HJ, Forbes PD, Davies RE, Cole C, Kelfkens G. Wavelength dependence of skin cancer induction by ultraviolet irradiation of albino hairless mice. *Cancer Res*. 1993;53(1):53-60

34. Atillasoy ES, Seykora JT, Soballe PW, et al. UVB induces atypical melanocytic lesions and melanoma in human skin. *Am J Pathol*. 1998;152(5):1179–1186

35. American Optometric Association. Statement on Ocular Ultraviolet Radiation Hazards in Sunlight. St Louis, MO: American Optometric Association; 1993

36. American Optometric Association. UV Protection. Available at: http://www.aoa.org/uv-protection.xml. Accessed April 3, 2011

37. Wong SC, Eke T, Ziakas NG. Eclipse burns: a prospective study of solar retinopathy following the 1999 solar eclipse. *Lancet*. 2001;357(9282):199–200

38. American Academy of Ophthalmology. Cataracts. Available at: http://www.aao.org/eyesmart/know/cataracts.cfm. Accessed April 3, 2011

39. Ullrich SE. Sunlight and skin cancer: lessons from the immune system. *Mol Carcinog*. 2007;46(8):629–633

40. Hollenbeak CS, Todd MM, Billingsley EM, Harper G, Dyer A, Lengerick EJ. Increased incidence of melanoma in renal transplant patients. *Cancer*. 2005;104(9):1962–1967

41. Ho WL, Murphy GM. Update on the pathogenesis of post-transplant skin cancer in renal transplant recipients. *Br J Dermatol*. 2008;158(3):217-224

42. Levine JA, Sorace M, Spencer J, Siegel D. The indoor UV tanning industry: a review of skin cancer risk, health benefit claims. *J Am Acad Dermatol*. 2005;53(6):1038–1044

43. Demko CA, Borawski EA, Debanne SM, Cooper KD, Stange KC . Use of indoor tanning facilities by white adolescents in the United States. *Arch Pediatr Adolesc Med*. 2003;157(9): 854-860

44. Cokkinides VE, Weinstock MA, O'Connell MC, Thun MJ. Use of indoor tanning sunlamps by US youth, ages 11-18 years, and by their parent or guardian caregivers: Prevalence and correlates. *Pediatrics*. 2002;109(6):1124-1130

45. International Agency for Research on Cancer Working Group on artificial ultraviolet (UV) light and skin cancer. The association of use of sunbeds with cutaneous malignant melanoma and other skin cancers: a systematic review. *Int J Cancer*. 2006;120(5):1116–1122

46. Karagas M, Stannard VA, Mott LA, Slattery MJ, Spencer SK, Weinstock MA. Use of tanning devices and risk of basal cell and squamous cell skin cancers. *J Natl Cancer Inst*. 2002;94(3): 224-226

47. International Agency for Research in Cancer. Sunbeds and UV Radiation. Available at: http://www.iarc.fr/en/media-centre/iarcnews/2009/sunbeds_uvradiation.php. Accessed April 3, 2011

48. National Conference of State Legislatures. Tanning restrictions for minors. A state-by-state comparison. Available at: www.ncsl.org/programs/health/tanningrestrictions.htm. Accessed April 3, 2011

49. Mayer JA, Hoerster KD, Pichon LC, Rubio DA, Woodruff SI, Forster JL. Enforcement of state indoor tanning laws in the United States. *Prev Chronic Dis*. 2008;5(4). Available at: http://www.cdc.gov/pcd/issues/2008/oct/07_0194.htm. Accessed April 3, 2011

50. Mosher CE, Danoff-Burg, S. Addiction to indoor Tanning. Relation to anxiety, depression, and substance use. *Arch Dermatol*. 2010;146(4):412-417

51. American Cancer Society. Skin Cancer Prevention and Early Detection. Available at: http://www.cancer.org/docroot/PED/content/ped_7_1_Skin_Cancer_Detection_What_You_Can_Do.asp?sitearea=&level. Accessed April 3, 2011

52. Centers for Disease Control and Prevention. Guidelines for school programs to prevent skin cancer. *MMWR Recomm Rep*. 2002;51(RR-4):1-16. Available at: www.cdc.gov/mmwr/preview/mmwrhtml/rr5104a1.htm. Accessed April 3, 2011

53. US Department of Health and Human Services. *Healthy People 2020*. Available at: http://www.healthypeople.gov/2020/topicsobjectives2020/objectiveslist.aspx?topicid=5. Accessed April 16, 2011.

54. National Council on Skin Cancer Prevention. *Skin Cancer Prevention Tips*. Available at: http://www.skincancerprevention.org/Tips/tabid/54/Default.aspx. Accessed April 3, 2011

55. Geller AC, Colditz G, Oliveria S, et al. Use of sunscreen, sunburning rates, and tanning bed use among more than 10 000 US children and adolescents. *Pediatrics*. 2002;109(6):1009-1014

56. US Federal Trade Commission. *FTC Consumer Alert. Sun-Protective Clothing: Wear It Well*. May 2001. Available at: http://www.ftc.gov/bcp/edu/pubs/consumer/alerts/alt094.shtm. Accessed April 3, 2011

57. Tuchinda C, Srivannaboon S, Lim HW. Photoprotection by window glass, automobile glass, and sunglasses. *J Am Acad Dermatol*. 2006;54(5):845–854

58. A new sunscreen agent. *Med Lett Drugs Ther*. 2007;49(1261):41–43

59. Prevention and treatment of sunburn. *Med Lett Drugs Ther*. 2004;46(1184):45–46

60. The Skin Cancer Foundation. Sunscreens Explained. Available at: http://www.skincancer.org/sunscreens-explained.html. Accessed April 3, 2011

61. US Food and Drug Administration. Questions and Answers: FDA announces new requirements for over-the-counter (OTC) sunscreen products marketed in the U.S. Available at: http://www.fda.gov/Drugs/ResourcesForYou/Consumers/BuyingUsingMedicineSafely/UnderstandingOver-the-CounterMedicines/ucm258468.htm. Accessed June 22, 2011

62. US Food and Drug Administration. Revised Effectiveness Determination; Sunscreen Drug Products for Over-the-Counter Human Use. Proposed Rule. Available at: http://www.gpo.gov/fdsys/pkg/FR-2011-06-17/pdf/2011-14769.pdf. Accessed June 22, 2011

63. Thompson SC, Jolley D, Marks R. Reduction of solar keratoses by regular sunscreen use. *N Engl J Med.* 1993;329(16):1147–1151

64. Naylor MF, Boyd A, Smith DW, Cameron GS, Hubbard D, Nelder KH. High sun protection factor sunscreens in the suppression of actinic neoplasia. *Arch Dermatol.* 1995;131(2):170–175

65. Green A, Williams G, Neale R, et al. Daily sunscreen application and betacarotene supplementation in prevention of basal-cell and squamous-cell carcinomas of the skin: a randomised controlled trial. *Lancet.* 1999;354(9180):723–729

66. Autier P, Dore JF, Cattaruzza MS, et al. Sunscreen use, wearing clothes, and number of nevi in 6- to 7-year-old European children. European Organization for Research and Treatment of Cancer Melanoma Cooperative Group. *J Natl Cancer Inst.* 1998;90(24):1873–1880

67. Autier P, Dore JF, Negrier S, et al. Sunscreen use and duration of sun exposure: a double-blind, randomized trial. *J Natl Cancer Inst.* 1999;91(15):1304–1309

68. Huncharek M, Kupelnick B. Use of topical sunscreens and the risk of malignant melanoma: a meta-analysis of 9067 patients from 11 case-control studies. *Am J Public Health.* 2002;92(7):1173–1177

69. Dennis LK, Beane Freeman LE, VanBeek MJ. Sunscreen use and the risk for melanoma: a quantitative review. *Ann Intern Med.* 2003;139(12):966–978

70. Green AC, Williams GM, Logan V, Strutton GM. Reduced melanoma after regular sunscreen use: randomized trial follow-up. *J Clin Oncol.* 2010;29:257-263

71. Jiang R, Roberts MS, Collins DM, Benson HAE. Absorption of sunscreens across human skin: an evaluation of commercial products for children and adults. *Br J Clin Pharmacol.* 1999;48(4):635-663

72. Calafat AM, Wong L-Y, Ye X, Reidy JA, Needham JL. Concentrations of the Sunscreen Agent Benzophenone-3 in Residents of the United States: National Health and Nutrition Examination Survey 2003–2004. *Environ Health Perspect.* 2008;116(7):893–897

73. Schlumpf M, Kypkec K, Vökt CC, et al. Endocrine active UV filters: developmental Toxicity and exposure through breast milk. *Chimia.* 2008;62:345–351

74. National Toxicology Program. NTP Technical Report on Toxicity Studies of 2-5Hydroxy-4-methoxybenzophenone (CAS Number: 131-57-7) Administered Topically and in Dosed Feed to F344/N Rats and B6C3F1 Mice. Research Triangle Park, NC: National Toxicology Program, National Institute of Environmental Health Sciences, US Department of Health and Human Services; 1992. Available at: http://ntp.niehs.nih.gov/ntp/htdocs/ST_rpts/tox021.pdf. Accessed April 3, 2011

75. Schlumpf M, Cotton B, Conscience M, Haller V, Steinmann B, Lichtensteiger W. In vitro and in vivo estrogenicity of UV screens. *Environ Health Perspect.* 2001;109(3):239–244

76. Wolff MS, Engel SM, Berkowitz GS, et al. Prenatal phenol and phthalate exposures and birth outcomes. *Environ Health Perspect.* 2008;116(8):1092–1097

77. Mancini AJ. Skin. *Pediatrics.* 2004;113(4 Suppl):1114–1119

78. American Academy of Ophthalmology. This Summer Keep an Eye on UV Safety. Available at: http://www.aao.org/newsroom/release/20090601a.cfm. Accessed April 3, 2011

79. American Optometric Association. Shopping Guide for Sunglasses. Available at: http://aoa.org/documents/SunglassShoppingGuide0810.pdf. Accessed April 3, 2011

80. Gilchrest BA. Sun protection and vitamin D: three dimensions of obfuscation. *J Steroid Biochem Mol Biol.* 2007;103(3-5):655–663

81. Holick MF. Vitamin D deficiency. *N Engl J Med.* 2007;357(3):266-281

82. Lim HW, Carucci JA, Spencer JM, Rigel DS, Commentary: a responsible approach to maintaining adequate serum vitamin D levels. *J Am Acad Dermatol.* 2007;57(4):594–595

83. Balk SJ; American Academy of Pediatrics, Council on Environmental Health, Section on Dermatology. Technical report: ultraviolet radiation: a hazard to children and adolescents. *Pediatrics.* 2011;127(3):e791-e817

84. Wagner CL; Greer FR; American Academy of Pediatrics, Section on Breastfeeding and Committee on Nutrition. Clinical report: prevention of rickets and vitamin D deficiency in infants, children, and adolescents. *Pediatrics.* 2008;122(5):1142-1152

85. Institute of Medicine. *Dietary Reference Intakes for Vitamin D and Calcium.* Washington, DC: National Academies Press; 2011

86. Abrams SA. Dietary guidelines for calcium and vitamin D: a new era. *Pediatrics.* 2011; 127(3):566-568

87. Weinstock MA. The struggle for primary prevention of skin cancer. *Am J Prev Med.* 2008; 34(2):171-172

88. American Academy of Pediatrics Council on Environmental Health and Section on Dermatology. Policy statement. Ultraviolet radiation: a hazard to children and adolescents. *Pediatrics.* 2011;127(3):588–597

89. National Toxicology Program. Executive Summary Dihydroxyacetone (96-26-4). Available at: http://ntp.niehs.nih.gov/index.cfm?objectid=6F5E9EA5-F1F6-975E-767789EB9C7FA03C. Accessed April 3, 2011

Chapter 42

Arts and Crafts

■ ■ ■ ■ ■ ■

Play activity and creative projects have many benefits and are critical to child development. This chapter discusses potential hazards from arts and crafts materials and ways to limit possibly toxic exposures. Simple interventions (such as hand washing, not eating while using art supplies, storing materials only in original labeled containers, and ensuring ventilation) will often prevent potentially toxic exposures.

Arts and crafts materials abound in homes, child care settings, schools, churches, and park and recreation facilities. Although there are some published case reports and reviews of occupationally related hazards for adult artists,[1–3] there is little peer-reviewed literature about toxic exposures from arts and crafts materials in children. Toxicity from specific arts and crafts materials typically becomes apparent only after reports are made public. Many arts and crafts products contain ingredients known to be hazardous. Parents, teachers, and adults and teenagers working with children may not be aware of the potential health hazards associated with these common materials. Dangerous chemicals found in art materials include metals, such as lead and manganese; solvents; and dusts or fibers.[4]

Lead, mercury, cadmium, and cobalt are found in paints, pastels, pigments, inks, glazes, enamels, and solder.[5] Legal bans on lead and other metals in paint do not apply to artists' paint, which is used in painting, drawing, ceramics, silk-screening, making stained glass, and other art activities that may involve children or adolescents.[2] Some papier-mâché products contain heavy metals from inks found in magazines. Hazardous organic solvents, such as turpentine, kerosene, mineral spirits, xylene, benzene, methyl alcohol, and formaldehyde are used in painting, silk-screening, and shellacking as well as in cleaning tools and preparing work surfaces.[6] Rubber cement, spray-on enamels, and spray-on fixatives are common products that also contain organic solvents.[7] Dusts and fibers containing materials such as asbestos, silica, talc, lead, cadmium, and mercury may be generated when using pastels, glazes, clay, and when reconstituting powdered pigments.

Physical hazards result from exposure to noise, dangerous mechanical and power tools, machinery and materials storage, and waste disposal practices. These are most likely to occur in industrial arts settings and often are regulated under Occupational Safety and Health Administration (OSHA) and US Environmental Protection Agency (EPA) rules.[8]

ROUTES OF EXPOSURE

The wide variety of arts and crafts materials used by children and adolescents permits the full spectrum of routes of exposure. The types of exposures depend on the activity, materials used, the age of the child, and environmental conditions such as ventilation. Inhalation is a major route of exposure for volatile organic solvents, dusts, and fibers. Exposure can occur during normal use, especially if ventilation is inadequate or necessary personal protective equipment is not available or properly used. Exposure can occur through inappropriate exploring of new materials by "sniff testing." Intentional inhalation, such as glue sniffing, can result in high-level exposure. Heating art work (as occurs during pottery glazing) can volatilize metals.

Unintentional ingestion is the route of exposure for many art hazards and may occur when common art materials are improperly stored in unlabeled or empty food containers. Even properly labeled art materials may be ingested by young or developmentally delayed children. Using homemade art as food or beverage containers can cause exposure if these products are contaminated. Ingestion also may occur through nail biting, thumb sucking, or other hand-to-mouth behaviors common in children. A potential source of toxicants in paint is "licking" the brush prior to dabbing it into paints. Cleaned used paint brushes may contain residual paint, and toxicity has been reported with this as an exposure source.[6]

Dermal absorption may occur from improper handling of hazardous art materials, accidental spills, or contact with cuts or abrasions. Exposure through the conjunctivae may occur from spills, splashes, and eye rubbing.

Arc welding used in sculpting potentially has the hazards of occupational welding, including ocular keratitis, respiratory tract irritation, inhalational exposure of metals, and metal fume fever (flulike symptoms 24 to 48 hours after inhaling metals, most commonly zinc).

Nonchemical Exposures

Physical hazards cause injury in several ways. Standards developed to protect adult workers from noise may be exceeded in secondary school industrial arts workshops, exposing children to noise levels that may cause hearing loss. Use of potentially dangerous equipment may result in cuts, crush injuries, fractures, punctures, or amputations. Power equipment may cause electrical injury or fires and can release carbon monoxide. Techniques requiring repetitive motion may cause tendonitis, carpal tunnel syndrome, or other injuries. Most of these hazards can be minimized through evaluations performed by industrial hygienists, engineering measures, and use of personal protective equipment.

SYSTEMS AFFECTED AND CLINICAL EFFECTS

Although relatively little is known about the effects on children of chronic low-level exposures to hazardous art materials, health problems in adult artists have been described. These experiences in adults raise the possibility that chronic low-level exposures to hazardous art materials could exacerbate or cause allergies, asthma, central and peripheral nerve damage, psychological and behavioral changes, respiratory damage, skin changes, or cancer.

Diagnostic Methods and Treatment

Diagnosis and treatment are specific to each type of exposure and illness.

Prevention of Exposure

Taking preventive measures may greatly reduce exposure to arts and crafts hazards. Subacute toxicity from long-term, low-level childhood exposure has not been studied or documented. Nonetheless, it is prudent to implement measures designed to prevent exposures that could be harmful. Some measures apply to all environments in which children use arts and crafts materials; others apply specifically to institutions. The California Office of Environmental Health Hazard Assessment (OEHHA) has developed guidelines on the safe use of arts and crafts materials for children that includes a list of products that should not be purchased for use by school-aged children (see Resources). Simple behavioral interventions (eg, do not lick paint brushes) and careful selection of art materials may eliminate much of the risk. For children, only materials certified to be safe should be selected (see Table 42.1). Materials should be properly labeled, purchased new or sealed in original containers with full instructions, and used with adult supervision according to manufacturers' instructions. The US Consumer Product Safety Commission (CPSC) considers a child to be anyone younger than 13 years or attending grade school or below. Adolescents are usually better able to follow directions, use precautions, and understand risks and are generally more able to use adult art materials and techniques.

Arts and crafts materials are labeled in a variety of ways. The familiar AP (Approved Product), CP (Certified Product), and HL Health Label (Non-Toxic) seals of the Art & Creative Materials Institute (ACMI) certify that an art material can be used by everyone, even children and adults who have impairments,

Table 42.1: Recommendations for Selecting Art Materials for Children Younger Than 13 Years
■ Read the label and instructions on all arts and craft materials.
■ Buy only products labeled "Conforms to ASTM D4236" and that bear the AP (Approved Product)/CP (Certified Product)/HL Health Label (Non-Toxic) seals of the Art & Creative Materials Institute.
■ Do not use materials labeled "Keep out of Reach of Children" or "Not for Use by Children."
■ Do not use materials marked with the words "Poison," "Danger," "Warning," or "Caution," or that contain hazard warnings on the label.
■ Do not use donated or found materials unless they are in the original containers with full labeling.

without risk of acute or chronic health hazards. This program covers approximately 80% of all children's art materials and approximately 95% of all fine art materials sold in the United States.

In 1983, the American Society for Testing and Materials (ASTM) developed a national voluntary standard, ASTM D4236, Labeling of Art Materials for Chronic Health Hazards. This standard requires that art materials must be evaluated by a toxicologist and, if labeling is required, conform to stringent labeling requirements that include identifying hazardous ingredients, risks associated with use, precautions needed to prevent harm, first aid measures, and sources of further information. All products certified by the Art & Creative Materials Institute have conformed to this standard since its inception. In 1990, the Labeling for Hazardous Art Materials Act went into effect. This act made the "voluntary" ASTM D4236 standard mandatory for all art materials imported or sold in the United States. This act, administered by the Consumer Product Safety Commission, requires that hazardous consumer products, including art materials, have warnings to "keep out of reach of children" (for acute health hazards) or that they "should not be used by children" (for chronic health hazards).

Occasionally, art materials available for purchase are improperly labeled. Crayons containing high levels of lead have been labeled "nontoxic." To make sure that an art material has been evaluated by a toxicologist, parents should look for the statement, "conforms to ASTM D4236" covering chronic health hazards and an Art & Creative Materials Institute seal for acute and chronic health hazards.[9]

It is important to ensure good ventilation in rooms used for arts and crafts activities (see Chapter 20). Proper storage and cleanup also are essential. Materials should only be stored in original, fully labeled containers. Appropriate cleanup at the end of an art session includes closing and storing containers, cleaning all tools, wiping down surfaces, and washing hands thoroughly. Adult art and hobby materials should be similarly labeled and stored out of children's reach. Half of all artists work in home studios, many of which are in living areas where children also live and may be exposed.

Close supervision of children during arts and crafts activities can prevent injuries and poisonings, ensure proper use of materials, and allow for the observation of adverse reactions. Eating or drinking should not occur while using art materials. Cuts and abrasions should be covered if they may come into contact with materials.

Prevention begins with selection of the safest materials. At district or state levels in public schools and other large institutions, central ordering can facilitate the selection of safe art materials.

Emergency protocols should be in place in case of an injury, poisoning, or allergic reaction. The local poison control center number should be prominently posted. Adequate flushing facilities should be provided in case of spills or eye splashes. Material Safety Data Sheets (MSDSs) should be available on-site for all hazardous materials that may be used in high school industrial arts classes. Adult supervisors should have proper first aid and emergency response skills and training.

Art safety education for all supervising adults and teenagers is desirable. Art activities are common in church schools, child care settings, preschools, elementary and secondary schools, hospitals, chronic care institutions, therapeutic facilities, and at art festivals. Art teachers should be thoroughly trained in safety for all techniques they use in the classroom. Children with special vulnerabilities should be identified and appropriate measures taken to protect their health. Children at higher risk include those with asthma and allergies who may be especially sensitive to exposures tolerated by children without these conditions. Children with physical, psychological, or learning disabilities may need special assistance in the use of some equipment or in understanding instructions and following safety techniques.[10]

Industrial arts programs should follow OSHA, EPA, and state guidelines for ventilation, physical plant, fire safety systems, and personal protective equipment. These programs for older children and young adults should have a formal health and safety component.

Frequently Asked Questions

Q *Are water-based art supplies always safe?*
A Some water-based, cold-water dyes are sensitizers. Long-term health effects have not been thoroughly studied. In general, water-based supplies are preferable, because they avoid the need for organic solvents. Accidental ingestion of even small amounts of organic solvents can be fatal. Coloring

agents used in paints and inks can contain toxic substances such as metals. It is best to wash hands after use and avoid ingestion (such as licking paint brushes).

Q   *Can I use glazed ceramic art to store food or beverages?*

A   Glazes may contain metals. Although lead content of glaze has been limited in dishes made in the United States for commercial sale, some glaze colors used for art projects may contain lead or other metals. These glazes may have labels recommending that they should not be used by children. Pottery made in foreign countries, particularly low or middle-income countries, may contain lead or other metals. Metal contamination has been reported from products made in Mexico and China. Hot foods or acidic foods or drinks stored in such glazed containers may result in leaching of metals found in glaze, resulting in exposure. Glazed ceramic art and pottery from outside the US should only be used for decoration, not for holding food or drinks.

Resources

American Industrial Hygiene Association
Phone: 703-849-8888; fax: 703-207-3561
Web site: www.aiha.org
E-mail: infonet@aiha.org
This organization gives guidance to institutions about designing and managing industrial arts facilities and programs.

Art & Creative Materials Institute (ACMI)
Phone: 781-293-4100; fax: 781-294-0808
Web site: www.acminet.org
The ACMI, an organization of art and craft manufacturers, develops standards for the safety and quality of art materials; manages a certification program to ensure the safety of children's art and craft materials and the accuracy of labels of adult art materials that are potentially hazardous; develops and distributes information on the safe use of art and craft materials; provides lists of certified products (those that are safe for children and adult art materials that may have a hazard potential) to individuals, to the US Consumer Products Safety Commission, state health agencies, and school authorities; and provides consultations for concerned individuals. The ACMI has access to toxicologists to answer questions about health concerns.

California Office of Environmental Health Hazard Assessment (OEHHA)
OEHHA has developed information to assist school personnel in selecting and using safe art and craft products in the classroom in a publication titled "Guidelines for the Safe Use of Art and Craft Materials" (updated October 2009). Available at: http://www.oehha.ca.gov/education/art/artguide.html

Public Interest Research Group (PIRG)

Phone: 202-546-9707; fax: 202-546-2461

Web site: www.pirg.org

E-mail: uspirg@pirg.org

Several state PIRGs have conducted surveys of art hazards in schools. Similar methodology was employed by all. Reports may be obtained from individual state groups.

US Consumer Product Safety Commission (CPSC)

Phone: 800-638-2772

Web site: www.cpsc.gov

The CPSC is responsible for developing and managing regulations to support the Labeling for Hazardous Art Materials Act and the Federal Hazardous Substances Act. The CPSC instigates actions on mislabeled products and/or misbranded hazardous substances (products whose labels do not conform to these acts). Actions may involve confiscations, product recalls, or other legal actions. The CPSC's Web site contains general product safety information and recent press releases. To report a dangerous product or product-related injury or illness, call CPSC's hotline at 800-638-2772 or e-mail info@cpsc.gov.

US EPA

Advice from EPA Region 2 on Arts and Crafts Safety Issues

www.epa.gov/Region2/children/k12/english/art-2of5.pdf

References

1. Dorevitch S, Babin A. Health hazards of ceramic artists. *Occup Med.* 2001;16(4):563-575
2. McCann MF. Occupational and environmental hazards in art. *Environ Res.* 1992;59(1): 139–144
3. Ryan TJ. Hart, EM, Kappler LL. VOC exposures in a mixed-use university art building. *AIHA J (Fairfax, Va).* 2002;63(6):703-708
4. Amdur MO, Doull J, Klaassen CD, eds. *Casarett and Doull's Toxicology: The Basic Science of Poisons.* 7th ed. New York, NY: McGraw Hill; 2007
5. Babin A, Peltz PA, Rossol M. *Children's Art Supplies Can Be Toxic.* New York, NY: Center for Safety in the Arts; 1992
6. Lesser SH, Weiss SJ. Art hazards. *Am J Emerg Med.* 1995;13(4):451–458
7. McCann M. *Artist Beware.* New York, NY: Lyons and Burford Publishers; 1992
8. McCann M. *School Safety Procedures for Art and Industrial Art Programs.* New York, NY: Center for Safety in the Arts; 1994
9. Lu PC. A health hazard assessment in school arts and crafts. *J Environ Pathol Toxicol Oncol.* 1992;11(1):12–17
10. Rossol M. The first art hazards course. *J Environ Pathol Toxicol Oncol.* 1992;11(1):28–32

Chapter 43

Asthma

■ ■ ■ ■ ■ ■

Asthma is a chronic respiratory disease characterized by bronchial hyperrespon-siveness, intermittent reversible airway obstruction, and airway inflammation.[1] This chapter will review factors that influence the development of asthma and then will focus on environmental triggers in children with asthma.

ASTHMA DEVELOPMENT

Genetic and environmental factors contribute to the development of asthma, and early life exposures may play an important role. It is likely that recent changes in children's environments have contributed to the increasing prevalence of asthma. Recent studies suggest that the neonatal immune system tends to favor an allergic (immunoglobulin E [IgE]-promoting) response to certain environ-mental allergens (eg, dust mite). This response is mediated in part through infant T helper cells that tend to release a series of cytokines that promote the development of an "allergic" B cell response—the generation of specific IgE—to certain environmental allergens. The end result of the T cell cytokine profile that favors an IgE response is termed a Th2 response. In contrast, as the immune system matures, naive T cells develop along a different path, releasing a mix of cytokines in response to exposure to environmental allergens that favor a Th1 response. It is postulated that exposures to environmental stimuli during early childhood could either perpetuate Th2 responses or shift the balance toward the expected Th1 response predominance, depending on the types of stimuli and/or an individual's genetic predisposition.[1,2] Proposed hypotheses on environmental factors that may favor the Th2 response include improved hygiene, changes in diet, changes in intestinal flora because of increased use of antibiotics, routine vaccination, increased exposure to allergens because of changes in housing and lifestyle, obesity and reduced physical activity, and changes in the prenatal environment.[3] The "hygiene hypothesis" postulates that early childhood infections (which promote a Th1 response) are becoming less frequent, favoring a persistent Th2 imbalance.[1,4] Observations that the presence of an older sibling and early child care attendance are associated with a reduced incidence of asthma support this hypothesis. The development of a Th2 (IgE) response to common environmental contaminants (eg, house-dust mite allergens, cockroach allergens, cat and possibly dog allergens) is strongly correlated with the development of childhood asthma.[2,5] The relationship between early life exposures and allergic sensitization is not completely understood. Some studies have suggested that exposure to pet allergens during infancy may be protective. Overall, the data show mixed results and are not compelling at this time.[4,6,7]

Associations between early exposure to airborne particulates or pollutant gases and childhood asthma development have also been suggested.[8]

ENVIRONMENTAL TRIGGERS OF ASTHMA

Major indoor triggers of asthma[9] include secondhand tobacco smoke (SHS), also known as environmental tobacco smoke; respiratory irritants such as volatile organic compounds (VOCs) and fragrances (see Chapter 20); animal and insect allergens (such as dander and cockroach antigen), and molds (Table 43.1). Although most agents that exacerbate asthma in children are inhaled, asthma may be exacerbated in some atopic individuals who touch (eg, latex) or ingest (eg, peanuts) certain products.

Outdoor air pollution also has been associated with asthma exacerbations[10,11] (see Chapter 21).

Indoor Environmental Triggers

Secondhand Tobacco Smoke

The prevalence of tobacco use and exposure to secondhand smoke has declined significantly, but more than 20% of US adults still used tobacco in 2009.[12] Children are among the most heavily exposed to secondhand smoke (see Chapter 40). Children whose mothers smoke have more wheezing symptoms and a higher incidence of lower respiratory tract illnesses compared with those whose mothers do not smoke.[13] The greatest effect seems to be related to maternal smoking during pregnancy and/or early infancy,[14] perhaps resulting from inflammatory stimuli on lung parenchyma during a period of rapid lung development and prolonged close exposure to the mother. Exposure to secondhand smoke is associated with an increase in asthma attacks, earlier asthma symptom onset, increased medication use, and a more prolonged recovery from acute attacks.[15,16] Maternal smoking of half a pack or more per day has been associated with an increased risk of developing asthma in children.[14] Acute short-term exposure to secondhand smoke has been demonstrated to increase bronchial

Table 43.1: Common Indoor and Outdoor Asthma Triggers

AGENT	MAJOR SOURCES
Indoor	
Secondhand tobacco smoke	Cigarettes, cigars, other tobacco products
Wood smoke	Fireplaces and wood-burning stoves
Molds	Floods, roof leaks, plumbing leaks, wet basements, air-conditioning units
Nitrogen oxides	Space heaters, gas-fueled cooking stoves
Odors or fragrances	Sprays, deodorizers, cosmetics, household cleaning products, pesticides
Volatile organic compounds	Building and insulation materials, cleaning agents, solvents, pesticides, sealants, adhesives, combustion products, molds
Dust mites	Bedding (pillows, mattress, box springs, bed linens), carpets, soft upholstered furniture, draperies, stuffed toys
Animals	Cat and dog dander and saliva, rodent urine
Cockroaches	Food and water, especially in kitchens and bathrooms
Outdoor	
Pollens	Seasonal release from flowering plants
Molds	Ubiquitous in soil, increased in wet environments and decaying organic matter (eg, wood chips)
Ozone (O_3)	Combustion sources (eg, motor vehicle exhaust, power plants)
Particulate matter (PM_{10}, $PM_{2.5}$, $PM_{1.0}$)	Combustion sources (eg, diesel engines, industry, wood burning)
Sulfur dioxide (SO_2)	Burning of coal (coal-fired power plants, other industrial sources)

PM_{10} indicates particulate matter less than 10 μm in aerodynamic diameter; $PM_{2.5}$, particulate matter less than 2.5 μm in aerodynamic diameter; $PM_{1.0}$, particulate matter less than 1 μm in aerodynamic diameter.

hyperreactivity, requiring as long as 3 weeks to recover baseline pulmonary function following exposure.[17,18]

Other Indoor Irritants

Other common sources of air pollutants that may be respiratory irritants include gas stoves and wood stoves, space heaters (gas or kerosene) and fireplaces, and furnishings and construction materials that release organic gases and vapors.[19]

Epidemiologic evidence for the role of these pollutants in exacerbating asthma is limited but suggests associations between exposures and asthma exacerbations.[19,20]

Gas stoves or ovens can generate high levels of nitrogen dioxide indoors, especially when there is inadequate ventilation or the gas stove is used as an ancillary heat source.[21] Poorly ventilated fireplaces can produce substantial levels of wood smoke indoors.

Volatile organic compounds and fragrances may induce acute asthma episodes in sensitive individuals.[22] The mechanism of action is unknown but presumed to be nonspecific irritation. Formaldehyde is emitted from many consumer products, including new carpets, paper products (eg, tissues, towels, and bags), urea-formaldehyde foam insulation, and glues used in plywood and pressed-board products. Formaldehyde is a known respiratory irritant in the occupational setting and a common air pollutant in the home (see Chapter 20).[19,23]

Allergenic Precipitants

Animal Allergens

Animal allergens are glycoproteins that often induce an IgE response in humans. These allergens usually are found in saliva, sebaceous glands (dog and cat), or sometimes in urine (rodents). Allergies to cow hair or horsehair and dander also have been reported, primarily through occupational exposures.[19] The spread of allergens in the environment has been studied primarily for cats; however, the pathway of spread is likely to be similar for other domestic furry animals.[19] Cat allergen-containing material dries and adheres to many surfaces (eg, animal fur or hair, bedding, and clothing) and can be transported to other environments via these sources. Once an animal enters the room, small airborne allergen-containing particles (diameter <5 μm) can be detected. These small particles remain suspended in the air for hours. Once allergen-containing particles are inhaled, they are easily deposited in distal airways. Clinical manifestations of animal allergy range from mild cutaneous symptoms, such as urticaria, to rhino-conjunctivitis to life-threatening bronchospasm and anaphylaxis.

Cats

The severity of allergic reactions to cats is greater than reactions to other common domestic pets. More than 6 million US residents have allergies to cats, and up to 40% of atopic patients demonstrate skin test sensitivity.[24] The major allergen *Fel d I* is present in high concentration in the saliva and sebaceous and anal glands of cats. The grooming habits of cats result in a large amount of saliva on the fur, and cat allergen can be spread via small airborne particles.[25] Children with cats can transmit cat allergens to schoolrooms, which may create an environment that can precipitate asthma in sensitized children.[26] Once a cat is removed from an indoor environment, the allergen may persist for many months in reservoirs, such as bedding.

Dogs

Dogs are the most common domesticated animal species found in US homes. Five percent to 30% of atopic patients have a positive skin test to the major allergen *Can f I*, although many do not demonstrate clinical symptoms or have positive bronchoprovocation tests.[27] There appears to be variation in clinical sensitivity to different dog breeds, and breed-specific allergens have been suggested.[28] Nevertheless, no dog breed is considered nonallergenic. As with cat allergen, the highest concentrations of *Can f I* are found in canine fur and dander.[28]

Rodents

People may be exposed to rodents if they are present as pests or pets in the home. Rat and mouse allergens are present primarily in their urine.[19] Through transfer, the fur and dander often contain high amounts of allergen. The prevalence of mouse allergen can be widespread in inner-city homes.[29] Among children with asthma living in inner cities, there was an association between mouse allergen in house-dust samples and sensitization to mouse allergen, especially among asthmatic children who exhibit atopy to multiple allergens on skin testing. Early mouse exposure has been associated with early wheeze and atopy later in life.[30]

Birds

In the occupational setting, hypersensitivity pneumonitis can be associated with antigens from bird excreta and proteinaceous materials found in dust dispersed from birds; however, it is unclear whether birds cause allergy and asthma.[19] Large quantities of dust mites have been documented in feathers, and dust mite allergen is the likely source of the allergic stimulus from feather-containing items in the home, including pillows, comforters, bedding, and down-filled clothes.[19]

Cockroaches

The incidence of cockroach hypersensitivity is related to the degree of infestation in the living environment, although nonresidential exposures (eg, schools) may cause allergy in individuals whose homes are not infested. Cockroach infestations are more common in warm, moist environments with readily accessible food sources. Although the highest allergen levels typically are found in the kitchen, significantly elevated concentrations of cockroach allergen also are found in bedrooms or television-watching areas, particularly if food is consumed in these places.

Numerous species of cockroaches have been described in the United States, and 3 predominant species have been associated with IgE antibody production. The German cockroach, *Blattella germanica,* is the source of 2 primary antigens, *Bla g 1* and *Bla g 2;* however, significant cross-reactivity exists between cockroach antigens. Cockroach allergens have been described as principal triggers of allergic rhinitis and asthma. Positive skin tests to cockroach antigens can be found in up to 60% of urban residents with asthma. Although several parts of the cockroach are allergenic, the whole body and feces seem to be more potent. Cockroach allergens may behave like the dust mite antigen; that is, they are carried on large particles that become airborne for short periods during active disturbance. Levels of allergen in places where children spend a significant amount of time may be most important. Inner-city children with asthma, cockroach allergy, and exposure to elevated levels of cockroach allergen in bedroom dust had more days of wheezing, more missed school days, and more emergency department visits and hospitalizations than did nonsensitized and/or nonexposed asthmatic children.[19,31] Additionally, hospitalization rates for children who were sensitized and exposed to excessive levels of cockroach allergen were nearly 3 times as high as for those with low exposure and sensitivity.

House-Dust Mites (*Dermatophagoides*)

House-dust mites probably play a major role in inducing asthma and triggering asthma exacerbations in sensitized children. Mite antigen commonly is found where human dander is found, and the principal allergens—*Der p I* and *Der p II*—are found in the outer membrane of mite fecal particles. Indoor environments that provide optimal growth conditions for *Dermatophagoides* species have a relative humidity greater than 55% and temperatures between 22°C and 26°C (71°F and 79°F), but dust mites can survive laundering at moderate temperatures. Under optimal conditions, mites proliferate on mattress surfaces, carpeting, and upholstered furniture, each of which contains a large amount of human dander, its primary food source. A gram of dust may contain 1000 mites and 250 000 fecal pellets. Pellet diameters range in size from 10 to 40 µm and, therefore, are not easily transported into the lower airway passages. Exposure occurs either by proximity of the nasopharyngeal mucosa to mite reservoirs (especially mattresses, pillows, carpets, bed linens, clothes, and soft toys) or to airborne antigen that is resuspended during house-cleaning activities.

Molds

Molds are most prominent in climates with increased ambient humidity, although some can grow in relatively dry areas. Species of common indoor molds (eg, *Aspergillus, Penicillium,* and *Cladosporium* species) require sufficient moisture for growth, and places where indoor mold growth is commonly found include household areas with high humidity (eg, basements, crawl spaces, ground floors, bathrooms, and areas with standing water, such as air-conditioner condensers) and areas with recent moisture damage. Carpeting, ceilings, and paneled or hollow walls also are common reservoirs.

Dampness and the presence of mold should be suspected when there is visible mold or mildew in the home, a moldy or musty smell, evidence of water condensation on windowsills (except immediately after showers or cooking in the kitchen), or the use of a humidifier. Many epidemiologic studies have documented an association between dampness and mold in the home and asthma symptoms.[19,32-39] Because dampness and visible mold growth could be indicators for dust mite allergen exposure, the relative contribution of molds versus other allergens (eg, house-dust mite) was not entirely clear. Several studies have documented, however, that the association between mold and asthma persists even after adjusting for levels of dust mite allergen.[40-42]

Miscellaneous Allergens

Latex

Latex may cause an allergic response either by direct contact or by inhalation of latex particles. Symptoms range from cutaneous eruption, sneezing, and bronchospasm to anaphylaxis.[43]

Widespread use of latex gloves and revised processing procedures, making the allergen more potent, may have contributed to the increase in reported cases. Most sensitivities occur in medical personnel, food service workers, or environmental service workers, although household exposures to balloons, gloves, condoms, and certain sporting equipment also may trigger allergic responses. Children with increased exposure to latex (eg, those with urogenital abnormalities, cerebral palsy, and preterm infants) are at increased risk of developing latex allergy. Up to one third of children with spina bifida have been reported to have positive skin tests to latex.[43]

Food

Many foods contain allergenic proteins that can trigger asthma or anaphylactic reactions in sensitized individuals. Peanuts, tree nuts, fish, shellfish, eggs, and milk are the most commonly associated foods.[44] Although oral ingestion typically is needed to elicit symptoms, contact with aerosolized particulates and oils that contain the offending antigens can induce symptoms in highly allergic individuals. In rare individuals, food additives, including sulfites and food coloring—especially tartrazine (a synthetic yellow dye) or cochineal (a red dye made of the dried and pulverized bodies of female cochineal insects)—also can be highly allergenic. Asthma symptoms are frequent among children experiencing anaphylaxis but are rarely the sole manifestations of food allergy.

Outdoor Environmental Triggers

Outdoor Air Pollution

Currently, more than 125 million Americans live in areas that fail to meet the 1997 National Ambient Air Quality Standards (NAAQS) for at least 1 of the criteria pollutants. Ozone and particulate matter are of special concern. Levels of these air pollutants are high enough in many parts of the United States to present respiratory hazards to children with asthma.

Ozone

Ambient (outdoor) ozone is formed by the action of sunlight on nitrogen oxides and reactive hydrocarbons (both of which are emitted by motor vehicles and industrial sources) under stable weather conditions. The levels tend to be highest on warm, sunny, windless days and often peak in the mid-afternoon.

During the warm season, ozone concentrations exceed the National Ambient Air Quality Standards in many urban and rural areas of the United States, with highest levels often being reached in suburban regions of major metropolitan areas.

Ozone is a powerful oxidant and respiratory irritant. Increased rates of hospitalization and acute visits for asthma exacerbations have been associated with high ozone days.[45,46] One study found an increased incidence of asthma associated with heavy exercise among children living in communities with high levels of ozone air pollution.[47]

Particulate Matter

Particulate matter is a heterogeneous mixture of airborne particles. In urban areas, motor vehicle exhaust (especially diesel), industry, and wood smoke are important sources of particulate pollution. Particulate pollution has been associated with asthma exacerbations and bronchitis symptoms in children with asthma. In addition to their irritant properties, diesel particulates may enhance the allergic response.

Sulfur Dioxide

Sulfur dioxide (SO_2) is a potent respiratory irritant that can cause asthma exacerbations. Principal sources of SO_2 include coal-fired power plants, paper and pulp mills, refineries, and other industries. Although ambient levels of SO_2 are below the national air quality standard in most areas of the United States, SO_2 levels can be increased in areas near these sources.

For additional information on health effects of outdoor air pollution, see Chapter 21.

Outdoor Allergens

Outdoor air contains a variety of allergens, most of which arise from plant pollens and mold spores. Exposures to high concentrations of tree, grass, and ragweed pollens that occur in the spring and late summer can induce respiratory symptoms, such as sneezing, rhinitis, and bronchospasm in sensitized children. Spores from mold, such as *Alternaria* and *Aspergillus* species, commonly are found in damp, wooded areas, including the wood chips often used as ground cover in playgrounds. These allergens also can cause acute and recurrent asthma exacterbations.[47,48] Outdoor exposure to mold spores has been implicated in fatal exacerbations of asthma.[49,50] Asthma attacks that occur during thunderstorms have also been linked to increased mold spores in the outdoor air.[51]

DIAGNOSIS

To establish a diagnosis of asthma, clinicians should take a detailed medical history. They should determine that the patient has a history of episodic symptoms of airflow obstruction or airway hyperresponsiveness. A physical examination should be performed, focusing on the upper respiratory tract, chest, and skin. Alternative diagnoses should be excluded.[3] Atopy and a family history of asthma and/or atopy are strong predictors of persistent asthma. Pulmonary function testing in children younger than 5 years is seldom reproducible. A response to a therapeutic trial of bronchodilator and/or anti-inflammatory medications frequently is helpful in confirming the diagnosis. Chest radiographs may reveal the presence of peribronchial thickening and hyperinflation, which may help to determine the chronicity of illness and also help to evaluate other diagnostic possibilities such as a congenital anomaly or foreign body. Baseline pulmonary function testing may demonstrate a decreased forced expiratory volume in 1 second (FEV_1), and a decreased mid-expiratory phase (FEV_{25-75}) compared with predicted norms. Prebronchodilator and postbronchodilator spirometry (>12% FEV_1 improvement), methacholine, exercise, or cold air bronchoprovocation (≥20% FEV_1 decrease) may help diagnose asthma in the patient with mild symptoms. Daily or diurnal variability in peak flow measurements also may help.

Determining the degree of atopy may be helpful in diagnosing asthma. Skin-prick test responses to inhaled antigens or specific foods may help to confirm suspected triggers. The ELISA assay generally is less sensitive than skin prick tests, although it may be more readily available and easily tolerated (but more expensive) when screening a patient for numerous potential sensitivities.

TREATMENT

The National Institutes of Health provide evidence-based guidelines discussing all aspects of asthma treatment.[3] Goals of treatment include preventing chronic and troublesome symptoms, maintaining normal pulmonary function, maintaining a normal quality of life, reducing the number of exacerbations, and minimizing emergency department visits and hospitalizations. Medications are categorized into 2 general classes: (1) long-term preventive medications that achieve and maintain control of persistent asthma; and (2) quick-relief medications that treat acute symptoms and exacerbations. The "step care" approach to asthma therapy emphasizes initiating higher-level therapy at the onset of treatment to control symptoms, and then "stepping down" the use of quick-relief medications followed by control medications. Preventive medications include inhaled corticosteroids and nonsteroid medications, such as leukotriene receptor antagonists, and long-acting beta-adrenergic agonists. Relief medications are largely inhaled rapid-acting adrenergic agonists.[3]

Uncontrolled asthma is a risk factor for severe anaphylaxis to food allergens. Management of asthma symptoms that occur as part of an anaphylactic reaction require the use of intramuscular epinephrine, rather than use of an inhaled adrenergic agonist.[52]

Allergen immunotherapy is available for many allergens and has had some success.[53] Immunotherapy should not take the place of efforts to control exposure to allergens, irritants (such as secondhand smoke), and other triggers.

MANAGEMENT OF ENVIRONMENTAL TRIGGERS OF ASTHMA

Reducing exposure to inhalant indoor allergens and irritants can improve asthma control.[3] Exposure reduction strategies are summarized in Table 43.2. Focusing on one allergen reduction strategy may be ineffective and generally, a multifaceted approach is required.[3] Multifaceted home environmental intervention strategies in combination with community health worker-based assessments and parent education can be cost-effective and represent an effective public health strategy, especially in inner-city communities.[3,54,55] These environmental interventions can be as effective as the use of inhaled corticosteroids in treating asthma symptoms.[3]

Control Measures for Allergens and Irritants

Avoiding environmental allergens and irritants is one of the primary goals of good asthma management. Skin testing or in vitro testing and counseling about appropriate environmental control strategies are recommended for all children with persistent asthma who are exposed to perennial indoor allergens.[3]

Most control measures have been directed at the control of chronic asthma symptoms and the prevention of asthma exacerbations.[54,56,57] Possible interventions to decrease the risk of developing asthma currently are being investigated.[3] To date, food allergen avoidance diets prenatally or postnatally have not been successful in decreasing the incidence of asthma. Randomized controlled trials are ongoing to evaluate the effect on asthma incidence of aggressive dust-mite control during pregnancy and early life.[57] Primary prevention of asthma should include efforts to reduce children's and adolescents' exposure to tobacco smoke. Pregnant women should not smoke and should avoid exposure to secondhand smoke.

Complete control of many of the environmental allergens is difficult, and multiple intervention strategies are recommended. Several reviews outline priorities for allergen avoidance.[3,19,57,58] Recommendations follow the basic principles of control of sources. Recommendations for aggressive and continual attention

Table 43.2: Reducing Exposures in the Home, School, and Child Care Setting*

ENVIRONMENTAL TRIGGERS	STRATEGIES TO REDUCE EXPOSURES
Animal dander	▪ Remove animal from indoor environment; at a minimum, keep animal out of the child's room ▪ Remove or limit animals
House-dust mites	**Recommended:** ▪ Encase mattress in an allergen-impermeable cover ▪ Encase pillow in an allergen-impermeable cover or wash it weekly ▪ Wash sheets and blankets on the child's bed in hot water weekly ▪ Water temperature of >130 °F (54°C) is necessary for killing mites; cooler water and detergent and bleach will still reduce live mites and allergen level ▪ Prolonged exposure to dry heat or freezing can also kill mites but does not remove allergen **Desirable:** ▪ Reduce indoor humidity to or below 60%, ideally 30%–50% ▪ Remove carpets from the bedroom ▪ Avoid sleeping or lying on upholstered furniture ▪ Remove carpets that are laid on concrete ▪ Select floor coverings at schools and child care settings on the basis of functional use
Cockroaches	▪ Use poison bait or traps to control insects; intensive cleaning is necessary to reduce reservoirs ▪ Do not leave food or garbage exposed ▪ Use integrated pest management methods
Pollens (from trees, grass, or weeds) and outdoor molds	▪ If possible, stay indoors with windows closed during periods of peak pollen exposure, which are usually during the midday and afternoon ▪ Run air conditioning on recirculation setting if possible ▪ At school and child care settings, schedule physical activities indoors when pollen or pollutant levels are excessive

continued on page 632

continued from page 631

Table 43.2: Reducing Exposures in the Home, School, and Child Care Setting,* *continued*	
ENVIRONMENTAL TRIGGERS	**STRATEGIES TO REDUCE EXPOSURES**
Indoor mold	▪ Fix all leaks and eliminate other sources of water intrusion ▪ Clean moldy surfaces and remove reservoirs of indoor and relevant outdoor mold ▪ Reduce indoor humidity to or below 60%, ideally 30%–50% ▪ Dehumidify basements if possible ▪ Ensure that exhaust fans or other sources of ventilation are used in areas of increased humidity (eg, bathrooms and kitchens) and that they are functioning effectively
Secondhand Smoke	▪ Advise parents and others in the home who smoke to stop smoking. Smoking outside the home will reduce but may not eliminate the child's exposure ▪ Advise the adolescent smoker to stop smoking or to smoke outside the home ▪ Promote tobacco-free schools and child care centers
Indoor/Outdoor Pollutants and Irritants	▪ Discuss ways to reduce exposures to: — Wood-burning stoves or fireplaces — Unvented gas stoves or heaters — Other irritants (eg, perfumes, cleaning agents, sprays) — Sources of volatile organic compounds (VOCs), such as new carpeting, particle board, painting

*Adapted from National Institutes of *Health Asthma Practice Guidelines*, 2007.[3]

to multiple reservoirs are especially relevant for children who require multiple medications to control their symptoms. Barriers to implementation of indoor environmental control strategies for low-income children with asthma recently have been evaluated.[55]

Secondhand Smoke and Other Indoor Irritants

Pediatricians should ask about children's exposure to secondhand smoke and counsel parents on smoking cessation and eliminating sources of smoke in the child's environment (see Chapter 40). There is no evidence that ventilation and air-cleaning methods decrease children's exposure to secondhand smoke.[19]

Adequate ventilation is imperative for indoor combustion appliances (eg, gas or kerosene space heaters, gas stoves, and wood-burning fireplaces or woodstoves). Gas or kerosene space heaters, often used in cold climates where they may be on for prolonged periods,[19] should not be used in unvented spaces because of the risk of carbon monoxide poisoning. Sealant coatings or coverings are sometimes applied over formaldehyde-containing materials to decrease emissions. Furniture, carpets, and building materials emit the highest levels of volatile organic compounds during the first months after manufacturing, and adequate ventilation should be supplied during and immediately after installation. Low-emission carpets, adhesives, and building materials are now commercially available, but there are no clinical studies comparing asthma exacerbations among children in homes with traditional versus low-emission carpets. Using alternative products that contain few or no volatile organic compounds or fragrances, such as paint and finishes with low levels of volatile organic compounds, non-aerosol and unscented cleaners, and cosmetics, should be encouraged.

Indoor Allergens

Animal Allergens

The preferred treatment for animal allergy is to avoid animals that provoke the reaction. Removing the animal from the home or keeping it outdoors (eg, in the garage) are strongly recommended. If removal is not possible or acceptable, efforts should be made to control all the sites where pet allergens accumulate as well as the source.[59] Other than service dogs, animals should be avoided or limited in schools and child care settings.[60]

Control of the major cat allergen *Fel d I* is difficult. Even if the cat is removed from the home, it may take more than 3 months to reduce allergen levels. Aggressive cleaning (eg, removing carpets and washing walls and furniture) may accelerate the process. Many cat-sensitive patients are exposed to cat allergens outside their home and should receive advice about avoiding these other settings.

If the cat remains in the home, measures should include restricting pets to one area and creating a "safe room" in the child's bedroom by not allowing pets into the room and keeping the door closed. Dense filter material may be placed over forced air outlets to trap airborne dander particles. Washing cats may decrease the amount of cat dander and dried saliva in the environment.[3,59]

Other methods include removing carpeting and heavily contaminated items, using high-efficiency particulate air (HEPA) filter vacuums and filters, regular damp mopping, weekly cat bathing, and washing cat-contaminated items. Many of these methods have been found to temporarily reduce airborne cat allergen levels by about 90%.[50,61] HEPA filters are effective for cat allergen only when used with the other measures.[19]

Avoiding early exposure to pets has been promoted to avoid sensitization. However, recent studies suggest that in some children, early contact with cats and dogs may, in fact, prevent allergy more effectively than avoiding these animals.[6,7,62] Further studies are needed to resolve this issue.

Dog allergens provoke significant bronchial hyperresponsiveness in people less often than do cat allergens. The decrease in response may be attributable to antigens that vary among breeds and among sources (dander, hair, saliva, and serum extracts) and because more dogs reside outside and better tolerate regular bathing. Guidelines recommended for minimizing cat allergen exposure should also be followed for minimizing dog allergen exposure.

Levels of airborne rodent urinary allergens have been reduced in most laboratory environments by regulations that mandate rapid room air exchanges and high-efficiency filters. No intervention strategies have been studied for people exposed to infestations in housing.

Cockroaches

Cockroaches may be found wherever water, heat, and organic material are present.[63] It is essential to minimize organic material on open surfaces to reduce infestation. Other measures include storing all foodstuffs in sealed containers, eliminating water sources, eating only in the kitchen, placing trash out daily, caulking all cracks around faucets and pipe fittings, and placing roach gel baits and bait stations in kitchens and bathrooms.[3,64] Boric acid can be used in areas not accessible to children. When considering using other pesticides, families must balance the risks of cockroaches, the severity of asthma, and the risks of pesticide use. The least toxic alternatives (ie, "Integrated Pest Management") for pest control should be employed (see Table 43.2 and Chapter 37). Families should avoid using over-the-counter "bug sprays," because they may cause toxic reactions.

Cockroach allergens are carried on particles similar in size to dust mite allergens. Therefore, exposure to cockroach allergens may be related to brief resuspension of settled dust. Concentrations of cockroach allergen are higher in the kitchen but often are found in bedrooms. The same physical barrier and cleaning interventions recommended for dust mite allergen should reduce exposure to cockroach allergen. Reducing cockroach allergen in infested homes decreases children's asthma symptoms and conplications.[65]

Dust Mites

Eliminating dust-mite exposure reduces symptoms and the degree of nonspecific bronchial hyperreactivity.[66] Because dust-mite allergen is carried on relatively large particles, exposure is mostly related to breathing allergen that is resuspended during activity. Encasing mattresses, pillows, and box springs in allergen-impermeable covers is the single most important avoidance measure to reduce dust-mite exposure. Plastic or vinyl covers are an economical choice for box springs but may be uncomfortable for use on mattresses and pillows. Vapor- or air-permeable covers that prevent the passage of allergens are available for a comparable price.[57,58] Clinical intervention trials have shown substantial allergen reduction and improvement in asthma symptoms with dust-mite allergen reduction methods (impervious pillow and mattress covers and weekly hot water washing of bed linens [>130°F or 54°C]). This is higher than the temperature of 120°F (49°C) recommended by the American Academy of Pediatrics as the maximum at which to set household water heaters; significant skin burns can be sustained within seconds of exposure to water at this temperature. As an alternative, water temperature could be increased temporarily during linen washing (ideally when the children are at school or asleep) and returned to a lower temperature once laundering is complete. One study suggests that normal laundering (adequate room, moderately warm water, and a variety of commercial laundry detergents) is sufficient to extract most dust mite and cat allergens from bedding.[67] Further studies are needed to determine whether there are any differences in clinical outcomes after different laundering conditions.

Alternatives to hot water washing that kill mites include drying bedding outside in the sun (dust mites are sensitive to sunlight), drying in a tumble dryer at 130°F (54°C) for at least 20 minutes, and placing soft toys in the freezer for 24 hours.[3,55] Dry cleaning of blankets kills mites but is less effective in removing allergens.[58]

Carpeting, a major source of mite antigen and proliferation, should be removed when possible, especially in the bedroom. A single vacuuming may decrease the dust-mite burden by only 35% for a carpeted surface but by 80% for a solid surface. If possible, upholstered furniture should be replaced with washable vinyl, leather, or wood. Window shades are preferable to curtains or venetian blinds. If curtains are used, they should be made of washable fabric. Blinds should be made of vinyl. Although acaricides (chemicals that kill mites) containing benzyl benzoate or tannic acid may reduce antigen levels on carpeting and upholstery, they must be reapplied every 3 months. Using acaricides is far less effective than removing carpet followed by regular damp mopping of hardwood or vinyl flooring. Therefore, many experts no longer recommend the use of acaricides in routine management of allergen avoidance.[3]

Because dust-mite allergen becomes airborne only during disturbances and falls rapidly, there is little opportunity for air cleaners to have an effect. Vacuum cleaners that incorporate a HEPA filter or double-thickness bag to prevent leakage of allergen may be helpful.[58]

Strategies to control humidity to limit growth of dust mites vary according to climate.[19,58] In humid climates (ie, at least 8 months per year with relative outdoor humidity ≥50%), controlling reservoirs for dust mites is key. Successful dehumidification of homes is very difficult in truly humid climates (eg, southeastern United States). Air conditioning to maintain indoor relative humidity below 50% requires tight housing and may be expensive to achieve. Air conditioning in the bedroom may be considered. In areas of moderate or seasonal humidity, mite growth may be strongly seasonal and growth can be substantially higher in areas of the house that maintain humidity (eg, carpets laid on a concrete slab). During dry seasons, opening windows for an hour per day will ensure removal of humidity from the house.[19] In dry climates (eg, the upper Midwest, the mountain states [altitude ≥5000 feet]) and the southwestern United States, growth of dust mites in homes is minimal unless the house is humidified.

Molds

Home remediation to reduce moisture sources is effective in decreasing asthma morbidity.[68,69] Because mold growth requires water, the water source must be eliminated to prevent and control mold growth. Sources of water include leaking roofs or pipes, prior flooding or rainwater, and condensation on pipes and ductwork within interior or exterior structure walls. To keep a home dry, exhaust fans in the kitchen and bathrooms should be in working order and used. Dehumidifiers can be considered for areas with consistently elevated humidity levels, with a target of <50% relative humidity. Dehumidifiers reduce ambient humidity but do not significantly reduce mold growth on surfaces in contact with groundwater.

Outdoor Air Pollution and Allergens

In communities with recognized periods of increased ozone, pediatricians should counsel patients with asthma and their parents about the health effects of ozone. Parents, physical education teachers, and coaches should consider modifying sports practice schedules on days with high ozone levels (see Chapter 21).

It is important to identify seasonal allergens that trigger a patient's asthma so the practitioner can initiate prophylactic antihistamine and/or anti-inflammatory therapies and/or recommend using air conditioning, if available. Staying indoors during the afternoon hours may help symptoms. Molds, especially *Alternaria* species, may be present outdoors year round in moderate climates but are greatly reduced following the onset of frost or recurrent freezing temperatures. Affected individuals should be instructed to follow pollution alerts for high pollen counts, especially during summer months.

Frequently Asked Questions

Q Do you recommend any special air filtration system for patients with asthma?
A Avoid room humidifiers and keep central furnace system humidification below 50% during winter months. Filters on central forced-air systems and furnaces should be changed periodically, according to manufacturers'

recommendations. Upgrading to a medium-efficiency filter (rated at 20%–50% efficiency at removing particles between 0.3 and 10 μm [MERV 8–12]) will improve air quality and is economical. (MERV stands for minimum efficiency reporting value. The MERV rating is the standard method for comparing the efficiency of air filters. The higher the MERV rating, the better the filter is at removing particles from the air.) Electrostatic filters/precipitators in central furnace and air-conditioning systems may be beneficial for airborne particles (eg, cat allergen) but only are effective when turned on. Avoid the use of air cleaners (usually labeled as "electrostatic") that generate ozone.

Room HEPA filters also may be beneficial. However, they only work in a single room, and the noise generated may not be acceptable. Preferably, they should be used in the child's bedroom but are of little benefit in reducing exposure to secondhand smoke.

Q *Do you recommend a special vacuum cleaner for patients with asthma?*

A Other strategies to reduce allergen exposure are more beneficial. However, an efficient vacuum cleaner that avoids resuspension of allergens may be useful for removing allergens, especially from hard surfaces. Leakage of allergen is minimized in vacuum cleaners that incorporate a double-thickness bag and have tight-fitting junctions within the cleaner; a HEPA filter is not always necessary, depending on vacuum design. Unfortunately, there is no certification process to guide consumers. Important features for an efficient vacuum cleaner have been reviewed.[58]

Q *How can we better prepare the house to prevent asthma attacks from occurring?*

A Quit smoking if you smoke, and eliminate children's exposures to secondhand smoke. Reduce dust mites, cockroaches, and home dampness or molds. Remove pets to which the child demonstrates specific allergy. If removing the pet is not possible, keep pets out of the bedroom and routinely perform allergen reduction measures (vacuuming, minimizing reservoirs of dander— eg, pillows). Consider using a vacuum cleaner that is efficient at cleaning and avoids resuspension of allergens (such as one equipped with a HEPA filter).

Q *Can odors of cooking foods cause an allergic reaction (eg, asthma) in susceptible patients?*

A Allergenic proteins aerosolized from foods during the cooking process may cause reactions in some patients. For example, a patient with a known anaphylactic or anaphylactoid response to peanuts may react to aerosolized peanut oil used for cooking. The presence of a positive skin-prick test or radioallergosorbent test (RAST) result or an elevated IgE level to a given food should not necessarily lead to an elimination diet, however, because only one third of individuals have an allergic response when challenged orally with the specific food. Children with a suspected reaction should be evaluated by an allergist.

Q Should I use a humidifier?

A Humidifiers should be avoided. A relative humidity of greater than 50% promotes the growth of dust mites and mold. If used, the humidifier must be cleaned frequently to prevent the growth of mold.

Q Are foam pillows safe for children or can they also be allergenic?

A All pillows, regardless of content, may serve as reservoirs for dust mites. An allergen-impermeable pillow cover should be used as a physical barrier between dust mite reservoirs in pillows and the child.

Q What can be done when a family lives in a multi-unit building where there are barriers to asthma control because of pest infestation and cigarette smoking in common areas?

A If families share concerns about issues such as pest control, mold problems, and cigarette smoking, they may want to organize as a group to alert management to their concerns for their children's health.

Q Should I worry about my young child swimming in a chlorinated pool?

A Recently, some studies have demonstrated that repeated exposure to chlorine byproducts among recreational swimmers may lead to lung damage.[70] In addition, some studies have been published on the issue of the possible harmful effects of swimming on a baby's respiratory health. Concerns are primarily with indoor chlorinated pools. Long-term studies will be needed to clarify this issue.

Resources

American Lung Association
Phone: 800-LUNG-USA
Web site: www.lungusa.org

Asthma and Allergy Foundation of America
Phone: 202-466-7643
Web site: www.aafa.org

Allergy & Asthma Network – Mothers of Asthmatics, Inc
Phone: 800-878-4403
Web site: www.aanma.org

California Indoor Air Quality Program
Infosheets: www.cal-iaq.org/iaqsheet.htm
Air cleaners: www.arb.ca.gov/research/indoor/aircleaners.htm

National Environmental Education Foundation
Phone: 202-833-2933
Web site: www.neefusa.org

National Institutes of Health, National Heart Lung and Blood Institute
Web site: www.nhlbi.nih.gov

National Heart Lung and Blood Health Information Center
Phone: 301-592-8573 (Public) or 1-800 877-8339 (Federal Relay Service)
Web site: www.nhlbi.nih.gov/health/infoctr/index.htm

US Environmental Protection Agency, Indoor Environments Division
IAQ Tools for Schools Program: www.epa.gov/iaq/schools
Asthma: www.epa.gov/asthma

**US Environmental Protection Agency, Transportation
and Air Quality Division.**
National Clean Diesel Campaign – Clean School Bus USA: www.epa.gov/
cleanschoolbus

University of California
Residential, Industrial, and Institutional Pest Control. 2nd ed. Pesticide
Application Compendium, Vol 2. Davis, CA: University of California; 2006.
Available at: www.ipm.ucdavis.edu/IPMPROJECT/ADS/manual_riipest-
control.html

References

1. Busse WW, Lemanske RF Jr. Asthma. *N Engl J Med.* 2001;344(5):350–362
2. Holgate ST. Pathogenesis of asthma. *Clin Exp Allergy.* 2008;38(6):872–897
3. National Institutes of Health, National Asthma Education Program. *Expert Panel Report 3 (EPR-3): Guidelines for the Diagnosis and Management of Asthma.* Bethesda, MD: National Institutes of Health, National Heart, Lung, and Blood Institute; 2007. Publication NIH 08-4051. Available at: www.nhlbi.nih.gov/guidelines/asthma/asthgdln.htm. Accessed April 2, 2011
4. Bufford JD, Gern JE. The hygiene hypothesis revisited. *Immunol Allergy Clin North Am.* 2005;25(2):247–262
5. Platts-Mills TA, Blumenthal K, Perzanowski M, Woodfolk JA. Determinants of clinical allergic disease. The relevance of indoor allergens to the increase in asthma. *Am J Respir Crit Care Med.* 2000;162(3 Pt 2):S128–S133
6. Platts-Mills TA. Paradoxical effect of domestic animals on asthma and allergic sensitization. *JAMA.* 2002;288(8):1012–1014
7. Celedon JC, Litonjua AA, Ryan L, Platts-Mills T, Weiss ST, Gold DR. Exposure to cat allergen, maternal history of asthma, and wheezing in first 5 years of life. *Lancet.* 2002;360(9335):781–782
8. Gehring U, Wijga AH, Brauer M, et al. Traffic-related air pollution and the development of asthma and allergies during the first 8 years of life. *Am J Respir Crit Care Med.* 2010;181(6):596-603
9. Gaffin JM, Phipatanakul W. The role of indoor allergens in the development of asthma. *Curr Opin Allergy Clin Immunol.* 2009;9(2):128-135
10. Etzel RA. How environmental exposures influence the development and exacerbation of asthma. *Pediatrics.* 2003;112(1 Pt 2):233–239

11. Yu O, Sheppard L, Lumley T, Koenig JQ, Shapiro GG. Effects of ambient air pollution on symptoms of asthma in Seattle-area children enrolled in the CAMP study. *Environ Health Perspect.* 2000;108(12):1209-1214

12. Centers for Disease Control and Prevention. Vital Signs: cigarette smoking among adults aged ≥18 years—United States, 2009. *MMWR.* 2010;59(35):1135-1140

13. Ehrlich RI, DuToit D, Jordaan E, et al. Risk factors for childhood asthma and wheezing. Importance of maternal and household smoking. *Am J Respir Crit Care Med.* 1996;154(3 Pt 1): 681–688

14. Martinez FD, Cline M, Burrows B. Increased incidence of asthma in children of smoking mothers. *Pediatrics.* 1992;89(1):21–26

15. Weitzman M, Gortmaker S, Walker DK, Sobol A. Maternal smoking and childhood asthma. *Pediatrics.* 1990;85(4):505–511

16. Abulhosn RS, Morray BH, Llewellyn CE, Redding GJ. Passive smoke exposure impairs recovery after hospitalization for acute asthma. *Arch Pediatr Adolesc Med.* 1997;151(2):135–139

17. Menon P, Rando RJ, Stankus RP, Salvaggio JE, Lehrer SB. Passive cigarette-smoke-challenge studies: increase in bronchial hyperreactivity. *J Allergy Clin Immunol.* 1992;89(2):560–566

18. American Thoracic Society, Committee of the Environmental and Occupational Health Assembly. Health effects of outdoor air pollution. *Am J Respir Crit Care Med.* 1996;153(1):3–50

19. Institute of Medicine. *Clearing the Air: Asthma and Indoor Air Exposures.* Washington, DC: National Academies Press; 2000

20. Delfino RJ. Epidemiologic evidence for asthma and exposure to air toxics: linkages between occupational, indoor, and community air pollution research. *Environ Health Perspect.* 2002;110(Suppl 4):573–589

21. Hansel NN, Breysse PN, McCormack MC, et al. A longitudinal study of indoor nitrogen dioxide levels and respiratory symptoms in inner-city children with asthma. *Environ Health Perspect.* 2008;116(10):1428-1432

22. Shim C, Williams MH Jr. Effect of odors in asthma. *Am J Med.* 1986;80(1):18–22

23. McGwin G, Lienert J, Kennedy JI. Formaldehyde exposure and asthma in children: A systematic review. *Environ Health Perspect.* 2009;118(3):313-317

24. Wood RA, Eggleston PA. Management of allergy to animal danders. *Pediatr Asthma Allergy Immunol.* 1993;7(1):13–22

25. Luczynska CM, Li Y, Chapman MD, Platts-Mills TA. Airborne concentrations and particle size distribution of allergen derived from domestic cats *(Felis domesticus).* Measurements using cascade impactor, liquid impinger, and a two-site monoclonal antibody assay for *Fel d I. Am Rev Respir Dis.* 1990;141(2):361–367

26. Almquist C, Wickman M, Perfetti L, et al. Worsening of asthma in children allergic to cats, after indirect exposure to cat at school. *Am J Respir Crit Care Med.* 2001;163(3 Pt 1):694–698

27. de Groot H, Goei KG, van Swieten P, Aalberse RC. Affinity purification of a major and a minor allergen from dog extract: serologic activity of affinity-purified *Can f I* and of *Can f I*-depleted extract. *J Allergy Clin Immunol.* 1991;87(6):1056–1065

28. Lindgren S, Belin L, Dreborg S, Einarsson R, Pahlman I. Breed-specific dog-dandruff allergens. *J Allergy Clin Immunol.* 1988;82(2):196–204

29. Phipatanakul W, Eggleston PA, Wright EC, Wood RA. Mouse allergen. I. The prevalence of mouse allergen in inner-city homes. The National Cooperative Inner-City Asthma Study. *J Allergy Clin Immunol.* 2000;106(6):1070–1074

30. Phipatanakul W, Celedon JC, Hoffman EB, Abdulkerim H, Ryan LM, Gold DR. Mouse allergen exposure, wheeze and atopy in the first seven years of life. *Allergy.* 2008;63(11): 1512-1518

31. Rosensteich DL, Eggleston P, Kattan M, et al. The role of cockroach allergy and exposure to cockroach allergen in causing morbidity among inner-city children with asthma. *N Engl J Med.* 1997;336(19):1356–1363

32. Peat JK, Dickerson J, Li J. Effects of damp and mould in the home on respiratory health: a review of the literature. *Allergy.* 1998;53(2):120–128

33. Bornehag CG, Blomquist G, Gyntelberg F, et al. Dampness in buildings and health. Nordic interdisciplinary review of the scientific evidence on associations between exposure to "dampness" in buildings and health effects (NORDDAMP). *Indoor Air.* 2001;11(2):72–86

34. Institute of Medicine. *Damp Indoor Spaces and Health.* Washington, DC: National Academies Press; 2004

35. American Academy of Pediatrics, Committee on Environmental Health. Policy statement: spectrum of noninfectious health effects from molds. *Pediatrics.* 2006 ;118(6):2582-2586

36. Mazur LJ; Kim J; American Academy of Pediatrics, Committee on Environmental Health. Technical report: spectrum of noninfectious health effects from molds. *Pediatrics.* 2006;118(6):e1909-e1926

37. Antova T, Pattenden S, Brunekreef B, et al. Exposure to indoor mould and children's respiratory health in the PATY study. *J Epidemiol Community Health.* 2008;62(8):708-714

38. Iossifova YY, Reponen T, Ryan PH, et al. Mold exposure during infancy as a predictor of potential asthma development. *Ann Allergy Asthma Immunol.* 2009;102(2):131-137

39. World Health Organization. *WHO Guidelines for Indoor Air Quality: Dampness and Mold.* Copenhagen, Denmark: World Health Organization; 2009

40. Nafstad P, Oie L, Mehl R, et al. Residential dampness problems and symptoms and signs of bronchial obstruction in young Norwegian children. *Am J Respir Crit Care Med.* 1998;157(2):410–414

41. Dales RE, Miller D. Residential fungal contamination and health: microbial cohabitants as covariates. *Environ Health Perspect.* 1999;107(Suppl 3):481–483

42. Seltzer JM, Fedoruk MJ. Health effects of mold in children. *Pediatr Clin North Am.* 2007;54(2):309-333

43. Landwehr LP, Boguniewicz M. Current perspectives on latex allergy. *J Pediatr.* 1996;128(3): 305–312

44. Sicherer SH, Sampson HA. Food allergy. *J Allergy Clin Immunol.* 2010;125(2 Suppl 2): S116-S125

45. White MC, Etzel RA, Wilcox WD, Lloyd C. Exacerbations of childhood asthma and ozone pollution in Atlanta. *Environ Res.* 1994;65(1):56–68

46. American Academy of Pediatrics, Committee on Environmental Health. Ambient air pollution: respiratory hazards to children. *Pediatrics.* 1993;91(6):1210–1213

47. McConnell R, Berhane K, Gilliland F, et al. Asthma in exercising children exposed to ozone: a cohort study. *Lancet.* 2002;359(9304):386–391

48. Licorish K, Novey HS, Kozak P, Fairshter RD, Wilson AF. Role of *Alternaria* and *Penicillium* spores in the pathogenesis of asthma. *J Allergy Clin Immunol.* 1985;76(6):819–825

49. O'Hollaren MT, Yunginger JW, Offord KP, et al. Exposure to an aeroallergen as a possible precipitating factor in respiratory arrest in young patients with asthma. *N Engl J Med.* 1991;324(6):359–363

50. Targonski PV, Perskey VW, Ramekrishnan V. Effect of environmental molds on risk of death from asthma during the pollen season. *J Allergy Clin Immunol.* 1995;95(5 Pt 1):955–961

51. Dales RA, Cakmak S, Judek S, et al. The role of fungal spores in thunderstorm asthma. *Chest.* 2003;123(3):745–750

52. Simmons FER. Anaphylaxis: recent advances in assessment and treatment. *J Allergy Clin Immunol.* 2009;124(4):625-636

53. Denning DW, O'Driscoll BR, Powell G, et al. Randomized controlled trial of oral antifungal treatment for severe asthma with fungal sensitization: The Fungal Asthma Sensitization Trial (FAST) Study. *Am J Respir Crit Care Med.* 2009;179(1):11-18

54. Wu F, Takaro TK. Childhood asthma and environmental interventions. *Environ Health Perpsect.* 2007;115(6):971-975

55. Krieger JK, Takaro TK, Allen C, et al. The Seattle-King County healthy homes project: implementation of a comprehensive approach to improving indoor environmental quality for low-income children with asthma. *Environ Health Perspect.* 2002;110(Suppl 2):311–322

56. Etzel RA. Indoor air pollution and childhood asthma: effective environmental interventions. *Environ Health Perspect.* 1995;103(Suppl 6):55–58

57. Tovey E, Marks G. Methods and effectiveness of environmental control. *J Allergy Clin Immunol.* 1999;103(2 Pt 1):179-191

58. Platts-Mills TA, Vaughan JW, Carter MC, Woodfolk JA. The role of intervention in established allergy: avoidance of indoor allergens in the treatment of chronic allergic disease. *J Allergy Clin Immunol.* 2000;106(5):787-804

59. de Blay F, Chapman MD, Platts-Mills TA. Airborne cat allergen (Fel d I). Environmental control with the cat in situ. *Am Rev Respir Dis.* 1991;143(6):1334-1339

60. American Academy of Pediatrics Committee on School Health, National Association of School Nurses. *Health, Mental Health, and Safety Guidelines for Schools.* Taras H, Duncan P, Luckenbill D, et al, eds. Elk Grove Village, IL: American Academy of Pediatrics; 2004

61. Sulser C, Schulz G, Wagner P, et al. Can the use of HEPA cleaners in homes of asthmatic children and adolescents sensitized to cat and dog allergens decrease bronchial hyperresponsiveness and allergen contents in solid dust? *Int Arch Allergy Immunol.* 2009;148(1):23-30

62. Kerkhof M, Wijga AH, Brunekreef B, et al. Effects of pets on asthma development up to 8 years of age: the PIAMA study. *Allergy.* 2009;64(8):1202-1208

63. Call RS, Smith TF, Morris E, Chapman MD, Platts-Mills TA. Risk factors for asthma in inner city children. *J Pediatr.* 1992;121(6):862-866

64. O'Connor GT, Gold DR. Cockroach allergy and asthma in a 30-year-old man. *Environ Health Perspect.* 1999;107(3):243-247

65. Morgan WJ, Crain EF, Gruchalla RS, et al. Results of a home-based environmental intervention among urban children with asthma. *N Engl J Med.* 2004;351(11):1068-1080

66. von Mutius E. Towards prevention. *Lancet.* 1997;350(Suppl 2):SII14-SII17

67. Tovey ER, Taylor DJ, Mitakakis TZ, De Lucca SD. Effectiveness of laundry washing agents and conditions in the removal of cat and dust mite allergen from bedding dust. *J Allergy Clin Immunol.* 2001;108(3):369-374

68. Kercsmar CM, Dearborn DG, Schluchter M, et al. Reduction in asthma morbidity in children as a result of home remediation aimed at moisture sources. *Environ Health Perspect.* 2006;114(10):1574-1180

69. Burr ML, Matthews IP, Arthur RA, Watson HL, Gregory CJ, Dunstan FD, Palmer SR. Effects on patients with asthma of eradicating visible indoor mould: A randomised controlled trial. *Thorax.* 2007;62(3):767-772

70. Uyan ZS, Carraro S, Piacentini G, Baraldi E. Swimming pool, respiratory health, and childhood asthma: should we change our beliefs? *Pediatr Pulmonol.* 2009;44(1):31-37

Chapter 44

Birth Defects and Other Adverse Developmental Outcomes

■ ■ ■ ■ ■ ■

Adverse developmental outcomes, including death, structural alterations (birth defects), functional impairments, and growth restriction,[1] can be produced by environmental chemicals.[2-7] These outcomes may be caused by maternal or paternal exposures, such as related to experiencing infections, medications, occupational or environmental pollutants,[8-11] and disasters (such as Hurricanes Rita, Katrina, and Ike and the World Trade Center collapse).[12]

Developmental disorders are recognized in approximately 3% of infants at birth, 6% of children at 1 year of age, and 12% of children at 7 years of age. Estimates of the proportion of adverse developmental outcomes related to various causes[7] have evolved as our understanding of development has progressed (Table 44.1).

Table 44.1: Estimates of the Etiology of Developmental Disorders[7]	
CAUSE OF DEVELOPMENTAL DISORDER	PERCENTAGE OF CHILDREN WITH DEVELOPMENTAL DISORDER AT BIRTH
Unknown	34%–70%
Multifactorial and interactions	20%–49%
Monogenic conditions	8%–20%
Chromosomal disorders	3%–10%
Environmental factors	2%–9%
Maternal diabetes	0.1%–1.4%
Medicinal products	0.2%–1.3%
Maternal infection	1.1%–2.0%

Most adverse developmental outcomes are of unknown etiology (>34%). Of the known causes, environmental factors are thought to represent few (<10%). However, "multifactorial and interactions" is the second most common category of etiological factors (>20%). "Multifactorial and interactions" refers to a model in which risk is a consequence of the reciprocal influence among environmental, social, and biological factors (Table 44.2). Thus, the effect of environmental factors on adverse developmental outcomes may be significantly underestimated.

ORIGINS OF BIRTH DEFECTS

Malformation

Some birth defects occur because an embryo or fetus is destined to develop abnormally. These are called malformations and include genetic as well as chromosomal disorders (Table 44.1). For certain malformations, environmental exposures can either increase or decrease the risk. For example, neural tube defects (NTDs) are an example of a multifactorial developmental disorder for which the risk is known to be decreased when folic acid supplementation is taken prior to conception.[13] Neural tube defects are the consequence of the reciprocal influence of genetic and nutritional factors with exposure to medications, chemicals, and environmental toxins (eg, fumonisin—a mycotoxin found on corn).[14–19] Neural tube defects have many causes in addition to deficiencies in folic acid.[20–23]

Developmental Outcomes

Examples of environmental exposures associated with birth defects and other developmental outcomes are summarized in Table 44.3. Much still remains to be understood about these sometimes controversial associations.[6] Length of gestation is included in Table 44.3, because preterm birth is a significant public health problem and there is evidence that gestational length is altered by some exposures.

Death

One consequence of chromosomal or genetic abnormalities is embryonic, fetal, or neonatal death. When pregnant experimental animals are treated with angiotensin-converting enzyme (ACE) inhibitors (used to treat hypertension), fetal death rates increase.[24] Similarly, increased fetal death rates (thought to be a consequence of reduction in renal blood flow) have been reported when pregnant women were treated with ACE inhibitors.[25] Death attributable to a congenital malformation has also been associated with certain paternal occupations.[9-11,26,27] Additionally, there are data linking a variety of environmental exposures with fetal and neonatal mortality.[28]

Table 44.2: Examples of Adverse Developmental Outcomes Produced by Interaction Among Environmental, Social, and Biological Factors				
ENVIRONMENTAL	**SOCIAL**	**BIOLOGICAL**	**DEVELOPMENTAL OUTCOME**	**REFERENCES**
Active smoking	Community reinforcement and peer pressure	Specific genes interact with tobacco smoke to increase risk of orofacial clefts	Orofacial clefting	29–31
Air pollution	Exposure to pollutants is based on race and socioeconomic status	Nutritional factors, which vary with race and socioeconomic status, are important in affecting birth weight	Birth weight, preterm birth, and perinatal mortality	6,32,33
Folic acid deficiency and exposures to environmental toxins, such as fumonisin	Preconception awareness and household socioeconomic status, dietary preferences (corn contaminated with fumonisin)	Specific genes, obesity, exposures to mycotoxins, use of medications that are anti-folate	Neural tube defects	13–17,20, 34–39

Structural Malformations

Approximately 50 chemicals and 15 infectious agents may produce human structural malformations.[2,4-7] This topic is extensively covered in traditional reviews.[2-5,29,40,41]

Functional Abnormalities

Functional abnormalities may be produced following adverse exposure during development. Many adult conditions and diseases are thought to have origins in fetal life.[42,43] For example, in utero lead exposure may result in lasting neurodevelopmental abnormalities.[44-46] Paternal or maternal lead exposure may increase the risk of spontaneous abortion as well as impair fetal growth and neurodevelopment. Because lead in maternal bone can be mobilized during pregnancy, exposures producing abnormal fetal development may have occurred many years prior to the pregnancy.[44] Chapter 31 contains more information about lead.

Table 44-3: Environmental Exposures Associated With Birth Defects and Other Developmental Outcomes

SITUATION OR TOXIC SUBSTANCE	BIRTH WEIGHT	LENGTH OF GESTATION	STRUCTURAL OR FUNCTIONAL DEFECT	DEATH
Agricultural work[47-52]	X		Total anomalous pulmonary venous return, anencephaly (both maternal and paternal exposures), ocular malformations, orofacial clefts	X (spontaneous abortion)
Benzene[53]	X		Neural tube defects and cardiac defects	
Carbon monoxide[54-56]	X			X
Chloroform and other trihalomethanes[57]	X		Central nervous system defects, oral cleft defects, and major cardiac defects	
Electronics assembly[26]	X			X (paternal exposure)
Hair dye[58]			Cardiac defects	
Hazardous waste[59]	X	X	Cardiac and circulatory defects, neural tube defects, hypospadias, gastroschisis	
Lead[44,60]	X	X	Total anomalous pulmonary venous return, neurodevelopmental impairment	X
Methylmercury[28,61,62]			Central nervous system defects, cerebral palsy, orofacial clefts	

Table 44-3: Environmental Exposures Associated With Birth Defects and Other Developmental Outcomes, *continued*

SITUATION OR TOXIC SUBSTANCE	BIRTH WEIGHT	LENGTH OF GESTATION	STRUCTURAL OR FUNCTIONAL DEFECT	DEATH
Paint/paint stripping[58]			Total anomalous pulmonary venous return, anencephaly	
Particulate matter[63,64]	X	X		
Pesticides[8,28,45,65-67]			Neurodevelopmental, childhood cancer	
Polychlorinated biphenyls[5,28,60,68]	X		"Yusho" syndrome, orofacial clefts, neurologic development, thyroid function disturbance, motor deficits	
Soldering[26]			Cardiac defects (paternal exposure)	
Solvents[69,70]	X		Anencephaly, gastroschisis, cardiac malformations	
Tetrachloroethylene[71]	X		Orofacial clefts	X
Trichloroethylene[58,70,72]			Central nervous system defects, neural tube defects, orofacial clefts	

Growth

Body size, birth weight, and rate of growth after birth may be indicators of insults that occur either during pregnancy and/or postnatal development. Because growth is influenced by many factors including nutrition, measures of growth are thought to be sensitive but not specific to chemical exposures. Prenatal exposure to tobacco smoke and alcohol increase fetal growth retardation and the incidence of low birth weight.[1,73,74]

SELECTED AGENTS AND THEIR HUMAN DEVELOPMENTAL CONSEQUENCES

Pregnancy represents a unique situation, because a mother's environmental exposures often reach the fetus. Consequently, understanding fetal dose and timing of exposure during pregnancy is critical for characterizing potential risks. Drugs and chemicals often result in adverse effects only during "critical periods" of development. Exposures outside of those critical periods may pose no risk of developmental disease.[2,5,7,40,41]

Anticonvulsants

The use of anticonvulsants by women of childbearing age illustrates the utility of preconception counseling as well as the risk-benefit analysis needed to determine the consequence of exposures during pregnancy.[7,75] Seizure disorders occur in approximately 800 000 US women of childbearing age (0.3%–0.5% of pregnant women), with 95% of women with epilepsy continuing anticonvulsant use during pregnancy.[75] Much attention has focused on the developmental effects produced by anticonvulsants. During a seizure, however, changes in the mother can also produce adverse developmental consequences.[75-77] Gene-environment interactions may play a significant role in developmental disorders observed in children whose mothers have seizure disorders. It appears, however, that the risk of developmental disorders is not increased in children of women with epilepsy who do not require medications for seizure control during pregnancy.

Most women with epilepsy need to continue anticonvulsant use during pregnancy to control seizures, which can be life threatening. Exposure to various anticonvulsants during pregnancy increases the risk of developmental disease two- to threefold. The risk of malformation varies substantially among the medications used to treat the various types of seizure disorders. Valproic acid use during the first 3 months of pregnancy is associated with an increased risk of major congenital malformations.[78] There is disagreement about the effects of seizure disorders on development.[76,79] Women with epilepsy who are of reproductive age should consume at least 0.4 mg/day of folic acid[80] (some recommendations for women with epilepsy suggest increasing the dose to 5 mg/day for at least 3 months prior to conception).[81,82]

Anticoagulants

The warfarin derivatives (coumarin, warfarin sodium) include anticoagulants that act by interrupting the vitamin K-dependent clotting factors and, thus, are used to treat coagulation disorders that occur among women of reproductive age.[83,84] Treatment is necessary, because untreated coagulation disorders can be life threatening. Use of warfarin derivatives results in an increased risk of developmental abnormalities, including underdevelopment of the nose, growth retardation, and vertebral abnormalities. Heparin use does not result in the same adverse fetal consequences of warfarin derivatives. Women with a coagulation disorder who are attempting to become pregnant often switch to heparin prior to conception and continue using it during pregnancy.

Cancer in Pregnancy

Treatment of cancer during reproductive ages in men and women raises concerns including impact on fertility, genetic effects increasing the risk of developmental disease in subsequent offspring, and risks should treatment be necessary during pregnancy. Radiotherapy and chemotherapy are associated with early menopause in women. The risk of developmental disease is increased when conception occurs during or shortly after treatment. If fertility is preserved, however, there is good evidence that the risk of developmental disease is no greater than in the general population.[7,85]

Environmental Exposures

Environmental exposures arise from pollutants in air, water, food, soil, consumer products, and other substances. Examples include secondhand tobacco smoke (SHS), air pollutants from motor vehicles and industrial facilities, pesticides, heavy metals, plasticizers, flame retardants, chemical byproducts of drinking water disinfection, and pharmaceuticals or other chemicals that that are incompletely removed during drinking water processing. The emotional and physical health of the mother is also included in the direct environment of the fetus.

Concern about fetal exposures to environmental hazards comes from an understanding that the fetus is sensitive during certain critical windows of development. Differing windows of vulnerability exist for many systems, including respiratory, immune, reproductive, nervous, cardiovascular, and endocrine systems. Exposures may affect general growth and may also result in later adverse outcomes, such as childhood- and adult-onset cancers[86] and other health effects including adult-onset diseases.[28,64,87]

Although fetal exposures to environmental hazards are often assumed to result from maternal exposures during pregnancy, fetal exposures to certain environmental chemicals can also be nonconcurrent with the maternal exposure (see Chapter 8). For certain persistent chemicals, such as dioxin, lead, and organochlorine pesticides, for example, the fetal exposure can occur from maternal body burdens resulting from exposures prior to conception. Paternal exposures may also contribute to fetal risk through mutagenic and epigenetic mechanisms involving the sperm; in some instances, the chemical can also be carried in the semen, with fetal exposure following conception.[9,10]

Although there are few data on the potential of most environmental exposures to produce developmental toxicity, contemporary epidemiologic techniques may be used to assess whether the exposure is likely to represent a developmental risk.[87] Data on selected chemicals and exposures are summarized in Table 44.4.

Tobacco Smoke

Many studies have demonstrated that infants born to smokers weigh less than infants born to nonsmokers, and maternal exposure to secondhand smoke is also considered a causal factor for reduction in birth weight,[88] although the evidence is only suggestive that it causes preterm birth. Evidence is accruing that prenatal tobacco exposure causes likely permanent brain changes that increase the likelihood of early and addictive nicotine use later in life.[89,90] The sensitization of the fetal brain to nicotine results in increased likelihood of addiction when the brain is exposed to nicotine at a later age. Studies of rodents[91] and primates[92] that were exposed prenatally to tobacco have demonstrated subtle brain changes that persist into adolescence and are associated with tobacco use and nicotine addiction.[93,94] Population-based human studies have demonstrated associations between prenatal tobacco exposure and early tobacco experimentation[95] as well as increased likelihood of tobacco use as an adolescent and adult.[96,97] Cigarette smoke consists of a mixture of thousands of substances including particulate matter, carbon monoxide, polycyclic aromatic hydrocarbons, lead, and cadmium (see Chapter 40), also generated as air pollutants by other sources.

Particulate Matter

Particulate matter is the mixture of solid particles and liquid droplets found in the air. Some particles are emitted directly from a source, such as construction sites, unpaved roads, fields, smokestacks, or fires. Others form from reactions in the atmosphere of chemicals such as sulfur dioxides and nitrogen oxides emitted from power plants, industries, and automobiles. See Chapter 21 for additional information about particulate matter.

Studies conducted in countries with relatively high levels of particulate matter have found limited evidence of an association with growth retardation.[28] Studies of preterm birth in the Czech Republic, China, southern California, Pennsylvania, and California have found associations between preterm birth and particulate matter. The associations tend to be relatively small, though typically statistically significant.[28]

Table 44.4: Select Environmental Exposures Associated With Adverse Developmental Outcomes

ENVIRONMENTAL EXPOSURE	DEVELOPMENTAL OUTCOME(S) OBSERVED	ESTIMATED RISK
Tobacco smoke[28,98]	Spontaneous abortion, stillbirth, birth weight, gestational length, orofacial clefts, sudden infant death syndrome (SIDS), certain birth defects	Clear evidence demonstrates that maternal smoking independently decreases birth weight and gestational length. Evidence also supports an association between maternal smoking and SIDS. It remains unclear whether maternal secondhand smoke exposure reduces birth weight and gestational length. Limited evidence supports an association between maternal active smoking and orofacial clefts, cardiac defects, spontaneous abortion, and stillbirth.
Particulate matter[6,64]	Birth weight, gestational length, cardiac defects, orofacial clefts	Evidence suggests there may be an association between particulate matter and birth weight and gestational length. Limited evidence supports an association between particulate matter and cardiac defects and orofacial clefts.
Pesticides[9,28,43,99]	Birth weight, gestational length, neurodevelopmental impact, spontaneous abortion	There is inadequate evidence linking maternal or paternal exposures to most pesticides and increased risk of spontaneous abortion, stillbirth, preterm birth, or growth restriction. Some data suggest an association between paternal exposure and spontaneous abortion. Limited evidence supports a relationship between maternal levels of DDT/DDE and preterm birth and growth restriction.

continued on page 652

continued from page 651

Table 44.4: Select Environmental Exposures Associated With Adverse Developmental Outcomes, *continued*

ENVIRONMENTAL EXPOSURE	DEVELOPMENTAL OUTCOME(S) OBSERVED	ESTIMATED RISK
Fumonisin (a mycotoxin found on corn and in corn flour)[14-17]	Neural tube defects	Neural tube defects along the US-Mexico border linked to consumption of corn contaminated with fumonisin. Fumonisin can produce neural tube defects in experimental animals (diminished by folic acid).
Methylmercury[62,63]	Brain damage	6% of infants in a Japanese fishing village in which seafood was contaminated demonstrated delayed developmental milestones and had cognitive, motor, visual, and auditory deficits.
Hypoxia[100,101]	Growth restriction, persistent ductus arteriosus	Functional closure of the patent ductus arteriosus is delayed in children living at altitudes >4 km. Asymptomatic pulmonary hypertension and other alterations of pulmonary hemodynamics also are increasingly found in these children.
Ethyl alcohol[73-102]	Brain damage, growth retardation, cardiac and joint defects	Clear evidence: 30% occurrence in infants of women with manifest chronic alcoholism.

DDT indicates dichlorodiphenyltrichloroethane; DDE, dichlorodiphenyldichloroethylene.

Pesticides

The agricultural sector accounts for more than 75% of the nation's total conventional pesticide use, suggesting that individuals engaged in agricultural work and/or residing in or near agricultural areas may be at greatest risk of exposure.[43,99]

Exposure to various pesticides has been correlated with preterm birth and reduced fetal growth.[28] A recent study on the effect of agricultural organo-phosphate pesticides found a significant positive association between maternal exposure and the occurrence of growth retardation. This finding is supported by studies of inner-city and minority populations, who are more likely to be exposed to indoor pesticides. In the first study, exposure of the fetus to chlorpy-rifos was inversely associated with birth weight.[103] The second study found that the inverse association between chlorpyrifos and birth weight was highly signifi-cant when limited to the newborn infants born before the US Environmental Protection Agency (EPA) banned residential use of this pesticide in 2000. Newborn infants born later had much lower exposure levels and, thus, did not exhibit a significant correlation between chlorpyrifos and birth weight.[104] Other studies of organophosphate metabolite concentrations and fetal growth have been less conclusive.[105,106]

Exposure to triazine and other herbicides, common contaminants of rural drinking water sources, may also lead to decreased fetal growth.[107,108]

Methylmercury

When inorganic mercury is dumped into seawater, aquatic organisms metabolize it to methylmercury. Methylmercury, an organic form of mercury, is fat soluble and concentrates in the fatty tissues of sea animals. When consumed by humans, it is concentrated in fat-rich tissues, including the brain. Two disastrous events provided information about the developmental effects of human exposures to methylmercury.[28] Iranians were exposed to methylmercury when they inadver-tently consumed seed grain that had been treated with methylmercury to repel rodents. Japanese villagers were exposed to methylmercury when they consumed fish and other aquatic species living in Minamata Bay. The bay was polluted with industrial releases of mercury that was converted to methylmercury. The mercury concentrated in the fatty tissue of fish. Children exposed in utero displayed marked neurodevelopmental effects.[62,63] See Chapter 32 for additional informa-tion about mercury.

Hypoxia

Several types of hypoxia may occur during pregnancy. In communities at high altitude, the amount of oxygen in the air is less than at sea level. Pregnancy complications related to oxygen deprivation are observed in these communities. Complications depend on the level, duration, and timing of the deprivation.

Lack of oxygen also results from carbon monoxide exposure, frequently a consequence of a faulty combustion device, such as an unventilated space heater. Carbon monoxide exposure, depending on level and duration, may produce headache, nausea, and ultimately unconsciousness. At the level producing unconsciousness, carbon monoxide can damage the fetus and affect the developing nervous system (see Chapter 25).

Ethyl Alcohol

Although alcohol has been used socially for thousands of years and its adverse effect on embryonic and fetal development had been suggested, it was not until the early 1970s that the impact on fetal development was explicitly defined.[102] Exposure to ethyl alcohol occurs as a consequence of ingestion in social settings but is considered to be an environmental exposure in the broadest sense. In some settings, occupational exposure can occur during the production of alcohol or products containing alcohol. Alcohol produces abnormal development of the face and central nervous system in a dose-dependent fashion across multiple species, including humans. It is not known what the safe dose of alcohol is during pregnancy or what the largest safe dose is during development.[102] Alcohol exposure is the most significant preventable cause of mental retardation during pregnancy.

CONCLUSIONS

Our understanding of birth defects and adverse developmental outcomes is changing; we are beginning to recognize that the impact of exposures during development may be recognized across the life of the individual into adulthood.[42,43] Birth defects are only one manifestation of developmental toxicity; others include death, growth restriction, and functional abnormalities. In addition, we now know that paternal exposures can result in adverse developmental outcomes in offspring.[9-11]

Testing systems are available to identify agents that are likely to cause human developmental disease. Clearly, the highest degree of certainty of the likelihood that a chemical, physical, or a biological agent is a human developmental toxicant comes from studies in which the agent is shown to produce developmental disease in human populations. However, human data are only available when exposure already has occurred and adverse developmental consequences have been discovered. Medical ethics does not allow clinicians and public health practitioners to wait until data in humans are available before evaluating the potential toxicity of a chemical and acting to limit or prevent exposure.

In all but a few cases, human epidemiologic research data are too sparse to support chemical risk assessments for developmental toxicity. However, experimental animal research data, in vitro experimental data, and theoretical data can be effectively used to identify potential developmental hazards. Thus, preliminary conclusions can be drawn about the likelihood that developmental disorders are attributable to drugs, environmental chemicals, or biological agents.

Given the number of known developmental toxicants relative to the number of agents that have been tested for developmental toxicity and the number of agents to which humans are exposed for which there are no developmental toxicity data, it is likely that additional developmental hazards will be identified.

NOTE: Portions of this chapter were adapted in part from: (1) Mattison DR. Developmental toxicology. In: Yaffe SJ, Aranda JV, eds. *Neonatal and Pediatric Pharmacology.* 4th ed. Philadelphia, PA: Lippincott Williams and Wilkins; 2010:130-143; (2) Stillerman KP, et al. Environmental exposures and adverse pregnancy outcomes: a review of the science. *Reprod Sci.* 2008;15(7):631-650; and (3) Giacoia G, Mattison D. Obstetric and fetal pharmacology. In: The Global Library of Women's Medicine. *Fetal Physiology.* London, England: Sapiens Global Library Ltd; 2008. Available at: http://www.glowm.com/index. html?p=glowm.cml/section_view&articleid=196. Accessed July 19, 2011.

Frequently Asked Question

Q *What can I do to ensure the healthiest possible pregnancy and to reduce the chance that my baby will have a birth defect?*

A Schedule a preconception visit with your doctor (or other clinician). Preconception health care is care that a woman of childbearing age receives before pregnancy; interconception care is care between pregnancies. A preconception visit can help you and your doctor to identify and treat health conditions that may adversely affect your pregnancy. These conditions include high blood pressure, diabetes, seizure disorders, and certain infections. The visit gives your clinician the opportunity to discuss important subjects, such as nutrition, weight, exercise, stress reduction, avoiding smoking and secondhand smoke exposure, avoiding alcohol, avoiding fish high in mercury, and avoiding recreational and occupational exposures that may pose risks. This is also an opportunity for your clinician to administer any missing vaccines and to make adjustments to any medications you are taking to ensure that they are the safest possible.

In addition to asking about your health history, your clinician will also ask about your partner's and family's health. If you or your partner have a history of birth defects or preterm births or if either of you has a high risk for a genetic disorder on the basis of family history, ethnic background, or age, your clinician may suggest that you see a genetic counselor.

Your clinician will suggest that you take 0.4 mg of folic acid daily to prevent certain types of birth defects. A higher dose of folic acid may be recommended in some situations, especially if you have already had a child with a certain kind of birth defect or if you are taking certain medications.

References

1. Stillerman KP, et al. Environmental exposures and adverse pregnancy outcomes: a review of the science. *Reprod Sci.* 2008;15(7):631-650
2. Shepard TH, Lemire RJ. *Catalog of Teratogenic Agents.* 12th ed. Baltimore, MD: The Johns Hopkins University Press; 2007
3. Schardein JL. *Chemically Induced Birth Defects.* 3rd ed. New York, NY: Marcel Dekker; 2000
4. Friedman JM, Polifka J. *Teratogenic Effects of Drugs. A Resource for Clinicians (TERIS).* 2nd ed. Baltimore, MD: The Johns Hopkins University Press; 2000
5. Kalter H. Teratology in the 20th century: environmental causes of congenital malformations in humans and how they were established. *Neurotoxicol Teratol.* 2003;25(2):131-282
6. Woodruff TJ, Parker JD, Darrow LA, et al. Methodological issues in studies of air pollution and reproductive health. *Environ Res.* 2009;109(3):311-320
7. Schaefer C, Peters P, Miller RK, eds. *Drugs During Pregnancy and Lactation. Treatment options and risk assessment Second Edition.* Amsterdam, The Netherlands: Elsevier; 2007
8. Winchester PD, Huskins J, Ying J. Agrichemicals in surface water and birth defects in the United States. *Acta Paediatr.* 2009;98(4):664-669
9. Cordier S. Evidence for a role of paternal exposures in developmental toxicity. *Basic Clin Pharmacol Toxicol.* 2008;102(2):176-181
10. Anderson, D. and M. Brinkworth, eds. *International Conference on Male-Mediated Developmental Toxicity.* Male-Mediated Developmental Toxicity. 2007, RSC Publishing: Cambridge, UK.
11. Anderson D. Male-mediated developmental toxicity. *Toxicol Appl Pharmacol.* 2005;207(2 Suppl):506-513
12. Xiong X, Harville EW, Mattison DR, Elkind-Hirsch K, Pridjian G, Buekens P. Exposure to Hurricane Katrina, post-traumatic stress disorder and birth outcomes. *Am J Med Sci.* 2008;336(2):111-1115
13. Rasmussen SA, Erickson JD, Reef SE, Ross DS. Teratology: from science to birth defects prevention. *Birth Defects Res A Clin Mol Teratol.* 2009;85(1):82-92
14. Greene ND, Copp AJ. Mouse models of neural tube defects: investigating preventive mechanisms. *Am J Med Genet C Semin Med Genet.* 2005;135C(1):31-41
15. Marasas WF, Riley RT, Hendricks KA, et al. Fumonisins disrupt sphingolipid metabolism, folate transport, and neural tube development in embryo culture and in vivo: a potential risk factor for human neural tube defects among populations consuming fumonisin-contaminated maize. *J Nutr.* 2004;134(4):711-716
16. Gelineau-van Waes J, Starr L, Maddox J, Aleman F, Voss KA, Wilberding J, Riley RT. Maternal fumonisin exposure and risk for neural tube defects: mechanisms in an in vivo mouse model. *Birth Defects Res A Clin Mol Teratol.* 2005;73(7):487-497
17. Missmer SA, Suarez L, Felkner M, et al. Exposure to fumonisins and the occurrence of neural tube defects along the Texas-Mexico border. *Environ Health Perspect.* 2006;114(2):237-241
18. Hernandez-Diaz S, Werler MM, Walker AM, Mitchell AA. Folic acid antagonists during pregnancy and the risk of birth defects. *N Engl J Med.* 2000;343(22):1608-1614
19. Hernandez-Diaz S, Werler MM, et al. Neural tube defects in relation to use of folic acid antagonists during pregnancy. *Am J Epidemiol.* 2001;153(10):961-968
20. Heseker HB, Mason JB, Selhub J, Rosenberg IH, Jacques PF. Not all cases of neural-tube defect can be prevented by increasing the intake of folic acid. *Br J Nutr.* 2008;102(2):1-8
21. Sayed AR, Bourne D, et al. Decline in the prevalence of neural tube defects following folic acid fortification and its cost-benefit in South Africa. *Birth Defects Res A Clin Mol Teratol.* 2008;82(4):211-216

22. Mosley BS, Cleves MA, et al. Neural tube defects and maternal folate intake among pregnancies conceived after folic acid fortification in the United States. *Am J Epidemiol.* 2009;169(1):9-17

23. Toepoel M, Steegers-Theunissen RP, Ouborg NJ, et al. Interaction of PDGFRA promoter haplotypes and maternal environmental exposures in the risk of spina bifida. *Birth Defects Res A Clin Mol Teratol.* 2009; 85(7):629-636

24. Tabacova S. Mode of action: angiotensin-converting enzyme inhibition—developmental effects associated with exposure to ACE inhibitors. *Crit Rev Toxicol.* 2005;35(8-9):747-755

25. Quan A. Fetopathy associated with exposure to angiotensin converting enzyme inhibitors and angiotensin receptor antagonists. *Early Hum Dev.* 2006;82(1):23-28

26. Sung TI, Wang JD, Chen PC. Increased risks of infant mortality and of deaths due to congenital malformation in the offspring of male electronics workers. *Birth Defects Res A Clin Mol Teratol.* 2009;85(2):119-124

27. Wong CM, Atkinson RW, Anderson HR, Hedley AJ, Ma S, Chau PY, Lam TH. A tale of two cities: effects of air pollution on hospital admissions in Hong Kong and London compared. *Environ Health Perspect.* 2002;110(1):67-77

28. Wigle DT, Arbuckle TE, Turner MC, Bérubé A, Yang Q, Liu S, Krewski D. Epidemiologic evidence of relationships between reproductive and child health outcomes and environmental chemical contaminants. *J Toxicol Environ Health B Crit Rev.* 2008;11(5-6):373-517

29. Shepard TH, Brent RL, Friedman JM, et al. Update on new developments in the study of human teratogens. *Teratology.* 2002;65(4):153-161

30. Shi M, Wehby GL, et al. Review on genetic variants and maternal smoking in the etiology of oral clefts and other birth defects. *Birth Defects Res C Embryo Today.* 2008;84(1):16-29

31. MacLehose RF, Olshan AF, Herring AH, Honein MA, Shaw GM, Romitti PA. Bayesian methods for correcting misclassification: an example from birth defects epidemiology. National Birth Defects Prevention Study. *Epidemiology.* 2009;20(1):27-35

32. Maantay J. Mapping environmental injustices: pitfalls and potential of geographic information systems in assessing environmental health and equity. *Environ Health Perspect.* 2002;110(Suppl 2): 161-171

33. de Medeiros AP, Gouveia N, Machado RP, et al. Traffic-related air pollution and perinatal mortality: a case-control study. *Environ Health Perspect.* 2009;117(1):127-132

34. Suarez L, Brender JD, Langlois PH, Zhan FB, Moody K. Maternal exposures to hazardous waste sites and industrial facilities and risk of neural tube defects in offspring. *Ann Epidemiol.* 2007;17(10):772-777

35. Schwarz EB, Sobota M, et al. Computerized counseling for folate knowledge and use: a randomized controlled trial. *Am J Prev Med.* 2008;35(6):568-571

36. Yang J, Carmichael SL, Canfield M, Song J, Shaw GM. Socioeconomic status in relation to selected birth defects in a large multicentered US case-control study. National Birth Defects Prevention Study. *Am J Epidemiol.* 2008;167(2):145-154

37. Brouns R, Ursem N, Lindemans J, et al. Polymorphisms in genes related to folate and cobalamin metabolism and the associations with complex birth defects. *Prenat Diagn.* 2008;28(6):485-493

38. Rasmussen SA, Chu SY, Kim SY, Schmid CH, Lau J. Maternal obesity and risk of neural tube defects: a metaanalysis. *Am J Obstet Gynecol.* 2008;198(6):611-619

39. Kjaer D, Horvath-Puho E, Christensen J, et al. Antiepileptic drug use, folic acid supplementation, and congenital abnormalities: a population-based case-control study. *BJOG.* 2008;115(1):98-103

40. Brent RL. How does a physician avoid prescribing drugs and medical procedures that have reproductive and developmental risks? *Clin Perinatol.* 2007;34(2):233-262

41. Brent RL. Environmental causes of human congenital malformations: the pediatrician's role in dealing with these complex clinical problems caused by a multiplicity of environmental and genetic factors. *Pediatrics.* 2004;113(4 Suppl):957-968

42. Grandjean P. Late insights into early origins of disease. *Basic Clin Pharmacol Toxicol.* 2008;102(2):94-99

43. Hanson MA, Gluckman PD. Developmental origins of health and disease: new insights. *Basic Clin Pharmacol Toxicol.* 2008;102(2):90-93

44. Bellinger DC. Teratogen update: lead and pregnancy. *Birth Def Res A Clin Mol Teratol.* 2005;73(6):409-420

45. Tyl RW, Crofton K, Moretto A, Moser V, Sheets LP, Sobotka TJ. Identification and interpretation of developmental neurotoxicity effects: a report from the ILSI Research Foundation/Risk Science Institute expert working group on neurodevelopmental endpoints. *Neurotoxicol Teratol.* 2008;30(4):349-381

46. Bjorling-Poulsen M, Andersen HR, Grandjean P. Potential developmental neurotoxicity of pesticides used in Europe. *Environ Health.* 2008;7:50

47. Weselak M, Arbuckle TE, Wigle DT, Walker MC, Krewski D. Pre- and post-conception pesticide exposure and the risk of birth defects in an Ontario farm population. *Reprod Toxicol.* 2008;25(4):472-480

48. Gonzalez BS, Lopez ML, Rico MA, Garduno F. Oral clefts: a retrospective study of prevalence and predisposal factors in the State of Mexico. *J Oral Sci.* 2008;50(2):123-129

49. Bretveld RW, et al. Reproductive disorders among male and female greenhouse workers. *Reprod Toxicol.* 2008;25(1):107-114

50. Batra M, Heike CL, Phillips RC, Weiss NS. Geographic and occupational risk factors for ventricular septal defects: Washington State, 1987-2003. *Arch Pediatr Adolesc Med.* 2007;161(1):89-95

51. Rull RP, Ritz B, Shaw GM. Validation of self-reported proximity to agricultural crops in a case-control study of neural tube defects. *J Expo Sci Environ Epidemiol.* 2006;16(2):147-155

52. Lacasana M, Vázquez-Grameix H, Borja-Aburto VH, et al. Maternal and paternal occupational exposure to agricultural work and the risk of anencephaly. *Occup Environ Med.* 2006;63(10):649-656

53. Wennborg H, Magnusson LL, Bonde JP, Olsen J. Congenital malformations related to maternal exposure to specific agents in biomedical research laboratories. *J Occup Environ Med.* 2005;47(1):11-19

54. Woodruff TJ, Darrow LA, Parker JD. Air pollution and postneonatal infant mortality in the United States, 1999-2002. *Environ Health Perspect.* 2008;116(1):110-115

55. Son JY, Cho YS, Lee JT. Effects of air pollution on postneonatal infant mortality among firstborn infants in Seoul, Korea: case-crossover and time-series analyses. *Arch Environ Occup Health.* 2008;63(3):108-113

56. Wang L, Pinkerton KE. Air pollutant effects on fetal and early postnatal development. *Birth Defects Res C Embryo Today.* 2007;81(3):144-154

57. Bove FJ, Fulcomer MC, Klotz JB, Esmart J, Dufficy EM, Savrin JE. Public drinking water contamination and birth outcomes. *Am J Epidemiol.* 1995;141(9):850-862

58. Wilson PD, Loffredo CA, Correa-Villaseñor A, Ferencz C. Attributable fraction for cardiac malformations. *Am J Epidemiol.* 1998;148(5):414-423

59. Fielder HM, Poon-King CM, Palmer SR, Moss N, Coleman G. Assessment of impact on health of residents living near the Nant-y-Gwyddon landfill site: retrospective analysis. *BMJ.* 2000;320(7226):19-22

60. Mendola P, Selevan SG, Gutter S, Rice D. Environmental factors associated with a spectrum of neurodevelopmental deficits. *Ment Retard Dev Disabil Res Rev.* 2002;8(3):188-197

61. Rice DC. Overview of modifiers of methylmercury neurotoxicity: chemicals, nutrients, and the social environment. *Neurotoxicology.* 2008;29(5):761-766

62. Grandjean P. Methylmercury toxicity and functional programming. *Reprod Toxicol.* 2007;23(3): 414-420

63. Wigle DT, Arbuckle TE, Walker M, Wade MG, Liu S, Krewski D. Environmental hazards: evidence for effects on child health. *J Toxicol Environ Health B Crit Rev.* 2007;10(1-2):3-39

64. Huynh M, Woodruff TJ, Parker JD, Schoendorf KC. Relationships between air pollution and preterm birth in California. *Paediatr Perinat Epidemiol.* 2006;20(6):454-461

65. Colborn T. A case for revisiting the safety of pesticides: a closer look at neurodevelopment. *Environ Health Perspect.* 2006;114(1):10-17

66. Weselak M, Arbuckle TE, Foster W. Pesticide exposures and developmental outcomes: the epidemiological evidence. *J Toxicol Environ Health B Crit Rev.* 2007;10(1-2):41-80

67. Infante-Rivard C, Weichenthal S. Pesticides and childhood cancer: an update of Zahm and Ward's 1998 review. *J Toxicol Environ Health B Crit Rev.* 2007;10(1-2):81-99

68. Yoshizawa K, Heatherly A, Malarkey DE, Walker NJ, Nyska A. A critical comparison of murine pathology and epidemiological data of TCDD, PCB126, and PeCDF. *Toxicol Pathol.* 2007;35(7):865-879

69. Thulstrup AM, Bonde JP. Maternal occupational exposure and risk of specific birth defects. *Occup Med (Lond).* 2006;56(8):532-543

70. Watson RE, Jacobson CF, Williams AL, Howard WB, DeSesso JM. Trichloroethylene-contaminated drinking water and congenital heart defects: a critical analysis of the literature. *Reprod Toxicol.* 2006;21(2):117-147

71. Beliles RP. Concordance across species in the reproductive and developmental toxicity of tetrachloroethylene. *Toxicol Ind Health.* 2002;18(2):91-106

72. Loffredo CA. Epidemiology of cardiovascular malformations: prevalence and risk factors. *Am J Med Genet.* 2000;97(4):319-325

73. Shea AK, Steiner M. Cigarette smoking during pregnancy. *Nicotine Tob Res.* 2008;10(2): 267-278

74. Rasmussen SA, Erickson JD, Reef SE, Ross DS. Teratology: from science to birth defects prevention. *Birth Defects Res A Clin Mol Teratol.* 2009;85(1):82-92

75. Uziel D, Rozental R. Neurologic birth defects after prenatal exposure to antiepileptic drugs. *Epilepsia.* 2008;49(Suppl 9):35-42

76. Battino D, Tomson T. Management of epilepsy during pregnancy. *Drugs.* 2007;67(18): 2727-2746

77. Holmes LB, Harvey EA, Coull BA, et al. The teratogenicity of anticonvulsant drugs. *N Engl J Med.* 2001;344(15):1132-1138

78. Jentink J, Loane MA, Dolk H, et al. Valproic acid monotherapy in pregnancy and major congenital malformations. EUROCAT Antiepileptic Study Working Group. *N Engl J Med.* 2010;362(23):2185-2193

79. Bromfield EB, Dworetzky BA, Wyszynski DF, Smith CR, Baldwin EJ, Holmes LB. Valproate teratogenicity and epilepsy syndrome. *Epilepsia.* 2008;49(12):2122-2124

80. Harden CL, Hopp J, Ting TY, et al. Practice parameter update: management issues for women with epilepsy—focus on pregnancy (an evidence-based review): obstetrical complications and change in seizure frequency: report of the Quality Standards Subcommittee and Therapeutics and Technology Assessment Subcommittee of the American Academy of Neurology and American Epilepsy Society. *Neurology.* 2009;73(2):126-132

81. Tomson T, Hiilesmaa V. Epilepsy in pregnancy. *BMJ.* 2007;335(7623):769-773

82. Walker SP, Permezel M, Berkovic SF. The management of epilepsy in pregnancy. *BJOG.* 2009;116(6):758-767

83. Cho FN. Management of pregnant women with cardiac diseases at potential risk of thromboembolism—experience and review. *Int J Cardiol.* 2008;136(2):229-232

84. Shannon MS, Edwards MB, Long F, Taylor KM, Bagger JP, De Swiet M. Anticoagulant management of pregnancy following heart valve replacement in the United Kingdom, 1986-2002. *J Heart Valve Dis.* 2008;17(5):526-532

85. Meirow D, Schiff E. Appraisal of chemotherapy effects on reproductive outcome according to animal studies and clinical data. *J Natl Cancer Inst Monogr.* 2005;(34):21-25

86. Selevan SG, Kimmel CA, Mendola P. Identifying critical windows of exposure for children's health. *Environ Health Perspect.* 2000;108(Suppl 3):451-455

87. Euling SY, Selevan SG, Pescovitz OH, Skakkebaek NE. Role of environmental factors in the timing of puberty. *Pediatrics.* 2008;121(Suppl 3):S167-S171

88. Office of the Surgeon General. *Women and Smoking: A Report of the Surgeon General.* Washington, DC: US Department of Health and Human Services, Public Health Service; 2001

89. Abreu-Villaça Y, Seidler FJ, Tate CA, Cousins MM, Slotkin TA. Prenatal nicotine exposure alters the response to nicotine administration in adolescence: effects on cholinergic systems during exposure and withdrawal. *Neuropsychopharmacology.* 2004;29 (5):879-890

90. Abreu-Villaça Y, Seidler FJ, Slotkin TA. Does prenatal nicotine exposure sensitize the brain to nicotine-induced neurotoxicity in adolescence? *Neuropsychopharmacology.* 2004;29(8):1440-1450

91. Nordberg A, Zhang XA, Fredriksson A, Eriksson P. Neonatal nicotine exposure induces permanent changes in brain nicotinic receptors and behaviour in adult mice. *Brain Res Dev Brain Res.* 1991;63(1-2):201-207

92. Slotkin TA, Seidler FJ, Qiao D, et al. Effects of prenatal nicotine exposure on primate brain development and attempted amelioration with supplemental choline or vitamin C: neurotransmitter receptors, cell signaling and cell development biomarkers in fetal brain regions of rhesus monkeys. *Neuropsychopharmacology.* 2005;30(1):129-144

93. Ernst M, Moolchan ET, Robinson ML. Behavioral and neural consequences of prenatal exposure to nicotine. *J Am Acad Child Adolesc Psychiatry.* 2001;40(6):630-641

94. Slotkin TA, Tate CA, Cousins MM, Seidler FJ. Prenatal nicotine exposure alters the responses to subsequent nicotine administration and withdrawal in adolescence: serotonin receptors and cell signaling. *Neuropsychopharmacology.* 2006;31 (11):2462-2475

95. Cornelius MD, Leech SL, Goldschmidt L, Day NL. Prenatal tobacco exposure: is it a risk factor for early tobacco experimentation? *Nicotine Tob Res.* 2000;2(1):45-52

96. Al Mamun A, O'Callaghan FV, Alati R, et al. Does maternal smoking during pregnancy predict the smoking patterns of young adult offspring? A birth cohort study. *Tob Control.* 2006;15(6):452-457

97. Roberts KH, Munafo MR, Rodriguez D, et al. Longitudinal analysis of the effect of prenatal nicotine exposure on subsequent smoking behavior of offspring. *Nicotine Tob Res.* 2005;7(5):801-808

98. Malik S, Cleves MA, Honein MA, et al. Maternal smoking and congenital heart defects. *Pediatrics.* 2008;121(4):e810-e816

99. Eskenazi B, Rosas LG, Marks AR, et al. Pesticide toxicity and the developing brain. *Basic Clin Pharmacol Toxicol.* 2008;102(2):228-236

100. Ornoy A. Embryonic oxidative stress as a mechanism of teratogenesis with special emphasis on diabetic embryopathy. *Reprod Toxicol.* 2007;24(1):31-41

101. Penaloza D, Sime F, Ruiz L. Pulmonary hemodynamics in children living at high altitudes. *High Alt Med Biol.* 2008;9(3):199-207

102. Henderson J, Gray R, Brocklehurst P. Systematic review of effects of low-moderate prenatal alcohol exposure on pregnancy outcome. *BJOG.* 2007;114(3):243-252

103. Perera FP, Rauh V, Tsai WY, et al. Effects of transplacental exposure to environmental pollutants on birth outcomes in a multiethnic population. *Environ Health Perspect.* 2003;111(2):201-205

104. Whyatt RM, Rauh V, Barr DB, et al. Prenatal insecticide exposures and birth weight and length among an urban minority cohort. *Environ Health Perspect.* 2004;112(10):1125-1132

105. Berkowitz GS, Wetmur JG, Birman-Deych E, et al. In utero pesticide exposure, maternal paraoxonase activity, and head circumference. *Environ Health Perspect.* 2004;112(3):388-391

106. Eskenazi B, Harley K, Bradman A, et al. Association of in utero organophosphate pesticide exposure and fetal growth and length of gestation in an agricultural population. *Environ Health Perspect.* 2004;112(10):1116-1124

107. Dabrowski S, Hanke W, Polanska K, Makowiec-Dabrowska T, Sobala W. Pesticide exposure and birthweight: an epidemiological study in Central Poland. *Int J Occup Med Environ Health.* 2003;16(1):31-39

108. Villanueva CM, Durand G, Coutté MB, Chevrier C, Cordier S. Atrazine in municipal drinking water and risk of low birth weight, preterm delivery, and small-for-gestational-age status. *Occup Environ Med.* 2005;62(6):400-405

Chapter 45

Cancer

■ ■ ■ ■ ■ ■

This chapter highlights some associations between certain environmental exposures in childhood and cancer risk. Childhood cancer is relatively rare, but in industrialized nations, it is the most common cause of death from disease and the second most common cause of death in children (after accidents). An estimated 10 700 new cancer cases were expected in 2010 in US children younger than 15 years.[1] Between 1992 and 2004, the overall incidence of cancer in patients younger than 20 years in the United States was 158 cases per million.[2] In contrast, 1.22 million cancers (excluding nonmelanoma skin cancers) are diagnosed annually among adults in the United States, corresponding to an average annual incidence rate of 3980 per million for all cancers.

The most common types of pediatric cancer are leukemias (27%) and central nervous system (CNS) malignancies (18%). Acute lymphocytic leukemia constitutes more than 75% of all pediatric leukemias and 21% of all pediatric cancers. The other childhood tumors consist of a heterogeneous group of malignancies, including Hodgkin (7%) and non-Hodgkin lymphoma (6%), neuroblastoma (5%), bone and soft tissue sarcomas (11%), germ cell tumors (7%), retinoblastoma (2%), Wilms tumors (4%), and others. The International Classification of Childhood Cancer was updated in 2005 and includes 12 major histologically based subtypes.[3]

The major categories and subtypes of childhood cancers have been evaluated for differences in age of onset, ethnic/racial, and gender-related characteristics.[2] For example, acute lymphocytic leukemia, the most common childhood cancer, has a peak incidence at 2 to 3 years of age; it is more common in males and white individuals in the United States. In contrast, osteosarcoma, a primary bone cancer, peaks during adolescence and is slightly more common in black individuals in the United States.[4] Ewing sarcoma, which also peaks during adolescence and young adulthood, is extremely rare in black people.[2] It is possible that genetic differences affecting carcinogen metabolism, immune function, growth, or other functional processes are important. Gender differences have been noted in certain types of childhood malignancies, including higher male-to-female ratios for Hodgkin disease, ependymomas, and primitive neuro-ectodermal tumors in contrast to other forms of CNS tumors.[2] A notable female predominance is apparent for thyroid carcinoma and for malignant melanoma in children and adolescents.

TIME TRENDS IN INCIDENCE AND MORTALITY

Public concern about possible increases in childhood cancer incidence in the United States led to recent analyses of childhood cancer time trends in incidence and mortality.[2,5,6] In a detailed evaluation of the trend patterns for cancers diagnosed among 14 450 children younger than 15 years from 1975 through 1995 in 9 population-based registries, a modest increase in the incidence of leukemia was largely attributable to an abrupt increase from 1983 to 1984; rates decreased from 1989 through 1995.[5] For CNS cancers, incidence increased modestly, although statistically significantly, from 1983 through 1986, but rates subsequently stabilized.

These findings were followed up in a study of trends in childhood cancer incidence between 1992 and 2004.[2] Thirteen registries representative of the US population were studied. In this time period, a modest, nonsignificant increase in the average annual incidence rate of all pediatric cancers was observed. As suggested in the earlier study, a modest increase (annual percentage change 0.7%) was noted in leukemia rates between 1992 and 2004. In this study, the rates for CNS tumors were stable, whereas increases in hepatoblastoma and melanoma were noted. Overall, there was no substantial change in incidence for the major pediatric cancers, and rates remained relatively stable from the mid-1980s through 2004.

The American Cancer Society estimated that approximately 1340 children younger than 15 years would die of malignancy in 2010.[1] Significant advancements in treatment of childhood cancers have led to an overall increase in the 5-year survival rate for all childhood cancers from 58.1% in 1975-1977 to 79.6% in 1996-2003. In the United States, approximately 1 in 640 adults between the ages of 20 and 39 years is a pediatric cancer survivor.[7]

INTERPRETING EPIDEMIOLOGIC STUDIES OF CHILDHOOD CANCER RISK

Designing and interpreting studies that attempt to evaluate environmental exposures and cancer risk are challenging, even for common adult-onset cancers.[8] The rarity of childhood cancer further adds to these challenges. Childhood cancers comprise a biologically and clinically heterogeneous group of disorders in which different environmental exposures and genetic risk factors may play a role. Careful definition of the specific disease types is very important when designing and interpreting studies of childhood cancer risk factors. For example, acute lymphocytic leukemia and acute myelocytic leukemia are leukemias with very different ages of onset and clinical outcomes. Even within acute lymphocytic leukemia, there are subtypes with differences in age of onset, outcomes, and chromosomal abnormalities in the leukemic cells. These different disease subtypes could have different etiologic factors.

To date, the majority of etiologic studies of childhood cancer have been relatively small case-control studies. These studies can be limited by statistical power, selection of controls, and recall bias. Longitudinal cohort studies that enroll healthy participants, follow them for years or even decades, and study disease outcomes are powerful studies that can elucidate risk factors. This approach has not been feasible in rare disorders, including childhood cancer. For example, even in a cohort of 1 million children, with a disease incidence of 1 in 2000 (similar to acute lymphocytic leukemia), only approximately 500 cases would occur. Clinical and biological heterogeneity would further reduce the power to find statistically meaningful associations. Investigators from around the world have formed the International Childhood Cancer Cohort Consortium that seeks to study childhood cancer etiology through combining data from existing birth cohorts.[9]

The method of exposure assessment should also be considered when etiologic studies are interpreted. Crude exposure assessments are often the only available data. For example, assessments are generally made of exposure to any type of pesticide versus studying the effects of one specific pesticide. Many chemicals are rapidly metabolized, making the evaluation of clinical specimens challenging. The timing of the exposure (preconception, prenatal, or postnatal) and the latency period between exposure and cancer development also are considerations. In the absence of environmental or biological measurements, it is difficult to interpret a child's exposure because exposure levels, or use may change over time as a result of growth, development, and behavioral changes. Finally, epidemiologic studies looking at many potential risk factors for childhood cancer might find at least one factor meeting the traditional definition of "statistically significant" ($P < .05$) by chance alone.

KEY FEATURES OF CARCINOGENESIS IN CHILDHOOD CANCERS

Although many chemical and physical agents are known to be associated with cancer risk in humans,[10] the etiology of most childhood malignancies is not known. Thus, the timing of an environmental exposure and its relationship to pediatric cancer risk cannot be directly measured. However, the latency period between a potential carcinogenic exposure and the onset of childhood cancer is relatively short in comparison with cancers in older adults. A relatively short latency period could exist for a carcinogenic exposure occurring during the prenatal period (such as the pregnant mother exposed to diagnostic x-rays) or postnatally (such as chemotherapy with epipodophyllotoxin drugs). The latency period may be longer for carcinogenic exposures occurring before conception (such as paternal cigarette smoking) that may increase the risk of childhood cancer in offspring. Latency periods are also longer for childhood exposures that may contribute to cancer in adulthood. The carcinogenicity of environmental agents may be enhanced or diminished by interaction with one another or by genetic influences.

ROUTES OF EXPOSURE

Exposures to known carcinogens such as radiation may occur directly through skin absorption, or may occur through ingestion (iodine-131 from fallout or accidents, such as the disaster at the Chernobyl, Ukraine, nuclear reactor or the explosion at the Fukushima nuclear reactor), injection (radioisotopes), or inhalation (radon decay products). Chemical and biological carcinogens may also be inhaled, ingested, or absorbed through the skin. These carcinogens occur in pollutants, tobacco products, naturally in the diet, or in medications. Occasionally, what is at first considered a therapeutic advance has eventually proved to have deleterious effects, including cancer, so practitioners must remain vigilant to the potential hazards of therapeutic innovations. In addition to exogenous agents, cancers also may result in children and adults from endogenous reactions, such as oxidation after ingestion, or other types of metabolic change. Several forms of exogenous chemical agents do not cause cancer until they undergo one or more endogenous chemical reactions.

Children are potentially exposed to environmental contaminants at higher levels than are adults. Young children spend more time on the floor or ground and put more things in their mouths. They also have a higher intake of food, water, and air per body unit of weight. Children have a higher surface-to-volume ratio than adults and, therefore, can absorb proportionally greater amounts of a contaminant. Developmentally disabled older children may be exposed to higher levels of environmental contaminants. These children may continue to put more things in their mouths for longer periods of time, may spend more time on the floor because of an inability to walk or because they engage in age-inappropriate behaviors and may fail to understand that some substances are dangerous.

BIOLOGICAL PROCESSES AND CLINICAL EFFECTS

Environmental carcinogens may act through several different mechanisms. Many carcinogens, such as ionizing radiation and certain chemotherapeutic medications, induce DNA damage.[11] Cellular processes usually repair the DNA damage, but occasionally, abnormal cellular proliferation and malignant transformation may result. Two major categories of cancer genes have been described. Oncogenes are a class of latent cancer genes that, when activated, transform normal cells to cancer cells. Tumor suppressor genes, the other main class of cancer genes, normally regulate development (eg, of the eye or kidney). When these genes are inactivated (mutated), they no longer regulate growth of the organ, and cancer develops (eg, retinoblastoma or Wilms tumor).

Carcinogens may also act by disrupting normal cellular proliferation in tissues of the fetus, developing child, or adult. Endocrine disrupters are exogenous agents that interfere with the mechanisms of natural hormones and may result in abnormal gene regulation or activation.[12,13] Disordered immune regulation, attributable to immunosuppressive agents or infection, is also associated with cancer risk. In this instance, immunosurveillance (which is responsible for the destruction of the earliest neoplastic cells) is reduced. The carcinogenic effect of a chemical is detectable when the dose is high or chronic, as in medicinal, occupational, or large accidental exposures. If an effect has been sought but not found after high exposures, it is unlikely to be found at lower ones.

RISK FACTORS

Some characteristic features of the major childhood cancer categories (and a limited number of subtypes) are shown in Table 45.1. More details about childhood cancer types and incidence can be found in the National Cancer Institute monograph and a 2008 update of childhood cancer incidence.[2,5] Although epidemiologic studies of childhood cancers have evaluated a large number of postulated risk factors, there are few known or suspected risk factor associations.[14] Familial and genetic factors seem to occur in no more than 5% to 15% of different categories of childhood cancer.[15,16] Some risk factors, such as exposure to ionizing radiation, have been established as causal. In moderate to high doses, ionizing radiation has been linked with increased risks of several types of pediatric cancers (acute lymphocytic leukemia, acute myelocytic leukemia, CNS tumors, malignant bone tumors, and thyroid carcinoma). Other risk factors have been linked with specific forms of childhood cancer. For example, treatment with alkylating agents has been linked to an increased risk of acute myelocytic leukemia in some children. An increased incidence of several types of childhood cancers is found in children with certain genetic syndromes or congenital disorders. Suggestive or limited data (the latter not shown in the tables) link certain maternal reproductive factors, parental occupational exposures, residential pesticides, cured meats, paternal smoking, and other exposures with increased risk of some types of childhood cancers.

Table 45.1: Overview of Childhood Cancer Risk Factors

CANCER TYPE	AGE PEAK	MALE: FEMALE RATIO	WHITE: BLACK RATIO	INCIDENCE (PER MILLION)	KNOWN RISK FACTORS	SUGGESTED RISK FACTORS
All cancer		1.1	1.4	157.9		
Hematologic						
—All leukemias		1.2	1.9	41.9	Birth weight >4000 g, ionizing radiation, sibling with leukemia, Down syndrome, inherited disorders (ataxia-telangiectasia, inherited bone marrow failure syndromes, Bloom syndrome, neurofibromatosis), treatment with chemotherapy for another cancer	Possible increased risk correlated with pesticide exposures
—Acute lymphocytic leukemia	2–4 y	1.3	2.4	31.9		Maternal fetal loss, maternal age >35 y during pregnancy, first born
—Acute myelocytic leukemia	Infancy	1.1	1.1	7.5		Parental occupational exposures such as benzene and pesticides
—Other/unspecified		1.3	0.8	2.4		

Table 45.1: Overview of Childhood Cancer Risk Factors, *continued*

CANCER TYPE	AGE PEAK	MALE: FEMALE RATIO	WHITE: BLACK RATIO	INCIDENCE (PER MILLION)	KNOWN RISK FACTORS	SUGGESTED RISK FACTORS
Hodgkin disease	Adolescence	1.0	1.4	11.7	Affected sibling, Epstein-Barr virus linked with some forms	
Non-Hodgkin disease	Adolescence	1.2	1.2	10.4	Immunosuppressive therapy, congenital immunodeficiency syndromes, HIV infection	
Central Nervous System						
— All CNS tumors	Infancy	1.2	1.3	27.6	Ionizing radiation, inherited disorders (neurofibromatosis, tuberous sclerosis, nevoid basal cell syndrome, Turcot syndrome, Li-Fraumeni syndrome)	Maternal diet during pregnancy (cured meats), sibling or parent with brain tumor
— Ependymoma		1.3	1.3	2.1		
— Astrocytoma		1.1	1.4	13.3		
— Primitive neuroecto-dermal tumor		1.4	1.5	6.6		
— Other gliomas		1.01	1.0	4.6		
— Other/unspecified		1.4	1.2	0.9		

continued on page 670

continued from page 669

Table 45-1: Overview of Childhood Cancer Risk Factors, *continued*

CANCER TYPE	AGE PEAK	MALE: FEMALE RATIO	WHITE: BLACK RATIO	INCIDENCE (PER MILLION)	KNOWN RISK FACTORS	SUGGESTED RISK FACTORS
Neuroblastoma	Infancy	1.1	1.2	7.3		Possible increased risk correlated with pesticide exposures, possible increased risk with maternal diuretic or oral contraceptive use
Bone Tumors						
— Osteosarcoma	Adolescence	1.34	0.9	4.7	Radiation therapy for cancer, inherited disorders (Li-Fraumeni syndrome, retinoblastoma, Rothmund-Thomson syndrome)	High birth weight, taller than peers
— Ewing sarcoma	Adolescence	1.6	9.7	2.3		Possible increased risk correlated with pesticide exposures
Soft Tissue Sarcomas						
— Rhabdomyosarcoma	Infancy	1.3	0.8	4.4	At least one congenital abnormality (up to one third of patients), inherited disorders (Li-Fraumeni syndrome, neurofibromatosis)	
— Other soft tissue sarcoma	Variable	1.1	1	6.6		

Table 45.1: Overview of Childhood Cancer Risk Factors, *continued*

CANCER TYPE	AGE PEAK	MALE: FEMALE RATIO	WHITE: BLACK RATIO	INCIDENCE (PER MILLION)	KNOWN RISK FACTORS	SUGGESTED RISK FACTORS
Wilms tumor	Infancy	0.8	0.9	5.3	Inherited disorders (WAGR [Wilms tumor, aniridia, genitourinary abnormalities, mental retardation], Beckwith-Wiedemann syndrome, Perlman syndrome, Denys-Drash syndrome)	Father employed as a welder or mechanic, possible increased risk correlated with pesticide exposures
Hepatic — Hepatoblastoma	Infancy	1.2	2.3	1.4	Inherited disorders (Beckwith Wiedemann syndrome, hemihypertrophy, familial adenomatous polyposis, Gardner syndrome)	
Germ Cell Tumors	Adolescence	1.5	1.9	11.5		
Thyroid Carcinoma	Adolescence	0.2	3.4	5.6	Ionizing radiation, inherited cancer predisposition syndromes (multiple endocrine neoplasia, familial polyposis)	

continued on page 672

continued from page 671

Table 45.1: Overview of Childhood Cancer Risk Factors, *continued*

CANCER TYPE	AGE PEAK	MALE: FEMALE RATIO	WHITE: BLACK RATIO	INCIDENCE (PER MILLION)	KNOWN RISK FACTORS	SUGGESTED RISK FACTORS
Melanoma	Adolescence	0.7	14.8	4.9	Ultraviolet radiation from sun, artificial sources (tanning salons), sunburns in childhood/ adolescence, number of nevi and dysplastic nevi, inherited disorders (xeroderma pigmentosum)	
Retinoblastoma	Infancy	1.0	1.0	3-4	Inherited disorders (mutations in retinoblastoma [RB] gene)	13q deletion syndrome

Physical Agents

Solar and Artificial Ultraviolet Radiation

A substantial proportion of all cancers in humans involve the skin. Skin cancers may be induced by ultraviolet radiation (UVR) from sun exposure.[17] Exposure to artificial sources of UVR, as occurs when teenagers visit tanning salons, also increases the risk of melanoma and other skin cancers. Because of the long latent period, skin cancers rarely occur in childhood, except when there is markedly heightened sensitivity, as in people with xeroderma pigmentosum, which has an inherent DNA repair defect, or in people with albinism because of the lack of pigment in the skin that protects against UVR damage. In the general population, individuals with darker pigmentation have lower risk of skin cancer. Maps of cancer mortality disclose that mortality attributable to malignant melanoma is significantly higher in the southern United States than in the northern United States. The incidence of melanoma has increased more rapidly than that of most cancers, and children and adolescents who experience repeated sunburns are at greater risk (see Chapter 41).[18,19]

Ionizing Radiation

Ionizing radiation (IR) is high-energy radiation that is strong enough to cause displacement of electrons and break chemical bonds. Exposure causes genotoxicity (DNA damage resulting from strand breaks and/or mutations) that can result in abnormal cell division and/or cell death. Ionizing radiation is a well-described carcinogen. Types of ionizing radiation exposure range from diagnostic radiation, such as x-rays, to nuclear power plant accidents. See Chapter 30 for more details.

Studies that began more than 50 years ago suggested a 1.6-fold excess of almost every type of cancer in children younger than 10 years after maternal exposure to diagnostic abdominal x-rays during pregnancy.[20] Subsequent epidemiologic studies confirmed these findings, but others did not.[21,22] The potential carcinogenic effects of postnatal diagnostic radiation exposure have been much less studied.[22] Large-scale data collection on pediatric exposure to diagnostic medical radiation began in the mid-1990s. Adolescents who underwent repeated exposure to diagnostic radiation examinations for scoliosis were documented to have an increased risk of breast cancer later in life.[23,24]

In recent years, computed tomography (CT) scans have been increasingly used in pediatric patients to aid in the diagnosis of a variety of illnesses. CT scanning[22,25] and pediatric interventional and fluoroscopic imaging modalities all expose patients to much higher levels of ionizing radiation than do x-rays. There are, however, no definitive data to suggest that multiple CT scans or fluoroscopic procedures increase childhood cancer risk. Large-scale studies have not yet been conducted. It is prudent to reduce exposure to diagnostic radiation whenever possible.[25-27]

Radiotherapy is associated with an increased risk of second primary cancers; treatment for Hodgkin disease, for example, has been associated with an excess of osteosarcoma, soft-tissue sarcoma, leukemia, skin cancer, and breast cancer.[28] Among children with some genetic disorders, such as hereditary retinoblastoma, the nevoid basal cell carcinoma syndrome, and ataxia telangiectasia, there is increased susceptibility to radiogenic cancers.

Numerous studies have been conducted on Japanese survivors of the atomic bombs. High rates of leukemia were initially noted in survivors, and approximately 30 years after the detonation, the rates of leukemia returned to baseline.[29] Initial studies of 807 Japanese atomic bomb survivors exposed in utero suggested that there was no excess of childhood cancer.[30] However, longer-term studies found an increased risk of breast cancer at younger ages in people younger than 20 years at the time of the bomb detonations.[31,32] Subsequent studies of solid cancer incidence in 2452 adult subjects exposed in utero identified 94 cancers, an increase over the expected number.[33] This study also evaluated 15 388 adult subjects who were younger than 6 years at the time of the detonation and found an increased risk of developing solid tumors.

In 1986, a partial meltdown at a nuclear reactor in Chernobyl, Ukraine, resulted in fallout of substantial amounts of radioactive isotopes, primarily in the Ukraine and Belarus, in neighboring countries, and to a lesser extent, throughout the world. In addition to the acute exposure, individuals were further exposed through food, milk, and water supplies. Increased rates of thyroid cancer in children, which is typically very rare, and in adults were found in several studies.[34] The incidence of leukemia following the accident did not increase in children or power plant workers involved in the cleanup.[35]

Nonionizing radiation

Nonionizing radiation refers to electromagnetic radiation that does not carry enough energy to cause displacement of electrons and break chemical bonds in living tissue. Nonionizing radiation includes static electric and magnetic fields, low-frequency electric and magnetic fields, radiofrequency electromagnetic fields (see Chapter 27), and microwaves.

Radiofrequency waves are generated as part of global telecommunications networks or as part of industrial processes utilizing this energy for heating. There are a number of studies of childhood cancer incidence and mortality in children living in the vicinity of radio and television broadcast towers, some of which suggested a small increase in leukemia risk.[36] Epidemiologic studies on electromagnetic fields and childhood leukemia have shown an increased risk of childhood leukemia with exposures above 0.3 to 0.4 microtesla (μT), compared with exposures below 0.1 μT.[36] On the basis of these studies, electromagnetic fields were classified as a possible carcinogen to humans.[37] A major shortcoming of these studies is that no experimental data from studies conducted in animals are currently available that would support the empirical association as observed in the epidemiologic studies. Selection bias is a concern in these studies, because subjects with low socioeconomic status have a higher likelihood of being exposed to electromagnetic fields, which may have led to an overestimation of the association. However, even if one assumes that the observed association is causal, the fraction of childhood leukemias attributable to magnetic field exposure is small—only approximately 2% to 4% in North America.

Asbestos

Exposure to asbestos fibers increases the frequency of lung cancer, especially in smokers, and after a latent period as long as 40 years, can cause mesothelioma.[38] The precise mechanism of asbestos-related carcinogenesis is still under investigation; postulated mechanisms include DNA damage attributable to free radicals generated by the fibers, alteration of proto-oncogene/tumor suppressor genes, and viral-host interactions. During the 1950s, schoolroom ceilings were routinely sprayed with asbestos, which deteriorated with time. As a result of recent public health initiatives, asbestos has been removed or walled off, but it is conceivable that mesothelioma may develop in adults exposed as school children, and those who smoke will have an increased risk of lung cancer (see Chapter 23).

Air Pollution

Air pollution is composed of a variable mixture of compounds that includes particulate pollutants, chemicals (eg, benzene), nitrogen oxides, carbon monoxide, and ozone (see Chapter 21). Levels of exposure vary on the basis of location, time of day, and season. At least 15 studies have been published on outdoor air pollution and childhood cancer risk. A 70% increased risk of all childhood cancer and of leukemia and CNS tumors separately was noted in 2 small case-control studies from the United States.[39] Increased childhood cancer risk was also noted with increased traffic density and nitrogen dioxide exposure in 2 other studies. However, 5 other larger studies of traffic-related exposures did not confirm these findings. Larger, prospective studies are needed and should include improved exposure assessment, characterization of cancer subtypes, and minimization of bias. So far, the weight of the epidemiologic evidence indicates that children exposed within their homes to traffic-related air pollution do not have an increased risk of developing childhood cancer.

Tobacco

Active smoking is a well-established cause of cancer. Studies on the health effects of secondhand smoke (SHS) exposure indicate an increase in the frequency of adult lung cancer among nonsmokers chronically exposed to the cigarette smoke of others. This effect is biologically plausible, given that there are known carcinogens in tobacco smoke. The risk of lung cancer is increased after exposure in childhood to secondhand smoke (also known as environmental tobacco smoke) from parents who smoke (see Chapter 40).[40] Smokeless tobacco causes oral cancer in young adults.[41] The habit of chewing tobacco has grown among high school students, who may view professional athletes as role models. The Council on Scientific Affairs of the American Medical Association has urged that restrictions applied to the advertising of cigarettes be applied to the advertising of snuff and chewing tobacco.[42] Pediatricians have an opportunity and responsibility to prevent tobacco-related cancers and other conditions.[43,44]

Environmental Chemical Exposures

Children are exposed to a wide range of chemical agents in residences, school, child care, and other environments. Environmental chemical exposures of particular concern include N-nitrosamines and nitrates; endocrine disrupters; pesticides; contaminants of drinking water, such as nitrates; mycotoxins, such as aflatoxin in peanuts; and hydrocarbons and solvents used in residences and other settings.

N-nitrosamines and Nitrates

N-nitrosamines and N-nitrosamides are the 2 major chemical groups that make up the N-nitroso compounds (NOCs).[45] N-nitrosamides are alkylating compounds that can lead to the formation of DNA adducts (new molecules that are created when a chemical binds or interacts with DNA), possibly resulting in carcinogenesis. The N-alkylnitrosoureas, one type of the N-nitrosamides, were found to induce brain tumors in the offspring of female rodents and monkeys. N-nitrosamines have been shown to induce tumors in several animal species. Exposure to N-nitroso compounds can occur via the diet, tobacco products, medications, and through work in occupations such as rubber, leather, and metal machining industries.

Maternal intake during pregnancy of cured meat, which contains high levels of N-nitroso compounds, was evaluated in case-control studies of childhood brain tumors. Two studies demonstrated statistically significant associations between high intake of cured meats and brain tumor risk, but 2 others were not able to demonstrate statistically significant associations.[46] Maternal use during pregnancy of hair coloring products, which also contain N-nitroso-related compounds, was not found to be consistently associated with childhood brain tumor risk.[47]

In view of the link between nitrate in drinking water and risk of cancer of the esophagus, stomach, colon, nasopharynx, bladder, prostate, and non-Hodgkin lymphoma (see Chapter 33), the International Agency for Research on Cancer

(IARC) has determined that ingested nitrate or nitrite under conditions that result in endogenous nitrosation is "probably carcinogenic to humans" (IARC cancer classification Group 2A).[48]

Endocrine Disrupters

Endocrine-disrupting compounds are defined as exogenous agents that change endocrine function and cause adverse effects at the level of the organism, its progeny, and/or subpopulations of organisms (see Chapter 28).[49] Diethylstilbestrol (DES) is an endocrine-disrupting compound that is also the only definitively established human transplacental chemical carcinogen.[50] DES is a synthetic estrogen that was used to prevent miscarriage from the late 1940s through the 1970s. It is now known to be associated with increased risk of vaginal clear cell carcinoma in young women whose mothers took DES during pregnancy. DES is also associated with increased rates of reproductive organ malformation and dysfunction in both male and female offspring.

The dioxin 2,3,7,8-tetrachlorodibenzo-p-dioxin (TCDD) is a highly toxic manmade compound that is also an endocrine-disrupting compound. It is a known human carcinogen, causing an increase in total cancer.[12] Rodent models suggest that altered mammary gland development and/or abnormal maternal estrogen or prolactin levels may contribute to its carcinogenic mechanism. Other endocrine-disrupting compounds are being evaluated as potential cancer risk factors. For example, di(2-ethylhexyl) phthalate, used in medical devices such as medical tubing, was recently evaluated by the International Agency for Research on Cancer and deemed to be "possibly carcinogenic to humans" (IARC cancer classification Group 2B).[51]

Pesticides

Pesticides are a heterogeneous group of chemicals with diverse mechanisms of action. As of 1997, the International Agency for Research on Cancer classified 26 pesticides as having sufficient evidence of carcinogenicity in animals and 19 having limited evidence in animals. Of these, 8 and 15, respectively, were still registered for use in the United States.[52] Many more were still in use in other countries, most notably the organochlorine insecticides. Exposures to pesticides can come from a variety of sources, including farming, manufacturing, and home and garden uses (see Chapter 37).

Most studies of childhood cancer and pesticide exposures have focused on risk of leukemia and brain tumors.[52,53] Although these case-control studies are limited by sample size, exposure assessment, and disease heterogeneity, the trends suggest a small increase in risk of leukemia and brain tumors with pesticide exposures. Increased risk of childhood cancer was suggested in an ecologic study (ie, a study in which the unit of observation is the population or community) that compared childhood cancer rates in regions of the United States with moderate to high levels of agricultural activity to regions with low agricultural activity.[54] It was postulated that children in regions of high agricultural activity would have higher pesticide exposures. This study suggested that counties with higher levels of agricultural activity had higher rates of childhood cancer. However, direct measurements of actual pesticide exposures were not conducted.

Future large, cohort studies of children are needed to further assess the risk that pesticide exposure may confer for childhood cancer. Until then, it appears prudent to continue to reduce and, if possible, eliminate pesticide exposure of children.

Hydrocarbons and Solvents

Hydrocarbons are organic compounds that include substances such as gasoline, paint thinner, solvents, trichloroethylene, and others. Benzene, a known human carcinogen, is used as an additive in motor fuels (see Chapter 29) and hobby glues and in the manufacture of plastics and is also formed by the incomplete combustion of fossil fuels. The dose-response relationship between benzene exposure and adult leukemia (especially acute myelocytic leukemia) risk has been well established in adults with occupational exposures.[10]

A few studies have been conducted of parental occupations, parental hobbies, and home projects that involve hydrocarbons and solvents in paints and plastic.[55] Some suggest an increased risk of childhood leukemia with these exposures, but most are limited by lack of information about the degree of exposure incurred by the child and the accuracy of the self-reported information. As with many other chemical exposures, there is much speculation about the role that a parental exposure (before conception, prenatally, or postnatally) could play in the development of childhood cancer.

Arsenic

Arsenic is a well-documented human carcinogen that is associated with the development of adult-onset cancer of the skin, lungs, bladder, and possibly liver (see Chapter 22).[56] It induces oxidative damage to DNA and has recently been shown to be an endocrine-disrupting compound. Arsenic crosses the placenta and has been associated with growth retardation and fetal loss. The long-term effects of arsenic exposure and childhood cancer risk are not well established.

Infection

Infectious agents also may contribute to childhood cancer risk.[57] Unless an infant is immunized shortly after birth, vertical transmission from infected mother to infant of hepatitis B virus (HBV) is common. More than 90% of infants infected perinatally with hepatitis B virus will develop chronic hepatitis B virus infection. Up to 25% of infants and older children who acquire hepatitis B virus infection will eventually develop hepatitis B virus-related hepatocellular carcinoma or cirrhosis. Immunization shortly after birth with hepatitis B vaccine and hepatitis B immune globulin, followed by routine administration of 2 additional doses of hepatitis B vaccine, will prevent chronic hepatitis B virus infection and consequences in most infants.[58]

In childhood, Burkitt lymphoma results from Epstein-Barr virus infection and is endemic in parts of Africa. It is rarely seen in North America and Europe, suggesting possible gene-environment interactions in susceptibility. Epstein-Barr virus is also associated with childhood Hodgkin lymphoma, nasopharyngeal carcinoma, and the majority of cases of post-transplant lymphoproliferative disorder. Infection with other agents raises risks of certain cancers in adults. They include Kaposi sarcoma in individuals infected with HIV, hepatitis C-associated liver cancer, and *Helicobacter pylori*-associated gastric cancer. Young women are at risk of cervical cancer caused by human papillomavirus (HPV). Human papillomavirus vaccine can be given to girls as early as 9 years of age and is universally recommended for girls and young women.[58] In 2009, the Advisory Committee on Immunization Practices of the Centers for Disease Control and Prevention (CDC) voted to recommend that CDC permit use of the quadrivalent human papillomavirus vaccine in boys and men ages 9 through 26 years but stopped short of universally recommending the vaccine in males.[59]

Several studies have found that children who have fewer recorded common infections (eg, upper respiratory tract infections) in the first year of life and less social contact (ie, through child care settings) are at increased risk of childhood leukemia.[57] Investigators hypothesize that early exposure to common childhood illnesses leads to a more "mature" immune system and that immune dysregulation may contribute to childhood leukemia risk. Further data are needed to fully understand these findings.

Diet

A variety of natural chemicals in food may be carcinogenic in people. These chemicals include aflatoxins, sassafras, cycasin, and bracken (their natural constituents are carcinogens), which can be found in peanuts, peanut butter, and many other foods, as well as protein pyrolysates produced when certain foods are cooked. Foods high in nitrates have been associated with cancer risk (see previous section on nitrates). Preliminary studies have associated maternal consumption of DNA topoisomerase II inhibitor-containing foods (including specific fruits and vegetables, soy, coffee, wine, tea, and cocoa) with increased risk of infant leukemia.[60] Some food constituents protect against cancer in experimental animals. Among these anticarcinogens are carotenoids, dietary fiber, and foods containing antioxidants.[61]

It has been difficult to derive strong evidence that individual components of the diet are carcinogenic in humans because of the long latent periods, the role of metabolic conversion, and possibly interactions that may potentiate or inhibit carcinogenesis. Laboratory experiments in animals and human correlational studies suggest that overeating contributes to cancer of the endometrium, and fats, in particular, contribute to cancer of the breast and colon.[62] The composition of the diet is believed to affect intestinal bacterial flora, which in turn produce carcinogenic metabolites through degradation of bile acids and cholesterol. High fiber content is believed to diminish the frequency of colon cancer by speeding transit time and, thus, diminishing contact between dietary carcinogens and intestinal mucosa.

Data from epidemiologic studies, clinical observations, and animal experiments are insufficient to allow for strong recommendations to be made about specific dietary factors. No harm would be done, however, and other health benefits might result from following the recommendations of several medical organizations about diet and cancer: reduce fat consumption from 40% to 30% of calories; include whole-grain cereals, citrus fruits, and green or yellow vegetables in the daily diet; limit consumption of salt-cured and smoke-cured foods and alcoholic beverages; and maintain optimal body weight.[61]

Parental Occupation

Since the mid-1970s, literature has implicated parental occupational exposures to potential carcinogens in the etiology of many types of childhood cancers.[14] Exposures have been studied before conception, prenatally, and postnatally. Agents such as ionizing radiation, asbestos, benzene, pesticides, and many others have been implicated in the etiology of childhood cancers. The strategy used to assess such exposures in most studies, however, has been limited to identifying job exposure from job titles on birth or death certificates or a job history obtained from one or, to a lesser extent, both parents. The relationship between specific jobs or parental occupational exposures and specific childhood cancers has often been inconsistent. The application of newer and more accurate methods to ascertain exposure is more likely to clarify the relationship of specific occupational exposures with specific forms of childhood cancer.

WHAT TO DO IF CLUSTERS ARE OBSERVED

Clusters of cancers occasionally occur within a neighborhood or school district, often by chance. It is possible that cancers may be environmentally induced (ie, the histories of the affected people reveal a large exposure in common, usually to a drug or occupational chemical).[63,64] In office practice, pediatricians can make novel observations about environmental or other causes of specific types of childhood cancers. If a cluster is suspected, the pediatrician should report this observation to the state health department. It is important to determine whether the cancers are of the same or related types. Cancers of the same type are more likely than diverse types to be induced by an environmental carcinogen. Cases should be excluded if the latent period is too short or if the neoplasm was present before the child resided, attended school, or was otherwise exposed in the area. If the exclusions do not dispel the clusters, an environmental epidemiologist from the state health department should be consulted.

An association between 2 events need not be causal. Establishing causality is enhanced by showing (1) a logical time sequence (ie, the presumed causal event preceded the effect); (2) specificity of the effect (ie, one type rather than multiple types of cancer caused by a given exposure); (3) a dose-response relationship; (4) biologic plausibility (ie, the new information is consistent with previous knowledge); (5) consistency with other observations about cause and effect (eg, determining whether the relationship of fat consumption to colon cancer rates is demonstrated in other countries); (6) the exclusion of concomitant variables (alternative explanations) in the analysis; and (7) disappearance of the effect when the cause is removed. Not all of these elements can be evaluated or will hold true for even the most fully studied effects of an environmental exposure. It is not the pediatrician's job to establish causality but to work with epidemiologists and health department to evaluate the situation.[65]

SEARCHING FOR CLUES TO CANCER CAUSES

In searching for clues to cancer causes, a careful history can provide important information. Family history ranks first. Ideally, the medical history for a child with cancer should include a recent pedigree showing illnesses and age of onset in each first-degree relative (parents, siblings, and children of the index case), as well as information about other relatives with cancer or other potentially related diseases, such as immunologic disorders, blood dyscrasias, or congenital malformations. Second, pediatricians should inquire about parents' occupations and other exposures (including smoking) before and during pregnancy and about the child's exposures to secondhand smoke, chemicals, radiation, and unusual infections. Other findings that may be important in determining the cause are coexistent disease (such as multiple congenital malformations), multifocal or bilateral cancer in paired organs (a possible clue to hereditary transmission), cancer of an unusual histologic type, cancer at an unusual age (eg, adult-type cancers in childhood), cancer at an unusual site, or marked overreaction to conventional cancer therapy (eg, acute reaction to radiotherapy for lymphoma in ataxia telangiectasia). This information, especially regarding family history, may be relevant to the risk of malignancy in relatives. Epidemiologists also can use this information to gain new understandings of the origins of childhood cancer.

Frequently Asked Questions

Q *What steps can I take to prevent cancer in my child?*

A The causes of most childhood cancers are unknown. Most cases of cancer occur in adulthood, and we still do not know how to decrease the chances of developing certain types of cancer in adulthood. Children should be encouraged not to smoke or use smokeless tobacco products. Adults should be encouraged to quit smoking; if they choose to keep smoking, they should never smoke indoors or in the car to prevent family members from being exposed to secondhand smoke. Children should not sunburn and should be encouraged to wear clothing and hats and to use sunscreen when outdoors. Teenagers should not be allowed to tan in tanning salons. Other important preventive measures include testing the home for radon and making sure no friable asbestos exists in the home.

Q *Why did neuroblastoma develop in my 3-month-old child?*

A Almost all childhood cancer in the United States occurs at random. In one study of 500 children, no cause of neuroblastoma could be found. A recent genome-wide association study identified a region on chromosome 2 that was associated with a 1.5- to 2-fold increased risk of neuroblastoma. We also know that damage to DNA occurs at a specific location in chromosome 1 in neuroblastoma, but rarely do we know what causes the mutation in this or other childhood cancers. Mutations may occur during normal reshuffling of genetic material. Usually, the damage is repaired and cancer does not develop, but unfortunately, this defense is sometimes breached.

Q *The cat's been sick. Could the cat have caused my child's leukemia?*

A Cats develop a similar disease caused by a virus, which they can transmit to other cats but not to humans. The same is true of chickens and cattle, in which a leukemia-like disease is virally induced. There is no evidence that pets transmit cancer to humans.

Q *Several children in our neighborhood have cancer. Could it be caused by the same thing?*

A Although most environmental causes of cancer in humans have been first recognized by the occurrence of a cluster of cases, such discoveries are infrequent and generally involve rare cancers attributable to heavy exposures to a carcinogen. The many types of cancer (more than 80) give rise to thousands of random clusters each year in the United States in neighborhoods, schools, social clubs, sports teams, and other groups of people. By focusing on the location of cases, an otherwise random clustering of cases may seem to be unusual. To establish a cause, however, more evidence than a cluster is needed, including a dose-response effect (the bigger the dose, the more frequent the effect) and biologic plausibility considering other knowledge about cancer. In most clusters, there are many different types of cancers and many different causes, rather than a single cause.

Q *Will my child with cancer give my other children cancer?*

A Cancer is not transmitted from one person to another. Occasionally, a genetic predisposition to specific cancers is transmitted from parents to children, which may have implications for other children in the family.

For example, retinoblastoma runs in families. Usually, signs of predisposition to hereditary cancer can be detected in the histories of families with genetic disorders. For children at risk, early detection and treatment can improve survival and well-being. Thus, few children die of retinoblastoma today.

Q *A member of our household smokes. Could that be the cause of my child's cancer?*

A There is no evidence that childhood cancer has been induced by exposure to secondhand smoke. Cancers in children younger than 15 years generally are of a different microscopic category from cigarette-induced cancers, and no evidence currently exists that the childhood types are inducible by secondhand smoke. On the other hand, adult cancers such as lung cancer, leukemia, and lymphoma have been associated with exposure to maternal smoking that occurs before the child reaches age 10 years.

Q *Is it possible that the drugs I took during pregnancy started my child's cancer?*

A Diethylstilbestrol (DES) is the only known medication given to pregnant mothers that is associated with increased cancer risk in their children. It has not been used since the 1970s and was associated primarily with vaginal clear cell adenocarcinoma in young women whose mothers took DES during pregnancy. Other drugs commonly used during pregnancy have not been shown to be carcinogenic in the offspring. Drugs that have been shown to present a risk of either malformations or a theoretical risk of cancer are generally avoided during pregnancy.

Q *I have heard that peanut butter may cause cancer. Is this true?*

A It is true that peanuts are often contaminated with molds producing aflatoxins, which are known carcinogens. The US Food and Drug Administration allows aflatoxins at low levels in nuts, seeds, and legumes, because they are considered "unavoidable contaminants." If a particular batch of peanut butter is tested and the concentration of aflatoxin is over the action level, it will be subject to a recall.

Q *Is childhood cancer increasing?*

A Overall, there has been no substantial change in the incidence for the major pediatric cancers since the mid-1980s in the United States. Modest increases in rates of certain types of childhood cancer (including the leukemias, brain/

central nervous system cancers) have been noted. The type and pattern of these increases over a short period suggest that the increases may reflect diagnostic improvements and/or reporting changes.

Q *Does living near a nuclear power plant increase my child's risk of cancer?*

A One study in Germany showed that children younger than 5 years with leukemia were more than twice as likely as a comparison group of children to live within 5 km of a nuclear power plant.[66] It is not clear whether this association is causal. Additional studies are needed to clarify the risk of living near a nuclear power plant.

Resources

National Cancer Institute
Phone: 800-4-CANCER
Web site: www.cancer.gov

CureSearch, Children's Oncology Group
Web site: www.childrensoncologygroup.org

Reference List

1. American Cancer Society. What is childhood cancer? Available at: http://www.cancer.org/Cancer/CancerinChildren/DetailedGuide/cancer-in-children-childhood-cancer. Accessed April 4, 2011
2. Linabery AM, Ross JA. Trends in childhood cancer incidence in the U.S. (1992-2004). *Cancer.* 2008;112(2):416-432
3. Steliarova-Foucher E, Stiller C, Lacour B, Kaatsch P. International Classification of Childhood Cancer, third edition. *Cancer.* 2005;103(7):1457-1467
4. Mirabello L, Troisi R, Savage SA. Osteosarcoma incidence and survival rates from 1973 to 2004: data from the surveillance, epidemiology, and end results program. *Cancer.* 2009;115(7):1531-1543
5. Linet MS, Ries LA, Smith MA, Tarone RE, Devesa SS. Cancer surveillance series: recent trends in childhood cancer incidence and mortality in the United States. *J Natl Cancer Inst.* 1999;91(12):1051-1058
6. Bleyer A, O'Leary M, Barr R, Ries LAG, eds. *Cancer Epidemiology in Older Adolescents and Young Adults 15 to 29 Years of Age, Including SEER Incidence and Survival: 1975-2000.* Bethesda, MD: National Cancer Institute; 2006. NIH Pub. No. 06-5767
7. Hewitt M, Weiner SL, Simone JV. *Childhood Cancer Survivorship: Improving Care and Quality of Life.* Washington, DC: The National Academies Press; 2003
8. Linet MS, Wacholder S, Zahm SH. Interpreting epidemiologic research: lessons from studies of childhood cancer. *Pediatrics.* 2003;112(1 Pt 2):218-232
9. Brown RC, Dwyer T, Kasten C, et al. Cohort profile: the International Childhood Cancer Cohort Consortium (I4C). *Int J Epidemiol.* 2007;36(4):724-730
10. Belpomme D, Irigaray P, Hardell L, et al. The multitude and diversity of environmental carcinogens. *Environ Res.* 2007;105(3):414-429
11. Anderson LM. Environmental genotoxicants/carcinogens and childhood cancer: bridgeable gaps in scientific knowledge. *Mutat Res.* 2006;608(2):136-156

12. Birnbaum LS, Fenton SE. Cancer and developmental exposure to endocrine disruptors. *Environ Health Perspect.* 2003;111(4):389-394

13. Soto AM, Vandenberg LN, Maffini MV, Sonnenschein C. Does breast cancer start in the womb? *Basic Clin Pharmacol Toxicol.* 2008;102(2):125-133

14. Bunin GR. Nongenetic causes of childhood cancers: evidence from international variation, time trends, and risk factor studies. *Toxicol Appl Pharmacol.* 2004;199(2):91-103

15. Pakakasama S, Tomlinson GE. Genetic predisposition and screening in pediatric cancer. *Pediatr Clin North Am.* 2002;49(6):1393-1413

16. Stiller CA. Epidemiology and genetics of childhood cancer. *Oncogene.* 2004;23(38):6429-6444

17. Leiter U, Garbe C. Epidemiology of melanoma and nonmelanoma skin cancer—the role of sunlight. *Adv Exp Med Biol.* 2008;624:89-103

18. American Academy of Pediatrics, Committee on Environmental Health. Ultraviolet radiation: a hazard to children and adolescents. *Pediatrics.* 2011;127(3):588-597

19. Strouse JJ, Fears TR, Tucker MA, Wayne AS. Pediatric melanoma: risk factor and survival analysis of the surveillance, epidemiology and end results database. *J Clin Oncol.* 2005;23(21):4735-4741

20. Bithell JF, Stewart AM. Pre-natal irradiation and childhood malignancy: a review of British data from the Oxford Survey. *Br J Cancer.* 1975;31(3):271-287

21. Schulze-Rath R, Hammer GP, Blettner M. Are pre- or postnatal diagnostic X-rays a risk factor for childhood cancer? A systematic review. *Radiat Environ Biophys.* 2008;47(3):301-312

22. Linet MS, Kim KP, Rajaraman P. Children's exposure to diagnostic medical radiation and cancer risk: epidemiologic and dosimetric considerations. *Pediatr Radiol.* 2009;39(Suppl 1):S4-S26

23. Hoffman DA, Lonstein JE, Morin MM, Visscher W, Harris BS, III, Boice JD Jr. Breast cancer in women with scoliosis exposed to multiple diagnostic x rays. *J Natl Cancer Inst.* 1989;81(17):1307-1312

24. Ronckers CM, Doody MM, Lonstein JE, Stovall M, Land CE. Multiple diagnostic X-rays for spine deformities and risk of breast cancer. *Cancer Epidemiol Biomarkers Prev.* 2008;17(3):605-613

25. Brody AS, Frush DP, Huda W, Brent RL. Radiation risk to children from computed tomography. *Pediatrics.* 2007;120(3):677-682

26. Goske MJ, Applegate KE, Boylan J, et al. The 'Image Gently' campaign: increasing CT radiation dose awareness through a national education and awareness program. *Pediatr Radiol.* 2008;38(3):265-269

27. Strauss KJ, Kaste SC. ALARA in pediatric interventional and fluoroscopic imaging: striving to keep radiation doses as low as possible during fluoroscopy of pediatric patients—a white paper executive summary. *J Am Coll Radiol.* 2006;3(9):686-688

28. Curtis RE, Freedman DM Ron E Ries LAG Hacker DG Edwards BK Tucker MA Fraumeni JF Jr, eds. *New Malignancies Among Cancer Survivors. SEER Cancer Registries, 1973-2000.* National Cancer Institute; 2008. NIH Publication No. 05-5302

29. Ichimaru M, Ishimaru T. Review of thirty years study of Hiroshima and Nagasaki atomic bomb survivors. II. Biological effects. D. Leukemia and related disorders. *J Radiat Res (Tokyo).* 1975;16(Suppl):89-96

30. Miller RW. Discussion: severe mental retardation and cancer among atomic bomb survivors exposed in utero. *Teratology.* 1999;59(4):234-235

31. Land CE, Tokunaga M, Koyama K, et al. Incidence of female breast cancer among atomic bomb survivors, Hiroshima and Nagasaki, 1950-1990. *Radiat Res.* 2003;160(6):707-717

32. Miller RW. Delayed effects of external radiation exposure: a brief history. *Radiat Res.* 1995;144(2):160-169

33. Preston DL, Cullings H, Suyama A, et al. Solid cancer incidence in atomic bomb survivors exposed in utero or as young children. *J Natl Cancer Inst.* 2008;100(6):428-436

34. Ron E. Thyroid cancer incidence among people living in areas contaminated by radiation from the Chernobyl accident. *Health Phys.* 2007;93(5):502-511

35. Howe GR. Leukemia following the Chernobyl accident. *Health Phys.* 2007;93(5):512-515

36. Schuz J. Implications from epidemiologic studies on magnetic fields and the risk of childhood leukemia on protection guidelines. *Health Phys.* 2007;92(6):642-648

37. International Agency for Research on Cancer. *IARC Monographs on the evaluation of carcinogenic risks to humans, Vol 80; non-ionizing radiation, part 1: static and extremely low-frequency (ELF) electric and magnetic fields.* Lyon, France: International Agency for Research on Cancer; 2002

38. Cugell DW, Kamp DW. Asbestos and the pleura: a review. *Chest.* 2004;125(3):1103-1117

39. Raaschou-Nielsen O, Reynolds P. Air pollution and childhood cancer: a review of the epidemiological literature. *Int J Cancer.* 2006;118(12):2920-2929

40. Boffetta P, Tredaniel J, Greco A. Risk of childhood cancer and adult lung cancer after childhood exposure to passive smoke: a meta-analysis. *Environ Health Perspect.* 2000;108(1):73-82

41. NIH State-of-the-Science Conference Statement on Tobacco Use: Prevention, Cessation, and Control. *NIH Consens State Sci Statements.* 2006;23(3):1-26

42. American Medical Association. Consolidation of AMA Policy on Tobacco and Smoking. Report 3 of the Council on Scientific Affairs (A04). Available at: http://www.ama-assn.org/ama/no-index/about-ama/13635.shtml. Accessed April 4, 2011

43. Best DB; American Academy of Pediatrics, Committee on Environmental Health, Committee on Native American Child Health, and Committee on Adolescence. Technical report—secondhand and prenatal tobacco smoke exposure. *Pediatrics.* 2009;124(5):e1017–e1044

44. American Academy of Pediatrics, Committee on Environmental Health, Committee on Substance Abuse, Committee on Adolescence, Committee on Native American Child Health. Policy statement—tobacco use: a pediatric disease. *Pediatrics.* 2009;124(5):1474–

45. Brambilla G, Martelli A. Genotoxic and carcinogenic risk to humans of drug-nitrite interaction products. *Mutat Res.* 2007;635(1):17-52

46. Dietrich M, Block G, Pogoda JM, Buffler P, Hecht S, Preston-Martin S. A review: dietary and endogenously formed *N*-nitroso compounds and risk of childhood brain tumors. *Cancer Causes Control.* 2005;16(6):619-635

47. Holly EA, Bracci PM, Hong MK, Mueller BA, Preston-Martin S. West Coast study of childhood brain tumours and maternal use of hair-colouring products. *Paediatr Perinat Epidemiol.* 2002;16(3):226-235

48. International Agency for Research on Cancer. *IARC Monographs on the Evaluation of Carcinogenic Risks to Humans. Volume 94: Ingested Nitrates and Nitrites, and Cyanobacterial Peptide Toxins.* Lyon, France: International Agency for Research on Cancer; 2010. Available at: http://monographs.iarc.fr/ENG/Monographs/vol94/mono94-1.pdf. Accessed April 4, 2011

49. US Environmental Protection Agency. Endocrine Disruptor Screening Program. Available at: http://www.epa.gov/endo/index.htm. Accessed April 4, 2011

50. Newbold RR. Lessons learned from perinatal exposure to diethylstilbestrol. *Toxicol Appl Pharmacol.* 2004;199(2):142-150

51. International Agency for Research on Cancer. *IARC Monographs on the Evaluation of Carcinogenic Risks to Humans. Volume 101: Some Chemicals in Industrial and Consumer Products, Some Food Contaminants and Flavourings, and Water Chlorination By-Products.* Lyon, France: International Agency for Research on Cancer; 2011

52. Zahm SH, Ward MH. Pesticides and childhood cancer. *Environ Health Perspect.* 1998;106 (Suppl 3):893-908

53. Infante-Rivard C, Weichenthal S. Pesticides and childhood cancer: an update of Zahm and Ward's 1998 review. *J Toxicol Environ Health B Crit Rev.* 2007;10(1-2):81-99

54. Carozza SE, Li B, Elgethun K, Whitworth R. Risk of childhood cancers associated with residence in agriculturally intense areas in the United States. *Environ Health Perspect.* 2008;116(4):559-565

55. Schuz J, Kaletsch U, Meinert R, Kaatsch P, Michaelis J. Risk of childhood leukemia and parental self-reported occupational exposure to chemicals, dusts, and fumes: results from pooled analyses of German population-based case-control studies. *Cancer Epidemiol Biomarkers Prev.* 2000;9(8):835-838

56. Vahter M. Health effects of early life exposure to arsenic. *Basic Clin Pharmacol Toxicol.* 2008;102(2):204-211

57. Greaves M. Infection, immune responses and the aetiology of childhood leukaemia. *Nat Rev Cancer.* 2006;6(3):193-203

58. American Academy of Pediatrics, Committee on Infectious Diseases. Red Book Online. Available at: http://aapredbook.aappublications.org. Accessed April 4, 2011

59. Centers for Disease Control and Prevention. FDA licensure of quadrivalent human papillomavirus vaccine (HPV4, Gardasil) for use in males and guidance from the Advisory Committee on Immunization Practices (ACIP). *MMWR Morb Mortal Wkly Rep.* 2010;59(20):630-632

60. Ross JA. Maternal diet and infant leukemia: a role for DNA topoisomerase II inhibitors? *Int J Cancer Suppl.* 1998;11:26-28

61. Key TJ, Schatzkin A, Willett WC, Allen NE, Spencer EA, Travis RC. Diet, nutrition and the prevention of cancer. *Public Health Nutr.* 2004;7(1A):187-200

62. Gonzalez CA, Riboli E. Diet and cancer prevention: where we are, where we are going. *Nutr Cancer.* 2006;56(2):225-231

63. Kingsley BS, Schmeichel KL, Rubin CH. An update on cancer cluster activities at the Centers for Disease Control and Prevention. *Environ Health Perspect.* 2007;115(1):165-171

64. Benowitz S. Busting cancer clusters: realities often differ from perceptions. *J Natl Cancer Inst.* 2008;100(9):614-615

65. Hill AB. The environment and disease: association or causation? *Proc R Soc Med.* 1965;58:295-300

66. Kaatsch P, Spix C, Schulze-Rath R, Schmiedel S, Blettner M. Leukaemia in young children living in the vicinity of German nuclear power plants. *Int J Cancer.* 2008;122(4):721-726

Chapter 46

Chelation for "Heavy Metal" Toxicity

■ ■ ■ ■ ■ ■

INTRODUCTION

This chapter refers specifically to the unnecessary use by some practitioners of chelation for so-called "heavy metal" toxicity. This chapter is not about chelation of patients who are iron-overloaded as a result of increased absorption (thalassemia intermedia) or chronic transfusion therapy. In these situations, chelation is approved and indicated.

The most frequently encountered off-label uses of chelation agents in the pediatric setting are for treatment of neurodevelopmental disorders, including attention-deficit/hyperactivity disorder (ADHD), autism spectrum disorders, and others. These disorders are difficult to diagnose and treat, resulting in frustrated families and clinicians. As a result, families may seek treatment outside of the usual medical system or ask their child's pediatrician for chelation therapy for heavy metal toxicity. It is important to understand and acknowledge the basis for these requests.

Heavy metal is a loosely defined term referring to metals with specific gravity of 5 or higher (although metalloids are sometimes called "heavy" as well), including copper, lead, zinc, cadmium, chromium, arsenic, mercury, and nickel.[1] The term may be used to mean that the metal is toxic when ingested or absorbed. Chelation is the treatment of heavy metal poisoning using agents that bind with a metal ion to form a complex with different chemical, biological, and/or physical properties. The resulting complexes are more easily removed or excreted from the body than the uncomplexed metal.[2] Ideal chelation agents are water soluble to enter the bloodstream, are stable, are able to reach physiological compartments in which metals accumulate, form nontoxic complexes with the metal, and

can be excreted without causing harm. Most chelation agents have some affinity for all metals; it is important to select the agent that is best suited to form
complexes with the metal of concern without depleting other essential minerals,
such as calcium and zinc.[3]

Chelation agents are classified mainly by their affinity for organic states.
Hydrophilic chelators enhance renal excretion of metals and do not cross
cellular walls well; as a result, they have limited effects on intracellular metal
concentrations. Lipophilic chelators decrease intracellular storage sites but may
redistribute toxic metals to other lipophilic compartments such as the brain.
Excretion rates may differ as well.[2]

ON-LABEL (APPROVED) USES OF CHELATION THERAPY

Chelation therapy is indicated for treatment of lead poisoning (for blood lead
levels ≥45 µg/dL) (see chapter 31). Although it is approved by the Food and
Drug Administration (FDA) for hemochromatosis, the treatment of choice for
hemochromatosis is blood donation. The frequency of chelation therapy for
elevated blood lead levels has decreased significantly as a result of the successful reduction of environmental lead sources. As a result, pediatricians in primary
care practice rarely encounter children for whom chelation therapy is indicated.

Pediatricians are strongly advised to consult experts and to weigh benefits
and harms of the disease and the treatment before initiating chelation therapy.
For specific exposures and treatments, a pediatrician experienced in managing
children with lead poisoning should be consulted—these can be found through
the American Academy of Pediatrics (AAP) Council on Environmental Health
or through lead poisoning prevention programs at state health departments
(http://www.cdc.gov/nceh/lead/grants/contacts/CLPPP%20Map.htm).

ADVERSE EFFECTS OF CHELATION AGENTS

Chelation therapy is associated with significant risks of morbidity and mortality,[4]
and there is increasing evidence of a lack of beneficial outcomes associated with
its use. Table 46.1 lists many of the adverse effects of general classes of agents
used for chelation. The primary guidance is "first, do no harm"; it is critical that
a harm-benefit analysis be performed prior to initiating treatment with chelation
agents, whether "off-" or "on-label."

Although chelation can promote excretion of heavy metals, most chelation
agents do not uniformly decrease the body burden of heavy metals.[4,5] Some
agents do not cross the blood-brain barrier efficiently; others do not enter
the intracellular space. Most are effective in binding with metals in the vascu-
lar system, which can cause release of metals from other compartments, resulting in an increase in blood levels of the target metal. Such an increase in
blood level can theoretically promote additional dispersion of the metal. Early

Table 46.1: Toxicities of Chelation Agents[2]

AGENT AND USES	TOXICITIES	NOTES
British anti-lewisite (BAL [2,3-dimercatopropanol], dimercaprol, and related agents, such as 2,3-dimercapto-1-propanesulfonic acid (DMPS) Arsenic, gold, mercury, lead (when combined with CaNa$_2$EDTA)	■ Adverse effects occur in 50% of subjects who receive 5 mg/kg intramuscularly (IM) ■ Increased systolic and diastolic arterial pressures, especially among adolescents (can be significant), with tachycardia (more common in younger children); nausea and vomiting; headache; burning sensation in lips, mouth, throat; feeling of throat, chest, or hand constriction; sterile abscesses at injection site; transient decline in percent polymorphonuclear leukocyte count ■ Children often develop fever, which abates with cessation of treatment ■ Toxicities are dose dependent ■ May cause hemolysis in patients with glucose-6-phosphate dehydrogenase deficiency	■ Dissociation of the metal-agent complex can occur, especially in acidic environments, such as urine. Release of metal into renal tissue can increase toxicity ■ Dosing challenging; requires small fractional doses to avoid high plasma concentrations ■ Should be given immediately after exposure; more effective in preventing inhibition of sulfhydryl enzymes than in reactivating them ■ IM only
Deferoxamine Iron, aluminum (dialysis patients)	■ Pruritus, wheals, rash, anaphylaxis, dysuria, abdominal discomfort, diarrhea, fever, leg cramps, tachycardia, cataract formation, neurotoxicity associated with long-term, high-dose use (typically for treatment of thalassemia major), including visual and auditory changes	

continued on page 692

continued from page 691

Table 46.1: Toxicities of Chelation Agents,[2] *continued*

AGENT AND USES	TOXICITIES	NOTES
Deferoxamine Iron, aluminum (dialysis patients) *continued*	▪ May cause renal failure, especially if patient is volume depleted (hydrate first) ▪ Contraindicated if renal insufficiency, anuria, pregnancy	▪ IM or intravenous (IV); IM preferred for acute iron poisoning, unless patient is in shock. IV use required if patient is in shock. ▪ Not recommended for treatment of primary hemochromatosis (treat with phlebotomy)
Disodium EDTA (Na_2EDTA)	▪ Hypocalcemic tetany can occur with too-rapid infusion ▪ Has caused death	
Edetate calcium disodium ($CaNa_2$EDTA) Lead, zinc, manganese, iron	▪ Renal toxicities; malaise and fatigue; thirst; chills, fever; headache; anorexia, nausea, and vomiting; transitory lowering of systolic and diastolic pressure; prolonged prothrombin time; T-wave inversion on electrocardiogram	▪ Bone lead stores preferentially chelated; after chelation, soft tissue lead is redistributed to bone ▪ Adequate renal function needed for therapy to be successful ▪ IV (associated with thrombophlebitis), IM (painful)
Pentetic acid (diethylenetriaminepentaacetic acid [DTPA])	▪ Investigational	▪ Limited use because of poor access to intracellular sites of metal stores

Table 46.1: Toxicities of Chelation Agents,[2] *continued*

AGENT AND USES	TOXICITIES	NOTES
Penicillamine (D-β,β-dimethylcysteine) Copper, lead, mercury, zinc, arsenic	■ Potential for anaphylaxis if used to treat penicillin-allergic patients ■ Long-term use associated with urticaria and maculopapular reactions, pemphigoid lesions, lupus erythematosus, dermatomyositis, collagen effects, skin dryness and scaling ■ Lymphopenia, aplastic anemia (sometimes fatal) ■ Renal toxicity, sometimes fatal ■ Bronchoalveolitis ■ Myasthenia gravis (long-term therapy) ■ Nausea, vomiting, diarrhea, dyspepsia, anorexia, loss of taste for sweet and salt (relieved by supplementation with copper)	■ Can be used orally; food, antacids, iron reduce absorption ■ Used to treat copper overload attributable to Wilson disease; cystinuria, rheumatoid arthritis
Succimer (2,3-dimercaptosuccinic acid) Lead, mercury, arsenic	■ Similar to BAL ■ Much less toxic than BAL	■ Orally administered
Trientine (triethylenetetramine dihydrochloride [cuprid]) Copper (especially attributable to Wilson disease)	■ Similar to penicillamine, decreased adverse-effect profile (and less effective)	

studies of mice treated with British anti-lewisite (BAL, 2,3-dimercatopropanol) showed increased distribution of mercury to the brain following treatment.[6-9] In some instances, chelation may actually cause more harm than no treatment. For example, lead stored in bone is relatively inert, as long as calcium intake is sufficient and bone stores of calcium are not resorbed to supply calcium.

There is no evidence that chelation reverses neurologic damage from lead poisoning. In a multisite, randomized, controlled trial, investigators studied the effect of chelation with 2,3-dimercaptosuccinic acid (DMSA or succimer) on neurodevelopmental outcomes of children aged 12 to 33 months whose blood lead levels were 20 to 44 µg/dL (levels for which chelation is not recommended). The blood lead levels of the children who had undergone chelation decreased, but 1 year following the start of chelation, the study found no differences between the blood lead levels of children who received chelation and those who received a placebo. Similarly, the trial was unable to show a difference between treated and untreated groups in neurodevelopmental outcomes at 7 years of age.[10,11]

Chelation agents are not selective for specific metals. This lack of selectivity is the cause of one of the most important adverse effects of chelation therapy—concomitant loss of essential metals and minerals, especially calcium and zinc, during treatment. Calcium and zinc are essential metals that can be depleted below critical limits, posing serious health threats to patients. Thus, the potential secondary targets of chelation agents must be identified prior to chelation. The agent most frequently implicated in deaths associated with chelation is edentate disodium (Na_2EDTA). The on-label indications for this agent are hypercalcemia and ventricular arrhythmias attributable to digitalis toxicity. Na_2EDTA use in children is contraindicated because of the high risk of hypocalcemia and fatal tetany. The chelation agent edentate disodium calcium ($CaNa_2EDTA$), which can be used for chelation, has a similar name. Despite the risks associated with Na_2EDTA, some pharmacies stock both types; confusion of the two has resulted in the death of at least 1 child.[12] Another child died after chelation with Na_2EDTA administered by a physician who regularly chelated adults as a treatment for atherosclerosis. The child's death was determined to be caused by acute cerebral hypoxic-ischemic injury, with secondary necrosis resulting from hypocalcemia.[12]

OFF-LABEL USES OF CHELATION AGENTS

In the United States, the FDA allows physicians to prescribe approved medications for purposes other than their intended indications—called "off-label" use. A growing number of practitioners of complementary and alternative medicine are using chelation agents to treat neurologic diseases, such as autistic spectrum disorders.

Exposure to high concentrations of heavy metals such as lead and mercury is associated with considerable toxicity (see Chapters 31 and 32); understanding of the harms associated with low but elevated concentrations is preliminary. Studies of lead-exposed children document adverse neurocognitive effects at blood levels below 10 μg/dL—the Centers for Disease Control and Prevention's "level of concern."[13-16] Comparable studies of the effects of mercury concentrations below the EPA "reference dose" have not been performed, although retrospective studies of children from populations with high fish intake suggest an inverse association of prenatal exposure to mercury and IQ.[17]

Similarly, our understanding of the benefits and harms of chelation therapy is incomplete. The evidence supporting chelation as an effective treatment for neurodevelopmental diseases is limited. Although chelation can lower the body's burden of heavy metals and slow or eliminate further decline associated with ongoing exposures, it has not been shown to reverse effects that have already occurred.[18-20] Evidence of harm from chelation is better described.[21] Because of ethical and logistical challenges of research in this field, many studies are limited to animal subjects or case reports in people. Because of ethical concerns, in 2008, the National Institutes of Health withdrew support for a study of chelation among children with autism spectrum disorders after preliminary results linked chelation to brain damage in rats.[22] Until these ethical concerns are resolved, studies will continue to be limited.

Autism Spectrum Disorders and Mercury

Thimerosal (sodium ethylmercury thiosalicylate, also known as merthiolate), an organic compound of ethylmercury, has been used in multidose vaccine vials to prevent bacterial and fungal contamination since it was patented in 1928.[23] As the number of childhood vaccinations increased, concerns arose that the amount of mercury to which infants were exposed as a result of delivery of multiple thimerosal-containing vaccines might reach toxic levels. As a result, the FDA reviewed the use of thimerosal in childhood vaccines and found no evidence of harm from its use as a vaccine preservative, other than local hypersensitivity reactions.[23] Despite the absence of evidence of harm attributable to thimerosal-containing vaccines, the US Public Health Service and the AAP recommended minimizing exposure to thimerosal-containing vaccines and eventual removal of thimerosal from vaccines.[24] Since 2001, all vaccines recommended for children 6 years and younger have contained no thimerosal or only "trace" or insignificant amounts (defined as a concentration of less than 0.0002%), with the exception of multidose vials of inactivated influenza vaccine.[23] Single-dose units of influenza vaccine formulated for pediatric use are thimerosal free. For more information, see www.fda.gov/cber/vaccine/thimerosal.htm.

In 2001, a group of parents of children with autism spectrum disorders published an article posing the idea that autism spectrum disorders are a "novel form of mercury poisoning"[25] in *Medical Hypotheses*, a nonpeer-reviewed journal that states it "…will publish radical ideas, so long as they are coherent and clearly expressed…"[26] Several other articles supporting the concept followed, many by the same authors of the original. The authors hypothesized that autism spectrum disorders were an expression of mercury toxicity resulting from thimerosal in vaccines. They cited evidence such as a similarity between the clinical signs of mercury toxicity and manifestations of autism spectrum disorders, temporal association between the increase in the prevalence of autism spectrum disorders and increased number of immunizations administered in early childhood, and higher levels of mercury in people with autism spectrum disorders than in people without.[25] Each of these claims has been addressed and refuted in the peer-reviewed literature.[27-29] In 2001, the Institute of Medicine published the findings of an extensive review concluding that no proof could be found linking thimerosal-containing vaccines and autism spectrum disorders, ADHD, speech or language delays, or other neurodevelopment disorders.[30] One of the arguments against the link is the unfortunate persistence of the increase in prevalence of autism spectrum disorders after the removal of thimerosal from childhood vaccines.[31]

Some clinicians promote the chelation of children with autism spectrum disorders to "detoxify" them of mercury and other metals. Most of these clinicians use $CaNa_2EDTA$; another agent reported is Bentonite clay, a naturally occurring clay marketed as a chelation agent for autism spectrum disorders and other childhood neurologic and behavioral diseases. According to a Web site on which the clay is sold, when mixed with water, the clay creates a negatively charged bath. The positive metals are purportedly drawn electrostatically through the pores and absorbed by the clay.[32]

Many clinicians who treat children with autism spectrum disorders using chelation cite case studies reporting improved cognitive function as evidence of therapeutic effect. One case series of 11 children (10 boys, 1 girl) with autism spectrum disorders treated for 2 to 7 months with leuprolide acetate (an antiandrogen) and *meso*-1,3,-dimercaptosuccinic acid was published in 2006.[33] This effort, which evaluated children before and after treatment, used an unvalidated 1-page tool, the "Autism Treatment Evaluation Checklist" (ATEC [Autism Research Institute, San Diego, CA]) to evaluate speech, language, communication, sociability, sensory and cognitive awareness, health, and physical behavior. The authors had a patent pending for a treatment for autism spectrum disorder at the time the results were published. The work is seriously flawed by the absence of a control group, the combination of 2 unproven therapies, and the unvalidated evaluation tool. Behaviors of children, including children with neurodevelopmental disorders, often improve with age; without a control group, age cannot be ruled out as a confounding factor. The combination of therapies in the absence of a control group also raises the possibility that the antiandrogen was responsible for affecting the children's behavior. The long-term effects of antiandrogens on prepubertal children are unknown.

Autism Spectrum Disorders and Lead

Evidence from case studies of autism spectrum disorders and lead is inadequate to draw any conclusions. One report[34] described 2 children who developed autism or autism-like symptoms following exposure to lead; both children received chelation therapy. Both children were reevaluated several years after treatment and found to have intellectual and functional impairments that did not fulfill the diagnostic criteria for autism spectrum disorders. Another case report of a child with symptoms of autism, ADHD, and a blood lead level of 42 µg/dL (below the level at which chelation is recommended[35]) showed decreased repetitive behaviors during chelation, but the behaviors returned once treatment was discontinued.[36] Other cases have been reported.[37]

Provocation

One technique used to demonstrate increased concentrations of heavy metals is "provocation" testing. Provocation analysis has been used to measure urinary excretion of metals after administration of a chelation agent, such as $CaNa_2EDTA$ or 2,3-dimercaptosuccinic acid; however, standard provocation levels in children have not been established. The theory behind provocation testing is circuitous: excretion of heavy metals following chelation is cited as evidence that the subject had an elevated body burden of heavy metals. One study using this technique reported significantly higher concentrations of mercury in the urine of 221 children with autism spectrum disorders following chelation, compared with urine collected from a group of 18 normal children who were tested for exposure to heavy metals but did not receive chelation.[38] The study was reported in the *Journal of American Physicians and Surgeons*, published by the Association of American Physicians and Surgeons, an organization that has campaigned against immunizations, government regulation of physicians, and Medicare.[39] A more recent study did not find increased heavy metal excretion after provocation in children with autism.[40]

RECOMMENDATIONS

Pediatricians should understand that appropriate uses of chelation are limited; Chapter 31 describes indications for chelation of children with lead poisoning. Families may ask pediatricians about the efficacy of off-label use of chelation agents to treat chronic neurodevelopmental diseases, such as autism spectrum disorders. The evidence base for the use of chelation to treat neurodevelopmental disorders is poor; many studies cited by clinicians who recommend chelation are poorly designed, have small sample sizes, and have conflicting results. It is important for pediatricians to be aware of the quality and quantity of the evidence cited in support of off-label uses of chelation.

1. Be ready to address chelation and heavy metal toxicities if parents of children with chronic health problems wish to learn more.
2. It is never prudent to dismiss parents' questions about chelation, because they may be considering it for their child. It is important to keep avenues for communication open.
3. Ask about chelation—as well as herbal products, vitamins, and other nonprescription drugs and treatments.
4. Learn about the misuses of chelation therapy and the harms and limited benefits to chelation.

Frequently Asked Question

Q *The parents of a 3-year old recently diagnosed with autism asked about chelation for heavy metal poisoning. They have information from a parent support group that suggests that chelation could help their child. What do I tell them?*

A Thank them for bringing the subject up with you. Emphasize the importance of open discussion of treatments they are considering for their child. Be supportive of the family's desire to find effective treatments. Acknowledge that medicine does not yet offer curative treatments for this condition.

Explore issues such as parental guilt and worries about prenatal exposures that may have contributed to development of autism. In particular, ask about environmental exposures about which parents may be concerned, including vaccines, anti-Rho D immunoglobin, diet, and stress. Address specific concerns about heavy metals, and emphasize possible exposures in your history taking. Does the child have a history of exposure to heavy metals? Can local sources of heavy metals, such as incinerators or power plants, be identified? Does the child have a history of pica? Does the child have a history of lead exposure? Does the family eat a lot of fish? What kinds of fish do they usually eat? Have the parents (or other household members) ever had jobs in which they were exposed to heavy metals?

Describe the strength of the evidence showing no association between exposure to heavy metals and autism spectrum disorders. Discuss the pitfalls of provocation testing.

If appropriate, discuss the risks of chelation, including identified risks such as hypocalcemia, effects on intelligence, toxicities of the drugs, potential harm from intravenous catheter placement, and others. Point out that children, including children with autism, continue to develop, and that uncontrolled studies may conclude that improvements in behaviors are attributable to treatment, when the improvements may actually be attributable to development.

Point out that continued research is being performed, and that you will be available to discuss new treatments in the future.

References

1. Duffus J. "Heavy Metals"—a meaningless term? *Pure Appl Chem.* 2002;74(5):793-807
2. Goyer R. Toxic effects of metals. In: Klaassen C, ed. *Casarett and Doull's Toxicology: The Basic Science of Poisons.* 5th ed. New York, NY: McGraw-Hill; 1995:694-696
3. Klaassen C. Heavy metal and heavy-metal antagonists. In: Gilman A, Rall T, Nies A, Taylor P, eds. *Goodman and Gilman's The Pharmacological Basis of Therapeutics.* New York, NY: Pergamon Press; 1990:1592-1614
4. Risher JF, Amler SN. Mercury exposure: evaluation and intervention the inappropriate use of chelating agents in the diagnosis and treatment of putative mercury poisoning. *Neurotoxicology.* 2005;26(4):691-699
5. Stangle DE, Strawderman MS, Smith D, Kuypers M, Strupp BJ. Reductions in blood lead overestimate reductions in brain lead following repeated succimer regimens in a rodent model of childhood lead exposure. *Environ Health Perspect.* 2004;112(3):302-308
6. Agency for Toxic Substances and Disease Registry. *Toxicological profile for Mercury.* Atlanta, GA: US Department of Health and Human Services, Public Health Service; 1999
7. Berlin M, Lewander T. Increased brain uptake of mercury caused by 2,3-dimercaptopropanol (BAL) in mice given mercuric chloride. *Acta Pharmacol Toxicol (Copenh).* 1965;22:1-7
8. Berlin M, Rylander R. Increased brain uptake of mercury induced by 2,3-dimercaptopropanol (BAL) in mice exposed to phenylmercuric acetate. *J Pharmacol Exp Ther.* 1964;146:236-240
9. Berlin M, Ullrebg S. Increased uptake of mercury in mouse brain caused by 2,3-dimercaptopropanol. *Nature.* 1963;197:84-85
10. Rogan WJ, Dietrich KN, Ware JH, et al. The effect of chelation therapy with succimer on neuropsychological development in children exposed to lead. *N Engl J Med.* 2001;344(19): 1421-1426
11. Dietrich KN, Ware JH, Salganik M, et al. Effect of chelation therapy on the neuropsychological and behavioral development of lead-exposed children after school entry. *Pediatrics.* 2004;114(1): 19-26
12. Centers for Disease Control and Prevention. Deaths associated with hypocalcemia from chelation therapy—Texas, Pennsylvania, and Oregon, 2003–2005. *MMWR. Morb Mortal Wkly Rep.* 2006;55(8):204-207
13. Lanphear BP, Hornung R, Khoury J, et al. Low-level environmental lead exposure and children's intellectual function: an international pooled analysis. *Environ Health Perspect.* 2005;113(7):894-899
14. Canfield RL, Henderson CR Jr, Cory-Slechta DA, Cox C, Jusko TA, Lanphear BP. Intellectual impairment in children with blood lead concentrations below 10 microg per deciliter. *N Engl J Med.* 2003;348(16):1517-1526
15. Canfield RL, Kreher DA, Cornwell C, Henderson CR Jr. Low-level lead exposure, executive functioning, and learning in early childhood. *Neuropsychol Dev Cogn Sect C Child Neuropsychol.* 2003;9(1):35-53
16. Centers for Disease Control and Prevention. *Preventing Lead Poisoning in Young Children.* Atlanta, GA: Centers for Disease Control and Prevention; 2005
17. Axelrad DA, Bellinger DC, Ryan LM, Woodruff TJ. Dose-response relationship of prenatal mercury exposure and IQ: an integrative analysis of epidemiologic data. *Environ Health Perspect.* 2007;115(4):609-615

18. Rogan WJ, Dietrich KN, Ware JH, et al. The effect of chelation therapy with succimer on neuropsychological development in children exposed to lead. *N Engl J Med.* 2001;344(19): 1421-1

19. Chisolm JJ Jr, Rhoads GG; Treatment of Lead-Exposed Children Trial Group. Dietrich KN, Ware JH, Salganick M, et al. Effect of chelation therapy on the neuropsychological and behavioral development of lead-exposed children following school entry. *Pediatrics.* 2004;114(1):19-26

20. Cao Y, Chen A, Jones RL, et al. Efficacy of succimer chelation of mercury at background exposures in toddlers: a randomized trial. *J Pediatr.* 2011;158(3):480.e1-485.e1

21. American Academy of Pediatrics, Committee on Children With Disabilities. Technical report: the pediatrician's role in the diagnosis and management of autistic spectrum disorder in children *Pediatrics.* 2001;107(5):e85

22. Boyles S. Chelation Study for Autism Called Off. *WebMD Health News.* September 18, 2008

23. Center for Biologics Evaluation and Research, US Food and Drug Administration. Thimerosal in Vaccines. Available at: http://www.fda.gov/cber/vaccine/thimfaq.htm. Accessed April 4, 2011

24. US Public Health Service, Department of Health and Human Services; and American Academy of Pediatrics. Thimerosal in vaccines: a joint statement of the American Academy of Pediatrics and the Public Health Service. *MMWR.Morb Mortal Wkly Rep.* 1999;48(26):563-565

25. Bernard S, Enayati A, Redwood L, Roger H, Binstock T. Autism: a novel form of mercury poisoning. *Med Hypotheses.* 2001;56(4):462-471

26. Aims and scope of the journal *Medical Hypotheses.* Available at: http://www.elsevier.com/wps/find/journaldescription.cws_home/623059/description#description. Accessed April 4, 2011

27. Nelson KB, Bauman ML. Thimerosal and autism? *Pediatrics.* 2003;111(3):674-679

28. Andrews N, Miller E, Grant A, Stowe J, Osborne V, Taylor B. Thimerosal exposure in infants and developmental disorders: a retrospective cohort study in the United kingdom does not support a causal association. *Pediatrics.* 2004;114(3):584-591

29. Verstraeten T, Davis RL, DeStefano F, et al. Safety of thimerosal-containing vaccines: a two-phased study of computerized health maintenance organization databases. *Pediatrics.* 2003;112(5):1039-1048

30. Institute of Medicine, Immunization Safety Review Committee. *Immunization Safety Review: Thimerosal-Containing Vaccines and Neurodevelopmental Disorders.* Stratton K, Gable A, McCormick M, eds. Washington, DC: National Academies Press; 2001. Available at: http://www.nap.edu/openbook.php?isbn=0309076366. Accessed April 4, 2011

31. Schechter R, Grether JK. Continuing increases in autism reported to California's developmental services system: mercury in retrograde. *Arch Gen Psychiatry.* 2008;65(1):19-24

32. Fighting autism with calcium bentonite clay. Available at: http://www.squidoo.com/fighting_autism. Accessed April 4, 2011

33. Geier DA, Geier MR. A clinical trial of combined anti-androgen and anti-heavy metal therapy in autistic disorders. *Neuro Endocrinol Lett.* 2006;27(6):833-838

34. Lidsky T, Schneider J. Autism and autistic symptoms associated with childhood lead poisoning. *J Applied Res.* 2005;5(1):80-87

35. Centers for Disease Control and Prevention. *Managing Elevated Blood Lead Levels Among Young Children: Recommendations from the Advisory Committee on Childhood Lead Poisoning Prevention.* Atlanta, GA: Centers for Disease Control and Prevention; 2002

36. Eppright TD, Sanfacon JA, Horwitz EA. Attention deficit hyperactivity disorder, infantile autism, and elevated blood-lead: a possible relationship. *Mo Med.* 1996;93(3):136-138

37. Accardo P, Whitman B, Caul J, Rolfe U. Autism and plumbism. A possible association. *Clin Pediatr (Phila).* 1988;27(1):41-44

38. Bradstreet J, Geier D, Kartzinel JJ, Adams JB, Geier MR. A case-control study of mercury burden in children with autistic spectrum disorders. *J Am Phys Surg*. 2003;8(3):76-79

39. Association of American Physicians and Surgeons, Inc. Available at: http://www.aapsonline.org. Accessed April 4, 2011

40. Soden SE, Lowry JA, Garrison CB, Wasserman GS. 24-hour provoked urine excretion test for heavy metals in children with autism and typically developing controls, a pilot study. *Clin Toxicol (Phila)*. 2007;45(5):476-481

Chapter 47

Chemical and Biological Terrorism

■ ■ ■ ■ ■ ■

HISTORY

Terrorism of all forms has the goal of producing injury, fear, or chaos in an effort to disable or intimidate a population. Recent terrorist acts have included, and at times targeted, child victims. In 2004, more than 750 children were among the 1100 hostages in the 3-day siege of a school in Beslan, North Ossetia, of the Russian Federation. Children have been among the victims in other well-known acts of terrorism, including release of the nerve agent sarin in the Tokyo subway system in 1995, the bombing of the Oklahoma City federal building in 1995, and the distribution of anthrax-containing letters through the US Postal Service in 2001.[1]

The release of chemical or biological agents could have a tremendous impact on children, adolescents, and on their environments.[1,2] There are physiologic, psychological, and developmental considerations unique to the pediatric population. If children were targeted directly, existing vulnerabilities within pediatric emergency medical services systems and hospitals would create extreme challenges to medical management, surge capacity, and care capabilities for ill and injured children.[3,4] Pediatricians should be prepared to consider the clinical issues that would arise after exposure to these agents as well as the safety of water and food supplies, and potential soil and air pollution. The principles of consequence management, designed to minimize morbidity and mortality after a chemical or biological agent release, must involve multiple pediatric disciplines including environmental health, emergency medicine, critical care, behavioral medicine, primary care, and infectious diseases. Response plans must address recognition, triage, diagnosis, and management. Moreover, an effective partnership between government agencies and pediatricians must be forged to promote preparedness and minimize the effects of terrorism on children.

Potential "weapons of mass destruction" may be formed from chemical, biological, radiological, nuclear, or explosive agents.[5] Chemical and explosive agents may be used as "weapons of opportunity," requiring limited planning or financial resources.[1,6] For example, an explosion involving a railcar carrying hazardous chemicals could result in contamination of a nearby community, causing major hardship and emotional distress.

Community planning, medication stockpiling, and preparation for chemical, biological, radiological, nuclear, or explosive events, especially for incidents that might involve numerous children, present daunting logistical challenges. As part of the network of health responders, pediatricians need to be able to answer questions, recognize signs of possible exposure to a chemical or biologic weapon, understand first-line response, and participate in disaster planning to ensure that the needs of children are addressed.[5] This chapter does not attempt to serve as a stand-alone reference on chemical or biological terrorism but instead provides an introduction to the topic, especially with regard to pediatric environmental health concerns; more information is available (see Resources).

AGENTS OF CONCERN

Chemical

A large number of chemicals may be used as terrorist weapons. They include nerve agents, cyanide, vesicants (chemicals that cause blistering), and pulmonary agents (Table 47.1).[7-11] The release of the nerve agent sarin in Japan demonstrated the ease with which a chemical agent can be dispersed and the resulting effects.[11] Relatively easy to manufacture, sarin, like all nerve agents, acts like an organophosphate pesticide, inhibiting the enzyme acetylcholinesterase. Victims of sarin exposure, therefore, present with a picture of cholinergic excess. Most common symptoms are miosis, nausea, and vomiting. More significant exposures produce lacrimation, salivation, and diarrhea. Moderate exposures to nerve agents result in stimulation of nicotinic receptors, with resulting muscle fasciculation and generalized weakness. Severe exposures produce central nervous system toxicity, manifested as seizures and coma. Death from sarin exposure results from respiratory failure or complications of central nervous system toxicity. Sarin also has unique chemical properties that enhance its toxicity. It is denser than air and settles close to the ground, in the breathing zone of children. Sarin is viscous and oily, leading to deposition on clothing and skin. It is readily absorbed through intact skin and through standard barriers (such as surgical gloves) used by health care personnel. Finally, because it can remain on clothing or skin until it is removed, sarin can secondarily affect anyone not wearing personal protective equipment while handling a contaminated victim. Sarin

Table 47.1: Potential Chemical Agents for Use in Terrorism	
CLASS	**EXAMPLES**
Nerve agents	Tabun Sarin Soman VX
Vesicants	Mustard gas Nitrogen mustard
Irritants/corrosives	Chlorine Bromine Ammonia
Choking agents	Phosgene
Cyanogens	Hydrogen cyanide
Incapacitating agents: central nervous system depressants, anticholinergics, lacrimators	3-Quinuclidinyl benzilate (BZ), capsaicin, cannabinoids, barbiturates

From the American Academy of Pediatrics.[1,2]

vapors can enter the ventilation system of a building or hospital, thereby affecting individuals throughout the structure.[12-14] Management of exposure to specific chemical weapons can be found in several reviews.[5,6,8,15,16]

Biological

Infectious agents or their toxins have been used as weapons. Unlike chemical agents, with which the release is usually obvious and casualties appear promptly, biological agents can be released covertly, with casualties appearing over a period of days, potentially leading to a significant delay in recognition and diagnosis.[17-19] Because of the time delay, victims typically become ill away from the site of exposure, and the epicenter of the release can be very difficult to identify. Victims of certain bioterror infections can, themselves, subsequently spread agents to diverse additional locations, analogous to the spread of severe acute respiratory syndrome (SARS).

According to the National Academy of Sciences, several dozen biological agents or toxins are potential candidates for use as bioweapons.[7] Included among these are agents that the Centers for Disease Control and Prevention (CDC) identifies as "category A agents" that:

- Can be easily disseminated or transmitted person-to-person;
- Cause high mortality, with potential for major public health impact;
- Have the potential for causing public panic and social disruption; and
- Require special attention for public health preparedness.

Table 47.2: Biological Weapons of Concern

CATEGORY A
Anthrax *(Bacillus anthracis)*
Smallpox *(Variola major)*
Tularemia *(Francisella tularensis)*
Plague *(Yersinia pestis)*
Botulinum (*Clostridium botulinum* toxin)
Viral hemorrhagic fevers (filoviruses [eg, Ebola, Marburg] and arenaviruses [eg, Lassa])

CATEGORY B
Q fever *(Coxiella burnetii)*
Brucellosis (*Brucella* species)
Glanders *(Burkholderia mallei)*
Melioidosis *(Burkholderia pseudomallei)*
Viral encephalitis (alphaviruses, Venezuelan equine encephalomyelitis, eastern equine encephalomyelitis, western equine encephalomyelitis)
Typhus *(Rickettsia prowazekii)*
Biotoxins (ricin, staphylococcal enterotoxin B)
Psittacosis *(Chlamydia psittaci)*
Food-safety threats (eg, *Salmonella* species, *Escherichia coli* O157:H7)
Water-safety threats (eg, *Vibrio cholerae, Cryptosporidium parvum*)

CATEGORY C
Emerging threat agents (eg, Nipah virus, hantavirus)
Multidrug-resistant tuberculosis
Tickborne encephalitis viruses
Tickborne hemorrhagic fever viruses
Yellow fever

From American Academy of Pediatrics and Centers for Disease Control and Prevention.[1,21]

The 6 category A agents are *Bacillus anthracis* (anthrax), *Yersinia pestis* (plague), *Variola major* (smallpox), *Francisella tularensis* (tularemia), *Clostridium botulinum* toxin, and filoviruses and arenaviruses (viral hemorrhagic fevers). Public health efforts have focused primarily on the category A agents; hospitals, pediatricians, and government agencies are being called on to improve preparedness (eg, by stockpiling and developing a distribution plan for antibiotics, vaccines, and antidotes).[7,20] Preparedness efforts should also address the potential risks posed by the many other agents, including those in categories B and C, but these are beyond the scope of this chapter.

Table 47.3: Factors Enhancing Children's Vulnerability to Biological Agents[23]	
FACTOR	**RELEVANT AGENTS**
Anatomic and physiologic differences ▪ Increased ratio of surface area to volume ▪ Skin more permeable ▪ Higher minute ventilation ▪ Breathing air closer to ground	▪ T-2 mycotoxins ▪ All aerosolized agents ▪ Denser aerosolized agents
Unique susceptibility/severity	▪ Smallpox, T-2 mycotoxins, VEE
Developmental considerations ▪ Dependent on others for care, more likely to lack knowledge or independent means to seek care or identify and avoid danger	▪ All agents

VEE indicates Venezuelan equine encephalitis.

PEDIATRIC IMPLICATIONS

Compared with adults, children may be especially susceptible to the effects of chemical and biological agents because of children's anatomic and physiologic differences and unique behavioral characteristics (see Table 47.3).[22,23] Because infants and children have an increased surface area-to-volume ratio compared with adults, greater skin permeability, higher minute ventilation, and breathing zones closer to the ground (where some agents may settle), they often are at higher risk of exposure to and absorption of many agents. Children often require different medical countermeasures, including different dosages, antibiotics, or antidotes. They have greater susceptibility to dehydration and shock from biological and chemical agents. Children often depend on others for care, and their developmental abilities and cognitive levels may impede their ability to escape danger. In addition, they cannot be easily or rapidly decontaminated in adult decontamination units. Children have unique psychological needs and vulnerabilities, and special management plans are needed in the event of mass casualties and evacuation. For all these reasons, emergency responders, medical professionals, and health care institutions require special expertise and training to ensure that children receive optimal medical and psychological care.

Certain groups may be especially vulnerable. Neonates and young infants are relatively immunocompromised compared with older children and adults. Preschool children have high hand-to-mouth activity and are also less likely than older children and adults to maintain personal hygiene (eg, cough etiquette and hand washing), thereby facilitating the spread of certain agents, particularly among similarly-aged children; older children and adolescents are more likely to engage in risk-taking behavior that may place them at higher risk.

Identification of Sentinel Events

Nuclear, incendiary, chemical, and explosive disasters are typically immediately recognized. Identifying a biological terrorist event stands in stark contrast. After the covert release of a biological agent, victims may present for medical care over several days; in the early phases of their illness, children and adults may seek medical attention with nonspecific complaints. Easily misdiagnosed, victims may then infect others (if the illness is communicable) before clinical manifestations become more characteristic. One cornerstone of effective planning is educating clinicians about agents used as biological weapons and the illnesses they produce.[24,25] An important component of a physician's role is biosurveillance or syndromic surveillance; the CDC has created a National Biosurveillance Strategy for Human Health that may be useful to pediatricians (http://sites. google.com/site/nbshh10).

A key principle of consequence management for biological terrorism is recognizing that pediatricians, in emergency departments, inpatient settings, and primary care settings, may be the first to encounter victims. Because early diagnosis and treatment substantially reduce the number of affected individuals, pediatricians and others who provide care to children must develop sufficient knowledge to recognize the first signal of a bioterrorist event. For example, skin lesions seen in initial cases of cutaneous anthrax in October 2001 (including the sole pediatric patient) were mistaken for spider bites. All physicians must acquaint themselves with the manifestations of diseases caused by the most common biological agents, including anthrax, plague, smallpox, botulism, and ricin.[6] Detailed descriptions of many biological agents are available in the AAP *Red Book* (http://aapredbook.aappublications.org). A physician who suspects a biological outbreak should immediately notify the local health department and ask for further assistance.

MANAGEMENT OF MASS CASUALTIES

In addition to producing large numbers of casualties, terrorist events produce an even larger number of patients with minor physical problems and well individuals with psychological distress. The latter groups may exceed the seriously injured or infected patients by ratios as high as 10:1. This ratio may be magnified in a pediatric population, because young children are unable to communicate effectively. Because they are concerned about possible exposure, parents are then likely to consult health care providers for symptoms or to request a thorough assessment even in the absence of signs or symptoms. Depending on the number of victims in each group (psychologically distressed, wounded, and severely injured), pediatric offices and emergency departments may become overwhelmed. After the release of the nerve agent sarin in Japan, patients came to emergency departments at a rate as high as 500 per hour, rapidly overwhelming hospital resources.[13] Moreover, because most patients came by foot, car, or taxi, there was no opportunity to perform out-of-hospital ("field") triage to separate healthy from contaminated patients. The principal lesson learned after that event was that office- and hospital-based emergency planning must include contingency plans for managing large numbers of victims ("surge-capacity" planning), with special attention to pediatric needs. An additional challenge arises when creating algorithms to facilitate assessment of young, preverbal children.

DECONTAMINATION, TREATMENT, AND PROPHYLAXIS

Protocols for treatment and postexposure prophylaxis of children exposed to chemical and biological weapons remain poorly developed. For example, some decontamination protocols for chemical agents have recommended a 10-minute shower with soap or diluted bleach.[10] In children, such a regimen risks hypothermia and serious skin or eye irritation. This can be minimized by using warmed water and with attention paid to timely drying, warming, and reclothing. It may be particularly difficult to decontaminate an exposed child or to interact with the child when a rescuer is wearing personal protective gear. The process may be made smoother and the child's anxiety and fear may be alleviated if a parent is present during the decontamination. It is important to incorporate these principles to develop appropriate pediatric decontamination protocols.[26,27]

Treatment of nerve-agent exposures includes supportive care and, when indicated, prompt administration of the antidotes atropine and pralidoxime. Auto-injectors that deliver premeasured doses of both medications can be life saving. This is especially true when large numbers of victims are exposed and first responders are in personal protective gear. In these situations, it is difficult to prepare timely and accurate medication doses based on weight using multidose vials; intravenous dosing in such situations also is impractical. The Food and Drug Administration (FDA) recently established pediatric dosing recommendations and labeling for pralidoxime. As of the end of 2010, however, auto-injectors allowing for rapid administration of both medications (atropine and pralidoxime) were not approved by the FDA for use in children. Such auto-injectors with pediatric-appropriate dosing are not available in the United States. The FDA has taken steps to encourage production and approval of these devices in the near future to address this pressing need. In the interim, consensus recommendations are available to guide the use of currently available auto-injectors for symptomatic children.[28]

In the case of biological weapons, recommendations for pediatric patients have been rudimentary, although some recommendations specific to children and pregnant women have been released.[23] The CDC Web site (www.bt.cdc. gov) contains recommendations for prophylaxis and treatment of children and pregnant women who have been exposed to or are suffering from anthrax.

Local supplies of antibiotics, antidotes, and other medical supplies may be quickly depleted. The CDC, under its Strategic National Stockpile program, oversees a national stockpile of materials for rapid delivery to local communities. Should an event occur, public health and government entities in states and cities have developed plans to rapidly request deployment of pharmaceuticals and equipment from the CDC Strategic National Stockpile for distribution to a point of care in the relevant jurisdiction. Unfortunately, because many medical countermeasures have not been evaluated or approved for use in children, these are not present in pediatric formulations or dosages within the Strategic National Stockpile.

Hospital administrators must consider how to protect hospitalized patients from an airborne release of chemical and biological weapons. Guidance has been prepared for protecting building environments from airborne chemical, biological, or radiologic attacks.[29]

BEHAVIORAL AND MENTAL HEALTH CONSEQUENCES

All forms of terrorism, including hoaxes, can produce significant psychological distress, which may persist long after any risk of adverse health effects has passed. However, the greatest potential for long-term or permanent emotional disturbances is found in mass casualty incidents resulting in injury or death. As the events of September 11, 2001, proved, children are at high risk of developing significant and persistent adjustment difficulties including acute stress reactions and post-traumatic stress disorder, anxiety, depression, and other mental health problems. In situations in which deaths have occurred, bereavement may be the predominant or concurrent challenge. Manifestations of adjustment difficulties after a terrorist event may include somatic complaints (eg, change in appetite, headache, abdominal pain, or malaise); fear, anxiety, or school avoidance; sadness or depression; difficulty concentrating and learning; regression; acting out or risk taking, including onset of or increase in alcohol or other substance use; and emotional withdrawal or avoidance of previously enjoyed activities. Sleep problems include trouble falling or staying asleep and nightmares (which are common in children).[22,30-35] After a terrorist event, pediatricians can educate parents about how to communicate with and support their children, limit their exposure to media reports, and recognize and seek treatment for adjustment reactions. Community-level disaster preparedness includes developing a network of mental health services to address psychological needs and developing ways to deliver psychological first aid, bereavement counseling, and other supportive services to large numbers of children, often in community sites such as schools.[4,34]

Planning by Government

Rapid, effective response to terrorist acts relies on the actions of a number of government agencies. State and local government agencies are essential collaborators in the process of disaster planning, especially as it relates to first responders. Planning for disasters at state and federal levels must consider the unique needs of children and families and should include input from pediatricians.

Depending on the type and impact of an event, responding federal agencies will likely include the US Department of Homeland Security/Federal Emergency Management Agency, the US Department of Health and Human Services, the CDC, the US Environmental Protection Agency, the US Department of Agriculture, and potentially a number of others. Acts of terrorism require not only the involvement of public health systems but also, as criminal acts, all branches of law enforcement, including the Federal Bureau of Investigation and state and local police. In contrast to natural disasters such as earthquakes, terrorism will require, in an unprecedented fashion, that these systems work together. By necessity, law enforcement agencies will need to work with public health agencies and health care providers to facilitate investigations (eg, collecting clothing and specimens as evidence, embargoing sensitive or classified information, interviewing victims). This process poses challenges for pediatricians, emergency physicians, nurses, and other health care providers.

COMMUNITY PLANNING

Disaster planning also takes place at the community level. Planning should be based on a thorough hazard vulnerability analysis, which takes into account unique characteristics, and henceforth vulnerabilities, of a community. An assessment of natural disaster and terrorism-based threats must consider where children may be located (eg, schools) and what their needs are, including children with special health care needs. Hazard vulnerability analysis and disaster planning should include input from pediatricians.

Important activities include identifying shelter facilities appropriate for children and families. These facilities must be large enough to care for large numbers of victims if a local area becomes uninhabitable. Alternate sites should be prepared to provide at least a 2- to 3-day supply of age-appropriate nutrition, water, toiletries, and other basic needs. Plans should ensure that mass care shelter environments are safe and secure for children and have appropriate access to essential services and supplies, such as infant formula and food suitable for infants and toddlers.[4]

Schools and child care facilities must be included in community-level planning, because children spend much of their time in these settings.[1,30,32] Schools may also be targets for such attacks, as exemplified by the Beslan school hostage crisis in the Russian Federation in 2004. Issues for planning in schools include establishing protocols for sheltering in place, lockdown, and/or rapid evacuation of children; identifying safe sites should a facility require immediate evacuation; developing mechanisms for notifying parents and reuniting them with their children as quickly as possible[36]; arranging care for children whose parents are incapacitated or unable to reach them; providing first aid; arranging for in loco parentis treatment of children when their parents cannot be reached; addressing how medical countermeasures can be administered to children as appropriate; and planning support strategies for children's adjustment to and recovery from disasters.

PEDIATRIC PLANNING FOR TERRORIST EVENTS

Children or adolescents may appear in pediatricians' offices or health centers after exposure. Pediatricians in these settings must (1) become knowledgeable about agents and their clinical manifestations and contribute to biosurveillance efforts; (2) become effective educators and communicators about chemical and biological agents and how these agents affect children (see Chapter 58); (3) become involved in local disaster planning to advocate for pediatric preparedness; (4) ensure that offices have emergency care plans and protocols that permit evaluation of victims, protect unaffected patients, and review the need for personal protective equipment; (5) develop surge-capacity protocols; (6) develop skills in providing psychological first aid and brief interventions for children who experience loss and crisis; and (7) develop and test office/practice plans for disasters to limit disruption of essential services provided to patients and families. For many of these tasks, pediatricians can adopt algorithms being developed by federal agencies or seek guidance from the American Academy of Pediatrics Children & Disasters Web site (http://www.aap.org/disasters). This site reviews or provides links to resources concerning evaluation and management of crisis events, provides guidance to prepare pediatricians and practices for disasters, and provides materials appropriate for families. Materials are available to help practices develop a written disaster plan (http://www.aap.org/disasters/practice.cfm).

Because pediatric residents are not adequately knowledgeable about this topic,[37] their education and training may be improved by including a curriculum in medical schools and pediatric residencies. An educational intervention in pediatric disaster medicine was conducted for pediatric and pediatric emergency medicine residents at a tertiary care teaching hospital. Participants increased their knowledge short-term and also showed moderate retention of information.[38]

Resources

American Academy of Pediatrics

Children, Terrorism & Disasters Web site: www.aap.org/disasters; www.aap.org/disasters/terrorism-biological.cfm; and www.aap.org/disasters/terrorism-chemical.cfm

Markenson D; Reynolds S; American Academy of Pediatrics, Committee on Pediatric Emergency Medicine and Task Force on Terrorism. Technical report: the pediatrician and disaster preparedness. *Pediatrics* 2006;117(2):e340-e362

Centers for Disease Control and Prevention

Emergency Preparedness and Response: http://emergency.cdc.gov

References

1. American Academy of Pediatrics, Committee on Environmental Health, Committee on Infectious Diseases. Chemical-biological terrorism and its impact on children. *Pediatrics.* 2006;118(3):1267-1278

2. American Academy of Pediatrics, Committee on Environmental Health, Committee on Infectious Diseases. Chemical-biological terrorism and its impact on children: a subject review. *Pediatrics.* 2000;105(3 Pt 1):662-670

3. Institute of Medicine, Committee on the Future of Emergency Care in the United States Health System. *Emergency Care for Children: Growing Pains.* Washington, DC: National Academies Press; 2006

4. National Commission on Children and Disasters. *2010 Report to the President and Congress.* Rockville, MD: Agency for Healthcare Research and Quality 2010. AHRQ Publication No. 10-M037. Available at: http://www.ahrq.gov/prep/nccdreport. Accessed April 6, 2011

5. American Academy of Pediatrics. *Pediatric Terrorism and Disaster Preparedness: A Resource for Pediatricians.* Foltin GL, Schonfeld DJ, Shannon MW, eds. Rockville, MD: Agency for Healthcare Research and Quality; 2006. AHRQ Publication No. 06(07)-0056

6. Macintyre A, et al. Weapons of mass destruction events with contaminated casualties: effective planning for health care facilities. *JAMA.* 2000;283(2):242-249

7. National Research Council. *Chemical and Biological Terrorism: Research and Development to Improve Civilian Medical Response.* Washington, DC: National Academics Press; 1999

8. US Army Medical Research Institute of Chemical Defense. *Field Management of Chemical Casualties Handbook.* Aberdeen Proving Ground, MD: US Army Medical Research Institute of Chemical Defense; 1996

9. Dunn M, Sidell F. Progress in medical defense against nerve agents. *JAMA.* 1989;262(5): 649-652

10. Holstege C, Kirk M, Sidell F. Chemical warfare. Nerve agent poisoning. *Crit Care Clin.* 1997;13(4):923-942

11. Okumura T, Takasu N, Ishimatsu S, et al. Report on 640 victims of the Tokyo subway sarin attack. *Ann Emerg Med.* 1996;28(2):129-135

12. Okumura T, Suzuki K, Fukuda A, et al. The Tokyo subway sarin attack: disaster management, part 1: community emergency response. *Acad Emerg Med.* 1998;5(6):613-617

13. Okumura T, Suzuki K, Fukuda A, et al. The Tokyo subway sarin attack: disaster management part 2: hospital response. *Acad Emerg Med.* 1998;5(6):618-624

14. Okumura T, Suzuki K, Fukuda A, et al. The Tokyo subway sarin attack: disaster management, part 3: national and international responses. *Acad Emerg Med.* 1998;5(6):625-628

15. *Pediatric Emergency Preparedness for Natural Disasters, Terrorism and Public Health Emergencies: A National Consensus Conference.* Markenson D, Redlener M, eds. New York, NY: National Center for Disaster Preparedness, Mailman School of Public Health, Columbia University; 2007. Available at: http://www.ncdp.mailman.columbia.edu/files/peds2.pdf. Accessed April 6, 2011

16. Shenoi R. Chemical warfare agents. *Clin Pediatr Emerg Med.* 2002;3:239-247

17. Christopher G, Berkowsky P. Biological warfare. A historical perspective. *JAMA.* 1997;278(5):412-417

18. Danzig R, Berkowsky P. Why should we be concerned about biological warfare? *JAMA.* 1997;278(5):431-432

19. Holloway H, Norwood AE, Fullerton CS, Engel CC Jr, Ursano RJ. The threat of biological weapons. Prophylaxis and mitigation of psychologic and social consequences. *JAMA.* 1997;278(5)425-427

20. Chung S, Shannon M. Hospital planning for acts of terrorism and other public health emergencies involving children. *Arch Dis Child.* 2005;90(12):1300-1307

21. Centers for Disease Control and Prevention. Emergency Preparedness and Response. Bioterrorism Agents/Diseases. http://emergency.cdc.gov/agent/agentlist-category.asp. Accessed April 6, 2011

22. Schonfeld D. Supporting children after terrorist events: potential roles for pediatricians. *Pediatr Ann.* 2003;32(3):182-187

23. Cieslak T, Henretig F. Bioterrorism. *Pediatr Ann.* 2003;32(3):154-165

24. Henretig F, Cieslak T, Eitzen EJ. Biological and chemical terrorism. *J Pediatr.* 2002;141(3): 311-326

25. Henretig F, et al. Medical management of the suspected victim of bioterrorism: an algorithmic approach to the undifferentiated patient. *Emerg Med Clin North Am.* 2002;20(2):351-364

26. Heon D, Foltin GL. Principles of pediatric decontamination. *Clin Pediatr Emerg Med.* 2009;10(3):186-194

27. New York City Department of Health and Mental Hygiene. *Pediatric Disaster Toolkit: Hospital Guidelines for Pediatrics During Disasters. Section 8 – Decontamination of the pediatric patient. 2006.* Available at: http://www.nyc.gov/html/doh/html/bhpp/bhpp-focus-ped-toolkit.shtml. Accessed April 6, 2011

28. Pediatric Emergency Preparedness for Natural Disasters, Terrorism and Public Health Emergencies: A National Consensus Conference. Garrett A, Redlener M, eds. New York, NY: National Center for Disaster Preparedness, Mailman School of Public Health, Columbia University; 2009. Available at: http://www.ncdp.mailman.columbia.edu/files/peds_consensus. pdf. Accessed April 6, 2011

29. Centers for Disease Control and Prevention. *Guidance for Protecting Building Environments from Chemical, Biological, or Radiological Attacks.* Washington, DC: National Institute for Occupational Safety and Health; 2002

30. Hagan JF Jr; American Academy of Pediatrics, Committee on Psychosocial Aspects of Child and Family Health, Task Force on Terrorism. Clinical report: psychosocial implications of disaster or terrorism on children: a guide for the pediatrician. *Pediatrics.* 2005;116(3):787-795

31. Burkle FJ. Acute-phase mental health consequences of disasters; implications for triage and emergency medical services. *Ann Emerg Med.* 1996;28(2):119-128

32. American Academy of Pediatrics, Committee on Pediatric Emergency Medicine, Committee on Medical Liability, Task Force on Terrorism. The pediatrician and disaster preparedness. *Pediatrics.* 2006;117(2):560-565

33. Pynoos R, Goenjian A, Steinberg A. A public mental health approach to the postdisaster treatment of children and adolescents. *Child Adolesc Psychiatry Clin North Am*. 1998;7(1): 195-210

34. Schonfeld D, Gurwitch R. Addressing disaster mental health needs of children: Practical guidance for pediatric emergency healthcare providers. *Clin Pediatr Emerg Med*. 2009;10(3): 208-215

35. Schonfeld D. Helping children deal with terrorism. In: Osborn L, DeWitt T, First L, Zenel J, eds. *Pediatrics*. Philadelphia, PA: Elsevier Mosby; 2005:1600-1602

36. Chung S, Shannon M. Reuniting children with their families during disasters: a proposed plan for greater success. *Am J Disaster Med*. 2007;2(3):113-117

37. Schobitz EP, Schmidt JM, Poirier MP. Biologic and chemical terrorism in children: an assessment of residents' knowledge. *Clin Pediatr (Phila)*. 2008;47(3):267-270

38. Cicero MX, Blake Eileen, Gallant N, et al. Impact of an educational intervention on residents' knowledge of pediatric disaster medicine. *Pediatr Emerg Care*. 2009;25(7):447-451

Chapter 48

Developmental Disabilities

■ ■ ■ ■ ■ ■

The developing central nervous system is exquisitely sensitive to environmental factors. Environmental factors that negatively affect central nervous
system development may manifest as disturbances in motor, cognitive, sensory,
behavioral, and/or social functioning that constitute developmental disabilities.
This chapter reviews why the developing central nervous system is vulnerable
to insults that result in developmental disabilities; how chemical, physical,
educational, and psychosocial aspects of the environment may contribute to
the development and expression of these conditions, especially in children
who live in circumstances of social and economic disadvantage; the clinical
features of several developmental disabilities; and steps that can be taken to
prevent, reduce, or mitigate developmental disabilities associated with environmental factors.

DEFINING "DEVELOPMENTAL DISABILITIES"

For the purposes of this chapter, a developmental disability is defined as a
neurologic condition that has origins in early life; is characterized by significant
developmental delays or differences in early childhood as a result of an insult
to the developing brain that manifests in one or more functional domains; and
requires timely identification, appropriate intervention, and medical, therapeutic, and psychosocial support to ensure optimal functioning of the child in the
community. This definition is more helpful in a clinical setting than the definition articulated in the Developmental Disabilities Act of 1977 (Section 1028]),
because it addresses etiology, neurologic nature and manifestations, and the
developmental dynamics involved.

CENTRAL NERVOUS SYSTEM DEVELOPMENT AND VULNERABILITIES

The central nervous system begins forming shortly after conception and continues developing into early adulthood. As a result, it remains vulnerable to environmental influences over a considerable period of time. In general, the earlier and more severe the insult to the developing brain, the more dramatic the outcome will be. The type of insult and the stage(s) during which it occurs are also important determinants of the extent and nature of the resulting developmental disability.[1]

On approximately day 18 of gestation, the neural plate invaginates and, over approximately 8 to 10 days, fuses to form the neural tube. At this point, neural crest cells begin to migrate; disturbances of migration result in a number of different conditions. Incomplete closure of the neural tube can result in brain and spinal cord abnormalities, including anencephaly, encephalocele, and spina bifida. Around the fourth week of gestation, the neural tube begins to differentiate into the forebrain, midbrain, and hindbrain. Neurons begin to proliferate and migrate. Insults occurring during these events can adversely affect neuronal number, location, and architecture.

The development of axonal sheaths (myelination) begins around the sixth month of gestation, peaks between birth and the first year of life, and continues into adulthood. Interference with this process negatively affects the speed and efficacy of electrical impulse transmission within the neuronal network.

Brain organization begins in mid-gestation and continues into the mid-20s. This process involves not only neuronal differentiation and synaptogenesis but also neuronal pruning through genetically programmed cell death (apoptosis). Periods of neuron exuberance followed by pruning occur prenatally, during the first 2 years of life, and during the prepubertal period and extending into adolescence. Disturbances in these processes can alter neurotransmitter production, release, and reuptake and can affect how the brain processes stimuli and coordinates tasks.

ETIOLOGIES

The etiologies of developmental disabilities can be roughly categorized as either primarily genetic or primarily environmental (the "nature versus nurture" paradigm). In many cases, however, it is not possible to determine a clear etiology. Humans are the product of a cascade of interactions between genes and the environment, so it may be preferable to think about "nature via nurture,"[2] also known as gene-environment interaction.[3]

GENETIC INFLUENCES

Many developmental disabilities stem from specific genetic or chromosomal abnormalities. Autosomal-recessive disorders, including inborn errors of metabolism (such as aminoacidopathies, lipoidoses, or mucopolysacchari-doses), are among the most serious, because they usually involve progressive neurodegeneration. Some genetic conditions are sex-linked, such as fragile X syndrome and Rett syndrome. Disorders of chromosome number include Down syndrome, caused by an extra chromosome 21. Microdeletion anomalies include velocardiofacial syndrome, with a microdeletion on chromosome 22q11, and Smith-Magenis syndrome, with a microdeletion on chromosome 17. Disorders of mitochondrial DNA, which are maternally transmitted via the mitochondria in the fertilized ovum, also result in a variety of neurologic disorders that may manifest in other family members to varying degrees.

Other developmental disabilities appear to involve a strong genetic pre-disposition, although the actual mechanism of inheritance is unclear. Spina bifida may have a genetic predisposition but can be prevented by ingesting adequate folic acid. Attention-deficit/hyperactivity disorder (ADHD) and autism may also fall into this category, because expression of these conditions is likely to involve complex interactions between 1 or more genes with environ-mental factors.

ENVIRONMENTAL INFLUENCES

Several environmental factors influence the manifestation of developmental disabilities. Stage of development, dosage and duration of exposure, and resil-ience are a few of the many variables that determine the nature and extent of disability. It is helpful to examine these factors in a temporal context (ie, before, during, or after birth).

Prenatal Environment

The developing central nervous system undergoes its most dramatic changes in embryonic and early fetal life. Therefore, it is much more vulnerable to adverse physical, chemical, and infectious agents transmitted through transplacental blood flow.

Alcohol

A range of neurologic and other problems collectively referred to as fetal alcohol spectrum disorders result from prenatal exposure to alcohol. Although chronic consumption of alcohol and binge drinking are especially likely to have adverse consequences on the central nervous system in utero, any prenatal alcohol exposure may result in harm.[4] In the US, approximately 4 million infants are born with prenatal alcohol exposure each year, and 1000 to 6000 infants are diagnosed with fetal alcohol syndrome. Fetal alcohol syndrome, the classic and more severe form of fetal alcohol spectrum disorders, is associated with physical anomalies, developmental disabilities, and significant behavioral problems that may be aggravated in infancy and early childhood by the very environmental factors that contributed to maternal substance abuse (eg, domestic violence, homelessness, family discord). Unlike many other conditions that give rise to developmental disabilities, fetal alcohol spectrum disorders are readily preventable.

Smoking

Maternal smoking during pregnancy—a common and preventable exposure—has long been associated with low birth weight, developmental delays, cognitive problems, learning disorders, and behavioral difficulties in children. Secondhand tobacco smoke inhaled by pregnant mothers and young children—another common, preventable exposure—is also associated with behavioral disorders (see Chapter 40).[5] As with alcohol exposure, the severity may vary, especially when the fetus is exposed to multiple teratogens.

Maternal use of drugs or medications

Prenatal use of "street" drugs, such as cocaine, methamphetamines, and cannabis, can cause neurologic symptoms in children, including inattention, impulsivity, and cognitive impairment.[6] Prescription medications, including the anticonvulsants phenytoin and valproic acid, may cause recognizable neurologic syndromes.[7]

Maternal illness and chronic conditions

The consequences of infections such as rubella, toxoplasmosis, cytomegalovirus, syphilis, herpes, and HIV vary, depending on the timing of infection. For example, the risk of congenital defects resulting from in utero rubella infection is inversely related to gestational age at the time of maternal infection. Congenital defects occur in more than 80% of infants infected in the first trimester; virtually no defects are found in infants infected after the first 16 weeks of gestation. The gestational age at the time of fetal infection also affects the distribution of congenital defects: infection in the first trimester is more likely to result in multiple congenital defects, whereas infection after 11 to 12 weeks of gestation is more likely to result in only deafness or retinopathy as clinical manifestations.[8] Investigators studying behavioral effects resulting from an epidemic of congenital rubella in the 1960s reported a higher-than-expected number of children with autism.[9] Other maternal illnesses during pregnancy may also affect fetal growth and development. Chronic conditions such as diabetes may be particularly problematic, especially if blood sugar is not well controlled. Women with phenylketonuria (PKU) who do not strictly adhere to their diets from preconception through pregnancy have an increased risk of delivering babies with neurologic impairment. Maternal stress, malnutrition, physical trauma secondary to domestic abuse, and illness also may adversely affect the fetus.

Exposure to environmental toxicants

Lead easily crosses the placenta and enters the fetal circulation. Because pregnancy is associated with a marked increase in maternal bone turnover, prenatal lead exposure can occur not only through current maternal environmental exposures but also through mobilization of the mother's accumulated stores of bone lead. Elevated maternal blood lead levels during pregnancy may result in effects on the fetus. Prenatal lead exposure can affect fetal DNA, which, in turn, may influence long-term epigenetic programming and disease susceptibility.[10]

Exposure during pregnancy to several commonly used chemicals may also result in developmental disabilities either by directly causing central nervous system damage or by modifying DNA and thereby predisposing a child to be more vulnerable to environmental toxicants. Prenatal exposure to pesticides such as organophosphates enhances the risk of memory deficits, poorer motor performance, and other conditions.[11] Polychlorinated biphenyls (PCBs) are mixtures of chlorinated compounds once used as cooling and insulating fluids in electronic components. They bioaccumulate in fat, so human exposure continues via fatty foods, including human milk. Prenatal exposure to (PCBs) can adversely affect neurologic functions such as planning efficiency, executive working memory, speed of information processing, verbal abilities, and visual recognition memory.[12] Polycyclic aromatic hydrocarbons are widely distributed air pollutants generated by motor fuel combustion, coal-fired power plants, tobacco smoking, and residential heating and cooking. High levels of these well-recognized human mutagens and carcinogens may have adverse effects on birth weight and cognitive development.[13]

A number of neurotoxicants may be introduced via drinking water. Although trace amounts of manganese are necessary for health and normal development, high levels of manganese (see Chapter 24) can damage the developing nervous system.[14] Prenatal and early childhood exposure to arsenic (see Chapter 22) can also adversely affect intellectual functioning.[14]

Limited Prenatal Care

Most significantly and more commonly, children born to women with limited access to appropriate prenatal care are at especially high risk of developmental disabilities. Prenatal care that includes education, screening, and appropriate prevention and management of maternal health problems can help reduce and even eliminate many risks.

THE PERINATAL ENVIRONMENT

The 2 most common perinatal events associated with developmental disabilities are hypoxic ischemic encephalopathy and cerebral hemorrhage. Preterm birth—frequently associated with lack of prenatal care as well as maternal alcohol use, tobacco use, and drug use—significantly increases the risk of perinatal vulnerability that contributes to developmental disabilities. Infants born preterm and with a low birth weight are significantly more likely than full-term infants of normal weight to have periventricular leukomalacia and intraventricular hemorrhage that result in serious neurologic impairment.[15] Preterm infants are also at risk of central nervous system complications as a result of difficulty maintaining body temperature, respiratory complications, hemodynamic fluxes, jaundice, susceptibility to infections, and significant vulnerability to the effects of medications and environmental toxicants.

To reduce the likelihood of morbidity and mortality, pregnancies associated with increased risk to the mother and infant should be closely monitored. Delivery should take place where expert obstetric and neonatal intensive care is available.

Postnatal Environments

A range of postnatal insults may contribute to developmental disabilities. Central nervous system damage may be caused by infection (eg, meningitis, encephalitis); injury associated with falls, motor vehicle crashes, drowning with varying outcomes (previously termed "near-drowning" or "dry drowning"), or child abuse; and chemical and physical agents found in soil, water, and air.

Heavy metal exposure may be associated with brain damage in early life. Lead has been recognized as a neurotoxicant in children for more than 100 years. Blood lead levels of 10 µg/dL and below have been shown to exert subtle influences on the developing central nervous system, with adverse effects on IQ, learning and behavior (see Chapter 31). Exposure to secondhand smoke in childhood is associated with behavioral problems and learning disabilities in school.[16]

Unfortunately, research on the neurologic effects of many chemicals is quite limited, so safe levels of exposure are often unknown. Because of this, few regulations have been implemented to reduce the potential effects of numerous chemicals on the developing brain.

The nutritional and psychosocial environments have significant influence on postnatal development. Children who have poor nutrition and those who receive inadequate sensory stimulation and nurturing in their early years are at higher risk of developmental delays and disabilities. Child maltreatment and other traumatic events may cause permanent changes in central nervous system structure and functioning that can manifest as developmental disabilities (see Chapter 52).

SPECIFIC DEVELOPMENTAL DISABILITIES

Developmental disabilities may be broadly categorized as motor, sensory, cognitive, or behavioral/psychological, although many involve multiple elements.

Historically, those relating to behavior or mood have been seen as "mental" or "psychological" rather than "physical" conditions. In recent years, research in molecular biology and epigenetics has begun to reveal how behavioral disorders such as ADHD and autism—and even conditions such as bipolar disorders and schizophrenia—may stem from complex interactions between genes and prenatal or early childhood environments.

Fig 48.1 demonstrates how prenatal, perinatal, and postnatal insults to the developing central nervous system may influence the development of mild and severe functional impairments. Some of these manifestations are discussed below.

Cerebral Palsy

Cerebral palsy describes a group of disorders affecting movement and posture as a result of insults to the developing fetal or infant brain.[18] The prevalence of cerebral palsy in the United States is approximately 3.6 cases per 1000 births.[19] Although motor impairment and associated orthopedic consequences are hallmarks of cerebral palsy, there are often also seizure disorders, sensory disorders, and disturbances of cognition, communication, perception, and behavior. Etiology, timing of insult, part(s) of the brain affected, and the severity of the injury determine the nature and severity of the clinical manifestation in each child.

Sensory Impairment

Sensory impairments can exist in isolation or be part of other conditions. Approximately 12 children in 10 000 have a hearing impairment originating congenitally or during early childhood.[20] Childhood hearing impairment may be genetic or be caused by infections, hyperbilirubinemia, head trauma, and exposure to aminoglycosides or other neurotoxicants. Childhood visual impairment also occurs in about 12 children per 10 000.[20] Preterm infants are at especially high risk of developing vision impairment secondary to retinopathy following exposure to high concentrations of oxygen and high ventilator pressure. Sensory impairments should be detected as early as possible to institute early interventions designed to ensure optimal functional outcome.

Sensory Integration Disorder

Sensory integration disorder, also known as "regulation disorders of sensory processing" and "sensory processing disorder," causes difficulties with processing visual, auditory, tactile, olfactory, and gustatory information as well as vestibular and proprioceptive data. Although sensory integration disorder is not included in the current *Diagnostic and Statistical Manual of Mental Disorders, Fourth Edition, Text Revision (DSM-IV-TR)*,[21] it is recognized as a distinct disorder in the *Diagnostic Classification of Mental Health and Developmental Disorders of Infancy and Early Childhood*[22] and *Greenspan's Infant and Early Childhood Mental*

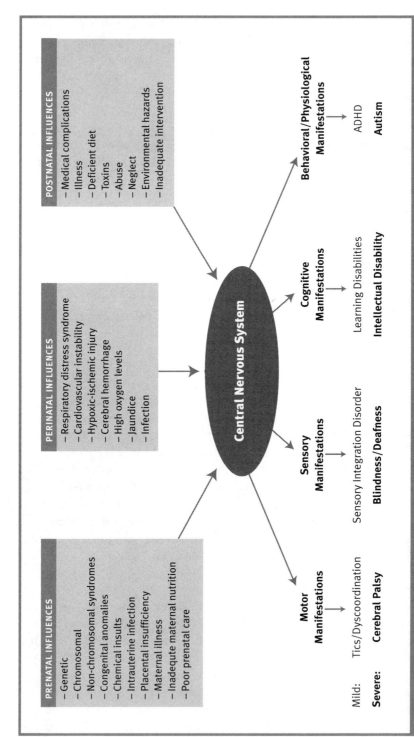

Fig 48.1: Etiologic Factors and Manifestations of Developmental Disabilities

PRENATAL INFLUENCES
– Genetic
– Chromosomal
– Non-chromosomal syndromes
– Congenital anomalies
– Chemical insults
– Intrauterine infection
– Placental insufficiency
– Maternal illness
– Inadequte maternal nutrition
– Poor prenatal care

PERINATAL INFLUENCES
– Respiratory distress syndrome
– Cardiovascular instability
– Hypoxic-ischemic injury
– Cerebral hemorrhage
– High oxygen levels
– Jaundice
– Infection

POSTNATAL INFLUENCES
– Medical complications
– Illness
– Deficient diet
– Toxins
– Abuse
– Neglect
– Environmental hazards
– Inadequate intervention

Central Nervous System

Motor Manifestations
Mild: Tics/Dyscoordination
Severe: Cerebral Palsy

Sensory Manifestations
Sensory Integration Disorder
Blindness/Deafness

Cognitive Manifestations
Learning Disabilities
Intellectual Disability

Behavioral/Physiological Manifestations
ADHD
Autism

Adapted from Rubin and Crocker 2006.[17]

Health.[23] Symptoms include unusual reactions to sensory stimuli; difficulty with perceptual processing; gross and fine motor dyscoordination and dyspraxia; heightened or reduced emotional reactivity; and difficulties with physiological functions, such as sleep, eating, and toileting as well as with language acquisition and development. Because sensory processing is a fundamental aspect of brain functioning, processing disorders may give rise to behavioral consequences that are seen in other developmental disabilities, such as hyperactivity associated with ADHD and behaviors associated with autism spectrum disorders.[24]

Intellectual Disability

Intellectual disability is characterized by significant limitations in intellectual functioning and in adaptive behavior that manifest before 18 years of age.[25] Intellectual disability has been estimated to occur in 1.2% to 1.6% of the US population.[26] An IQ of 70 or below is the measure considered indicative of intellectual disability; however, actual functioning with regard to conceptual skills (language, literacy, time, numbers, self-direction), social skills (communication, social problem-solving, rule compliance, personal boundaries, avoidance of victimization), and practical skills (activities of daily living, occupational skills, health care, travel/transportation, schedules/routines, safety, money management, telephone use) must be considered before making the diagnosis of intellectual disability.[25]

The term "intellectual disability" has replaced "mental retardation," because the former emphasizes "an ecologic perspective that focuses on the person-environment interaction and recognizes that the systematic application of individualized supports can enhance human functioning."[27] The *DSM-IV-TR*[21] and the *International Classification of Diseases, Ninth Revision, Clinical Modification (ICD-9-CM)*[28] describe 4 degrees of mental retardation/intellectual disability based on IQ scores: mild (50-55 to 70-75); moderate (35-40 to 50-55); severe (20-25 to 35-40); and profound (less than 20-25). These categories may be eliminated (or at least significantly modified) in the forthcoming *Diagnostic and Statistical Manual of Mental Disorders, Fifth Edition*.[29] Intellectual disability is often associated with other neurologic, medical, and functional disorders. The etiology determines the pattern and severity of symptoms, which, in turn, determines the impact on health and well-being.[17] The precise mechanisms by which environmental toxicants affect cognitive functioning are often unclear, especially in children with multiple risk factors.

Learning Disabilities

Learning disabilities (also sometimes referred to as "learning differences" or "learning challenges") are characterized by impairments related to reading, mathematics, or written expression that significantly interfere with academic achievement or negatively affect activities of daily living.[21] They are often associated with cognitive processing deficits involving visual perception, language, attention, and memory. Approximately 4.6 million children 3 to 17 years of age (7.5%) have been diagnosed with at least one learning disability.[30]

Although learning disabilities are present at a very young age, they are not usually recognized until the child reaches school age and experiences academic difficulties. If a child is having difficulty with learning at school, he or she should undergo a thorough history and physical examination to look for any medical factors that may affect learning, such as obstructive sleep apnea related to large tonsils or adenoids; poor vision and/or hearing; environmental exposures to lead or mercury; or emotional factors, such as family strife or difficulties with peers. Once medical and emotional factors have been addressed, psychoeducational or neuropsychological testing can be used to assess the child's academic strengths and weaknesses, suggest strategies that parents and teachers can use to support the child, and inform the development of an appropriate individualized educational plan for the child.

ADHD

ADHD is perhaps the most common neurobehavioral developmental disorder. Estimates of the prevalence of ADHD in school-aged children range from 2% to 18% in community samples.[31] The cardinal feature of ADHD is a persistent pattern of inattention and distractibility, with or without impulsivity and hyperactivity, that is constant and manifests in more than one environment (eg, home and school).[32] This should be differentiated from simple exuberance and occasional inattentiveness. The hyperactivity manifested by many, but not all, children with ADHD may be viewed by parents and teachers as evidence of laziness, willfulness, emotional disturbance, ineffective discipline, or lack of ability, rather than as a neurologically based disorder that can be treated. Children with ADHD often also have coexisitng conditions, such as learning disabilities.[33]

Appropriate diagnosis and treatment is critical to ensure that each child reaches his or her full potential and functions comfortably in home, school, and social settings. Because children with other emotional, psychosocial, and psychiatric problems (eg, anxiety disorders) may present with some ADHD symptoms, a detailed physical, psychosocial, academic, and environmental history should be taken. Medication, combined with behavioral therapy, can be highly effective in treating primary symptoms and may positively affect associated emotional, social, and educational performance. Close monitoring of the child and family are critical, especially when starting and titrating medication.[32] If the child does not respond to the combination of medication and behavioral therapy, the family should be referred to a developmental pediatrician or to a center specializing in developmental disabilities or a child psychiatrist where necessary and appropriate.

Studies of families have revealed a genetic pattern in how ADHD manifests. In some cases, specific genes have been linked to the disorder.[34] Environmental factors include maternal smoking during pregnancy, preterm birth, cerebral hypoxic ischemia, alcohol exposure, viral infections, and endocrine disorders.[35] Lead poisoning may be a contributing factor. Children growing up and living in circumstances of social and economic disadvantage, including those living in older, poorer neighborhoods, are at high risk of developing ADHD because of their increased risk of lead exposure as well as psychosocial and other environmental factors.[36] Because ADHD is less likely to be properly diagnosed and treated in disadvantaged children, they are also more likely to experience long-term, negative psychological and social consequences as well as adverse educational outcomes (eg, high grade retention and dropout rates).[37]

Autism Spectrum/Pervasive Developmental Disorders

Autism spectrum disorders, also known as pervasive developmental disorders, represent a spectrum of related neurodevelopmental disorders characterized by a constellation of developmental and behavioral characteristics:

- Significant, qualitative difficulty in reciprocal social interaction skills;
- Significant, qualitative difficulty in communication skills; and/or
- Insistence on adhering to routines or restrictive, repetitive, and stereotyped behavior, interests, and activities.[21,38]

Historically, autism spectrum disorders have been poorly understood. The term "autism" was coined in the 1940s by Kanner to emphasize the affected child's focus on the self rather than the social world.[39] This term was not, however, immediately adopted by the larger psychiatric community. In the first 2 editions of the *Diagnostic and Statistical Manual of Mental Disorders*, autism spectrum disorders were considered to be variants of childhood psychosis or schizophrenia. The third edition of the *Diagnostic and Statistical Manual of Mental Disorders* allowed for slightly better diagnostic refinement, as it included autism as a separate diagnosis. The *DSM-IV* and its revisions recognized several additional pervasive developmental disorders[21]: Asperger syndrome was distinguished from the classic picture of autism by a lack of delay or deviance in early language development. Pervasive Developmental Disorder (of Childhood) was a term originally coined to distinguish the classic picture of autism from a less dramatic presentation. Under the current nomenclature, the diagnosis "pervasive developmental disorder not otherwise specified" (PDD-NOS) is applied when children exhibit pervasive developmental anomalies but do not meet criteria for any of the other diagnoses.[40] The terminology continues to evolve, as evidenced by the consideration of the Neurodevelopmental Disorders Workgroup of the forthcoming *Diagnostic and Statistical Manual of Mental Disorders, Fifth Edition* to consolidate autistic disorder, Asperger syndrome, and PDD-NOS into one diagnostic category of autism spectrum disorders.

Understanding the epidemiology of autism spectrum disorders has been complicated by these taxonomical and definitional changes. The well-documented increase in the prevalence of autism in recent years is attributed, in significant part, to increased case identification resulting from greater public awareness and professional understanding of autism spectrum disorders. A recent report gives a point-prevalence of 110 per 10 000—approximately 1 child in 90 or 1.1% of the population.[41] The number of children affected underscores the importance of exploring the etiologies of autism spectrum disorders, identifying children with autism spectrum disorders early in life, and providing appropriate, consistent treatment to improve long-term outcomes.

Many people continue to pose questions about how environmental factors may have contributed to the increased prevalence of autism spectrum disorders. There have been many articles in the scientific literature and the popular press regarding possible links between autism and vaccines. A great deal of attention focused on whether autism could be triggered by exposure to the measles-mumps-rubella (MMR) vaccine or by exposure to thimerosal, an ethylmercury-based preservative previously used in several childhood vaccines (but not MMR vaccine).[42] In 2004, the Institute of Medicine conducted an extensive review of the literature and concluded that no existing evidence supported a causal relationship between the MMR vaccine or thimerosal and autism, although further study was warranted.[43] Many more studies are needed to elucidate any relationships between environmental factors and autism and to identify possible mechanisms, such as gene-environment interactions.

Accumulating data suggest that autism may have a genetic component.[44] This is demonstrated in twin studies.[45] Anecdotally, detailed family histories of children with autism spectrum disorders that include questions about patterns of behavior and social interaction among relatives frequently reveal information suggesting that a tendency and propensity for autism-like traits is inheritable. Studies have begun to reveal particular genes associated with autism, but there has been no consistency.[46] Conditions subsumed under the diagnostic label of autism (or autism spectrum disorders) represent a heterogeneous group of conditions that have a common set of developmental and behavioral features. Autism spectrum disorders have been associated with several genetic syndromes—most notably fragile X but also Down syndrome, tuberous sclerosis, and others.[47] This suggests that autism spectrum disorders are likely to result from multiple genetic, environmental, and gene-environment interactions rather than from a single genetic factor or etiologic agent.

Screening and diagnostic tools are available to clinicians who suspect that a child has features of autism.[38] Genetic testing (including fragile X analysis, extended-band chromosomal analysis, and microarray analysis) is frequently performed. Neurologic workup with magnetic resonance imaging, electroencephalography, and metabolic studies for inborn errors of metabolism should be performed if clinically indicated. Assessing blood lead levels in children with ADHD and autism spectrum disorders, especially those with pica, is often warranted, because these conditions may mask or coexist with lead poisoning. Other testing for metals and neurotoxicants is not recommended unless indicated after conducting a thorough environmental health history. Children with suspected autism spectrum disorders can be referred to a developmental specialist or developmental center for evaluation and treatment or directly for appropriate therapies if availability or accessibility of diagnostic resources is limited.

SOCIAL AND ECONOMIC FACTORS

Children who grow up in environmental circumstances of social and economic disadvantage are more likely to have developmental disabilities.[48] Maternal risk factors include poverty, low socioeconomic status, mental illness, substance abuse, and living in communities where environmental hazards are plentiful and resources are limited. Prenatal and perinatal risk factors—such as preterm birth, low birth weight, central nervous system abnormalities, and prolonged hospitalizations that can drain family resources and interfere with parent-infant bonding—also contribute to adverse developmental outcomes.

For many children, the environmental risks are compounded during their early years. Poverty remains one of the most complex and far-reaching risk factors, because it affects so many aspects of the life of a child. In 2006, approximately 1 in 5 US children younger than 6 years and 16% of children ages 6 to 17 years lived in poverty.[49] The rate for children of all ages living in single female-headed families was 42%. During that same year, approximately 17% of children (12.6 million) lived in households with food insecurity (defined as a condition existing when people lack sustainable access to enough safe, nutritious, and socially acceptable food for a healthy and productive life). Children who were impoverished were also more likely to have a blood lead level of 10 µg/dL or greater. Children living in poverty are 1.7 times more likely to be born at a low birth weight.[48] Moreover, living in low-income areas decreases children's access to appropriate educational, health care, and habilitative services. Too often, children and their families are trapped in a cycle of disadvantage and disability (see Fig 48.2) that is difficult to escape unless interrupted by outside social forces (see Chapter 52) or the extraordinary efforts of individuals and families.

Children in low-income countries may be at especially high risk of developmental disabilities (see Chapter 14). Major risk factors include specific genetic diseases, a higher frequency of births to older mothers, consanguinity, micronutrient deficiencies, and infections.[51] Toxic exposures are also important risk

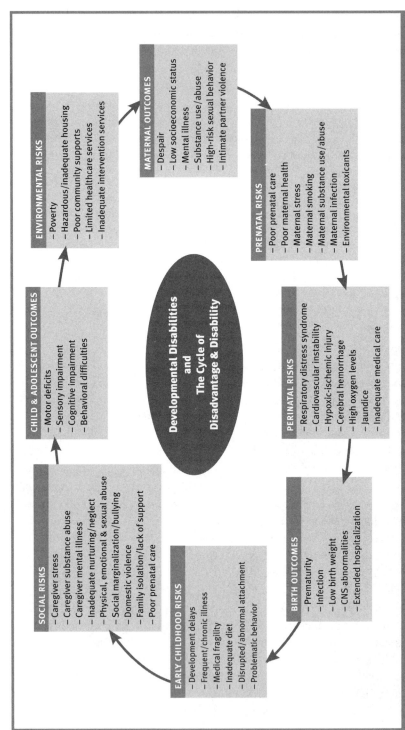

Developmental Disabilities and The Cycle of Disadvantage & Disability

MATERNAL OUTCOMES
- Despair
- Low socioeconomic status
- Mental illness
- Substance use/abuse
- High-risk sexual behavior
- Intimate partner violence

ENVIRONMENTAL RISKS
- Poverty
- Hazardous/inadequate housing
- Poor community supports
- Limited healthcare services
- Inadequate intervention services

PRENATAL RISKS
- Poor prenatal care
- Poor maternal health
- Maternal stress
- Maternal smoking
- Maternal substance use/abuse
- Maternal infection
- Environmental toxicants

CHILD & ADOLESCENT OUTCOMES
- Motor deficits
- Sensory impairment
- Cognitive impairment
- Behavioral difficulties

PERINATAL RISKS
- Respiratory distress syndrome
- Cardiovascular instability
- Hypoxic-ischemic injury
- Cerebral hemorrhage
- High oxygen levels
- Jaundice
- Inadequate medical care

SOCIAL RISKS
- Caregiver stress
- Caregiver substance abuse
- Caregiver mental illness
- Inadequate nurturing/neglect
- Physical, emotional & sexual abuse
- Social marginalization/bullying
- Domestic violence
- Family isolation/lack of support
- Poor prenatal care

EARLY CHILDHOOD RISKS
- Development delays
- Frequent/chronic illness
- Medical fragility
- Inadequate diet
- Disrupted/abnormal attachment
- Problematic behavior

BIRTH OUTCOMES
- Prematurity
- Infection
- Low birth weight
- CNS abnormalities
- Extended hospitalization

Fig 48.2: Developmental disabilities and the cycle of disadvantage and disability.

Adapted from Rubin et al 2007.[50]

factors, although their contributions are not well documented. Displacement by natural and man-made disasters (eg, war) can result in physical, chemical, and psychological effects on a child's brain development and functional outcome. Unfortunately, data on epidemiology, etiology, screening, and intervention services are often lacking.[52]

REDUCING ENVIRONMENTAL RISKS ASSOCIATED WITH DEVELOPMENTAL DISABILITIES

Preconception and Prenatal Counseling

Clinicians counseling women who are pregnant or likely to become pregnant should help them to identify risk factors such as using tobacco, drinking alcohol, and using teratogenic medications or other drugs. Clinicians should stress the importance of daily intake of folic acid during the childbearing years.[53] Women should also be asked about exposure to pesticides, lead, and other metals as well as secondhand smoke, mold, and other forms of air pollution. Pregnant women should be encouraged to receive regular prenatal care and given information about sleep, stress reduction, and exercise. They should be counseled about nutrition and dietary recommendations related to fish consumption as well as the benefits of breastfeeding.

Role of the Pediatrician

Because pediatricians see children frequently in the first and second years of life, they are well positioned to identify delays and unusual patterns of a child's development and behavior. It is important for pediatricians to ask questions about the family history, occupations of parents, and environmental risk factors, especially the age of the home and about smoking. When indicated, referrals should be made for neurologic, genetic, metabolic, or toxicologic workups and for developmental evaluations and therapies.

Early detection of developmental issues and subsequent referral to early intervention and other specialty services can positively affect the child's development and the family's stability and harmony. Primary care follow-up includes monitoring the child for appropriate development, identifying and mitigating ongoing risks, making appropriate referrals, and helping coordinate services. The importance of responding to parental concerns cannot be overemphasized.

Frequently Asked Questions

Q   *How should I respond when parents express concern about having their child vaccinated because of a possible connection between vaccination and autism?*

A   First, acknowledge the parents' concern and desire to do their best to promote their child's health. Second, explain the research findings relating to the known benefits and potential risks of vaccination. Parents may have little understanding of the potentially serious outcomes, including death, that childhood vaccinations prevent. Many may have little understanding of the scientific method and may find it difficult to weigh the relative weight of information published in peer-reviewed journals versus that published in self-help books or on the Internet. Ultimately, parents must make an informed decision about their child's health care.

Q *How should I respond when parents ask about alternative treatments for autism?*

A It is common for parents to search for medical information and information about nonstandard treatments. Some alternative treatments may have a valid scientific basis, but others rely on unproven claims and testimonials. Parents may ask about having their child undergo expensive "biomedical" or "environmental" testing to determine whether they have been exposed to environmental hazards that might contribute to developmental problems. Often, such testing is offered by private companies that also sell special remedies or supplements that have not been studied or documented to be of benefit. Pediatricians should be generally familiar with these treatment alternatives to help parents understand the potential risks that may be involved, especially with unproven and sometimes potentially dangerous treatments, such as chelation (see Chapter 46). When talking with parents, it is important to avoid being judgmental, because this can interfere with the doctor-family relationship.

Resources

ADHD assessment and treatment guidelines are available from the American Academy of Pediatrics (www.aap.org/healthtopics/adhd.cfm) and the American Academy of Child & Adolescent Psychiatry (www.aacap.org). Both organizations offer information for parents and teachers. Another excellent general resource is the Children and Adults with Attention-Deficit/Hyperactivity Disorder (CHADD) website, www.chadd.org.

Autism assessment and treatment guidelines are available on the AAP's Web site (www.aap.org/healthtopics/autism.cfm). An Autism Tool Kit for professionals is available through the site.

Bibliography

1. Rice D, Barone S. Critical periods of vulnerability for the developing nervous system: Evidence from humans and animal models. *Environ Health Perspect.* 2000;108(Suppl 3):511-533
2. Ridley M. *Nature Via Nurture: Genes, Experience and What Makes Us Human.* New York, NY: Harper Collins; 2003
3. Centers for Disease Control and Prevention, Office of Genetics and Disease Prevention. Gene-Environment Interaction Fact Sheet. Atlanta, GA: Centers for Disease Control and Prevention; August 2000. Available at: http://www.ashg.org/pdf/CDC%20Gene-Environment%20 Interaction%20Fact%20Sheet.pdf. Accessed April 6, 2011

4. Bertrand J, Floyd RL, Weber MK. Guidelines for identifying and referring persons with fetal alcohol syndrome. *MMWR Recomm Rep.* 2005;54(RR-11):1-10

5. Herrmann M, King K, Weitzman M. Prenatal tobacco smoke and postnatal secondhand smoke exposure and child neurodevelopment. *Curr Opin Pediatr.* 2008;20(2):184-190

6. Huizink AC, Mulder EJH. Maternal smoking, drinking or cannabis use during pregnancy and neurobehavioral and cognitive functioning in human offspring. *Neurosci Biobehav Rev.* 2006;30(1):24-41

7. Moore SJ, Turnpenny P, Quinn A, et al. A clinical study of 57 children with fetal anticonvulsant syndromes. *J Med Genet.* 2000;37(7):489-497

8. Maldonado YA. Rubella virus. In: Long SS, Pickering LK, Prober CG, eds: *Principles and Practice of Pediatric Infectious Diseases.* 3rd ed (rev reprint). New York, NY: Churchill Livingstone; 2009

9. Chess S. Autism in children with congenital rubella. *J Autism Child Schizophr.* 1971;1:33-47. Available at: http://www.neurodiversity.com/library_chess_1971.pdf. Accessed April 6, 2011

10. Pilsner RJ, Hu H, Ettinger A, et al. Influence of prenatal lead exposure on genomic methylation of cord blood DNA. *Environ Health Perspect.* 2009;117(9):1466–1471

11. Rauh VA, Garfinkel R, Perera FP, et al. Impact of prenatal chlorpyrifos exposure on neurodevelopment in the first 3 years of life among inner-city children. *Pediatrics.* 2006;118(6):e1845-e1859

12. Boucher O, Muckle G, Bastien CH. Prenatal exposure to polychlorinated biphenyls: a neuropsychologic analysis. *Environ Health Perspect.* 2009;117(1):7-16

13. Perera FP, Rauh V, Whyatt RM, et al. Effect of prenatal exposure to airborne polycyclic aromatic hydrocarbons on neurodevelopment in the first 3 years of life among inner-city children. *Environ Health Perspect.* 2006;114(8):1287-1292

14. Wright RO, Amarasiriwardena C, Woolf AD, Jim R, Bellinger DC. Neuropsychological correlates of hair arsenic, manganese, and cadmium levels in school-age children residing near a hazardous waste site. *Neurotoxicology.* 2006;27(2):210-216

15. Vohr BR, Wright LL, Dusick AM, et al. Kaplan neurodevelopmental and functional outcomes of extremely low birth weight infants in the National Institute of Child Health and Human Development Neonatal Research Network, 1993-1994. *Pediatrics.* 2000;105(6):1216-1226

16. Best DB; American Academy of Pediatrics, Committee on Environmental Health, Committee on Native American Child Health, and Committee on Adolescence. Technical report—secondhand and prenatal tobacco smoke exposure. *Pediatrics.* 2009;124(5):e1017–e1044

17. Rubin IL, Crocker AC. *Delivery of Medical Care for Children and Adults with Developmental Disabilities.* 2nd ed. Baltimore, MD: Paul H. Brookes; 2006

18. Bax M, Goldstein M, Rosenbaum P, et al. Proposed definition and classification of cerebral palsy, April 2005. Executive Committee for the Definition of Cerebral Palsy Proposed Definition and Classification of Cerebral Palsy. *Dev Med Child Neurol.* 2005;47(8):571–576

19. Yeargin-Allsopp M, Braun KV, Doernberg NS, et al. Prevalence of cerebral palsy in 8-year-old children in three areas of the United States in 2002: a multisite collaboration. *Pediatrics.* 2008; 121(3):547-554

20. Centers for Disease Control and Prevention. *Metropolitan Atlanta Developmental Disabilities Surveillance Program (MADDSP).* Atlanta, GA: Centers for Disease Control and Prevention; 2000. Available at: http://www.cdc.gov/ncbddd/dd/ddsurv.htm. Accessed April 6, 2011

21. American Psychiatric Association. *Diagnostic and Statistical Manual of Mental Disorders, Fourth Edition, Text Revision (DSM-IV-TR).* Washington, DC: American Psychiatric Association; 2000

22. Zero to Three. *Diagnostic Classification of Mental Health and Developmental Disorders of Infancy and Early Childhood, Revised (DC:0-3R).* Washington, DC: Zero to Three; 2005

23. Greenspan SI, Wieder S. *Infant and Early Childhood Mental Health: A Comprehensive Developmental Approach to Assessment and Intervention.* Washington, DC: American Psychiatric Association; 2005

24. Belmonte MK, Cook EH Jr, Anderson GM, et al. Autism as a disorder of neural information processing: directions for research and targets for therapy. *Mol Psychiatry.* 2004;9(7):646-663

25. Luckasson R, Borthwick-Duffy S, Buntinx WHE, et al. *Mental Retardation: Definition, Classification, and Systems of Supports.* 10th ed. Washington, DC: American Association on Mental Retardation; 2002

26. Bhasin TK, Brocksen S, Avchen RN, Braun KVN. Prevalence of four developmental disabilities among children aged 8 years—Metropolitan Atlanta Developmental Disabilities Surveillance Program, 1996 and 2000. *MMWR Surveill Summ.* 2006;55(SS-01):1-9

27. American Association on Intellectual and Developmental Disabilities. *FAQ on Intellectual Disability.* Available at: http://www.aamr.org/content_104.cfm. Accessed April 6, 2011

28. Centers for Medicare and Medicaid Services, National Center for Health Statistics. *International Classification of Diseases, Ninth Revision, Clinical Modification (ICD-9-CM).* Washington, DC: Government Printing Office; 2010

29. Swedo S. *Report of the DSM-V Neurodevelopmental Disorders Work Group.* Washington, DC: American Psychiatric Association; 2009. Available at: http://psych.org/MainMenu/Research/DSMIV/DSMV/DSMRevisionActivities/DSM-V-Work-Group-Reports/Neurodevelopmental-Disorders-Work-Group-Report.aspx. Accessed April 6, 2011

30. Bloom B, Cohen RA, Freeman G. Summary health statistics for U.S. children: National Health Interview Survey, 2008. National Center for Health Statistics. *Vital Health Stat.* 2009;10(244):1-90

31. Rowland AS, Lesesne CA, Abramowitz AJ. The epidemiology of attention-deficit/hyperactivity disorder (ADHD): a public health view. *Ment Retard Dev Disabil Res Rev.* 2002;8(3):162-170

32. American Academy of Pediatrics, Subcommittee on Attention-Deficit/Hyperactivity Disorder and Committee on Quality Improvement. Clinical practice guideline: treatment of the school-aged child with attention-deficit/hyperactivity disorder. *Pediatrics.* 2001;108(4):1033-1044

33. Pastor PN, Reuben CA. Diagnosed attention deficit hyperactivity disorder and learning disability: United States, 2004–2006. *Vital Health Stat.* 2008;10(237):1-14

34. Goos LM, Crosbie J, Payne S, Schachar R. Validation and extension of the endophenotype model in ADHD patterns of inheritance in a family study of inhibitory control. *Am J Psychiatry.* 2009;166(6):711-717

35. Millichap JG. Etiologic classification of attention-deficit/hyperactivity disorder. *Pediatrics.* 2008;121(2):e358-e365

36. Rowland AS, Umbach DM, Stallone L, Naftel J, Bohlig EM, Sandler DP. Prevalence of medication treatment for attention deficit–hyperactivity disorder among elementary school children in Johnston County, North Carolina. *Am J Public Health.* 2002;92(2):231-234

37. Eiraldi RB, Mazzuca LB, Clarke AT, Power TJ. Service utilization among ethnic minority children with ADHD: a model of help-seeking behavior. *Adm Policy Ment Health.* 2006;33(5):607-622

38. Johnson CP; Myers SM; American Academy of Pediatrics, Council on Children With Disabilities. Identification and evaluation of children with autism spectrum disorders. *Pediatrics.* 2007;120(5):1183-1215

39. Kanner L. Autistic disturbances of affective contact. *Nervous Child.* 1943;2:217-250

40. Volkmar FR, Klin A. Issues in the classification of autism and related conditions. In: Vokmar FR, Paul R, Klin A, Cohen DJ, eds. *Handbook of Autism and Pervasive Developmental Disorders. Vol 1: Diagnosis, Development, Neurobiology, and Behavior.* 3rd ed. Hoboken, NJ: Wiley; 2005: 5-41

41. Kogan MD, Blumberg SJ, Schieve LA, et al. Prevalence of parent-reported diagnosis of autism spectrum disorder among children in the US, 2007. *Pediatrics.* 2009;124(5):1395-1403

42. Peacock G, Yeargin-Allsopp M. Autism spectrum disorders: prevalence and vaccines. *Pediatr Ann.* 2009;38(1):22-25

43. Institute of Medicine. *Immunization Safety Review: Vaccines and Autism.* Washington, DC: National Academies Press; 2004

44. Nishiyama T, Notohara M, Sumi S, Takami S, Kishino H. Major contribution of dominant inheritance to autism spectrum disorders (ASDs) in population-based families. *J Hum Genet.* 2009;54(12):721-726

45. Betancur C, Leboyer M, Gillberg C. Increased rate of twins among affected sibling pairs with autism. *Am J Hum Genet.* 2002;70(5):1381-1383

46. Geschwind DH. Autism: many genes, common pathways? *Cell.* 2008;135(3):391-395

47. Moss J, Howlin P. Autism spectrum disorders in genetic syndromes: implications for diagnosis, intervention and understanding the wider autism spectrum population. *J Intellect Disabil Res.* 2009;53(10):852-873

48. Institute of Medicine. *From Neurons to Neighborhoods: The Science of Early Childhood Development.* Shonkoff JP, Phillips DA, eds. Washington, DC: National Academies Press; 2000

49. Federal Interagency Forum on Child and Family Statistics. *America's Children in Brief: Key National Indicators of Well-Being.* Washington, DC: US Government Printing Office; 2008

50. Rubin IL, Nodvin JT, Geller RJ, Teague WG, Holzclaw BL, Felner EI. Environmental health disparities and social impact of industrial pollution in a community—the model of Anniston, AL. *Pediatr Clin North Am.* 2007;54(2):375-398

51. Durkin M. The epidemiology of developmental disabilities in low-income countries *Ment Retard Dev Disabil Res Rev.* 2002;8(3):206-211

52. Maulik PK, Darmstadt GL. Childhood disability in low- and middle-income countries: overview of screening, prevention, services, legislation, and epidemiology. *Pediatrics.* 2007;120(Suppl 1):S1-S55

53. Centers for Disease Control and Prevention. Recommendations to improve preconception health and health care—United States. A Report of the CDC/ATSDR Preconception Care Work Group and the Select Panel on Preconception Care. *MMWR Recomm Rep.* 2006;55 (RR-6):1-23. Available at: http://www.cdc.gov/mmwr/preview/mmwrhtml/rr5506a1.htm. Accessed April 6, 2011

Chapter 49

Drug (Methamphetamine) Laboratories

■ ■ ■ ■ ■ ■

Amphetamines and methamphetamines are stimulants that affect the central and the sympathetic nervous systems. Methamphetamine (the chemical name for which is desoxyephedrine) is the *N*-methyl homologue of amphetamine. Illicit methamphetamine ("meth") manufacturing often occurs in homes in which children live, potentially exposing them to toxic chemicals. Children living at a clandestine methamphetamine lab site may be subjected to fires and explosions. They are at risk of unintentional ingestion of methamphetamine with resulting toxicities. Their caregivers' hazardous lifestyle includes the presence of firearms, pornography, and social problems. Homes may be substandard, may lack plumbing, and may have code violations with hazardous conditions. Children often are witnesses to violence. They often suffer abuse and neglect and lack of food. Thus, when these children are removed from methamphetamine lab sites, their care is coordinated among medical, social work, and law enforcement professionals. Pediatricians may be asked to do a medical evaluation of children from such homes or of parents who use methamphetamine and are rendered unable to care for their children.

Amphetamine was first synthesized in 1887, but it was not tested in animal models until 1910. It was first commercially available in 1931 as the nasal spray Benzedrine, a racemic *d, l* form of amphetamine. The first amphetamine tablet appeared in 1937 and was used to treat narcolepsy. Because of its euphoric, stimulating, and appetite-suppressing effects, amphetamine use became widespread during the 1930s and 1940s and was used by foreign armies in World War II.[1]

Methamphetamine was first synthesized in 1919 by a Japanese chemist. In the late 1970s, biker gangs began to manufacture methamphetamine, primarily using the phenyl-2-propanone method. Manufacturing via another method, ephedrine reduction, began to occur in trailer parks and mobile homes and was more commonly found in rural areas. In the Midwestern United States, makeshift "mom and pop" labs produce relatively small amounts of methamphetamine. Labs capable of producing more than 10 pounds of methamphetamine ("superlabs") are more common in California and are controlled by California- and Mexico-based criminal groups.[2] The market for methamphetamine has been sustained by drug-trafficking organizations. Mexico is now the primary source for methamphetamine, and large-scale methamphetamine production is increasing in Canada. To avoid law enforcement officials, labs are mobile. A single batch of methamphetamine may be produced in several stages, with each stage occurring at a different location. Labs can be active, in the process of active chemical reactions; set-up, ready for manufacture but having no chemical reactions; boxed, stored for transit; or former labs, in which all reaction vessels have been removed.[3]

Methamphetamine exists as a powder resembling granulated crystals or as a rock form called "ice," the smokable version that came into use in the 1980s. Methamphetamine can be heated to form a vapor that is smoked, snorted, orally ingested, or injected. The "rush" results from the release of high levels of dopamine into the brain, which is almost instantaneous if methamphetamine is smoked or injected, occurs after about 5 minutes if it is snorted, and occurs after about 20 minutes if orally ingested.[4]

The major action of amphetamines is to cause the release of monoamines from storage sites in axon terminals, increasing the concentration of these amines in the synaptic cleft. Amphetamines are taken into the neurons, enter the neurotransmitter storage vesicles, and block the transport of dopamine into these vesicles. This results in intracellular and extravesicular accumulation of dopamine. The dopamine may undergo oxidation, producing toxic, reactive chemicals such as oxygen radicals, peroxides, and hydroxyquinones. Amphetamines also cause the release of serotonin and norepinephrine.[5] Methamphetamine inhibits the reuptake of norepinephrine, dopamine, and serotonin into the presynaptic terminals, which causes postsynaptic hyperstimulation of alpha-1 and beta-1 receptors.[6]

The primary site of metabolism is in the liver by aromatic hydroxylation, N-demethlyation (to form the metabolite amphetamine), and deamination. Acidic urine enhances excretion, leading to a shorter half-life, while basic urine slows excretion and prolongs half-life.[7] The elimination half-life varies from 12 to 34 hours.

CHEMICALS INVOLVED IN MANUFACTURE

Clandestine manufacturing methods ("cooks") generally start with pseudo-ephedrine or phenylacetic acid as the precursor and require the combination and addition of several other household chemicals as reagents. These chemicals include acids, bases, and organic solvents as well as lithium, red phosphorus, or iodine, depending on the method of synthesis. The older amalgam method started with phenylacetic acetic to generate phenyl-2-propanone. Lead acetate was used in one of the first steps. Methylamine and mercuric chloride were used in the second step to generate methamphetamine.[8] This method may result in mercury and lead contamination at the cook site.[9]

Current production methods involve the chemical reduction of ephedrine or pseudoephedrine to produce methamphetamine chloride. There are 3 different processes commonly used to accomplish this reduction. Two of these processes (red phosphorus and hypophosphorous acid) are similar in their use of phosphorus and iodine. The third process is the Birch reduction, or anhydrous ammonia method, commonly found in agricultural communities where anhydrous ammonia is used as a fertilizer. All 3 methodologies utilize hydrogen chloride gas that is typically generated using sulfuric acid and sodium chloride (rock salt) to precipitate methamphetamine hydrochloride. The classes of chemicals used to produce methamphetamine by the above processes and their major adverse effects are listed in Table 49.1.

A complete list of chemicals may be found in the Drug Enforcement Agency's "Guidelines for Law Enforcement for the Cleanup of Clandestine Drug Laboratories."[10] The Drug Enforcement Agency estimates that for every pound of methamphetamine manufactured, 5 to 6 pounds of toxic waste may be generated.

ROUTES OF EXPOSURE

Exposure to methamphetamine, the chemicals used in its production and their by-products is commonly by inhalation or dermal contact. Adolescents may intentionally abuse methamphetamine. Children may also unintentionally ingest methamphetamine manufactured in drug labs.

SOURCES OF EXPOSURE

Children may be exposed through primary or secondary sources, depending on the status of the laboratory. An active or recently active laboratory poses hazards, primarily from inhalation. Once these primary sources are removed, secondary sources include solvent spills and upholstered furniture, drapes, carpet, and wallboard that have absorbed solvent vapors and volatile contaminants. These chemicals may be rereleased during cleanup. Nonvolatile compounds, such as the hydrochloride salt of methamphetamine, are possible

Table 49.1: Chemical Components of Methamphetamine Labs and Risks

CHEMICAL CLASS	ROUTE OF EXPOSURE	ADVERSE EFFECTS
Anhydrous ammonia	Inhalation	Eye, nose, throat irritation, dyspnea, wheezing, chest pain, pulmonary edema
	Dermal	Skin burns, vesiculation, frostbite[11]
Acids and bases	Inhalation	Pneumonitis, pulmonary edema
	Dermal	Caustic burns
	Ingestion	Gastric perforation, esophageal burns with later strictures, nausea, vomiting
Solvents	Inhalation and ingestion	Liver and kidney damage, bone marrow suppression, headache
	Inhalation	Respiratory irritation, central nervous system depression or excitation, aspiration[12]
Iodine	Inhalation	Respiratory distress, mucus membrane irritation[13]
	Ingestion	Corrosive gastritis
Phosphorus	Ingestion	Gastrointestinal tract irritation, liver damage, oliguria
Red phosphorus		Flammable
Potential: phosphine gas	Inhalation	Ocular irritation, nausea, vomiting, fatigue, chest pain, headache, fatal respiratory effects, seizures, coma[14]

skin contaminants.[15] In one study, investigators sampled former clandestine lab sites immediately after entry by law enforcement personnel. Controlled cooks were performed in these inactive labs to simulate exposures during illicit methamphetamine manufacturing and to identify chemicals that were present. Methamphetamine was detected on multiple surfaces, including refrigerators, microwaves, and ceiling fans. Methamphetamine was detected on surfaces after experimental cooks via the anhydrous ammonia,[16] red phosphorus, and hypophosphorous methods. The median methamphetamine particle diameter was <0.1 µm, a respirable size that may penetrate the lungs and the bloodstream. Sequential sampling up to 24 hours after simulated red phosphorus cooks in a 1-story home yielded higher levels of airborne methamphetamine with increasing activity, such as walking and vacuuming. This may represent probable resuspension from contaminated surfaces.[17] Surface iodine was detected after red phosphorus and hypophosphorous cooks. Hydrochloric acid was released during all cook methods, with extraction phase levels close to the "Immediately Dangerous to Life and Health" level of 50 parts per million (ppm) as defined by the US National Institute for Occupational Safety and Health. Ammonia was detected after an experimental anhydrous cook.

Products of passive exposure to methamphetamine were assessed via simulating single and multiple sessions of smoking varying amounts of methamphetamine in a hotel room. Study authors assumed that a person smoking methamphetamine would absorb 67% to 90% of the drug.[18] They found that an average smoke of approximately 100 mg of methamphetamine results in airborne methamphetamine concentrations from 37 to 123 $\mu g/m^3$. These will likely result in surface deposition levels in the vicinity of the smoke approaching 0.07 $\mu g/100\ cm^2$. As more smoking occurs, levels may exceed 5 $\mu g/100\ cm^2$.

These studies highlight the risk of exposure to methamphetamine or other chemicals during and after an active cook, passive smoking, or inhabiting a former cook site.

SYSTEMS AFFECTED

The lungs, central nervous system, and skin are most affected.

CLINICAL EFFECTS

Acute Effects

The most significant health risk related to methamphetamine production is acute injury secondary to massive chemical exposure via inhalation and contact with the skin and eyes. Thus, when a clandestine lab is raided, the team members wear special protective gear, including a self-contained breathing apparatus and chemical-resistant suits, gloves, and boots. The majority of exposures reported from clandestine lab incidents were from inhalation. These were reported in adult first responders who were not wearing proper personal protective equipment, such as respirators.[3,19] Data specific for children's exposures via inhalation and dermal contact are very limited.

Pediatric exposures result primarily from acute poisoning from unintentional ("accidental") methamphetamine ingestions. Children generally presented to an emergency department or were reported to a poison control center. Diagnosis was usually made after the results of toxicologic analyses were known. Central nervous and cardiovascular system effects predominated. In the larger case series, the most common presenting symptom was agitation. Eighty-two percent of a series[20] of children younger than 6 years reported to the California Poison Control Center and 50% of another[21] series of children younger than 13 years brought to an urban emergency department presented with agitation. Eighty-nine percent of a series of patients with an average age of 19 months presented

Table 49.2: Reported Signs and Symptoms of Acute Methamphetamine Ingestion in Children[6,20-26]	
SYSTEM	**FINDINGS**
Central nervous: mental status	Irritability Agitation Inconsolability with and without crying Hyperactivity Delirium
Central nervous: movement	Ataxia Constant movement Seizure Flailing movements of head, neck, and extremities Involuntary side-to-side head turning
Ocular	Roving eye movements Cortical blindness
Central and peripheral nervous	Hyperthermia
Cardiovascular	Tachycardia Hypertension Myocarditis
Gastrointestinal tract	Vomiting Esophagitis
Respiratory tract	Respiratory distress Hypoxia
Musculoskeletal	Rhabdomyolysis
Cutaneous/orofacial	Burns of lips, tongue
Metabolic	Decreased serum bicarbonate Hyperkalemia, Hepatic and renal failure

with crying.[27] Other central nervous system findings included irritability, seizures, or abnormal movements. Cardiovascular findings were tachycardia and hypertension. Other organ systems may be affected (Table 49.2). One 14-year-old patient developed multisystem organ failure and secondary hyperthermia after intentional abuse of methamphetamine.[22]

Chronic Exposure

Only data on chronic adult users are available. Chronic methamphetamine abusers may exhibit anxiety, confusion, insomnia, mood disturbances, and violent behavior. They may display psychotic features such as paranoia, visual and auditory hallucinations, and delusions such as the sensation of insects crawling under their skin. Repetitive motor activity, weight loss, and severe dental problems may occur.[28] Choreoathetoid movement disorders, acute and chronic cardiomyopathy, acute aortic dissections, arterial aneurysms, pulmonary hypertension, hepatocellular damage, and acute renal failure have been reported.[29] No data are available about the health risks of longer-term exposures in children living in currently or previously contaminated home settings.

MANAGEMENT OF CHILDREN EXPOSED TO METHAMPHETAMINE LABS

Children removed from methamphetamine labs require comprehensive medical, social work, developmental, and psychological evaluations. An evaluation for abuse includes attention to possible physical, sexual, and emotional abuse. An evaluation for neglect includes assessing their medical, dental, and educational needs as well as basic needs for food, clothing, and shelter.

The National Alliance for Drug Endangered Children, established in 2000, authored the national protocol for the medical evaluation of children found in drug labs, along with reference fact sheets (available at www.nationaldec.org).[30] Management of these children involves decontamination, medical evaluation, and toxicologic evaluation.

Decontamination

Full decontamination according to standard protocols is indicated (if the child is medically stable) where there has been significant chemical exposure, such as in an explosion or fire. Basic life support measures take precedence over decontamination. Rescuers should take measures to avoid injury to themselves. In cases with significant chemical exposure (as evidenced by a chemical smell on the person or by clothes with chemical stains), the child should have the chemicals removed at the scene by removing clothes. These clothes are then given to law enforcement agents. The child should be cleansed with running water and soap when this can be done without causing trauma. An asymptomatic child who is removed from a laboratory and has no signs of obvious chemical contamination is unlikely to present a significant danger to other individuals. It is suggested that the child's clothing be removed as soon as is reasonably safe. Although it is unlikely that significant amounts of methamphetamine or other chemicals will be transferred from clothing, a cloth placed over vehicle seats may be used for further protection. Toys and objects should be left at the home.[31]

Medical Evaluation

A child must be transported to the closest emergency department if there has been an explosion at the lab site or if the child has respiratory distress, burns, lethargy, or somnolence. Decontamination may be required on-site or during transportation. The emergent evaluation suggested by the National Alliance for

Drug Endangered Children national protocol focuses on the child's respiratory and neurologic status along with the usual assess-ments of temperature, blood pressure, respirations, and pulse.

Toxicologic Evaluation

The authority over drug laboratory and federal drug testing programs resides with the Division of Workplace Programs in the Substance Abuse and Mental Health Services Administration (SAMSHA), a division of the US Department of Health and Human Services.

Examination of the urine is the preferred method to detect acute exposure to methamphetamine. It is best obtained within 8 to 12 hours of removal from the laboratory site. The commonly used initial screening test for amphetamines (methamphetamine and amphetamine) is an immunoassay with a commonly used federal workplace cutoff of 1000 nanograms (ng)/mL that was lowered by SAMSHA to 500 ng/mL in 2010.

This may not detect small concentrations found in children, and thus, the referring laboratory should be informed of the pediatric source of the specimen. If the amount detected is above the cutoff, then confirmation by gas chromatography-mass spectrometry is indicated and should be requested. False-negative and false-positive results may occur. Isomer resolution by further toxicologic analysis can distinguish between the l–isomer and the d–isomer more commonly found in illicit preparations.[32]

TREATMENT OF ACUTE METHAMPHETAMINE TOXICITY

Because there is no antidote for methamphetamine, treatment of methamphetamine toxicity in children is based on symptoms and should be managed in consultation with a pediatric toxicologist or poison control center. Agitation in pediatric patients hospitalized in an intensive care unit was successfully treated with parenteral benzodiazepines, alone or in combination with haloperidol.[27] A monitored setting was recommended, as haloperidol has been associated with prolongation of the QT interval. Haloperidol was not recommended if children had seizures.

REMEDIATION

Methamphetamine residues may be found at former makeshift lab sites and may pose risks to future residents. Remediation standards are usually legislated, and vary by state. Several state regulations regarding methamphetamine contamination of residences are based on the detection limit of methamphetamine. The State of Colorado assessed several states' technology-based cleanup standards for their health-protectiveness,[9] and then selected 0.5 mg /100 cm^2 as the final clean-up standard for methamphetamine residues. California published

2 research papers addressing remediation. The first attempted to identify a subchronic daily reference dose of methamphetamine. The subchronic daily reference dose is an estimate of daily exposure for a subchronic duration (up to 10% of a lifespan) that will not have deleterious effects in the general population, including sensitive subpopulations such as children, during a lifetime (http://www.epa.gov/IRIS/help_gloss.htm#s). Methodology detailed in the paper results in a subchronic daily reference dose of 0.3 µg/kg/day.[33] The second paper[15] uses the daily reference dose established in the first to suggest a risk-based cleanup standard of 1.5 µg/100 cm². The State of Washington Department of Health has information about remediation available (www.doh.wa.gov/ehp/ts/CDL). At the federal level, the Methamphetamine Remediation Research Act of 2007, Pub L No. 110-143, provides for establishing voluntary guidelines based on scientific knowledge for the remediation of former methamphetamine laboratories. The Act also addresses the need for research on the effects of methamphetamine on former residents, particularly children.

REGULATION

The Controlled Substance Act of 1970 regulated the manufacture of methamphetamine, restricting its availability. The Federal Chemical Diversion and Trafficking Act of 1988 placed phenyl-2-propanone and other chemicals on the controlled-substance list, making it more difficult to obtain precursors for the phenyl-2-propanone method. The National Methamphetamine Drug Assessment of 2008 noted that domestic production of methamphetamine decreased dramatically since 2004. In April 2004, Oklahoma enacted House Bill 2167 regulating the sale of pseudoephedrine; other states followed suit. In September 2006, the federal Combat Methamphetamine Epidemic Act of 2005 took effect. Provisions include limiting, in grams, the retail sale of pseudoephedrine, ephedrine, and phenylpropanolamine; specifying placement of these compounds behind the counter; and establishing the recording of sales in logbooks. Individual states have added requirements such as a prescription requirement for pseudoephedrine products. These actions, along with sustained law enforcement pressure, have decreased domestic methamphetamine production. However, 5080 methamphetamine clandestine laboratory incidents were still reported in 2007.[34]

Children removed from methamphetamine labs or from parents who are chronic users of methamphetamine are victims of child abuse and/or neglect. Several states have established their own Alliances for Drug Endangered Children (www.nationaldec.org/statesites.html). Pediatricians can provide a medical home for these children and help to coordinate and advocate for services needed.

Frequently Asked Questions

Q *What are the long-term effects when children live in a methamphetamine manufacturing environment?*

A There is no long-term information available. Neglect by caregivers appears to be the primary concern, and a complete developmental assessment would be indicated.

Q *How can I find out if the home I moved into was a former clandestine laboratory?*

A The Drug Enforcement Administration maintains a list of former clandestine laboratories that can be accessed at http://www.usdoj.gov/dea/seizures/index.html.

Q *What should I do to have my children evaluated if I find my home was a former site?*

A A comprehensive pediatric health assessment is indicated. Referrals to specialists are based on symptoms. Local agencies should be contacted to verify that proper remediation was completed.

Resources For Professionals

New York State Department of Health
Web site: www.nyhealth.gov/diseases/aids/harm_reduction/crystalmeth/docs/meth_literature_index.pdf.
Ongoing comprehensive site for methamphetamine literature references.

Drug Enforcement Agency: Guidelines for Law Enforcement for the Cleanup of Clandestine Drug Laboratories
Web site: www.usdoj.gov/dea/resources/redbook.pdf

Legislation
National Alliance for Model State Drug Laws (NAMSDL)
Web site: www.namsdl.org

Decontamination
National Jewish Research and Medical Center
Web site: http://health.utah.gov/meth/html/decontamination/AdditionalResources.html

Resources For Parents

National Alliance for Drug Endangered Children
Web site: www.nationaldec.org
Parents can contact them directly with questions. Frequently asked questions can also be accessed at www.nationaldec.org/resourcecenter/faqs.html.

References

1. Beebe K, Walley W. Smokable methamphetamine ("ice"): an old drug in a different form. *Am Fam Physician*. 1995;51:449-453

2. United States Department of Justice, National Drug Intelligence Center. *Methamphetamine Drug Threat Assessment*. Johnstown, PA: US Department of Justice; March 2005. Document ID No. 2005-Q0317-009

3. Burgess JL, Barnhart S, Checkowar H. Investigating Clandestine Drug Laboratories: Adverse Medical Effects in Law Enforcement Personnel. *Am J Ind Med*. 1996;30(4):488-494

4. Rawson RA, Gonzalez RG, Brethen P. Methamphetamine: current research findings and clinical challenges. *J Subst Abuse Treat*. 2002;23(2):145-150

5. Sadock BJ, Sadock V, eds. Kaplan and Sadock's Comprehensive Textbook of Psychiatry. 8th ed. Philadelphia, PA: Lippincott Williams and Wilkins; 2005:1191-1192

6. Ruha AM, Yarema M. Pharmacologic treatment of acute pediatric methamphetamine toxicity. *Pediatr Emerg Care*. 2006;22(12):782-785

7. Huestis MA, Cone EJ. Methamphetamine disposition in oral fluid, plasma, and urine. *Ann N Y Acad Sci*. 2007;1098:104-121

8. Burgess JL, Chandler D. Clandestine drug laboratories. In: Greenburg MI, ed. *Occupational, Industrial and Environmental Toxicology*. 2nd ed. Philadelphia, PA: Mosby Inc; 2003:746-764

9. Hammon TL, Griffin S. Support for selection of a methamphetamine cleanup standard in Colorado. *Regul Toxicol Pharmacol*. 2007;48(1):102-114

10. US Drug Enforcement Administration. *Guidelines for Law Enforcement for the Cleanup of Clandestine Drug Laboratories*. Washington, DC: US Drug Enforcement Administration; 2005. Available at: www.usdoj.gov/dea/resources/redbook.pdf. Accessed October 13, 2010

11. Centers for Disease Control and Prevention. Anhydrous ammonia thefts and releases associated with illicit methamphetamine production 16 states, January 2000-June 2004. *MMWR Morb Mortal Wkly Rep*. 2005;54(14):359-361

12. Amdur MO, Klassen CD, Doull J, Casarett LJ, eds. *Casarett and Doull's Toxicology: The Basic Science of Poisons*. 4th ed. New York, NY: Pergammon Press; 1991

13. Oishi, SM, West KM, Stuntz S. *Drug Endangered Children Health and Safety Manual*. Los Angeles, CA: The Drug Endangered Children Resource Center; 2000

14. Lineberry TW, Bostwick JM. Methamphetamine abuse: a perfect storm of complications. *Mayo Clin Proc*. 2006;81(1):77-84

15. Salocks CB. *Assessment of Children's Exposure to Surface Methamphetamine Residues in Former Clandestine Methamphetamine Labs, and Identification of a Risk-Based Cleanup Standard for Surface Methamphetamine Contamination*. Sacramento, CA: California Environmental Protection Agency; 2009. Available at: http://www.oehha.ca.gov/public_info/public/kids/pdf/ExposureAnalysis022709.pdf. Accessed October 13, 2010

16. Martyny JW, Arbuckle SL, McCammon CS Jr, et al. Chemical exposures associated with clandestine methamphetamine laboratories. *J Chem Health Safety*. 2007;14(4):40-52

17. VanDyke M, Erb N, Arbuckle S, Martyny J. A 24-hour study to investigate persistent chemical exposures associated with clandestine methamphetamine laboratories. *J Occup Environ Hyg*. 2009;6(2):82-89

18. Martyny J, Arbuckle SL, McCammon CS, Erb N, Van Dyke M. Methamphetamine contamination on environmental surfaces caused by simulated smoking of methamphetamine. *J Chem Health Safety*. 2008; 15(5):25-31

19. Witter RZ, Martyny JW, Mueller K, Gottschall B, Newman LS. Symptoms experienced by law enforcement personnel during methamphetamine lab investigations. *J Occup Environ Hyg*. 2007;4(12):895-902

20. Matteucci MJ, Auten JD, Crowley B, Combs D, Clark RF. Methamphetamine exposures in young children. *Pediatr Emerg Care.* 2007;23(9):638-640

21. Kolecki P. Inadvertent methamphetamine poisoning in pediatric patients. *Pediatr Emerg Care.* 1998;14(6):385-387

22. Prosser JM, Naim M, Helfaer M. A 14 year old girl with agitation and hyperthermia. *Pediatr Emerg Care.* 2006;22(9):676-679

23. Gospe SM Jr. Transient cortical blindness in an infant exposed to methamphetamine. *Ann Emerg Med.* 1995;26(3):380-382

24. Nagorka AR, Bergensen PS. Infant methamphetamine toxicity posing as scorpion envenomation. *Pediatr Emerg Care.* 1998;14(5):350-351

25. Farst K. Methamphetamine exposure presenting as caustic ingestions in children. *Ann Emerg Med.* 2007;49(3):341-343

26. Horton KD, Berkowitz Z, Kaye W. The acute health consequences to children exposed to hazardous substances used in illicit methamphetamine production, 1996 to 2000. *J Child Health.* 2003;1:99-108

27. Ruha AM, Yarema M. Pharmacologic treatment of acute pediatric methamphetamine toxicity. *Pediatr Emerg Care.* 2006;22(12):782-785

28. National Institute on Drug Abuse. Research Report Series: *Methamphetamine Abuse and Addiction.* Bethesda, MD: National Institute on Drug Abuse; April 1998; Reprinted January 2002; Revised September 2006. NIH Publication No. 06-4210

29. Albertson TE, Derlet RW, Van Hoozen BE. Methamphetamine and the expanding complications of amphetamines. *West J Med.* 1999;170(4):214-219

30. National Alliance for Drug Endangered Children. *National Guidelines for Medical Evaluation of Children Found in Drug Labs.* Available at: http://www.nationaldec.org/goopages/pages_downloadgallery/download.php?filename=13258.pdf&orig_name=40.pdf. Accessed October 13, 2010

31. National Alliance for Drug Endangered Children. *Guidelines for Methamphetamine January 2006.* Available at: http://www.nationaldec.org/goopages/pages_downloadgallery/download.php?filename=9250.pdf&orig_name=6.pdf. Accessed October 13, 2010

32. Dasgupta A, ed. *Critical Issues in Alcohol and Drugs of Abuse Testing.* Washington, DC: American Association for Clinical Chemistry Press; 2009

33. Salocks C. Development of a Reference Does (RfD) for Methamphetamine. Sacramento, CA: California Environmental Protection Agency, Office of Environmental Health Hazard Assessment, Integrated Risk Assessment Branch; 2007. Available at: http://www.oehha.ca.gov/public_info/public/kids/meth022609.html. Accessed October 13, 2010

34. National Seizure System. Total of all meth clandestine laboratory incidents. Available at: www.usdoj.gov/dea/concern/map_lab_seizures_2007p.html. Accessed October 13, 2010

Chapter 50

Emerging Technologies and Materials

■ ■ ■ ■ ■ ■

Emerging technologies, new chemicals, and novel discoveries have shaped and reshaped the lives of children. Ongoing discoveries create new industries or reshape existing ones. Automobiles and commercial aviation revolutionized transport. Refrigeration has brought fresh fruits in winter. New building materials and motor fuels have made possible modern cities and their suburbs. Breakthroughs in microelectronics and physics produced desktop computing and the Internet. Continuing advances in information and communication technology, biotechnology, and nanotechnology are rapidly changing methods of social interaction, medical treatments, and data evaluation strategies.

Some technologies have profoundly benefited children's health. For example, vaccines and antibiotics have helped control major communicable diseases and chemotherapeutic agents have made possible the cure of many childhood cancers. Emerging technologies also have, however, been responsible for disease, death, and environmental degradation. Many of these episodes have resulted in severe injury to children. Two sequences of events mark many of these tragedies and continue today to powerfully shape the context of pediatric environmental health: (1) the enthusiastic introduction and wide dissemination of many thousands of new technologies, new chemicals, and new products; and subsequently (2) the belated discovery that some of these apparently beneficial technologies pose threats to children's health and the environment that were neither imagined nor in any way sought before their introduction.

Classic examples of technologies, chemicals, and medications initially hailed as beneficial but later found to cause great harm include the addition of lead

Table 50.1: Production Volumes of Newer Synthetic Chemicals	
CHEMICAL	**ANNUAL PRODUCTION, POUNDS (YEAR)**
Bisphenol A	2.3 billion (2004)
Diethylhexyl phthalate	200 million (2002)
Brominated flame retardants	118.9 million (2001)
Perfluorinated compounds	4 million (2000)

to paint and later to gasoline (Chapter 29), asbestos (Chapter 23), dichloro-diphenyltrichloroethane (DDT) (Chapter 35), thalidomide, polychlorinated biphenyls (PCBs) (Chapter 35), diethylstilbestrol (DES) (Chapter 44), and the ozone-destroying chlorofluorocarbons (CFCs). A recurrent theme in each of these examples was that commercial introduction and wide dissemination of the new technology, chemical, or medication preceded any systematic effort to assess potential toxicity.

Examples of more recent chemicals that became widespread before any assessment of their potential hazards and that are now of substantial concern include bisphenol A (Chapter 38), phthalates (Chapter 38), brominated flame retardants, and perfluorinated compounds. All of these materials are produced in extremely high volumes (Table 50.1) and are used in myriad consumer products and widespread in children's environments. Only now, decades after their introduction, are their possible hazards to children's health beginning to be assessed.

Early warnings that emerging technologies might pose hazards to children's health and the environment have frequently been ignored. As a result, efforts to control exposures and to prevent injuries to children have often been delayed, sometimes for decades.[1] In some instances, industries with deeply vested commercial interests in protecting markets for hazardous technologies have actively opposed efforts to understand and control children's exposures to these materials. These industries have used highly sophisticated disinformation campaigns to confuse the public, and they have directly attacked heroic pediatricians and environmental scientists who called attention to the risks of emerging technologies. Such has been the case with lead, mercury, and tobacco and is happening today with chlorinated solvents and organophosphate pesticides.[2]

The pace of scientific discovery in the past 50 years has been more rapid than in any previous time in human history. This age of scientific discovery has resulted in the emergence of hundreds of new technologies, the synthesis of tens of thousands of new chemicals, and the release into the environment of millions of new products.

Chemical production has increased drastically in the past half century (Fig 50.1). Today, there are more than 80 000 chemicals registered for commercial use with the US Environmental Protection Agency (EPA). Most of these chemicals are new synthetics, and nearly all have been invented in the past 50 years. They did not exist previously in nature.[3]

Children are most at risk of exposure to the 3000 synthetic chemicals produced in quantities of more than 1 million pounds per year. The EPA classifies these materials as high-production-volume (HPV) chemicals. High-production-volume chemicals are widespread in the modern environment. They are found in a great array of consumer goods, cosmetics, medications, motor fuels, and building materials. They are detectable in much of the United States in air, food, and drinking water.

Measurable quantities of several hundred high-production-volume chemicals are routinely found in the blood and urine of virtually all Americans.[4] Elevated concentrations of high-production-volume chemicals are seen also in the milk of nursing mothers and the cord blood of newborn infants.[5]

REGULATORY STRATEGY

In the United States, emerging technologies generally are not subject to premarket evaluations of potential toxicity before their introduction to commerce. Thus,

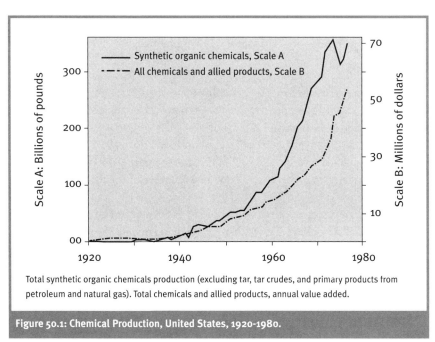

Total synthetic organic chemicals production (excluding tar, tar crudes, and primary products from petroleum and natural gas). Total chemicals and allied products, annual value added.

Figure 50.1: Chemical Production, United States, 1920-1980.

Reprinted with permission from Davis DL, Magee BH. Cancer and industrial chemical production. *Science.* 1979;206(4425):1356, 1358

information on potential toxicity is publicly available for only about half of the 3000 high-production-volume chemicals, and information on developmental toxicity or capacity to harm infants and children is available for fewer than 20% of high-production-volume chemicals.[3] Failure to test technologies for potential toxicity puts children at risk daily of exposure to technologies whose potential for hazard is virtually unknown.

The Toxic Substances Control Act (TSCA) was intended, at the time of its passage in 1976, to be pioneering legislation that would require premarket evaluation of all new chemicals for potential toxicity. The Toxic Substances Control Act was also intended to require retroactive testing of industrial chemicals already in commerce. However, the Toxic Substances Control Act never fulfilled these intentions, because the law did not provide EPA with a means to obtain sufficient information on the safety or health effects of chemicals as is needed to establish appropriate regulation. Therefore, existing technologies are presumed to be safe and emerging technologies and new materials may be released and presumed to be safe due to a paucity of available information.[6] The US EPA has published a list of principles for reform of chemicals management legislation.[7]

EMERGING TECHNOLOGIES OF CURRENT INTEREST: TWO CASE STUDIES

Two technologies currently in early stages of commercial introduction—nanotechnology and methylcyclopentadienyl manganese tricarbonyl (MMT) used as a fuel additive—illustrate the strengths and weaknesses of current efforts to address the potential hazards of emerging technologies.

Nanotechnology

Nanotechnology is a novel, rapidly emerging technology based on the precisely engineered assembly of atoms and molecules to produce nanoparticles, nanotubules, and a wide array of molecular-scale nanodevices, such as pumps and switches. A nanometer (nm) is one-billionth of a meter. By definition, a nanomaterial must have at least one dimension measuring 100 nm or less. Nanomaterials are, therefore, of the same size range as virus particles, DNA, and protein molecules.

Worldwide investment in nanotechnology has exploded and in 2008 was reported to total $8 billion. Approximately 400 nanotechnology-based consumer products—cosmetics, inorganic sunscreens (zinc oxide and titanium dioxide), pharmaceuticals, electronics, and fuel cells—have already been introduced to the market.[8]

Nanomaterials have extraordinarily high surface-to-volume ratios and unique chemical and physical properties. These characteristics raise the possibility that nanomaterials may interact with cells and organisms in novel ways quite different from those of their parent materials. Carbon nanotubules, for example, appear to be far more hazardous than the graphite from which they are manufactured.[9]

Knowledge of the potential toxicity of nanomaterials is scant. Knowledge of their possible toxicity to early human development is virtually nil. Hints of potential toxicity are, however, beginning to emerge and are cause for concern.[10] Emerging data suggest, for example, that nanoparticles may be able to produce toxic effects as a consequence of their ability to enter cells. Small size enhances cell entry and appears to be a major determinant of toxicity. Once within cells, nanoparticles appear to be able to cause injury through several mechanisms, among them oxidative stress, lipid peroxidation, and protein misfolding. Protein misfolding is of concern, because it is associated with neuronal degeneration and with degeneration of insulin-producing beta cells in the pancreas. Nanotubules, by contrast, because they are predominantly fibrous, do not enter cells, but instead remain in the extracellular spaces, where they can induce chronic inflammation. In a recent pilot study in mice, carbon nanotubules produced pathogenic effects similar to those caused by asbestos.[9]

This information suggests the need to exercise considerable caution in adopting nanotechnology and in introducing nanomaterials into the environment. Several expert advisory groups have called for prudent assessment of the potential hazards of nanotechnology before further dissemination.[8]

Methylcyclopentadienyl manganese tricarbonyl

MMT is an organic compound of manganese proposed for use as a fuel additive to replace tetraethyl lead. MMT is added to gasoline to enhance octane. The manufacturer of MMT is aggressively pressing for its adoption in nations worldwide. Use of MMT in the United States, although not legally banned, has, to date, been minimal. Since 1976, Canada has used MMT in gasoline, and attempts by the Canadian government to restrict MMT use, prompted by perceived harm to pollution-control devices, failed under free-trade agreement law.[11] Premarket toxicity testing of MMT has been scant.

Concern has arisen about the potential of MMT to cause neurotoxicity. In occupationally exposed adults, manganese is a known cause of parkinsonism.[12] Prenatal exposures to manganese in drinking water have been associated with delayed attainment of milestones and neurodevelopmental neurotoxicity in children.[13] The potential consequences of population-wide exposure to manganese emitted into the environment through combustion of MMT in motor fuels are little studied and poorly understood. Information is especially lacking on potential consequences of MMT exposure in pregnant women and young children.

In light of the growing evidence that MMT may pose threats to human health and the environment, the International Commission on Occupational Health (ICOH) and the Collegium Ramazzini, 2 international, nongovernmental bodies, have urged that addition of MMT to gasoline be halted in all nations pending further assessment of potential hazard.[14] This call for a ban on MMT was specifically intended to prevent a recurrence of the worldwide tragedy of tetraethyl lead (Chapter 31). This recommendation has already persuaded several countries, most notably China, to postpone adoption of MMT.

As these case studies illustrate, the introduction of new technologies is accompanied by a host of important health-related questions. Under current US regulations, society has borne much of the costs of evaluating chemical safety, cleaning up hazards created by chemicals, and supporting people who have been injured. A shift to industry bearing the responsibility to determine whether their chemical or material is safe before marketing is needed. The strategy to demonstrate lack of harm (or that benefits outweigh harms) before marketing is termed the "Precautionary Principle" (see Chapter 57). The Precautionary Principle has recently been introduced into national and international law.[15] The MMT case study exemplifies an application of the Precautionary Principle.

In 2007, the European Union began implementation of a new chemical regulatory system termed REACH (Registration, Evaluation, Authorization and Restriction of Chemical substances). REACH places responsibility on industry to evaluate and manage chemical risks and provide safety information on the substance before it can be marketed. This information is placed in a central database managed by the European Chemicals Agency, and further testing, regulation, and enforcement of regulations of suspicious chemicals is managed by the European Chemicals Agency as well. The extent of required testing depends on the volume of chemical production; high-volume chemicals intended for consumer products will require closer scrutiny than low-volume materials. Successful implementation of the European REACH regulations holds promise that chemicals with unacceptable risks will be withheld from introduction and that strategies to reduce harms from other chemicals will be developed and applied to protect societal and individual health.

Resources

Technology Review published by Massachusetts Institute of Technology (www.technologyreview.com). Reviews emerging communications, biomedical, energy, and materials technologies.

References

1. Gee D. Late lessons from early warnings: toward realism and precaution with endocrine-disrupting substances. *Environ Health Perspect.* 2006;114(S-1):152–160
2. Michaels D. *Doubt Is Their Product: How Industry's Assault on Science Threatens Your Health.* London, England: Oxford University Press; 2008
3. Goldman LR. Chemicals and children's environment: what we don't know about risks. *Environ Health Perspect.* 1998;106(Suppl 3):875–880

4. Centers for Disease Control and Prevention. *Fourth National Report on Human Exposure to Environmental Chemicals.* Atlanta, GA: Centers for Disease Control and Prevention; 2009. Available at: http://www.cdc.gov/exposurereport. Accessed October 14, 2010

5. Environmental Working Group. *Body Burden—The Pollution in Newborns. A Benchmark Investigation of Industrial Chemicals, Pollutants and Pesticides in Umbilical Cord Blood.* Washington, DC. Environmental Working Group; 2005

6. American Academy of Pediatrics, Council on Environmental Health. Chemical-management policy: prioritizing children's health. *Pediatrics.* 2011;127(5):983-990

7. US Environmental Protection Agency. Essential Principles for Reform of Chemicals Management Legislation. Washington, DC: Environmental Protection Agency; 2009. Available at: http://www.epa.gov/oppt/existingchemicals/pubs/principles.html. Accessed March 12, 2011

8. Balbus JM, Maynard AD, Colvin VL, et al. Meeting report: hazard assessment for nanoparticles—report from an interdisciplinary workshop. *Environ Health Perspect.* 2007;115(11):1664-1659

9. Poland CA, Duffin R, Kinloch I, et al. Carbon nanotubes introduced into the abdominal cavity of mice show asbestos-like pathogenicity in a pilot study. *Nature Nanotechnol.* 2008;3(7):423-428

10. Howard CV. The anticipated spectrum of human disease from exposure to novel nanoparticles (abstr). Presented at Ramazzini Days 2008 Conference: New Chemicals, Nanotechnology and Health Protection: Confronting the Challenges of the 21st Century; Carpi, Italy; October 24-26, 2008

11. Walsh MP. The global experience with lead in gasoline and the lessons we should apply to the use of MMT. *Am J Ind Med.* 2007;50(11):853–860

12. Lucchini RG, Albini E, Benedetti L, et al. High prevalence of Parkinsonian disorders associated to manganese exposure in the vicinities of ferroalloy industries. *Am J Ind Med.* 2007;50(11): 788-800

13. Wasserman GA, Liu X, Parvez F, et al. Water manganese exposure and children's intellectual function in Araihazar, Bangladesh. *Environ Health Perspect.* 2006;114(1):124-129

14. Landrigan P, Nordberg M, Lucchini R, et al. International Workshop on Neurotoxic Metals: lead, mercury, and manganese—from research to prevention. The Declaration of Brescia on prevention of the neurotoxicity of metals June 18, 2006. *Am J Ind Med.* 2007;50(10):709-711

15. Grandjean P, Bailar JC, Gee D, et al. Implications of the Precautionary Principle in research and policy-making. *Am J Ind Med.* 2004;45(4):382-385

Chapter 51

Environmental Disasters

■ ■ ■ ■ ■ ■

Environmental health problems can accrue after a number of catastrophic events. Such events can range from natural disasters, such as earthquakes, floods, hurricanes, tornadoes, and wildfires, to human-made disasters, such as the release of methyl isocyanate in Bophal, India, the release of the dioxin 2,3,7,8-tetrachloro-dibenzodioxin in Seveso, Italy, and the release of millions of gallons of crude oil into the Gulf of Mexico in 2010. The terrorist events leading to the destruction of the World Trade Center buildings in September 2001, released a large cloud of toxic materials, resulting in respiratory illnesses in many first responders and people living in the proximity of the disaster. Follow-up investigations of victims, including first responders and children, have revealed evidence of long-term illness as a result of this unprecedented event. Whether intentional or natural, environmental disasters can result in significant morbidity and mortality. As events such as Hurricanes Rita and Katrina, the 2010 earthquake in Haiti, and the 2011 earthquake and subsequent tsunami in Japan have shown, children and adolescents are often disproportionately affected in a disaster.

OVERVIEW OF LOCAL COMMUNITY, STATE AND FEDERAL ROLES DURING RESPONSE

Local communities and states have the largest role in disaster preparedness and response; it is the federal government, however, that funds a significant proportion of preparedness activities and drives requirements for readiness. The National Response Framework, released in 2008, provides guiding principles for response preparation by all response entities and provides a unified national response plan to disasters and emergencies from the smallest incident to the largest catastrophe.[1]

The National Response Framework defines roles and structures of entities involved with response; establishes essential processes for requesting and receiving Federal assistance; and summarizes key capabilities and emergency support functions (see Table 51.1 for terms). The emergency support functions most pertinent to medical response include emergency support function 6, which directs the Federal Emergency Management Agency (FEMA) to lead activities relating to mass care, emergency assistance, and human services; emergency support function 8, which directs the US Department of Health and Human Services to lead the public health and medical response; emergency support function 9, which addresses urban search and rescue activities and is led jointly by the US Department of Homeland Security (including the Federal Emergency Management Agency and the US Coast Guard), the Department of the Interior/National Parks Service, and the Department of Defense/US Air Force; and emergency support function 10, which directs the US Environmental Protection Agency (EPA) to coordinate, integrate, and manage the overall federal effort to detect, identify, contain, decontaminate, clean up, dispose of, or minimize discharges of oil or releases of hazardous materials or prevent, mitigate, or minimize the threat of potential releases. There is nothing in the National Response Framework that specifically addresses the needs of children, pregnant women, or families with children.

Because of the many similarities between terrorist events and natural disasters, the principle of the "all-hazards approach" has become the foundation of response to either type of incident. In this approach, public health and emergency management authorities responsible for developing disaster response protocols develop and implement guidelines that can be adapted to human-made disasters, terrorist incidents (which are exceedingly rare in the United States) or natural disasters, which are inevitable. The development of adaptable and scalable systems promotes efficiency, reduces costs, and may eliminate system redundancy. The basis of the all-hazards approach is found in the Incident Command System (and its hospital counterpart, the Hospital Incident Command System). The Incident Command System, initially created in the 1970s to improve response to natural disasters, such as fires, has gone on to become the unifying mechanism for disaster response. The Incident Command System is based on the principle that with disasters of any type, there should be a fixed response mechanism, fixed roles, and a common terminology. The Incident Command System has been adapted around the world. All individuals (including first responders, hospital workers, and volunteers) who might be called on to respond to a disaster are advised to obtain Incident Command System training to respond more effectively during a disaster (see Resources).[2]

Response to disasters begins locally. When a disaster strikes, it is first responders who arrive on the scene to provide an initial assessment to local

Table 51.1: Terminology		
ENTITY	**ACRONYM**	**RESPONSIBILITY**
National Response Framework	NRF	Provides guiding principles for response preparation by all response entities and provides a unified national response plan
Federal Emergency Management Agency	FEMA	Part of Department of Homeland Security, leads activities relating to mass care, emergency assistance, and human services
Incident Command System	ICS	This is an organizational framework that guides the application of on-scene disaster management
Hospital Incident Command System	HICS	An incident command system designed for use by hospitals in emergency and nonemergency situations
Disaster Medical Assistance Teams	DMAT	A team of professionals and paraprofessionals organized to provide rapid-response medical services during a disaster
■ Homeland Security Grants Program ■ Urban Areas Security Initiative ■ Metropolitan Medical Response System ■ National Healthcare Preparedness Program	 UASI MMRS	Grants programs to areas for hazard planning and preparedness

officials. Such assessments focus on the extent of the incident, the numbers of casualties, anticipated numbers of casualties, property damage, and resources needed to treat and transport victims. Medical issues are addressed by local emergency medical services, local health care facilities and providers, and local public health agencies. The local government sets up an emergency operations center and determines whether the incident exceeds or is expected to exceed local capabilities. For incidents beyond local capacity, local officials can request aid from other local governments within the state and from the state government. The Stafford Act provides for federal support of local communities during major disasters. Local communities are responsible for ensuring that any planning or preparation done in anticipation of a disaster response include consideration of the needs of children and families.[3]

The state governor is responsible for activating the state emergency operations center; the state emergency operations center assesses the extent of the damage and the scope of casualties to determine whether response needs have exceeded state capabilities. If so, the governor then requests aid through the Emergency Management Assistance Compact or through other interstate agreements. The governor can request a presidential declaration, and if the event is anticipated, such as with a hurricane, the federal government can predeploy response assets to the expected disaster area. National-level activities are coordinated by the Federal Emergency Management Agency, a part of the Department of Health and Human Services. When the president declares an emergency or disaster, federal response teams and other resources are deployed, and a joint field office is set up to provide unified coordination of response resources. The EPA, for example, may be requested to assess and advise on possible exposures to toxic contaminants. A federal medical asset available to an affected area includes the disaster medical assistance teams of the National Medical Disaster System, which also includes plans and processes for moving patients between facilities. These teams are limited, however, by the amount of time for deployment and set-up as well as the number of teams available. Although most disaster medical assistance teams may not have been provided with specific training in the care or transportation of children,[4] there are currently 2 pediatric-specific teams, and the American Academy of Pediatrics (AAP) is working with the National Medical Disaster System to determine a mechanism for pediatric training.

Before a disaster, the federal government supports a number of state and local preparedness activities. The federal government provides financial resources through grant programs, such as the Homeland Security Grants Program, Urban Areas Security Initiative, Metropolitan Medical Response System, and the National Healthcare Preparedness Program. Through grant programs, the federal government sets requirements and promotes best practices. The federal government also provides guidance to states and territories for disaster preparedness and response activities and funds research on medical countermeasure development, development of detection and response technologies, and best practices. The federal government also stockpiles medications, equipment, and supplies to supplement state and local caches.[4] These stockpiles should, but often do not, have adequate resources for children.

THE DISASTER CYCLE

Although all disasters are unique because of differences in notice, severity, location, socioeconomic conditions, and baseline health of the affected population, there are patterns to all disasters that can be described in a disaster cycle model. The disaster cycle occurs in phases. The "interdisaster period" occurs between disasters. The "prodromal" period occurs when a disaster is imminent (eg, hurricane in the Gulf of Mexico). For some disasters, however, there is no warning (eg, an earthquake) but only an "impact," which varies in length of time depending on the incident. The phase after impact is the "rescue" phase, during which the actions of first responders are most critical to saving lives. It is during the "recovery" phase that coordinated efforts bring the population back to its normal state.[5]

Measures to prevent and prepare for disasters occur during the interdisaster phase. Such measures may include moving people from the vicinity of an active volcano or from areas known to be susceptible to severe flooding. Mitigation measures that aim to reduce the likely impact of a disaster can also occur during this period as well as during other phases. Examples of mitigation measures include applying stringent building codes in earthquake-prone areas, augmenting levees in flood zones, and instituting warning systems for tsunamis.[6]

Successful response depends on adequate training of first responders, prompt institution of incident command, and effective coordination between emergency services, public health authorities, and the health care system. All disasters remain local in scope until the local community becomes overwhelmed. It is critical that local communities undertake robust planning and preparedness activities during the interdisaster phase of the disaster cycle to mitigate the effects of disasters. Recovery depends on adequate planning, the baseline resiliency of the community, effective coordination of basic services, and the provision of mental health services.

EXAMPLES OF DISASTERS

Tornadoes and Hurricanes

Natural disasters can be somewhat predictable, because they tend to cluster geographically or temporally. For example, certain geographic regions are more susceptible to tornadoes and hurricanes. During spring 2011, multiple tornadoes in the southern United States killed more than 300 people, and in May 2011, a single tornado killed more than 100 people in Missouri. In recent years, the United States and its neighbor nations also suffered the effects of severe hurricanes, including Hurricanes Katrina (2005) and Andrew (1992). Both were devastating to the infrastructure of the affected states and uncovered shortcomings in the nation's capabilities to withstand disasters, including the lack of preparedness for the care of children and adolescents. Many homes were lost after Hurricane Katrina, and occupants of trailers provided by the Federal Emergency Management Agency and used for temporary housing after the hurricane experienced problems with respiratory illness. Levels of formaldehyde were elevated in some of these trailers, raising concerns about exposures to residents.[7] The health care infrastructure experienced severe long-term disruptions. Many school buildings were destroyed or damaged so severely that they could not be reoccupied for long periods. Environmental equity issues arose after the hurricane, because the disaster disproportionately affected the poor, being that the more vulnerable areas within the community were populated by those with less means. As a result of these problems and others, the lives of children and adolescents were disrupted for months to years, with potential effects on their development and mental health. Anticipating these effects and developing mitigation measures before, during, and after disasters are key to preventing similar devastation in the future.

Earthquakes

Earthquakes can be devastating and costly, especially in less wealthy nations that may not have building codes to protect occupants. Mortality can be very high depending on the magnitude and location of the quake. Many children died after the 2008 earthquake in the Sichuan province of China, in part because of a failure to ensure consistent implementation of protective building codes for schools. Earthquakes are a potential problem in many places within the United States, such as California, Idaho, Utah, the Pacific Northwest, and areas in the Midwest. Mitigation measures in earthquake-prone areas include developing and implementing special building codes so that buildings can sustain high forces and remain intact.[8]

Notable earthquakes, such as the 2010 earthquake in Haiti and the 2011 earthquake off the coast of Japan, have killed thousands to hundreds of thousands of people and damaged infrastructure, with economic costs well into the billions of dollars.[2] Rescue efforts are complicated by the danger posed by damage created by the quake, the difficulty in extricating victims, and the time limits to finding victims who are savable. Most of the morbidity and mortality seen in earthquakes results from physical injuries, although this can include secondary wound infections and long-term disability. Additional morbidity and mortality may result from radiation leaks, as occurred after the nuclear power plant in Fukushima, Japan, was damaged.

Floods

Floods are perhaps the most common of natural disasters, accounting for approximately 30% of disasters worldwide. Twenty-five to 50 million Americans live or work in flood plains, and another 110 million live in coastal areas. Flash floods are especially dangerous to people living in flood-prone zones; most deaths attributable to flash floods are caused by drowning. Otherwise, floods are usually not directly associated with loss of life but can cause much destruction and disruption and potentially cause widespread disease, because flood waters often contain human or animal waste. Flood water may also be contaminated with toxic substances that may have been stored in homes and other sites. Failure to promptly remove water-damaged items after floods can lead to growth of mold in buildings and possible respiratory or chronic disease problems.[9,10] Access to clean drinking water is a major concern after a flood; disinfecting drinking water by boiling or chlorination or by providing alternate sources may be needed.[8]

The World Trade Center Disaster

Tens of thousands of children and adolescents living or attending school in or near lower Manhattan were exposed to the World Trade Center disaster. The terrorist attack on the World Trade Center caused combustion of more than 90 000 L of jet fuel at temperatures greater than 1000°C. The resulting atmospheric plume and subsequent collapse of the 2 World Trade Center towers generated thousands of tons of particulate matter containing cement dust, glass fibers, lead, asbestos, polycyclic aromatic hydrocarbons, polychlorinated biphenyls (PCBs), organochlorine pesticides, polychlorinated furans, and dioxins.[11] The majority of studies of World Trade Center-related health effects have been conducted on rescue workers who were often exposed to high levels of debris, dust, fumes, and smoke. These studies show high rates of respiratory and gastrointestinal tract problems and high rates of disability.[12]

The World Trade Center Health Registry, established to evaluate physical and psychological effects of the disaster, collected information on 3184 children who were younger than 18 years on September 11, 2001. Many children, especially those exposed to higher amounts of toxins (such as the dust cloud), experienced respiratory symptoms immediately after the event.[12] Children younger than 5 years had a higher-than-expected prevalence of reported asthma compared with national estimates.[13] A new diagnosis of asthma in all age groups was higher than expected in children exposed to the dust cloud.[13] Follow-up is needed to determine whether the increases in asthma will be sustained. Other commonly reported symptoms among children enrolled in the registry included heartburn, lower respiratory tract symptoms, and sinus problems.[13]

Exposure to the disaster was associated with effects on birth outcomes.[14-16] One study examined 187 pregnant women within or near the World Trade Center on or immediately after the attacks. Compared with a nonexposed group, those acutely exposed experienced a twofold increase in the risk of delivering a small-for-gestational age baby. There were no increases in miscarriages, preterm birth, or low birth weight infants. The authors suggested that the detrimental effects might have been mediated through exposure to polycyclic aromatic hydrocarbons or particulate matter.[14]

Researchers followed a subset of children born to World Trade Center-exposed pregnant women to measure cognitive and motor development using the Bayley-II scales of child development. There was a significant interaction between polycyclic aromatic hydrocarbon-DNA adducts and in utero exposure to secondhand smoke on the mental development index score when the children were 3 years old. Neither adducts alone nor secondhand smoke exposure alone were significant predictors of cognitive development.[17] An adduct is a species formed by the union of 2 species (usually molecules) held together by a covalent bond.

Mental health issues have been identified in children exposed to the World Trade Center disaster. A study of New York City schoolchildren conducted in the first 6 months after the attack found that approximately 1 in 10 children surveyed had symptoms of probable post-traumatic stress disorder (11%), major depressive disorder (8%), separation anxiety disorder (12%), and panic attacks (9%) and that 15% had symptoms of agoraphobia (fear of going out or taking public transportation).[18] Children more likely to experience symptoms were either directly affected by the disaster, had parents who were directly affected, or had previously suffered from post-traumatic stress disorder or depression. Another study of 115 lower Manhattan preschool children found that children who had a history of trauma exposure before the disaster and subsequently experienced trauma related to the World Trade Center attack had an increased risk of significant behavioral problems. These findings suggested that children with prior trauma exposure may be in particular need of mental health services.[19] Specific additional risk factors for psychological morbidity following the attacks of September 11, 2001 included community violence and poverty, feeling less protected by the government, and loss of psychosocial resources.[20]

SPECIAL SUSCEPTIBILITY OF CHILDREN IN DISASTERS

Children have several vulnerabilities during and after disasters. They have specific physical vulnerabilities in disasters because of their size, physiology, and development. Because children are smaller in stature than adults, they may be more vulnerable to injury and drowning in floods and to toxic effects of chemical agents, because many of these are heavier than air and, therefore, exist in higher concentrations closer to the ground. The same is true for radiation exposure in the case of a radiological-nuclear blast event. Children have a larger ratio of skin surface area to body mass compared with adults and, therefore, may absorb more toxicants per unit body mass through their skin. They have a higher respiratory rate, which increases their exposure to aerosolized or gaseous agents. Children are at increased risk of dehydration because of higher fluid needs. Children are often especially susceptible to, and may be reservoirs for, the spread of influenza and other transmissible infections. Because children are immature developmentally, they may not have the motor skills to escape a disaster or the judgment to remove themselves from harm.[21] Children are also more curious about their environment and are, therefore, more likely to touch potentially contaminated surfaces and place objects or their fingers in their mouths.

Children and adolescents may be separated from their caregivers in a disaster. After Hurricanes Rita and Katrina in 2005, more than 5000 children were separated from their parents and guardians. Because of the lack of a well-established system for reunification, some of these pediatric victims were separated from their caregivers for as long as 18 months.[22]

Facilities may not have adequate pediatric equipment to care for neonates, infants, and older children or for children with special needs. Resources may not be allocated with children in mind. These and other consequences of disasters have emphasized the importance of including children and adolescents in disaster planning. Congressional legislation was enacted to ensure that the needs of children and adolescents are met after disasters (eg, the Addressing the Disaster Needs of Children Act of 2007).

THE PSYCHOSOCIAL NEEDS OF CHILDREN AND ADOLESCENTS DURING AND AFTER DISASTERS

The Institute of Medicine released a report in 2006 on the state of emergency care in the United States, which concluded that children and adolescents are among those with the highest risk of psychological trauma, including significant behavioral difficulties, after a disaster.[21] Some of these disorders include: agoraphobia, separation anxiety, conduct disorder, and depression.[23] Risk factors for developing mental health problems include a previous history of mental health issues, direct exposure to the disaster, lower socioeconomic status, loss of a family member, and living with a parent with significant post-traumatic stress reactions.

In the aftermath of a disaster, medical first responders and other health care providers need to provide psychological first aid to children, adolescents, and families. Further, pediatric and other health care providers need to conduct a brief assessment for the presence of adjustment problems and other risk factors for subsequent difficulties to provide rapid and effective triage for mental health issues.[24] The manner in which a child or adolescent reacts to a disaster depends on factors including the nature and extent of the disaster and the child's or adolescent's direct involvement, preexisting vulnerabilities and coping skills, age, and developmental/cognitive level.[25,26]

Common immediate reactions in children after a disaster include[24]:

- Development of fears;
- Development of worries and anxieties;
- Sadness and tearfulness;
- Regressive behavior;
- Social regression;
- Difficulty concentrating and focusing;
- Physical symptoms such as headaches or stomachaches; and
- Exacerbations of underlying disorders (especially stress-induced disorders).

First responders and health care providers have the potential to alleviate some of a child's reactions by initiating psychological first aid, which should be provided broadly to those impacted by the disaster. Psychological first aid is the practice of recognizing and responding to people who have been affected by a disaster to provide help with feelings of stress resulting from their situations.[27]

Immediately after medical stabilization and evaluation, it is recommended that the physician assess the child for adjustment reactions. Psychological first aid includes offering emotional support, providing information and education, encouraging the practice of positive coping, recognizing when more help is needed, and assisting people to get this extra help. It is critical to identify children who are at risk of longer-term mental health issues. Children at higher risk include those who have a family member or friend who has died; who have been exposed to injury, death, or destruction; who have the perception that their life was in jeopardy; who have been separated from parents or other caregivers; who have existing mental health problems; and whose parents have difficulty coping. Children with dissociative symptoms, intense grief, extreme cognitive impairment resulting from the disaster with confusion, impaired decision making, and significant somatization also are at higher risk.[24]

SUMMARY

Children are particularly vulnerable to both physical and psychological harm from disasters. Pediatric health care providers can educate themselves about disaster preparedness and participate in the planning for, and the management and recovery from, disasters.

Frequently Asked Questions

Q   *Where can pediatric clinicians learn more about disaster preparedness and receive training to act locally in the event of a disaster?*

A   The Centers for Disease Control and Prevention has a Clinical Outreach and Communication Activity (http://www.bt.cdc.gov/coca). Clinicians can sign up to receive e-mails, participate in conference calls, and participate in online and other types of training. Also, the Federal Emergency Management Administration operates the Emergency Management Institute (http://training.fema.gov), which provides online and in-person training about the Incident Command System and other topics.

Q   *How can pediatric clinicians work locally on disaster preparedness?*

A   Many local health departments have established volunteer Medical Reserve Corps units. Medical Reserve Corps units are community based and function as a way to locally organize and utilize volunteers who want to donate their time and expertise to prepare for and respond to emergencies and promote healthy living throughout the year. Pediatricians can interface with their local health departments and emergency operations centers to make sure that the needs of children are considered in community disaster planning. They should also ensure that their own practices and institutions are prepared.

Q *Where can pediatric clinicians find information to give to parents about disasters?*

A The American Academy of Pediatrics Disaster Web site has materials that clinicians can share with parents (http://www.aap.org/disasters/index.cfm).

Q *After the Gulf oil spill, where can I go to find information about the long-term effects of the oil on a child?*

A Very little is currently understood about the potential long term effects of the Gulf oil spill on children. Some basic information is available at http://www.aoec.org/PEHSU/documents/oil_spill_information_for_health_professionals_8_2010.pdf.

Resources

American Academy of Pediatrics, Children and Disasters
Web site: www.aap.org/disasters/index.cfm

Centers for Disease Control and Prevention,
Emergency Preparedness and Response
Web site: www.bt.cdc.gov

Federal Emergency Management Agency
Web site: www.fema.gov

National Commission on Children and Disasters
Web site: www.childrenanddisasters.acf.hhs.gov

Natural Disasters and Weather Emergencies –
US Environmental Protection Agency
Web site: www.epa.gov/naturalevents

State Offices and Agencies of Emergency Management
Web site: www.fema.gov/about/contact/statedr.shtm

References

1. Federal Emergency Management Agency, NRF Resource Center. Available at: http://www.fema.gov/emergency/nrf. Accessed April 6, 2011
2. Federal Emergency Management Agency, NIMS Resource Center. Available at: http://www.fema.gov/emergency/nims. Accessed April 6, 2011
3. Robert T. Stafford Disaster Relief and Emergency Assistance Act, as Amended and Related Authorities. FEMA 592, June 2007. Washington, DC: Federal Emergency Management Agency; 2007. Available at: http://www.fema.gov/pdf/about/stafford_act.pdf. Accessed April 6, 2011

4. Adirim T. Protecting children during disasters: the federal view. *Clin Pediatr Emerg Med.* 2009;10(3):164-172

5. Noji EK. *The Public Health Consequences of Disasters.* 1997; New York: Oxford University Press.

6. Waeckerle JF. Disaster Planning and Response. *N Engl J Med.* 1991;324(12):815-821

7. Centers for Disease Control and Prevention. FEMA-Provided Travel Trailer Study. http://www.cdc.gov/nceh/ehhe/trailerstudy/default.htm. Accessed April 6, 2011

8. Agency for Health Care Research and Quality. Pediatric Terrorism and Disaster Preparedness. A Resource for Pediatricians. Available at: http://www.ahrq.gov/research/pedprep/resource.htm. Accessed April 6, 2011

9. Hajat S, Ebi KL Kovats S, Meene B, Edwards S, Haines A. The human health consequences of flooding in Europe and the implications for public health: a review of the evidence. *Appl Environ Health Sci Public Health.* 2003;1(1):13-21

10. Janerich DT, Stark AD, Greenwald P, Burnett WS, Jacobson HI, McCusker J. Increased leukemia, lymphoma, and spontaneous abortion in Western New York following a flood disaster. *Public Health Rep.* 1981;96(4):350-356

11. Landrigan PJ, Lioy PJ, Thurston G, et al. Health and environmental consequences of the World Trade Center disaster. *Environ Health Perspect.* 2004;112(6):731-739

12. Cone J, Perlman S, Eros-Sarnyai M, et al. Clinical guidelines for children and adolescents exposed to the World Trade Center disaster. The New York City Department of Health and Mental Hygiene. *City Health Information.* 2009;28(4):29-40

13. Thomas PA, Brackbill R, Thalji T, et al. Respiratory and other health effects reported in children exposed to the World Trade Center disaster of 11 September 2001. *Environ Health Perspect.* 2008;116(10):1383–1390

14. Berkowitz GS, Wolff MS, Janevic TM, Holzman IR, Yehuda R, Landrigan PJ. The World Trade Center disaster and intrauterine growth restriction. *JAMA.* 2003;290(5):595-596

15. Lederman SA, Rauh V, Weiss L, et al. Effects of the World Trade Center event on birth outcomes among term deliveries at three lower Manhattan hospitals. *Environ Health Perspect.* 2004;112(17):1772-1778

16. Perera FP, Tang D, Rauh V, et al. Relationship between polycyclic aromatic hydrocarbon-DNA adducts and proximity to the World Trade Center and effects on fetal growth. *Environ Health Perspect.* 2005;113(8):1062-1067

17. Perera FP, Tang D, Rauh V, et al. Relationship between polycyclic aromatic hydrocarbon-DNA adducts, environmental tobacco smoke, and child development in the World Trade Center cohort. *Environ Health Perspect.* 2007;115(10):1497-1502

18. Hoven CW, Duarte CS, Lucas CP, et al. Psychopathology among New York City public school children 6 months after September 11. *Arch Gen Psychiatry.* 2005;62(5):545-552

19. Chemtob CM, Nomura Y, Abramovitz RA. Impact of conjoined exposure to the World Trade Center attacks and to other traumatic events on the behavioral problems of preschool children. *Arch Pediatr Adolesc Med.* 2008;162(2):126-133

20. Calderoni ME, Alderman EM, Silver EJ, Bauman LJ. The mental health impact of 9/11 on inner-city high school students 20 miles north of Ground Zero. *J Adolesc Health.* 2006;39(1): 57-65

21. Institute of Medicine. *Emergency Care for Children: Growing Pains.* Washington, DC: National Academies Press; 2007. Available at: http://www.nap.edu/catalog.php?record_id=11655. Accessed April 6, 2011

22. American Academy of Pediatrics. Hurricane Katrina, children, and pediatric heroes: hands-on stories by and of our colleagues helping families during the most costly natural disaster in US history. *Pediatrics.* 2006;117(5 Suppl):S355-S460

23. Hoven CW, Duarte CS, Mandell DJ. Children's mental health after disasters: the impact of the World Trade Center attack. *Curr Psychiatr Rep*. 2003;5(2):101-107

24. Schonfeld DJ, Gurwitch RH. Addressing disaster mental health needs of children: practical guidance for pediatric emergency care providers. *Clin Pediatr Emerg Med*. 2009;10(3):208-215

25. Madrid PA, Grant R, Reilly MJ, et al. Challenges in meeting immediate emotional needs: short-term impact of a major disaster on children's mental health: building resiliency in the aftermath of Hurricane Katrina. *Pediatrics*. 2006;117(5 Pt 3):S448-S453

26. Gurwitch RH, Kees M, Becker SM, et al. When disaster strikes: responding to the needs of children. *Prehosp Disaster Med*. 2004;19(1):21-28

27. American Red Cross. *Foundations of Disaster Mental Health*. Washington, DC: American Red Cross; 2006

Chapter 52

Environmental Equity

■ ■ ■ ■ ■ ■

Children in poor or ethnic minority communities frequently suffer disproportionately from the effects of environmental pollution. Children from poor or
minority families often live in neighborhoods with poor air quality and occupy
homes that are substandard, placing them at risk from exposure to multiple
environmental hazards.[1-8] Although these risks are much greater than those
experienced by their wealthier counterparts, racial differences often persist
across economic strata.[9] Additionally, poor communities are relatively powerless
compared with their more affluent neighbors and have fewer resources to
protect their children from the environmental risks present.

Disparities in the burdens of illness and death experienced by minority
groups, such as African American, Hispanic, Asian and Pacific Islander, and
American Indian/Alaska Native individuals, compared with white individuals
and with the US population as a whole, have existed since the government began
tracking health outcomes. Current research suggests that health disparities are
produced by both environmental (eg, physical, chemical, or biological agents to
which individuals are exposed in a multitude of settings, including home, school,
and workplace) and social (eg, individual and community level characteristics,
such as socioeconomic status, education, psychosocial stress, coping resources,
and support systems; residential factors; cultural variables; and institutional and
political factors, such as racism and classism) forces.[9] Moreover, environmental
justice advocates have encouraged scientists and regulators to view the "environment" holistically, by considering the effects that socioeconomic and other
social factors have on exposure to environmental hazards and resulting health
outcomes. Eliminating these disparities is a major goal of Healthy People 2020,
the nation's health agenda for this decade and beyond.[10] Achieving this national

health goal will require interventions that address both social and physical environmental factors. Public health advocates and local/state health departments are beginning to recognize the connections between physical and social environments. They are focusing more on "social determinants" of health (eg, poverty and racism)—instead of individual level behavior change approaches—to develop better strategies to eliminate health disparities and achieve health equity.[11,12]

DISPARITIES IN MORTALITY AND MORBIDITY

Racial and ethnic differences in birth outcomes and the prevalence and severity of many childhood diseases are well recognized. It is postulated that the elevated and/or cumulative exposures to environmental pollutants combined with material deprivation, low social position, psychosocial stress, and preexisting health conditions experienced by people of ethnic minorities and low-income populations increase the probability of environmentally induced illness and injury, thereby contributing to observed disparities in health status. Although the specific mechanisms through which social and physical environmental factors interact and produce the differences in morbidity and mortality among race/ethnic groups are not well understood, there is no doubt that these environmental factors play a role in differences in health outcomes. Recent studies show that social factors may lead to increased sensitivity or vulnerability to the adverse health effects of environmental toxicants such that these social factors are acting as effect modifiers (eg, enhancing the toxic effects) of exposures to environmental contaminants.[13,14] This is an emerging area of environmental health research.

Infant Mortality

Infant mortality is generally viewed as good indicator of community health, representing full integration of intrinsic biological factors with environmental and social factors distributed throughout every facet of life.[15] Since the early 1900s, the infant mortality rate in the United States has always been higher for African American and American Indian infants than for white infants.[16,17] Substantial racial and ethnic disparities continue. Non-Hispanic African American and American Indian/Alaska Native infants have consistently had a higher infant mortality rate than that of any other racial or ethnic groups.[18] For example, in 2004, the mortality rate for non-Hispanic African American infants was 13.6 infant deaths per 1000 live births and for American Indian/Alaska Native infants was 8.4, both higher than the that among white, non-Hispanic (5.7), Hispanic (5.5), and Asian/Pacific Islander (4.7) infants.[18] Infant mortality rates also vary within racial and ethnic populations. For example, among Hispanic people in the United States, the infant mortality rate for 2004 ranged from 4.6 deaths per 1000 live births for infants of Cuban origin to a high of 7.8 for Puerto Rican infants.[18] The reasons for the racial disparities are not fully understood. Sudden infant death syndrome (SIDS) is a major contributor to excess infant mortality in nonwhite groups. The rate of deaths from SIDS is higher among Alaska Native, American Indian, and black infants.[19,20] In addition to race/ethnicity, important environmental risk factors for SIDS include prone sleep position, maternal smoking during pregnancy, postnatal exposure to secondhand smoke, and (possibly) exposure to outdoor air pollution.[21-23]

Low Birth Weight

Low birth weight is an important predictor of infant morbidity and mortality. African American women are twice as likely as white women to deliver a low birth weight infant, even within the same category of educational attainment (eg, college education).[15,24] Lack of education and low-income status are also associated with low birth weight.[25] Cigarette smoking affects birth weight by causing intrauterine growth retardation.[26,27] These and other risk factors during pregnancy, however, do not adequately account for persistent racial disparities.[25,28] Exposure to environmental contaminants also contributes to the increased risk of having a low birth weight infant. A number of studies have found associations between low birth weight and proximity to landfills and other land-based environmental hazards,[29-32] air pollution,[33-37] and pesticides.[38] Studies[35,38] indicate that interactions of multiple contaminants, including polycyclic aromatic hydrocarbons, pesticides (chlorpyrifos), and secondhand smoke are associated with low birth weight, decreased head circumference, and decreased birth length among African American (nonsmoking) women in Harlem. In a study on air pollution and birth outcomes in Connecticut and Massachusetts, researchers found that the risk of low birth weight associated with exposure to fine particle air pollution particulate matter ($PM_{2.5}$) was higher for infants of black mothers than those of white mothers.[33]

Asthma

Puerto Rican, African American, and Cuban American children in the United States have a higher prevalence of asthma than do white children.[39] African American children are twice as likely as white children to have asthma.[39] African American individuals younger than 24 years are 3 to 4 times more likely to be hospitalized for asthma. Asthma is a complex disease with a number of causes. Racial and ethnic differences in the burden of asthma may be related to social and economic status, access to health care, and exposure to environ-mental triggers.[40] Approximately 13% of non-Hispanic African American children were reported to currently have asthma, compared with 8% of non- Hispanic white children and 9% of Hispanic children. Disparities exist within the Hispanic population, such that 20% of Puerto Rican children were reported to currently have asthma, compared with 7% of children of Mexican origin.[41]

Infant Pulmonary Hemorrhage

Clusters of cases of acute pulmonary hemorrhage were reported among infants in Cleveland, Chicago, and Detroit.[42-44] Most infants in these clusters were black. It is not known whether race is a risk factor for infant pulmonary hemorrhage or whether race is associated with socioeconomic status or with the prevalence of other specific risk factors, for which race may be a marker.[45]

DISPARITIES IN EXPOSURE

Air Pollution Exposure

Children of minority populations may experience greater exposure to polluted indoor and outdoor air. Indoors, they may have greater exposures to secondhand smoke, dust mites, molds, and cockroaches.[46-47] They also may live in neighborhoods with substandard outdoor air quality. For instance, 50% of all white children in the United States live in counties where the ozone concentrations exceed the national standard, whereas 60% of black children, 67% of Hispanic children, and 66% of Asian or Pacific Islander children live in counties with exceedingly high ozone concentrations. Higher percentages of black, Hispanic, and Asian or Pacific Islander American children than white children reside in counties where air quality exceed standards for $PM_{2.5}$ and carbon monoxide (see Table 52.1).[48]

Exposure to Contaminants in Food

Individuals of ethnic minority groups may be exposed to certain chemical contaminants in the food supply because of dietary habits. Individuals from American Indian/Alaska Native, Asian or Pacific Islander American, and subsistence fishing communities may be at much greater health risk from contaminants in fish.[49-53] For example, in their survey of fishing behavior and consumption along the New York-New Jersey harbor estuary, Burger et al found that African American people had the highest consumption rate of locally caught fish; Hispanic people had the second-highest rate.[50] White people, more than other groups, engaged in catch and release—they did not eat their catch and had lower consumption rates.[50] American Indian people are also differentially exposed to toxicants because of traditional dietary patterns involving consumption of locally caught fish and game.[52-55] Asian or Pacific Islander American people may consume 10 times more fish and shellfish than the average US person.[56] As a result, Asian or Pacific Islander American children may be more exposed to contaminated seafood than the general population. A recent analysis that used national data found that mercury concentrations among Asian

Table 52.1: Percentage of Children Living in Counties in Which Air Quality Standards Were Exceeded, by Race/Ethnicity, 2005

	ALL RACES/ ETHNICITIES	WHITE NON-HISPANIC	BLACK NON-HISPANIC	AMERICAN INDIAN/ ALASKA NATIVE NON-HISPANIC	ASIAN OR PACIFIC ISLANDER NON-HISPANIC	HISPANIC
Ozone 8-hour standard	55.00%	50.00%	60.00%	31.00%	66.00%	67.00%
PM_{10}	5.90%	4.90%	4.00%	7.30%	10.00%	9.60%
$PM_{2.5}$	25.00%	19.00%	36.00%	6.90%	27.00%	33.00%
Carbon monoxide	0.02%	0.02%	0.14%	0.20%	0.16%	0.12%
Lead	0.07%	0.12%	0.01%	0.02%	0.01%	0.01%
Sulfur dioxide	0.00%	0.00%	0.00%	0.00%	0.00%	0.00%
Nitrogen dioxide	0.00%	0.00%	0.00%	0.00%	0.00%	0.00%
Any standard	60.00%	37.00%	66.00%	33.00%	76.00%	71.00%

PM_{10} indicates particulate matter less than 10 µm in aerodynamic diameter; $PM_{2.5}$, particulate matter less than 2.5 µm in aerodynamic diameter.
Source: US Environmental Protection Agency, Office of Air and Radiation, Aerometric Information Retrieval System.

and Pacific Islander American women were statistically higher than those of other racial/ethnic groups.[57] This has implications for children's health, because exposure to methylmercury in utero can cause damage to the fetal central nervous system, resulting in impaired cognitive and motor skills.[58] These results were corroborated by a biomonitoring study in New York City showing racial disparities in blood mercury concentrations among Asian individuals, specifically foreign-born Chinese adults residing in New York City.[59] This study prompted the New York City Department of Health and Mental Hygiene to issue an advisory to health care providers to encourage healthy fish consumption among their patients. However, it is difficult for communities to make decisions about good dietary choices when information is not available regarding mercury concentrations (or other contaminants) in foods, particularly foods sold in specialty shops or ethnic food shops.

Lead

Despite recent large decreases in blood lead concentrations, there are persistent racial, ethnic, and income disparities in blood lead concentrations. An African American child who lives in poverty has 4 times the chance of having elevated blood lead concentration as does a white child who does not live in poverty.

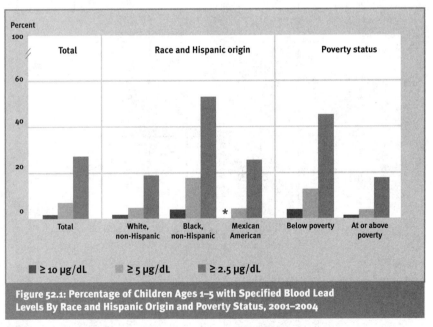

Figure 52.1: Percentage of Children Ages 1–5 with Specified Blood Lead Levels By Race and Hispanic Origin and Poverty Status, 2001–2004

Taken from Interagency Forum
*Data not shown. Estimate is considered unreliable (relative standard error is greater than 40 percent).
Note: Data for 2001–2004 are combined.
Source: Centers for Disease Control and Prevention, National Center for Health Statistics, National Health and Nutrition Examination Survey. Available at: http://www.childstats.gov/americaschildren/phenviro4.asp.

Table 52.2: Percentage of Children 1–5 Years of Age With Blood Lead Levels (BLLs) ≥10 µg/dL and Weighted Geometric Mean (GM) by Year Housing Built and Selected Characteristics

CHARACTERISTIC	YEAR HOUSING BUILT			TOTAL	
	BEFORE 1946 %	1946–1973 %	AFTER 1973 %	%	GM BLL (µg/dL)
Race/Ethnicity					
Black/non-Hispanic	21.9	13.7	3.4	11.2	4.3
Mexican American	13.0	2.3	1.6	4.0	3.1
White, non-Hispanic	5.6	1.4	1.5	2.3	2.3
Income					
Low	16.4	7.3	4.3	8.0	3.8
Middle	4.1	2.0	0.4	1.9	2.3
High	0.9	2.7	0.0	1.0	1.9
Urban status					
Population ≥1 million	11.5	5.8	0.8	5.4	2.8
Population <1 million	5.8	3.1	2.5	3.3	2.7
Total	8.6	4.6	1.6	4.4	2.7

Source: Centers for Disease Control and Prevention. Update: blood lead levels—United States, 1991–1994. *MMWR Morb Mortal Wkly Rep.* 1997;46(7):141-146

About 17% of non-Hispanic African American children, 4% of non-Hispanic white children, and 4% of Mexican American children had blood lead concentrations ≥5 µg/dL in 2001–2004 (see Fig 52.1).[18] In 2001-2004, African American children had the highest median blood lead concentration of 2.5 µg/dL, compared with 1.5 µg/dL for white children and 1.6 for Mexican American children.[48] Lead exposure in disadvantaged populations is thought to be related to older substandard housing (see Table 52.2). Although lead-based paints were banned for use in housing in 1978, 38 million housing units in the United States still have lead-based paint and high levels of lead-contaminated dust.[60]

Some Hispanic families use traditional ceramic ware for cooking and food storage, which has lead in the glazing that can leach into the food. Other sources include ethnic or folk remedies that contain lead, such as "greta," a traditional Mexican laxative, "azarcon," used to treat an upset stomach, and "litargirio," used as a deodorant. Imported makeup, such as "surma" or "kohl," is used primarily by individuals of Asian, African, or Middle Eastern descent. It is also applied to the umbilical stump of newborn infants. Although kohl may be made by hand using recipes that do not contain lead, commercial kohl makeup may have very high lead concentrations and pose a serious threat to human health. One study found that the use of kohl was a potential cause of elevated blood lead concentrations in Saudi school children,[61] suggesting that the cosmetic use of kohl may be a significant source of exposure to lead in children. Children can ingest kohl after rubbing their eyes and then licking their fingers.

Herbal medicine products may also be a source of lead exposure, and their use may vary by ethnic group. In one study, 70 Ayurvedic products from Boston area markets were analyzed (Ayurvedic medicine, or "ayurveda," is a system of health that has been practiced in India for more than 5000 years). Almost 20% contained lead, ranging from 5 µg/g to 37 000 µg/g per sample. The majority of these herbal medicine products contain one or more heavy metals that are toxic to adults and children.

Pesticide Exposure

More than 3 decades ago, several surveys reported that levels of dichlorodiphen-yltrichloroethane (DDT) and its metabolites (in fat or blood) were higher in black people than in white people.[62] In a community in Florida, DDT and dichlorodiphenyldichloroethylene (DDE, a degradation product of DDT) concentrations in blood were significantly lower in the affluent groups than in the low-income groups, for both black and white people. However, in comparable income groups, black people had higher DDT concentrations than did white people.[62]

Children of farm workers may accompany their parents to the fields, live in housing contaminated by direct pesticide spray or drift from nearby fields, and work in the fields themselves.[63,64] Farm workers can bring home pesticides on their shoes, clothes, and skin and then transfer them to their children, food, and home environment. Studies in California and Washington State suggest potential for higher residential exposure to some pesticides for children of farm workers as opposed to children of non-farm workers. In a recent study in Washington State among farm workers in the pome fruit industry (apples and pears), urinary concentrations of dimethyl pesticide metabolites from children of farm workers were significantly correlated with their parent's metabolite concentrations and with house-dust concentrations of the pesticides.[65] The authors concluded that results provide support for take-home pathway for pesticide exposures among farm worker children.

Concern about disparities in exposure to pesticides extends beyond the farm to impoverished children who live in urban areas. Home pesticide use tends to be more frequent and concentrated in densely populated urban areas. Pesticide use is especially high in multifamily housing with buildings that are in poor repair.[66] In 2004, some 71 000 children in the United States were poisoned by or exposed to household pesticides.[67] There were 15 000 rodenticide exposures involving children 6 years and younger. Many of these incidents occurred in the inner city among low-income minority residents.[67]

Ineffective pest control in low-income urban housing may lead to use of illegal pesticides. For example, in New York City, 9% of all households report using the pesticide Tempo.[68] Although Tempo is legal to use in agricultural settings, it is not legal to use in homes, because residents do not have access to the protective clothing worn and equipment used by agricultural workers. Other pesticides that should not be used in homes include "Chinese" chalk and Tres Pasitos, because they contain harmful chemicals that are toxic to people, especially children. To read more about these illegal pesticide products, visit http://www.epa.gov/opp00001/health/illegalproducts/index.htm.

Rituals

In certain ethnic groups, rituals may be potential sources of exposure to environmental contaminants. For example, some Hispanic American people who practice Santeria may sprinkle elemental mercury in the house, possibly resulting in elevated concentrations of mercury in the indoor air (see Chapter 32). Lead and other toxic metals are used in some Latin American and Asian traditional medicines, such as Ayurvedic medicines, that are given to children (see Chapter 19).

Exposure to Drinking Water Contaminants

Many small, rural, or low-income neighborhoods do not have access to safe and affordable drinking water supplies. Some water contamination problems may disproportionately affect certain racial or socioeconomic populations. Examples include lead exposure from deteriorating pipes/solder in older homes and fertilizer runoff into rural water supplies. Federal standards for drinking water quality (treatment and monitoring) do not apply to small private systems, many of which are domestic wells. These small private systems serve approximately 43.5 million people in the United States. Many of these systems are in rural and agricultural areas and may be at increased risk from nitrate and fecal contamination as well as from pesticides and other chemicals. Water quality data are not routinely collected from private wells; this situation presents a significant limitation to understanding children's exposures.

Waste Sites

Hazardous waste sites are often located disproportionately in minority neighborhoods. A 1987 report by the United Church of Christ's (UCC) Commission for Racial Justice revealed that 3 of the 5 largest hazardous waste landfills in the United States were in African American or Hispanic neighborhoods and that the mean percentage of residents of minority groups in areas with toxic waste sites was twice that in areas without toxic waste sites.[69] In 1994, in recognition of the disproportionate impact of environmental hazards on low-income communities, President Clinton issued an Executive Order seeking to achieve environmental justice.[70] The UCC report was recently updated and confirms earlier findings and also shows that disproportionate sitings of hazardous waste facilities have increased.[71] In 2000, neighborhoods within 3 kilometers (1.8 miles) of commercial hazardous waste facilities contained 56% people of minorities, whereas nonhost areas contained 30% people of minorities. Thus, percentages of people of minorities as a whole are 1.9 times greater in host neighborhoods than in nonhost areas.[71]

PRACTICAL RECOMMENDATIONS FOR CLINICIANS

Children in poverty face an array of formidable challenges. Environmental health sciences education is an essential tool for achieving environmental equity and protecting children. Pediatricians must work together to protect children, especially those living in low-income or minority communities, from environmental threats to their health.

Advocating for the health and well-being of children from ethnic minority groups requires knowledge of the unique environmental risks of the neighborhood or community, a high index of suspicion for environmental causes of disease, and a willingness to work with local health officials to sort out public health issues and make appropriate referrals. The pediatrician should consider doing the following:

- Build a network to learn about environmental concerns within the community. Meet and establish relationships with the local, county, or state environmental health unit.
- Actively learn the history of environmental illness that has affected various ethnic and minority groups within your practice. The special problems may vary between urban and rural settings and between racial and minority groups. Look for patterns of disease and exposures among your patients to help identify areas for policy change. Ask parents and community leaders for their perceptions of environmental exposure and disease.
- Tailor the environmental history to local conditions, risks, and concerns.
- Consider local cultural practices that may lead to environmental exposures and risk for illness. These may range from subsistence fishing in waters contaminated with polychlorinated biphenyls (PCBs) to use of unusual substances in cooking, home building, and home remedies.
- Speak out on behalf of these children before local, state, and national groups. Reframe the debate about health disparities by focusing more on health equity and away from individual behavior as the cause and solution.

Resources

Kaiser Family Foundation Health Disparities Report: A Weekly Look at Race, Ethnicity and Health

Web site: kaisernetwork.org/daily_reports/rep_disparities.cfm

DiversityData, Harvard School of Public Health

Web site: www.DiversityData.org

This Web site gives information about how people of different racial/ethnic backgrounds live includes comparative data about housing, neighborhood conditions, residential integration, and education.

Unnatural Causes

Web site: www.unnaturalcauses.org

A TV documentary series and public outreach campaign on the causes of socioeconomic racial/ethnic inequities in health.

National Association of County and City Health Officials

Roots of Health Inequity. Available at: www.naccho.org/topics/justice/roots.cfm

Hofrichter R, Bhatia R, eds. *Tackling Health Inequities Through Public Health Practice: Theory to Action.* 2nd ed. New York, NY: Oxford University Press; 2010

National Center on Minority Health and Health Disparities, National Institutes of Health

Web site: ncmhd.nih.gov

National Alliance for Hispanic Health

Web site: www.hispanichealth.org

National Council of La Raza

Web site: www.nclr.org

African American Health Care and Medical Information

Web site: www.blackhealthcare.com

African American Health Network, National Medical Association

Web site: www.aahn.com

Asian American and Pacific Islander Web sites

Web site: www.asianamerican.net/org_main.html

Asian and Pacific Islander Health Forum

Web site: www.apiahf.org

South Asian Health Forum
Web site: www.sahf.net

The Coalition for Asian American Children and Families (CACF)
Web site: www.cacf.org

American Indian Health
Web site: www.americanindianhealth.nlm.nih.gov

Indian Health Service
Web site: www.ihs.gov

References

1. Powell DL, Stewart V. Children. The unwitting target of environmental injustices. *Pediatr Clin North Am*. 2001;48(5):1291–1305

2. Dilworth-Bart JE, Moore CF. Mercy mercy me: social injustice and the prevention of environmental pollutant exposures among ethnic minority and poor children. *Child Dev*. 2006;77(2):247-265

3. American Lung Association. Urban air pollution and health inequities: a workshop report. *Environ Health Perspect*. 2001;109(Suppl 3):357-474

4. Perera FP, Rauh V, Tsai WY, et al. Effects of transplacental exposure to environmental pollutants on birth outcomes in a multiethnic population. *Environ Health Perspect*. 2003;111(2):201-205

5. Institute of Medicine. *Toward Environmental Justice: Research, Education, and Health Policy Needs*. Washington, DC: National Academies Press; 1999

6. Morello-Frosch R, Pastor M, Sadd J. Integrating environmental justice and the precautionary principle in research and policy making: the case of ambient air toxics exposures and health risks among schoolchildren in Los Angeles. *Annals AAPSS*. 2002;584:47-68

7. Evans GW, Kantrowitz E. Socioeconomic status and health: the potential role of environmental risk exposures. *Annu Rev Public Health*. 2002;23:303-331

8. Krieger J, Higgins DL. Housing and health: time again for public health action. *Am J Public Health*. 2002;92(5):758-768

9. Gee GC, Payne-Sturges DC. Environmental health disparities: a framework integrating psychosocial and environmental concepts. *Environ Health Perspect*. 2004;112(17):1645-1653

10. US Department of Health and Human Services. *Healthy People 2020. Disparities*. Available at: http://healthypeople.gov/2020/about/DisparitiesAbout.aspx. Accessed June 18, 2011

11. National Association of County and City Health Officials. *Tackling Health Inequities Through Public Health Practice: A Handbook for Action*. Washington, DC: National Association of County and City Health Officials; 2006

12. World Health Organization. *Commission on Social Determinants of Health*. Geneva, Switzerland: Interim Statement of the Commission on Social Determinants of Health, World Health Organization; 2007

13. Rauh VA, Whyatt RM, Garfinkel R, et al. Developmental effects of exposure to environmental tobacco smoke and material hardship among inner-city children. *Neurotoxicol Teratol*. 2004;26(3):373-385

14. Weiss B, Bellinger DC. Social ecology of children's vulnerability to environmental pollutants. *Environ Health Perspect*. 2006;114(10):1479-1485

15. Kington RS, Nickens HW. Racial and ethnic differences in health: recent trends, current patterns, future directions. In: *America Becoming: Racial Trends and Their Consequences.* Washington, DC: National Academy of Sciences; 2003:253-310

16. MacDorman MF, Atkinson JO. Infant mortality statistics from the linked birth/infant death data set—1995 period data. *Mon Vital Stat Rep.* 1998;46(6 Suppl 2):1–22

17. Grossman DC, Baldwin LM, Casey S, Nixon B, Hollow W, Hart LG. Disparities in infant health among American Indians and Alaska Natives in US metropolitan areas. *Pediatrics.* 2002;109(4):627–633

18. Federal Interagency Forum on Child and Family Statistics. *America's Children: Key National Indicators of Well-Being.* Washington, DC: Federal Interagency Forum on Child and Family Statistics, US Government Printing Office; 2007 http://www.childstats.gov/pdf/ac2007/body.pdf

19. Irwin KL, Mannino S, Daling J. Sudden infant death syndrome in Washington State: why are Native American infants at greater risk than white infants? *J Pediatr.* 1992;121(2):242–247

20. Oyen N, Bulterys M, Welty TK, Kraus JF. Sudden unexplained infant deaths among American Indians and whites in North and South Dakota. *Paediatr Perinat Epidemiol.* 1990;4(2):175–183

21. American Academy of Pediatrics, Task Force on Infant Positioning and SIDS. Positioning and SIDS. *Pediatrics.* 1992;89(2 Pt 1):1120–1126

22. MacDorman MF, Cnattingius S, Hoffman HJ, Kramer MS, Haglund B. Sudden infant death syndrome and smoking in the United States and Sweden. *Am J Epidemiol.* 1997;146(3):249–257

23. Woodruff TJ, Grillo J, Schoendorf KC. The relationship between selected causes of postneonatal infant mortality and particulate air pollution in the United States. *Environ Health Perspect.* 1997;105(6):608–612

24. Montgomery LE, Carter-Pokras O. Health status by social class and/or minority status: implications for environmental equity research. *Toxicol Ind Health.* 1993;9(5):729-773

25. Lu MC, Halfon N. Racial and ethnic disparities in birth outcomes: a life-course perspective. *Matern Child Health J.* 2003;7(1):13-30

26. Kramer MS. Determinants of low birth weight: methodological assessment and meta-analysis. *Bull World Health Organ.* 1987;65(5):663-737

27. Misra DP, Nguyen RH. Environmental tobacco smoke and low birth weight: a hazard in the workplace? *Environ Health Perspect.* 1999;107(Suppl 6):897-904

28. Fuller KE. Low birth-weight infants: the continuing ethnic disparity and the interaction of biology and environment. *Ethn Dis.* 2000;10(3):432-445

29. Baibergenova A, Kudyakov R, Zdeb M, Carpenter DO. Low birth weight and residential proximity to PCB-contaminated waste sites. *Environ Health Perspect.* 2003;111(10):1352-1357

30. Elliott P, Briggs D, Morris S, et al. Risk of adverse birth outcomes in populations living near landfill sites. *BMJ.* 2001;323(7309):363-368

31. Shaw GM, Schulman J, Frisch JD, Cummins SK, Harris JA. Congenital malformations and birthweight in areas with potential environmental contamination. *Arch Environ Health.* 1992;47(2):147-154

32. Vrijheid M. Health effects of residence near hazardous waste landfill sites: a review of epidemiologic literature. *Environ Health Perspect.* 2000;108(Suppl 1):101-112

33. Bell ML, Ebisu K, Belanger K. Ambient air pollution and low birth weight in Connecticut and Massachusetts. *Environ Health Perspect.* 2007;115(7):1118-1124

34. Maisonet M, Bush TJ, Correa A, Jaakkola JJ. Relation between ambient air pollution and low birth weight in the Northeastern United States. *Environ Health Perspect.* 2001;109(Suppl 3):351-356

35. Perera FP, Rauh V, Whyatt RM, et al. Molecular evidence of an interaction between prenatal environmental exposures and birth outcomes in a multiethnic population. *Environ Health Perspect.* 2004;112(5):626-630

36. Rogers JF, Thompson SJ, Addy CL, McKeown RE, Cowen DJ, Decoufle P. Association of very low birth weight with exposures to environmental sulfur dioxide and total suspended particulates. *Am J Epidemiol.* 2000;151(6):602-613

37. Wang X, Ding H, Ryan L, Xu X. Association between air pollution and low birth weight: a community-based study. *Environ Health Perspect.* 1997;105(5):514-520

38. Perera FP, Rauh V, Tsai WY, Kinney P, Camman D, Barr D. Effects of transplacental exposure to environmental pollutants on birth outcomes in a multiethnic population. *Environ Health Perspect.* 2003;111(2):201-205

39. Akinbami LJ. The state of childhood asthma, United States, 1980-2005. *Adv Data.* 2006 Dec 12;(381):1-24

40. Asthma and Allergy Foundation of America and National Pharmaceutical Council. *Ethnic Disparities in the Burden and Treatment of Asthma.* Washington, DC: Asthma and Allergy Foundation of America; January 2005. Available at: www.aafa.org. Accessed August 25, 2010

41. Federal Interagency Forum on Child and Family Statistics. *America's Children: Key National Indicators of Well-Being.* Washington, DC: Federal Interagency Forum on Child and Family Statistics, US Government Printing Office; 2007

42. Centers for Disease Control and Prevention. Acute pulmonary hemorrhage/hemosiderosis among infants—Cleveland, January 1993–November 1994. *MMWR Morb Mortal Wkly Rep.* 1994;43(48):881–883

43. Centers for Disease Control and Prevention. Acute pulmonary hemorrhage among infants— Chicago, April 1992–November 1994. *MMWR Morb Mortal Wkly Rep.* 1995;44(4):67, 73–74

44. Pappas MD, Sarnaik AP, Meert KL, Hasan RA, Lieh-Lai MW. Idiopathic pulmonary hemorrhage in infancy. Clinical features and management with high frequency ventilation. *Chest.* 1996;110(2):553–555

45. Dearborn DG, Smith PG, Bahms BB, et al. Clinical profile of 30 infants with acute pulmonary hemorrhage in Cleveland. *Pediatrics.* 2002;110(3):627–637

46. Sarpong SB, Hamilton RG, Eggleston PA, Adkinson NF Jr. Socioeconomic status and race as risk factors for cockroach allergen exposure and sensitization in children with asthma. *J Allergy Clin Immunol.* 1996;97(6):1393–1401

47. US Environmental Protection Agency. *National Survey on Environmental Management of Asthma and Children's Exposure to Environmental Tobacco Smoke.* Washington, DC: US Environmental Protection Agency; 2004. Available at: http://www.epa.gov/smokefree/healtheffects.html. Accessed August 25, 2010

48. US Environmental Protection Agency. Body burdens. In: *America's Children and the Environment (ACE).* Available at: http://www.epa.gov/envirohealth/children/body_burdens/bb_tables_2006. htm#B1. Accessed August 25, 2010

49. Arquette M, Cole M, Cook K, et al. Holistic risk-based environmental decision making: a Native perspective. *Environ Health Perspect.* 2002;110(Suppl 2):259-264

50. Burger J. Consumption patterns and why people fish. *Environ Res.* 2002;90(2):125-135

51. Burger J, Gaines KF, Boring CS, et al. Metal levels in fish from the Savannah River: potential hazards to fish and other receptors. *Environ Res.* 2002;89(1):85-97

52. Schell LM, Hubicki LA, DeCaprio AP, et al. Organochlorines, lead, and mercury in Akwesasne Mohawk youth. *Environ Health Perspect.* 2003;111(7):954-961

53. Fitzgerald EF, Hwang SA, Deres DA, Bush B, Cook K, Worswick P. The association between local fish consumption and DDE, mirex, and HCB concentrations in the breast milk of Mohawk women at Akwesasne. *J Expo Anal Environ Epidemiol.* 2001;11(5):381-388

54. Harper BL, Flett B, Harris S, Abeyta C, Kirschner F. The Spokane Tribe's multipathway subsistence exposure scenario and screening level RME. *Risk Anal.* 2002;22(3):513-526

55. Judd NL. Are seafood PCB data sufficient to assess health risk for high seafood consumption groups? *Hum Ecol Assess.* 2003;9(3):691-707

56. Judd NL. Consideration of cultural and lifestyle factors in defining susceptible population for environmental disease. *Toxicology.* 2004;198:121-133

57. Hightower JM, O'Hare A, Hernandez GT. Blood mercury reporting in NHANES: identifying Asian, Pacific Islander, Native American, and multiracial groups. *Environ Health Perspect.* 2006;114(2):173-5.

58. US Environmental Protection Agency. *Health Effects of Mercury.* Washington, DC: US Environmental Protection Agency; 2007; Available at: www.epa.gov/hg/effects.htm. Accessed August 25, 2010

59. McKelvey W, Gwynn RC, Jeffery N, et al. A biomonitoring study of lead, cadmium, and mercury in the blood of New York City adults. *Environ Health Perspect.* 2007;115(10): 1435-1441

60. Jacobs DE, Clickner RP, Zhou JY, et al. The prevalence of lead-based paint hazards in U.S. housing. *Environ Health Perspect.* 2002;110(10):A599-A606

61. Al-Awamy BH. Evaluation of commonly used tribal and traditional remedies in Saudi Arabia. *Saudi Med J.* 2001;22(12):1065-1068

62. Davies JE, Edmundson WF, Raffonelli A, Cassady JC, Morgade C. The role of social class in human pesticide pollution. *Am J Epidemiol.* 1972;96(5):334–341

63. Arcury TA, Grzywacz JG, Barr DB, Tapia J, Chen H, Quandt SA. Pesticide urinary metabolite levels of children in eastern North Carolina farmworker households. *Environ Health Perspect.* 2007;115(8):1254-1260

64. Curwin BD, Hein MJ, Sanderson WT, et al. Pesticide dose estimates for children of Iowa farmers and non-farmers. *Environ Res.* 2007;105(3):307-315

65. Coronado GD, Vigoren EM, Thompson B, Griffith WC, Faustman EM. Organophosphate pesticide exposure and work in pome fruit: evidence for the take-home pesticide pathway. *Environ Health Perspect.* 2006;114(7):999-1006

66. Whyatt RM, Camann DE, Kinney PL, et al. Residential pesticide use during pregnancy among a cohort of urban minority women. *Environ Health Perspect.* 2002;110(5):507-514

67. American Association of Poison Control Centers. 2004 Poison Center Survey. Available at: http://www.aapcc.org/. Accessed August 25, 2010

68. New York City Department of Health and Mental Hygiene. Pests can be controlled… safely. *NYC Vital Signs.* 2005;4(3):1-4. Available at: http://www.nyc.gov/html/doh/downloads/pdf/survey/survey-2005pest.pdf. Accessed August 25, 2010

69. Commission for Racial Justice, United Church of Christ. *Toxic Wastes and Race in the United States: A National Study of the Racial and Socioeconomic Characteristics of Communities with Hazardous Waste Sites.* Cleveland, OH: United Church of Christ; 1987

70. Presidential Executive Order 12898: Federal Actions to Address Environmental Justice in Minority Populations and Low-Income Populations. 59 FR 7629 (1994)

71. Bullard R, Mohai P, Saha R, Wright B. *Toxic Wastes and Race at Twenty: 1987-2007. Grassroots Struggles to Dismantle Environmental Racism in the U.S.* Cleveland, OH: United Church of Christ, Justice and Witness Ministries; 2007

Chapter 53

Ethical Issues in Environmental Health Research

■ ■ ■ ■ ■ ■

Ethical issues in environmental health research encompass the overall topic of biomedical ethics, the subset of biomedical research ethics, and a further subset related to such research involving children. Furthermore, consideration of ethical issues related to research in public health, of which research in environmental health is itself a subset, is different from consideration of biomedical research on individual subjects, whether children or adults. An overarching principle of research involving children is that children are a vulnerable population and that they require special consideration. In particular, the cognitive abilities of children—their understanding of the nature of a research protocol and its implications for future effects on them, and their ability to advocate for themselves—are age dependent, creating special challenges for the conduct of research studies. There are many unanswered questions about risks to children from exposures to hazards in the environment. There is a need for high-quality, ethically performed research to answer these questions. The United States is in the early phase of a large prospective study of children's health and the environment—the National Children's Study (www.nationalchildrensstudy.gov). It is important that the highest ethical standards be applied to this and all other research on children's health. This chapter illustrates some of the major challenges that must be addressed when conducting environmental health research involving children and offers guidelines for judging the ethical soundness of proposed environmental research protocols that involve children. Other sources offer a more complete review of the ethical issues in biomedical research, public health research, and research involving children.[1-3]

HISTORY

The discussion of ethical issues in medicine can be traced to the time of Hippocrates. Considerations of ethical issues related to biomedical and public health research is a post-World War II phenomenon.

As a result of the Nazi medical war crimes and the unethical research carried out in the United States (eg, the Tuskegee syphilis study, in which black men with syphilis were left untreated and uninformed about their treatment options, and the Willowbrook hepatitis study, in which children were placed in a situation in which it was anticipated that they would become infected with hepatitis virus to study the efficacy of gamma globulin in preventing the infection), in 1974, Congress passed the National Research Act, which established the National Commission for the Protection of Human Subjects of Biomedical and Behavioral Research ("the National Commission").[4-7] In 1977, the National Commission published a report and recommendations on research in children in which it outlined conditions under which the participation of children in research would be ethically acceptable and conditions under which participation may be authorized by the participants and their parents.[8] In 1978, the National Commission published the Belmont Report, titled *Ethical Principles and Guidelines for the Protection of Human Subjects of Research.*[9] This led to the formulation of Title 45, Code of Federal Regulations, Part 46 (45 CFR 46), also known as the Common Rule.[10] The Common Rule is a short name for "The Federal Policy for the Protection of Human Subjects" and was adopted as policy by a number of federal agencies in 1991. This has been modified to include special oversight for children and special access to research for children (Table 53.1).[11] In addition, the American Academy of Pediatrics and the Academic Pediatric Association have provided recommendations about research involving children.[12-15]

Concerns about ethical issues in environmental health research involving children came to the forefront with a research project undertaken by the staff of the Kennedy Krieger Institute in Baltimore, MD. The Kennedy Krieger Institute study was designed to compare different approaches for reducing the risk of lead poisoning in dwelling units. Lawsuits were filed against the researchers and Kennedy Krieger Institute, alleging that children in the study sustained lead poisoning or were put at risk of lead poisoning because the research protocol required that some of the dwellings not be fully abated. In 2001, in the case of *Grimes vs Kennedy Krieger Institute*, a court in Maryland rendered a preliminary opinion that nontherapeutic research on children was inappropriate. The court later seemed to step back from its ruling, and the Maryland legislature passed legislation to allow nontherapeutic research.[16-18]

In 2004, another controversy erupted that underscored the need for more discussion and debate about ethical issues related to research on children's health and the environment. The US Environmental Protection Agency (EPA) proposed the Longitudinal Study of Young Children's Exposures in their Homes to Selected Pesticides, Phthalates, Brominated Flame Retardants, and Perfluorinated Chemicals. This was also known as the Children's Health Environmental Exposure Research Study (CHEERS).[19] The study proposed tracking the use of pesticides by families with young children. For a number of reasons, the study came under severe criticism in the professional and lay press—it seemed to target poor families, and some perceived that the study would encourage parents to use pesticides, contrary to EPA guidelines. Another criticism was that the study was partly funded by the American Chemistry Council, an industry association that represents pesticide manufacturers and other chemical companies. Ultimately, the study was never begun.

Regulatory Structure

Subpart A of 45 CFR 46 provides guidelines for the ethical conduct of research on humans funded by the federal government but also should be followed in research funded privately (Tables 53.1 and 53.2). An institutional review board (IRB) has the responsibility to ensure that researchers implement these guidelines in a particular research project. An IRB is usually, but not always, a locally constituted committee composed of scientists and nonscientists established to protect the rights and welfare of the human research subjects to be enrolled in a research project. The nature, responsibilities, and procedural requirements of the IRB are clearly delineated in the Code of Federal Regulations. However, the IRB has certain latitude to modify or waive compliance with usual procedures. For instance, research that presents minimal risk to participants and meets other specific requirements can receive expedited review by an IRB, including waiver of informed consent.[10] For all other research, the IRB must closely examine and approve research protocols to ensure that:

- Risks to participants are minimized to the extent possible;
- Risks posed by research participation are reasonable in relation to potential benefits;
- Participants are selected equitably;
- Informed consent is obtained in accordance with national guidelines and federal, state, and local regulations;
- Measures are taken to protect the privacy of participants; and
- If research involves vulnerable populations, such as children, additional safeguards are implemented.

Guidance for those additional safeguards for children can be found in Subpart D of the Common Rule. Researchers must be more vigilant about risks to which children might be exposed during the research (Table 53.2). The IRB can approve a pediatric research protocol even if it is not likely to provide

Table 53.1: Allowable Categories of Research Involving Children Under Subpart D: 45 CFR 46

CATEGORY (CFR)	POTENTIAL RISK	POTENTIAL BENEFIT	PARENTAL CONSENT	CHILD ASSENT[a]
46.404	No greater than minimal	Not necessarily	1 parent	Yes
46.405	Justified by potential benefit	Sufficient to justify the risks	1 parent	Yes
	Risk/benefit balance is at least as favorable as that presented by available alternatives			
46.406	Minor increase over minimal risk	No potential for direct benefit	2 parents	Yes
	Intervention or procedure is similar to subject's naturally occurring situations			
		Likely to yield generalizable knowledge of vital importance to understanding or ameliorating the condition being studied		
46.407[b]		Not otherwise approvable but which 1. has the potential to further the understanding, prevention, or alleviation of a serious problem affecting health or welfare of children; or 2. Follows sound ethical principles	2 parents	Yes

CFR indicates Code of Federal Regulations.
Adapted from Diekema 2006.[11]
[a] Can be waived for children of certain ages if the IRB determines that the research holds the potential to benefit the child and is only available in the research context, or the child cannot be reasonably consulted.
[b] This category of research also requires that the IRB determine that the research provides a reasonable opportunity to further understanding, prevention, or alleviation of a serious problem affecting the health and welfare of children, and approval by the secretary of the Department of Health and Human Services.

Table 53.2: Guidelines for Judging the Ethical Soundness of Environmental Health Research Protocols Involving Children (Derived From Subpart D: 45 CFR 46)

An appropriate research protocol should consider and disclose the following:

1. The purpose of the research;

2. The expected duration of the child's involvement;

3. A description of procedures to be followed and identification of any experimental procedures;

4. A description of any reasonably foreseeable risks or discomforts to the subject;

5. A description of any reasonably expected benefits to the subject or others;

6. A disclosure of appropriate alternative procedures that may be advantageous to the subject;

7. A description of the extent to which the confidentiality of records will be maintained;

8. An explanation as to whether any compensation is provided or what treatments are available if injury occurs;

9. An explanation of whom to contact with questions about the research;

10. A statement that enrollment is voluntary and that refusal to enroll or to continue to participate, once enrolled, will not result in a loss of benefits the child is otherwise entitled to;

11. Information about the nature of the risk or hazard being studied;

12. Assurance that the subject will be informed of any significant findings discovered during the study that might influence their willingness to continue to participate;

13. Circumstances when the subject may be terminated from the study by the investigator without the consent of the subject; and

14. While reimbursement of study participants for out-of-pocket expenses is appropriate, care must be taken to ensure that any tokens of appreciation or payments for time and inconvenience are not sufficient to influence a parent's or child's decision to participate or not to participate in the study.

direct benefit to pediatric participants if (1) a study may yield generalizable knowledge about the medical disorder or condition; or (2) the study "presents an opportunity to understand, prevent, or alleviate a serious condition affecting the health or welfare of children."[10] These are the types of exceptions likely to be found in issues related to environmental health. Furthermore, consent for participation must include permission from one or both parents or a guardian and, when age-appropriate, the assent of the child, depending on the nature of the study.[1,20,21] Permission from only one parent is sufficient when research does not involve more than minimal risk; if it involves greater than minimal risk, it must present the prospect of direct benefit to the child. Permission from both parents is required for any research that exceeds minimal risk and does not offer the prospect of direct benefit to the participant.[10] Certain research protocols cannot be approved at the local IRB level alone and must be referred to the Department of Health and Human Services. The IRB can waive the acquisition of parental signed consent under certain conditions.[10]

Although much public health and environmental health research is about or involves communities, federal regulations do not provide guidance on community-wide research except to insure that participants are selected equitably and the risks and benefits of the research must be equitably distributed among the participants. There is a mechanism to involve communities in approving research, but it is generally reserved for protocols in which consent cannot be obtained (such as trauma/resuscitation protocols). (See subsequent discussion of community involvement and oversight.)

Environmental research often seeks information about early life exposures. Therefore, enrollment and protection of women who may become pregnant, who are pregnant at the time of enrollment, or who become pregnant after enrollment is another issue for the IRB to consider. In nontherapeutic research involving women who are pregnant, the fetus must not be exposed to more than minimal risk. Furthermore, because data collected during research or tissue stored in biobanks may be available for years, environmental research should specifically address protecting the privacy of the child including into his or her majority.

THE INSTITUTIONAL REVIEW BOARD

For research projects undertaken in academic institutions, the IRB that reviews the proposal is housed in the same institution. In part, this ensures that the IRB brings local sensibilities into the consideration of the proposal. However, in some instances, researchers may seek approval from IRBs that are independent of academic institutions and that may not be local. This may be a particularly relevant issue in research involving communities (discussed in subsequent part of this chapter).

The Common Rule defines the responsibilities of the IRB to interpret the federal regulations and apply them to individual research projects. Before research can be conducted, protocols and consent forms must be reviewed and approved by an IRB to ensure compliance with all federal, state, and local laws and regulations. IRBs are responsible for ensuring that research protocols meet specific requirements as described earlier, including that the research is ethical and the protocol will be conducted in an ethical manner. The members of the IRB, in the aggregate, must possess the expertise to evaluate and oversee the research. This includes expertise in child health and in environmental health research. Thus, the typical university-based IRB, which is usually constituted to evaluate university-based research, may not have the appropriate representation to adequately evaluate and oversee research involving communities. (See subsequent discussion of community advisory boards or environmental health and community review boards.)

CHILDREN'S INFORMED CONSENT: A SPECIAL CIRCUMSTANCE

The Nuremberg Code, which was written in response to inhumane Nazi human experimentation, explicitly states that informed consent is "absolutely essential" to the ethical conduct of research to ensure that the research participant's involvement is not based on "force, fraud, deceit, duress, overreaching, or other ulterior forms of constraint or coercion."[22] Because informed consent is the primary mechanism by which we respect the autonomy of research participants, children present a unique challenge, because below a certain age, they do not possess the developed rationality that would make such consent informed and, thereby, legitimate. Thus, we rely on the proxy judgments of children's parents or legal guardians to offer permission on their behalf, because we assume that parents are in the best position to make choices in line with the child's interests, emerging values, and commitments.

Thus, in addition to parental consent, researchers must request child assent when the IRB deems that the child is capable of providing it based on age, maturity, and psychological state. Assent refers to a "child's voluntary affirmative agreement to participate in research"[10] and, like parental consent, requires the active agreement of the child to participate and not just a failure to object to participation.

The form of assent and information provided will vary depending on the child's maturity. When there is no prospect of direct benefit from participation, children have the right to dissent and to have that dissent respected.

PRIVACY

Information that is collected about children for research purposes may require more than conventional privacy protections, especially for longitudinal studies. Outcomes that may not manifest until years later require long-term data storage and analysis of data, years after a pregnancy is completed or a child is grown. Data cannot be completely deidentified, because they will need to be linked with subsequently collected data. Given the lapses between data collection periods and children's developing abilities to understand their rights, the privacy rights of children who are participating in longitudinal studies are best protected by viewing parental permission and child assent as an ongoing process that is repeated at appropriate intervals.[23,24] Researchers must also consider the issue of whether and when to obtain consent from children who were enrolled in a trial and who have now turned 18 years of age and from whom data continue to be collected and used.

COMMUNITY INVOLVEMENT IN RESEARCH—COMMUNITY "CONSENT"

The primary responsibility of IRBs is to protect individual research participants. Public health and some environmental health research involve communities. The Common Rule does not address research performed in which communities are participants. Such research has the potential to harm as well as help its participants, including the members of the community. To protect the community and its members and to consider unique issues that arise when communities are the subject of research, some have suggested the creation of community advisory boards or environmental health and community review boards.[26]

An environmental health and community review board combines the fundamental responsibilities and ethical precepts of the traditional IRB with an expanded ethical construct of dignity, veracity, sustainability, and justice and an added focus on community (see Table 53.3).[25] Dignity incorporates the concept of autonomy with the notion of a right to understand the research and the outcomes of the research. Veracity reflects transparency, indicating that all relevant facts have been revealed, thus allowing the community to make a decision about what is good (beneficence) and what protects them from harm (nonmaleficence). Sustainability means that businesses and individuals within the community are likely to thrive as a result of participating in the research. In this context, the notion of justice is expanded to encompass the community and extends beyond the self-interest of an individual or individual business.

REPORTING RESULTS

There is considerable controversy and uncertainty about whether to report individual results of environmental contamination or body burden to study subjects. The National Bioethics Advisory Commission[27] recommends disclosing individual results only when the findings have been scientifically validated

---

Table 53.3: Proposed Criteria for Conducting a Randomized Controlled Trial Concerning an Environmental Hazard Involving Children[25]

1. Tests questions about a widely disseminated and persistent pollutant;
2. Tests questions that cannot be answered in adults;
3. Evaluates the safety or efficacy of unproven environmental interventions;
4. Evaluates the uncertain causal relationship of an exposure and a disease;
5. Includes an adequate sample size to test the hypothesis;
6. Includes mechanisms for communicating research findings to participants;
7. Involves the community in the design and implementation of the study; and
8. Includes mechanisms to ensure that legal guardians and participants are fully informed about the rationale for the trial.

and confirmed; the findings have significant implications for the subject's health concerns; and a course of action to ameliorate or treat these concerns is readily available. Some ethicists, however, argue that respect for research participants requires investigators to provide individual results to study participants, except in unusual circumstances.

Most environmental health researchers and community advocates would agree that results of commonly used clinical tests or biomarkers that conform to the National Bioethics Advisory Commission's criteria, such as blood lead concentration and skin allergy testing, should be reported promptly to families. There is, however, considerable uncertainty about reporting individual test results for biomarkers or environmental samples that are not performed in Clinical Laboratory Improvement Amendments (CLIA)-approved laboratory settings, that are not typically used in the clinical setting, or that have uncertain clinical indications. Most commonly, research results performed in non-CLIA settings are not returned to participants, because the results have no clear clinical indication. At a minimum, researchers must adhere to what was promised in the informed consent.

Resource

Panel to Review the National Children's Study Research Plan. Ethical procedures and community engagement. In: *The National Children's Study Research Plan: A Review*. Washington, DC: National Academies Press; 2008:121-130. Available at: http://www.nap.edu/catalog.php?record_id=12211. Accessed October 15, 2010

References

1. Institute of Medicine, Committee on Clinical Research Involving Children, Board on Health Sciences Policy. *The Ethical Conduct of Research Involving Children*. Field MJ, Behrman RE, eds. Washington, DC: The National Academies Press; 2004
2. Ross LF. *Children in Medical Research: Access Versus Protection (Issues in Biomedical Ethics)*. Oxford, England: Oxford University Press; 2006
3. Kodish E. *Ethics and Research with Children. A Case-Based Approach*. Oxford, England: Oxford University Press; 2005
4. Advisory Committee on Human Radiation Experiments. *The Human Radiation Experiments*. Oxford, England: Oxford University Press; 1996
5. Faden RR. Human-subjects research today: final report of the advisory committee on human radiation experiments. *Acad Med*. 1996;71(5):482-483
6. Krugman S. The Willowbrook hepatitis studies revisited: ethical aspects. *Rev Infect Dis*. 1986;8(1):157-162
7. Rothman DJ. Research ethics at Tuskegee and Willowbrook. *Am J Med*. 1984;77(6):A49
8. National Commission for the Protection of Human Subjects of Biomedical and Behavioral Research. Report and Recommendations: Research Involving Children. Washington, DC: National Commission for the Protection of Human Subjects of Biomedical and Behavioral Research; 1977. Available at: http://bioethics.georgetown.edu/pcbe/reports/past_commissions/ Research_involving_children.pdf. Accessed October 15, 2010

9. National Institutes of Health. Belmont Report on Ethical Principles and Guidelines for the Protection of Human Subjects of Research. Bethesda, MD: National Institutes of health, Office on Human Subjects Research; 1979. Available at: http://ohsr.od.nih.gov/guidelines/belmont. html. Accessed October 15, 2010

10. Department of Health and Human Services. Guidance Document for 45 CFR 46 (2005). Available: http://www.hhs.gov/ohrp/humansubjects/guidance/45cfr46.htm. Accessed October 15, 2010

11. Diekema DS. Conducting ethical research in pediatrics: A brief historical overview and review of pediatric regulations. *J Pediatr*. 2006;149(1 Suppl):S3-S11

12. American Academy of Pediatrics, Committee on Bioethics. Institutional ethics committees. *Pediatrics*. 2001;107(1):205–209

13. American Academy of Pediatrics, Committee on Bioethics. Informed consent, parental permission, and assent in pediatric practice. *Pediatrics*. 1995;95(2):314-317

14. American Academy of Pediatrics, Committee on Native American Child Health and Committee on Community Health Services. Ethical considerations in research with socially identifiable populations. *Pediatrics*. 2004;113(1 Pt 1):148–151

15. Etzel RA; Ambulatory Pediatric Association, Research Committee. Policy statement: ensuring integrity for research with children. *Ambul Pediatr*. 2005;5(1):3–5

16. *Ericka Grimes v Kennedy Krieger Institute Inc* and *Myron Higgins, a minor, etc, et al v Kennedy Krieger Institute Inc*. Available at: http://www.courts.state.md.us/opinions/coa/2001/128a00.pdf. Accessed October 15, 2010

17. Phoenix JA. Ethical considerations of research involving minorities, the poorly educated and/or low-income populations. *Neurotoxicol Teratol*. 2002;24(4):475–476

18. Pinder L. Commentary on the Kennedy Krieger Institute lead paint repair and maintenance study. *Neurotoxicol Teratol*. 2002;24(4):477–479

19. US Environmental Protection Agency. Children's Health Environmental Exposure Research Study. Washington, DC: US Environmental Protection Agency; 2005. Available: http://www.epa.gov/cheers/. Accessed October 15, 2010

20. American Academy of Pediatrics, Committee on Drugs. Guidelines for the ethical conduct of studies to evaluate drugs in pediatric populations. *Pediatrics*. 1995;95(2):286

21. Wendler D. Protecting subjects who cannot give consent: toward a better standard for "minimal" risks. *Hastings Cent Rep*. 2005;35(5):37-43

22. National Institutes of Health, Office on Human Subjects of Research. Nuremberg Code. Available at: http://ohsr.od.nih.gov/guidelines/nuremberg.html. Accessed October 15, 2010

23. Fisher CB. Privacy and ethics in pediatric environmental health research—part I: genetic and prenatal testing. *Environ Health Perspect*. 2006;114(10):1617–1621

24. Fisher CB. Privacy and ethics in pediatric environmental health research—part II: protecting families and communities. *Environ Health Perspect*. 2006;114(10):1622–1625

25. Gilbert SG. Supplementing the traditional institutional review board with an environmental health and community review board. *Environ Health Perspect*. 2006;114(10):1626–1629

26. Institute of Medicine, Board on Children, Youth, and Families and Behavioral and Social Sciences and Education. *Ethical Considerations for Research on Housing-Related Health Hazards Involving Children*. Lo B, O'Connell ME, eds. Washington, DC: National Academies Press; 2005

27. National Bioethics Advisory Commission. *Research Involving Human Biological Materials: Ethical Issues and Policy Guidance. National Children's Study*. Rockville, MD: National Bioethics Advisory Commission; 2006. Available at: http://nationalchildrensstudy.gov. Accessed October 15, 2010

Chapter 54

Global Climate Change

■ ■ ■ ■ ■ ■

INTRODUCTION

"Warming of the climate system is unequivocal, as is now evident from observations of increases in global average air and ocean temperature, widespread
melting of snow and ice, and rising global mean sea level."[1] Scientists[1] and
governments[2] concur that the earth is warming. Global climate change is accelerating, and human activities are the main cause. A glossary of climate change
terms can be found at http://www.epa.gov/climatechange/glossary.html. Adverse
human health and ecosystem consequences are anticipated,[3] and some are
already being measured. Children represent a particularly vulnerable group likely
to suffer disproportionately from both direct and indirect adverse health effects
from climate change.[4-8]

The greenhouse effect is necessary to life on earth. Without heat-trapping
greenhouse gases, such as water vapor, carbon dioxide, and other natural
components of the atmosphere, the earth would be a lifeless, frozen planet.
Since the onset of the industrial age, human activity has drastically enhanced
the greenhouse effect by rapidly adding large amounts of greenhouse gases to
the atmosphere. Three greenhouse gases—carbon dioxide, methane, and nitrous
oxide—are responsible for approximately 88% of the anthropogenic influences
enhancing the greenhouse effect and have increased 36%, 155%, and 19%,
respectively, since 1750 (the beginning of the industrial era).[5] The rate of
increase of atmospheric greenhouse gases is accelerating, up 22.7% between
1990 and 2006.

Carbon dioxide is the most important greenhouse gas (Fig 54.1), accounting for more than 63% of human-enhanced increases and more than 91% of

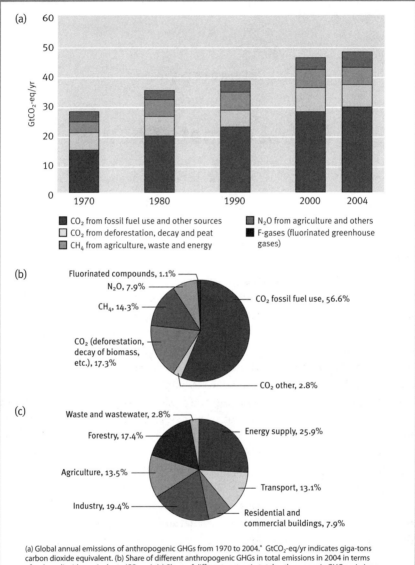

(a) Global annual emissions of anthropogenic GHGs from 1970 to 2004.* GtCO₂-eq/yr indicates giga-tons carbon dioxide equivalent. (b) Share of different anthropogenic GHGs in total emissions in 2004 in terms of carbon dioxide equivalents (CO₂-eq). (c) Share of different sectors in total anthropogenic GHG emissions in 2004 in terms of CO₂-eq (Forestry includes deforestation).

*Includes only carbon dioxide (CO₂), methane (CH₄), nitrous oxide (N₂O), hydrofluorocarbons (HFCs), perfluorocarbons (PFCs) and sulphurhexafluoride (SF6), whose emissions are covered by the United Nations Framework Convention on Climate Change (UNFCCC). These GHGs are weighted by their 100-year Global Warming Potentials, using values consistent with reporting under the UNFCCC.

Fig 54.1. Global anthropogenic greenhouse gas (GHG) emissions

the increase in the past 5 years.[5] Most carbon dioxide emissions are from the burning of fossil fuels, such as coal, oil, and natural gas. Rising carbon dioxide is also related, to a lesser extent, to deforestation, which eliminates an important carbon sink. Carbon sinks, also known as greenhouse gas sinks, are reservoirs that absorb or take up released carbon from another part of the carbon cycle. The 4 major sinks on the planet are the atmosphere, the terrestrial biosphere (including trees and freshwater systems), oceans, and sediments. Currently, the atmosphere contains more than 380 parts per million (ppm) carbon dioxide (compared with approximately 280 in 1750), higher than it has been in at least 650 000 years.[1] The rate of increase is accelerating, up from 1.5 parts per million per year in the 1990s to 2.0 parts per million per year in 2006 because of increased burning of fossil fuels.[5]

The importance of the magnitude of greenhouse gas emissions is linked to the rate of release. In the distant geologic past, similar concentrations of atmospheric carbon dioxide have occurred, but they accumulated over many thousands of years, allowing for the slow, global biogeochemical cycles to adjust to the increases. Current emissions are being added to the atmosphere at 300 times this rate.[9,10] This confluence of speed and quantity of emissions has created the current, unprecedented rapid climate change. Although there is no longer any doubt that the Earth's climate is warming, there remains uncertainty about how rapid and extensive that change will be.

The Intergovernmental Panel on Climate Change (IPCC) is an international body of scientists formed by the World Meteorological Organization and the United Nations Environment Programme and tasked with evaluating the state-of-the-art science regarding climate change science and projected effects. Formed in 1988, the scientists developed a suite of scenarios for different levels of mitigation and adaptation in response to anthropogenic global climate change. For this work, Intergovernmental Panel on Climate Change investigators shared the Nobel Peace Prize with former US Vice President Al Gore in 2007. The Intergovernmental Panel on Climate Change functions by scientific consensus; thus, its projections are generally considered conservative.

The Intergovernmental Panel on Climate Change's scenarios predict that temperatures and sea level will continue to increase throughout the 21st Century. Even if greenhouse emissions were abruptly reduced to zero, the planet would continue to warm for decades until the energy stored in the system could equilibrate.[1] The possibility of reaching a tipping point at which abrupt, large, and irreversible change could be superimposed on current trends adds both urgency and further ambiguity to the situation. In this context, it is critical to understand that current human activities are accelerating climate change and that future human activities will affect their trajectories.

Tipping Points and Tipping Elements in Climate Change

A tipping point is a critical threshold at which a tiny perturbation can qualitatively alter the state of a system. A tipping element is a large-scale component of the Earth system that may pass a tipping point. A recent analysis based on a literature review after the 4th report of the Intergovernmental Panel on Climate Change and analysis by a broad spectrum of climate experts has defined and identified a short list of policy-relevant tipping elements and their approximate tipping points.[11] Only tipping elements that are affected by human activity and amenable to policy intervention on a 100-year time scale (the maximum human lifetime and span of political forward thinking) and that would result in large, qualitative, and potentially irreversible global change on a 1000-year time scale (the length of most civilizations) were considered. Two elements—loss of Arctic sea ice and partial disintegration of the Greenland ice sheets—are dangerously close to, if not already past, their tipping points. Five others—loss of the west Antarctic ice sheet, loss of boreal forests, loss of Amazonian rainforests, intensification of El Niño, and increase in west African monsoons—represent an intermediate likelihood of being surpassed during this century. With the exception of increased west African monsoons (that support vegetation and improve carrying capacity [the number of individuals who can be supported in a given area within natural resource limits] in parts of Africa), these tipping elements, if passed, will make the Earth less hospitable to human life by amplifying warming, damaging ecosystems, reducing biodiversity, raising sea level, and increasing drought. Although the 4th Intergovernmental Panel on Climate Change consensus analysis suggests that the worst ramifications of climate change can be averted if the average temperature is stabilized at 2°C to 2.5°C above 1990 levels, a subsequent estimate suggests that the tipping points for both Arctic sea ice loss and Greenland ice sheet loss will occur at or below +2°C. Additional independent scientific analyses utilizing data produced since the 4th report of the Intergovernmental Panel on Climate Change suggest that the timetable of reaching peak greenhouse gas emissions by 2015 and a reduction of 80% by 2050 may not be sufficient to avert major consequences from anthropogenic climate change.[12]

CLIMATE CHANGE – ASSOCIATED HEALTH EFFECTS IN CHILDREN

Because of their physical, physiologic, and cognitive immaturity, children are often more vulnerable to adverse health effects from environmental hazards compared with adults (see Chapter 3). As the climate changes, some existing environmental hazards will worsen and other new ones will emerge. Anticipated direct health consequences from climate change include increased morbidity and mortality from extreme weather events and weather disasters, higher rates of climate-sensitive infectious diseases, more air pollution-related disease and premature mortality, and more cases of heat stroke and heat-related death.[4] Within all of these categories, children have increased vulnerability compared with most other groups. These direct health threats are discussed in the next section, with an emphasis on children in the United States. Indirect threats are discussed briefly in the subsequent section.

DIRECT CLIMATE CHANGE – ASSOCIATED HEALTH THREATS TO CHILDREN

Extreme Weather Events and Weather Disasters

The Intergovernmental Panel on Climate Change predicts that it is "likely" or "very likely" that climate change will cause increased frequency and intensity of extreme weather events and weather disasters.[1] Often, these events are divided into floods, storms, and droughts. Floods represented 43% of weather-related disasters between 1992 and 2001 and are the most frequent weather-related disaster. Although less prevalent, droughts and associated famines are the most deadly weather-related disasters.[3] Industrialized nations, such as the United States, have systematically increased the risk to populations from flood events by developing coastlines and flood plains. In the United States, hurricanes and tornadoes are often the most dramatic and visible weather disasters. Evidence suggests that the frequency of category 4 and 5 hurricanes has increased over the past 30 years, but the observation period is still too short to attribute this change to increased sea surface temperature and climate change with high confidence.[13]

The health consequences associated with extreme weather events include death, injury, increases in infectious diseases, and post-traumatic mental health and behavior problems. Few studies have specifically examined such consequences in children. Globally, 66.5 million children annually were affected by natural disasters between 1990 and 2000.[14] Children everywhere are at risk of injury and death from storms and floods. In the industrialized world, infectious disease outbreaks follow natural disasters when water purification and sanitation systems are disrupted and people are unusually crowded in temporary shelters. These outbreaks are usually mild and well controlled, in contrast to the aftermath of similar catastrophes in developing nations, where disease outbreaks can be deadly. Mosquitoborne and other vectorborne illnesses may also be increased when storms or floods create large amounts of standing water suitable for breeding. Mental and emotional distress documented in children and adolescents after weather disasters include post-traumatic stress disorder and high rates of sleep disturbance, aggressive behavior, sadness, and substance use or abuse.[4] Children may lose or be displaced from their homes, lose precious or favorite belongings, or even experience injury to or death of a loved one. Some studies suggest that children have more persistent symptoms than adults who experience the same disaster, but further studies specific to children's experience are required. Community support services and early therapeutic intervention and postdisaster counseling can significantly reduce the medium- and long-term mental health burden in children. Experiences with Hurricane Katrina demonstrated that there were difficulties with tracking children's whereabouts, keeping children and caregivers together, and meeting the special medical needs of hospitalized infants and children.[15] Changes in zoning laws and stricter property insurance laws are adaptation methods that may influence where people choose to rebuild and create new developments, thereby affecting the size of the population at risk during coastal storms.

Infectious Diseases

Globally, infectious diarrhea is the second leading cause of death in young children; waterborne gastroenteritis is projected to increase under conditions of global warming. Currently, the World Health Organization (WHO) estimates that approximately 1.62 million children younger than 5 years die annually of diarrhea, with most cases attributable to contaminated water.[16] Although children in developed countries are unlikely to die of waterborne infections, they may suffer increased diarrheal and other types of infectious illness linked to climate change.[4] Events associated with El Niño (a periodic variation of temperature of the surface of the tropical Pacific Ocean that causes extreme weather, such as floods and droughts, in many regions of the world) serve as a model for global warming by altering weather for periods of several years in the direction of a hotter climate. During El Niño events, rates of hospitalizations of children for diarrhea increase. In one study, the rate of hospitalizations of children for diarrhea increased 8% per degree centigrade of temperature increase. Waterborne disease outbreaks in the United States exhibit a positive correlation with excess precipitation events, which are likely to increase with climate change; over a 45-year period, 68% of waterborne illness outbreaks have been associated with precipitation above the 80th percentile. Foodborne illness correlates positively with ambient temperature and is also likely to increase as the climate warms.[4,17,18]

Vectorborne infections are also affected by climate change. Both hosts (eg, rodents, insects, snails) and pathogens (eg, bacteria, viruses, parasites) can be sensitive to climatic variables, such as temperature, humidity, and rainfall. The ability to predict disease rates related to climate change is complicated by additional variables such as topography, land use, urbanization, human population distribution, level of economic development, and public health infrastructure.[19] There is no easy formula that predicts climate change-related infection risk with confidence. Many countries are working on early warning systems that help forecast increased infection risk.

Two vectorborne infections, malaria and dengue fever, already contribute significantly to the global burden of disease; the incidence of both diseases is expected to increase under a changing climate. Malaria and dengue fever are more dangerous to children than to adults. According to the World Health Organization, malaria causes nearly 250 million illnesses annually and more than 1 million deaths.[20] More than 3 billion people live in malaria-prone areas today. That number is likely to increase as climate change causes expansion of the range of host mosquitoes to higher altitudes and higher latitudes and as warmer temperatures speed the development of the parasite within the host vector.[21-25] Because they lack specific immunity, children experience disproportionately high levels of morbidity and mortality from malaria; 75% of malaria deaths occur in children younger than 5 years. Dengue fever currently threatens 2.5 billion people, but that number could increase to 6 billion as the climate warms and populations increase.[26] When dengue progresses to hemorrhagic fever, the untreated case-fatality rate is more than 20%. Children younger than 15 years are the most vulnerable to poor outcomes from dengue fever.

In the United States, vectorborne diseases, such as Lyme disease, West Nile virus, Western Equine encephalitis, and Eastern Equine encephalitis, are expected to be affected by climate change. The vectors of these diseases will likely increase in abundance and distribution under a changing climate.[27] The geographic distribution of *Ixodes* species ticks, the vector for Lyme disease, is already expanding with climate change.[28] Children 5 to 14 years of age (and adults 50 to 59 years of age) are more likely than the general population to contract the illness. Warmer temperatures increase replication of West Nile virus within its mosquito vector and promote natural selection of a more infectious strain.[29] Children, who spend more time outdoors than adults, may be at increased risk of exposure. Adaptations such as window screens, air conditioners, use of effective insect repellants, and vector-control programs can prevent infection.[30] Human adaptation has the capacity to significantly reduce the ultimate global disease burden.[26]

Air Pollution

Air pollutants such as fine particulates, nitrogen oxides, sulfur oxides, and ozone are likely to increase as countries adapt to hotter temperatures by using more energy to drive air conditioning and fans. If growing energy demands are met by burning more fossil fuels, ambient (outdoor) air pollution and greenhouse gas emissions will worsen. Children are especially vulnerable to short-term illness and long-term damage from ambient air pollution, because their lungs are developing and growing, they breathe at a higher rate than adults, and they spend more time outdoors engaging in vigorous physical activity.[31] Air pollutants cause respiratory and asthma hospitalizations, school absences, increased respiratory symptoms, and decrements in lung function. Formation of ozone, in particular, increases with increasing temperature, even without increases in the precursor primary pollutants (volatile organic hydrocarbons and oxides of nitrogen).[32] Children who are active in outdoor sports in communities with high ozone levels are at increased risk of developing asthma.[31] Additionally, high levels of particulate matter and other copollutants affect the ability of children's lungs to grow whether or not children have asthma. Rates of preterm births, low birth weight, and infant mortality are increased in communities with high levels of particulate air pollution.

A second change in air quality is the temperature-related increase in pollen production and other aeroallergens and mycotoxins.[4,33] Increased temperature can cause increases in amounts of pollens produced and can also affect the spatial distribution and density of plants, fungi, and molds. Some data suggest that plant products become more allergenic in higher levels of carbon dioxide and higher ambient temperatures. These changes may affect the incidence, prevalence, and severity of asthma, atopy, and other respiratory disease in children.[4,34] Some investigators argue that part of the current global increase in childhood asthma can be explained by increased exposure to aeroallergens driven by climate change.[35]

Thermal Stress

The Intergovernmental Panel on Climate Change concludes that with climate change, we are "virtually certain" to experience warmer days and warmer nights and that it is "very likely" that there will be an increase in the frequency of heat waves.[1] Fewer cold-related deaths are expected in a warmer world, but it is not known whether this will offset the expected increase in heat-related deaths.[26] Populations living in temperate climates, such as the United States and Europe, are likely to be hard hit initially, because global warming is most dramatic in these latitudes and there has been little time for these populations to acclimatize to changes in temperature. Observations on heat and mortality have been reported for decades and have gained recent attention with the heat waves of 2003 in Europe and of 2006 in Europe and North America. Heat-related deaths and hospitalizations are most common in the elderly. One study found that infants and young children may represent a second, albeit smaller, high-risk group,[36] but effects on children have not been adequately studied. Additionally, children spend more time outside, especially playing sports in the heat of the afternoon, putting them at increased risk of heat stroke and heat exhaustion.[37] Increased outdoor time during hot weather may also put children at higher risk of ultraviolet radiation-related skin damage, including basal cell carcinoma and malignant melanoma.[38] Some data indicate that heat-related mortality in the United States has decreased in recent years, in part associated with the increasing percentage of homes using air conditioning. More study is needed to determine the most cost-effective and efficient ways of preventing excess heat-related deaths through adaptation and acclimatization.

LONG-TERM AND INDIRECT CLIMATE CHANGE — ASSOCIATED HEALTH THREATS TO CHILDREN

Long-term and indirect effects on children's health from climate change will depend on both the extent of climate change over the next decades and the kinds of mitigation and adaptations strategies that are adopted now. How quickly and comprehensively greenhouse gas emissions can be stabilized and then reduced will have a significant effect on the rate and degree of warming, but even the most optimistic scenarios describe a 1°C to 2°C increase by the end of the century.[1] Food availability may be affected as land and ocean food productivity patterns shift.[39] More foods may be contaminated by mycotoxins.[40,41] Water availability may change, becoming much reduced in some regions, including during summer in the snow run-off dependent American west coast.[42] Coastal populations will be forced to move because of rises in sea level, and massive forced migrations are conceivable, driven by abrupt climate change, natural disasters, or political instability resulting from the unavailability of resources. Further, the world population is expected to grow by 50% to 9 billion by 2050, placing additional stresses on ecosystem services and increasing the demand for energy, fresh water, and food.[43] As long-term and indirect factors as well as more proximal climate-change associated health threats evolve, social and political institutions will need to respond with aggressive mitigation strategies and flexible adaptation strategies to preserve and protect public health, particularly for sensitive populations.

SOLUTIONS TO CLIMATE CHANGE: MITIGATION AND ADAPTATION STRATEGIES

The strategies to address the effects of climate change are known as mitigation and adaptation. Mitigation works to reduce the causes of climate change and is equivalent to primary prevention in pediatrics and public health. Specific strategies include reducing emissions through energy efficiency and using renewable energy sources,[44] increasing carbon sinks by forest preservation and reforestation, and developing greenhouse gas capture and sequestration technologies (Table 54.1). Adaptation involves developing public health strategies to minimize adverse health outcomes anticipated from climate change, the equivalent of secondary and tertiary prevention in pediatrics and public health. These strategies include improving disease surveillance and reporting, improving weather forecasting and early warning systems, advancing emergency management and disaster preparedness programs, developing and disseminating appropriate vaccines and medicines, and increasing public health education

Table 54.1: Examples of Mitigation Strategies*

	INTERNATIONAL	NATIONAL AND STATE	COMMUNITY	BUSINESSES, NONPROFIT ORGANIZATIONS, PROFESSIONAL SOCIETIES	INDIVIDUALS
Reduce Emissions and Increase Use of Renewable Energy Sources	■ Impose carbon emissions caps by treaty ■ Support clean, renewable technologies in developing countries ■ Support research and development and use of clean, renewable fuels ■ Promote energy conservation	■ Create greenhouse gas inventory ■ Impose carbon emissions caps at national and/or state levels ■ Increase solar, wind, energy-efficient biofuels, and other renewable sources ■ Invest in research and development and use of clean, renewable fuels ■ Raise corporate average fuel efficiency standards for vehicles ■ Promote energy conservation ■ Augment public transportation options	■ LEED† (Leadership in Energy and Environmental Design)-certify public buildings ■ Require energy audits and renovations for all public buildings ■ Install efficient lighting in public spaces ■ Reward businesses and home owners for energy efficiency ■ Maximize public transport, ticket idling cars, tax individual parking spaces, create bike lanes, enforce high-occupancy vehicle lanes ■ Develop sustainability awards ■ Promote energy conservation	■ Initiate energy audits of office ■ Work toward LEED certification† ■ Reward carpoolers or employees using public transport or walking/biking to work ■ Promote energy conservation ■ Buy Energy Star office equipment ■ Support telecommuting and flexible hours ■ Maximize video and teleconference meetings ■ Consider buying carbon offsets for travel to meetings‡	■ Drive less, use public transport, carpool ■ Use vehicles with highest gas mileage ■ Perform energy audits of home or business and make associated changes ■ Buy Energy Star appliances ■ Buy local foods ■ Engage in energy conservation efforts ■ Switch to compact fluorescent bulbs ■ Reduce waste

Table 54.1: Examples of Mitigation Strategies*, continued

	INTERNATIONAL	NATIONAL AND STATE	COMMUNITY	BUSINESSES, NONPROFIT ORGANIZATIONS, PROFESSIONAL SOCIETIES	INDIVIDUALS
Increase (Protect) Sinks	▪ Arrest deforestation ▪ Restore forests and wilderness	▪ Identify, protect, restore carbon sinks ▪ Protect national forests and wilderness areas	▪ Plant trees ▪ Reward construction of green roofs ▪ Build parks and green space	▪ Increase green space ▪ Put plants and trees in parking areas	▪ Plant trees and shrubs ▪ Support parks and greenways
Carbon Trapping and Sequestration	▪ Support research and development	▪ Support research and development	▪ Support research and development	▪ Support research and development	▪ Support through personal investments

*This table is not exhaustive. Many strategies are proposed and overlap among sectors. Additional information can be found at the following Web sites: http://www.grida.no/climate/ipcc_tar/wg3/index.htm, http://epa.gov/climatechange/wycd/index.html, and http://www.princeton.edu/~cmi/.

†The Leadership in Energy and Environmental Design (LEED) Green Building Rating System is a nationally accepted benchmark for the design, construction, and operation of high-performance green buildings. LEED gives building owners and operators the tools they need to have an immediate and measurable impact on their building's performance. LEED promotes a whole-building approach to sustainability by recognizing performance in 5 key areas of human and environmental health: sustainable site development, water savings, energy efficiency, materials selection, and indoor environmental quality.

‡Reduction of greenhouse gas production can be accomplished by buying carbon offsets whereby an individual or business can pay to reduce or remove GHG production in that company's name. For example, if a company agrees to buy 10 tons of carbon offsets, the seller guarantees that 10 fewer tons of GHG will enter the atmosphere.

Reprinted from Shea KM, American Academy of Pediatrics, Committee on Environmental Health. Global climate change and children's health. *Pediatrics.* 2007;120(5):e1359-e1367.[5]

and preparedness. Adaptation must involve policy and legislative actions, engineering responses, and personal behavior changes.

Effective implementation of mitigation and adaptation strategies requires actions from the global to local levels by governments, corporations, communities, and individuals. Furthermore, climate change is part of generalized global change, which includes population growth, land use, economic change, and evolving technology; all have effects on individual and public health. Any solutions that address climate change must be developed within the context of overall sustainable development (the use of resources by the current generation to meet current needs while ensuring that future generations will be able to meet their needs). Protecting the health of current and future generations requires that health professional undergo a fundamental shift in thinking; pediatricians, as advocates for children's health, can be leaders in a move away from a traditional focus on disease prevention to a broader, more integrated focus that encompasses environmental sustainability as synonymous with health. Preventing or minimizing the effects of climate change on children's health is beyond the control of individual pediatricians. Pediatricians can, however, play important public roles as advocates by individual example and through community and AAP chapter participation, political involvement, or collective advocacy at local, state, and national levels (Table 54.2).[45,46]

Frequently Asked Questions

Q *What impact can individual actions have on a problem as overwhelming as global climate change?*

A Forty-five percent of carbon dioxide emissions globally are a result of individual actions and choices. In the United States, that number is about 60%. Carbon dioxide emissions come from creating electricity to power homes and businesses and driving personal vehicles. Food choices, particularly beef, add to the individual "carbon footprint" and are amenable to change. Collectively, changes made to reduce individual carbon emissions through energy conservation and efficiency not only will have global impact but also are a necessary part of effective greenhouse gas mitigation strategies. Individuals can also speak out to peers and policy makers to increase awareness about the health impacts of climate change, and exercise influence through the media, consumer choices, and voting.

Q *How much time do we have before it is too late to do anything about climate change or avoid catastrophic climate change?*

A No one can say for sure, but the scientific consensus from the Intergovernmental Panel on Climate Change is that greenhouse gas emissions must peak by 2015 and be reduced by 80% by 2050 in order to avert the most dangerous consequences of climate change. This may

Table 54.2. Responding to Climate Change: A "Starter List" of What Health Professionals Can Do*

ADAPTING TO CLIMATE CHANGE

In your practice

- Maximize immunizations

- Educate your families on use of heat, air-quality, and ultraviolet radiation indices

- Identify and report unusual diseases or disease patterns

Working with local public health officials

- Engage in disaster preparedness and response planning

- Develop low toxicity approaches to vectorborne disease threats

- Augment surveillance of climate-related infectious diseases

In your community/region

- Protect local drinking water sources

- Support local, organic agriculture

- Advocate for greener energy power sources

MINIMIZING FUTURE CLIMATE CHANGE THROUGH REDUCING GREENHOUSE GAS EMISSIONS

In your practice

- "Green" your office and hospital; if building, use the Green Guide for Health Care and consider Leadership in Energy and Environmental Design (LEED) certification

- Institute policies to reward coworkers who bike/walk/carpool/use public transport (eg, more flexible work hours to accommodate public transportation schedules)

- Develop educational materials and signage about reducing greenhouse gas emissions

- Educate patients and families about actions to reduce climate change

- Educate medical students and residents on climate-related health problems

- Explore ways to do more by phone and electronically (continuing medical education, videocamera consultations)

- Acknowledge that pediatricians are generally perceived as trusted experts and that modeling sustainable lifestyles impacts coworkers and patients

In your home

- Switch to compact fluorescent bulbs or light-emitting diode (LED) lights if possible

- Turn equipment off at the power source when not in use

- Adjust your thermostat up in the summer and down in the winter

continued on 810

continued from page 809

Table 54.2. Responding to Climate Change: A "Starter List" of What Health Professionals Can Do*, *continued*

MINIMIZING FUTURE CLIMATE CHANGE THROUGH REDUCING GREENHOUSE GAS EMISSIONS

In your home, *continued*

- Do an energy audit

- Set computers to use existing features to automatically shift to lower power states or to turn off after extended periods of inactivity

- Eat lower on the food chain, local, organic, and in season when possible

- Reduce red meat intake, substitute vegetable proteins or fish

In your travels

- Walk and bike more

- Change to a more fuel-efficient car

- Carpool

- Consider public transport

- Minimize and consolidate long-distance travel

In your community

- Speak locally about health reasons to reduce greenhouse gas emissions

- Ask your mayor to sign the "mayor's pledge," become a Sierra Club "cool city"

- Offer expert testimony and write op-eds and letters to the editor on health threats from climate change

- Engage medical students and residents in advocacy for the planet

- Participate fully as a citizen—vote, educate elected officials, volunteer, run for public office

* Adapted from Shea KM, Balk SJ. Climate Change and Children's Health: What Health Professionals Need to Know and What We Can Do About It. Available on the Collaborative for Health and the Environment web site (http://www.healthandenvironment.org/?module=uploads&func=download&fileId=418).

be too generous a time frame according to some experts. Regardless, actions at all levels and in all regions should be underway now.

Q *Why should pediatricians be involved in climate change issues?*

A Pediatricians speak for children, a vulnerable and politically powerless constituency. Children cannot take the individual and political actions needed now that will define the climate and affect their health in the future. The history of pediatrics is one of advocacy for the rights and

International Agreements: The Kyoto Protocol and Beyond

The Kyoto Protocol is an international agreement among countries, worldwide, to limit emissions of greenhouse gases. The Kyoto Protocol aims to limits carbon dioxide, methane, hydrofluorocarbons, perfluorocarbons, and sulphur hexafluoride. It came into force in 2005 and requires 55 industrialized countries to reduce their greenhouse gas emissions to target levels 5.2% below those of 1990. If unable to, they must buy emission credits from countries that are under these levels.

At negotiations on climate change in Copenhagen in 2009, the countries of the world failed to reach a legally binding agreement to limit warming to no more than 2°C. The United States, China, Brazil, India, and South Africa did, however, agree to set a mitigation target to limit warming to no more than 2°C and, importantly, to take action to meet this objective. Another negotiation took place in Mexico in 2010, and established a "Green Climate Fund," to channel financial resources to developing countries and a registry to help developing countries match their projects with available international support. The climate change negotiations will continue in Durban, South Africa, in 2011.

health of children; working to mitigate and adapt to climate change is consistent with that history.

Q   *What practical actions can pediatricians take to fight climate change?*

A   Table 54.2 and the AAP policy statement "Global Climate Change and Child Health"[47] contain concrete actions and recommendations for pediatricians. Pediatricians and other pediatric health care professionals can work to reduce emissions in their personal and professional lives, support political changes to prepare for and lessen future climate change, and work with local and regional public health officials to develop strong, locally relevant adaptive strategies to minimize the health consequences from climate change.[48,49]

Q   *How should considerations about climate change be incorporated into pediatric practice?*

A   All patients and families can be taught about climate-related health conditions and given instruction on how to minimize personal exposures and risks. For example, parents and children should understand how to access, interpret and use local air quality and ultraviolet indices, daily pollen counts and heat advisories. Families should be encouraged to develop disaster response plans for the extreme weather events and weather disasters likely to occur in their locale. Regardless of whether or not pediatricians incorporate the recommendations into anticipatory guidance, they should remember that as health care providers they serve as important lifestyle role models and the choices they are seen making in their practices can educate and impact the behavior of others.

Resources

CLIMATE CHANGE SCIENCE

Intergovernmental Panel on Climate Change
Web site: www.ipcc.ch

US Climate Change Science Program
Web site: www.climatescience.gov

CLIMATE CHANGE SOLUTIONS

Carbon Mitigation Initiative at Princeton University
Web site: www.princeton.edu/~cmi/resources/stabwedge.htm

Environmental Defense Fund
Fight Global Warming: What You Can Do:
www.fightglobalwarming.com/page.cfm?tagID=135

Green Guide for Health Care
Web site: www.gghc.org

Medical Alliance to Stop Global Warming
Web site: www.psr.org/environment-and-health/global-warming/medical-alliance-global-warming.html

National Resources Defense Council
Solving Global Warming: It Can Be Done:
www.nrdc.org/globalWarming/solutions/default.asp

Sierra Club
10 Things You Can Do to Fight Global Warming:
www.sierraclub.org/globalwarming/tenthings

Stop Global Warming
Take Action: www.stopglobalwarming.org/sgw_takeaction.asp

Union of Concerned Scientists
Global Warming: What You Can Do: Ten Personal Solutions:
www.ucsusa.org/global_warming/solutions/ten-personal-solutions.htm

US Environmental Protection Agency

Energy Star: Protect Our Environment for Future Generations:
www.energystar.gov

US Green Building Society

Leadership in Energy and Environmental Design:
www.usgbc.org/DisplayPage.aspx?CategoryID=19

World Health Organization

www.who.int/globalchange/en/index.html

World Wildlife Federation

What You Can Do to Switch off Global Warming:
www.panda.org/about_wwf/what_we_do/climate_change/what_you_can_
do/index.cfm

References

1. Intergovernmental Panel on Climate Change. Climate Change 2007: Synthesis Report. Summary for Policy Makers. Available at: http://www.ipcc.ch/pdf/assessment-report/ar4/syr/ar4_syr_spm.pdf. Accessed April 7, 2011

2. G8 Summit Documents. Declaration of Leaders Meeting of Major Economies on Energy Security and Climate Change. Hokkaido Toyako, Japan. 7-9 July 2008. Available at: http://www.g8.utoronto.ca/summit/2008hokkaido/2008-climate.html. Accessed April 7, 2011

3. McMichael AJ, Woodruff RE, Hales S. Climate change and human health: present and future risks. *Lancet*. 2006;367(9513):859-869

4. Bunyavanich S, Landrigan CP, McMichael AJ, Epstein PR. The impact of climate change on child health. *Ambul Pediatr*. 2003;3(1):44-52

5. Shea KM; American Academy of Pediatrics, Committee on Environmental Health. Technical report: Global climate change and children's health. *Pediatrics*. 2007;120(5):e1359-e1367

6. Sheffield PE, Landrigan PJ. Global climate change and children's health: Threats and strategies for prevention. *Environ Health Perspect*. 2011;119(3):291-298

7. Tillett T. Climate change and children's health: Protecting and preparing our youngest. *Environ Health Perspect*. 2011;119(3):a132

8. Bernstein AS, Myers SS. Climate change and children's health. *Curr Opin Pediatr*. 2011;23(2):221-226

9. World Meterologic Organization World Data Centre for Greenhouse Gases. *Greenhouse Gas Bulletin: The State of Greenhouse Gases in the Atmosphere Using Global Observations up to December 2006*. No 3. November 2007. Available at: http://gaw.kishou.go.jp/wdcgg/products/bulletin/Bulletin2006/ghg-bulletin-3.pdf. Accessed April 7, 2011

10. National Climatic Data Center, National Oceanic and Atmospheric Administration. Global Warming: Frequently Asked Questions. Available at: http://www.ncdc.noaa.gov/oa/climate/globalwarming.html Accessed 27 October 2008. Accessed April 7, 2011

11. Lenton TM, Held H, Kriegler E, et al. Tipping elements in the Earth's climate system. *Proc Natl Acad Sci*. 2008;105(6):1786-1793

12. Hansen J, Sato M, Reudy R, et al. Dangerous human-made interference with climate: a GISS model E study. *Atmos Chem Phys*. 2007;7:2287-2312.

13. Webster PJ, Holland GJ, Curry JA, Chang JR. Changes in tropical cyclone number, duration and intensity in a warming environment. *Science.* 2005;309(5742):1844-1846

14. Penrose A, Takaki M. Children's rights in emergencies and disasters. *Lancet.* 2006;367(9511):698-699

15. Johnson C, Redlener I. Hurricane Katrina, children, and pediatric heroes. Hands-on stories by and of our colleagues helping families during the most costly natural disaster in US history. *Pediatrics.* 2006;117(Suppl 2):S355-S460

16. World Health Organization. Water, Sanitation, and Hygiene Links to Health. Geneva, Switzerland: World Health Organization; 2004. Available at: http://www.who.int/water_sanitation_health/publications/facts2004/en/index.html. Accessed April 7, 2011

17. Kovats RS, Edwards SJ, Hajat S, Armstrong BG, Ebi KL, Menne B. The effect of temperature on food poisoning: a time-series analysis of salmonellosis in ten European countries. *Epidemiol Infect.* 2004;132(3):443-453

18. Fleury M, Charron DF, Holt JD, Allen OB, Maarouf AR. A time series analysis of the relationship of ambient temperature and common bacterial enteric infections in two Canadian provinces. *Int J Biometerol.* 2006;50(6):385-391

19. Sutherst RW. Global change and human vulnerability to vector-borne diseases. *Clin Microbiol Rev.* 2004;17(1):136-173

20. World Health Organization. World Malaria Report 2008. Available at: http://www.who.int/malaria/wmr2008/. Accessed 27 October 2008.

21. Bouma MJ. The El Niño southern oscillation and the historic malaria epidemics on the Indian subcontinent and Sri Lanka: an early warning system for future epidemics? *Trop Med Int Health.* 1996;1(1):86-96

22. Cullen JR. An epidemiological early warning system for malaria control in northern Thailand. *Bull World Health Organ.* 1984;62(1):107-114

23. Ruiz D, Poveda G, Velez ID, et al. Modelling entomological-climatic interactions of Plasmodium falciparum malaria transmission in two Colombian endemic-regions: Contributions to a national malaria early warning system. *Malaria J.* 2006;5:66

24. Thomson MC, Connor SJ. The development of malaria early warning systems for Africa. *Trends Parasitol.* 2001;17(9):438-445

25. Epstein RP, Mills E, eds. *Climate Change Futures; Health, Ecological and Economic Dimensions.* Boston, MA: The Center of Health and the Global Environment, Harvard Medical School; November 2005

26. McMichael A, Githeko A. Human health. In: McCarthy JT, Canziani OF, Leary NA, Dokken DJ, White KS, eds. *Climate Change 2001: Impacts, Adaptations, and Vulnerability.* Geneva, Switzerland: Intergovernmental Panel on Climate Change; 2001:453-485. Available at: http://www.grida.no/climate/ipcc_tar/wg2/pdf/wg2TARchap9.pdf. Accessed April 7, 2011

27. US Climate Change Science Program, Subcommittee on Global Change Research. *Analyses and Effects of Global Change on Human Health and Welfare and Human Systems.* (SAP 4.6) Washington, DC: US Environmental Protection Agency; 2008. Available at http://www.climatescience.gov/Library/sap/sap4-6/final-report/sap4-6-final-all.pdf. Accessed April 7, 2011

28. Lindgren E, Tälleklin L, Polfeldt T. , Impact of climatic change on the northern latitude limit and population density of the disease-transmitting European tick *Ixodes ricinus. Environ Health Perspect.* 2000;108(2):119-123

29. Kilpatrick AM, Meola MA, Moudy RM, Kramer LD. Temperature, viral genetics, and the transmission of West Nile virus by *Culex pipiens* mosquitoes. *PLoS Pathog.* 2008;4(6):e1000092. Available at: http://www.plospathogens.org/article/info%3Adoi%2F10.1371%2Fjournal.ppat.1000092 Accessed April 7, 2011

30. Reiter P, Lathrop S, Bunning M, et al. Texas lifestyle limits transmission of Dengue fever. *Emerg Infect Dis.* 2003;9(1):86-89

31. American Academy of Pediatrics, Committee on Environmental Health. Ambient air pollution: health hazards to children. *Pediatrics.* 2004;114(6):1699-1707

32. Knowlton K, Rosenthal JE, Hogrefe C, et al. Assessing ozone-related health impacts under a climate change. *Environ Health Perspect.* 2004;112(15):1557-1563

33. D'Amato G, Cecchi L. Effects of climate change on environmental factors in allergic respiratory disease. *Clin Exp Allergy.* 2008;38(8):1264-1274

34. Shea KM, Truckner RT, Weber RW, Peden DB. Climate change and allergic disease. *J Allergy Clin Immunol.* 2008;122(3):443-453

35. Beggs PJ, Bambrick HJ. Is the global rise of asthma an early impact of anthropogenic climate change? *Environ Health Perspect.* 2005;113(8):915-919

36. Centers for Disease Control and Prevention. Heat-related deaths—four states, July–August 2001, and United States, 1979–1999. *MMWR Morb Mortal Wkly Rep.* 2002;51(26):567-570

37. American Academy of Pediatrics, Committee on Sports Medicine and Fitness. Climatic heat stress and the exercising child and adolescent. *Pediatrics.* 2000;106(1 Pt 1):158-159

38. American Academy of Pediatrics, Council on Environmental Health and Section on Dermatology. Ultraviolet radiation: a hazard to children and adolescents. *Pediatrics.* 2011;127(3):588-597

39. Slingo JM, Challinor AJ, Hoskins BJ, Wheeler TR. Introduction: food crops in a changing climate. *Philos Trans R Soc Lond B Biol Sci.* 2005;360(1463):1983-1989

40. Paterson RRM, Lima N. How will climate change affect mycotoxins in food? *Food Res Int.* 2010;43:1902-1914

41. Wu F, Bhatnagar D, Bui-Klimke T, et al. Climate change impacts on mycotoxin risks in US maize. *World Mycotox J.* 2011;4:79-93

42. Barnett TP, Adam JC, Lettenmaier DP. Potential impacts of a warmer climate on water availability in snow-dominated regions. *Nature.* 2005;438(7066):303-309

43. United Nations Population Division. World Population Prospects: the 2006 revision. Available at: http://esa.un.org/unpp/ Accessed April 7, 2011

44. Smith KR, Jerrett M, Anderson HR, et al. Public health benefits of strategies to reduce greenhouse-gas emissions: health implications of short-lived greenhouse pollutants. *Lancet.* 2009;374(9707):2091-2103

45. Gruen RL, Campbell EG, Blumenthal D. Public roles of US physicians: community participation, political involvement, and collective advocacy. *JAMA.* 2006;296(20):2467-2475

46. Rushton FE Jr; American Academy of Pediatrics, Committee on Community Health Services. The pediatrician's role in community pediatrics. *Pediatrics.* 2005;115(4):1092-1094

47. American Academy of Pediatrics, Committee on Environmental Health. Global climate change and child health. *Pediatrics.* 2007;120(5):1149-1152

48. Frumkin H, Hess J, Luber G, Malilay J, McGeehin M. Climate change: the public health response. *Am J Public Health.* 2008;98(3):435-445

49. Jackson R, Shields KN. Preparing the US health community for climate change. *Annu Rev Public Health.* 2008;29:57-73

Chapter 55

Multiple Chemical Sensitivity

■ ■ ■ ■ ■ ■

DEFINITION

Multiple chemical sensitivity, also known as "environmental illness" or "idiopathic environmental intolerance," is a highly controversial condition. There is overlap between the syndrome and other ill-defined conditions, such as fibromyalgia, chronic fatigue syndrome, sick building syndrome, and Gulf War syndrome. Although it most commonly is seen in adults, conditions attributed to multiple chemical sensitivity are reported to occur in children and adolescents.[1,2] To respond to parental concerns, pediatricians should be familiar with the condition.

Multiple chemical sensitivity has been defined as an acquired, chronic disorder characterized by recurrent symptoms, referable to multiple organ systems, occurring reproducibly in response to exposure to many chemically unrelated compounds at doses far below those established in the general population to cause harmful effects.[3,4] No single test or physiologic function correlates with multiple chemical sensitivity; the symptoms improve when the incitants are removed. In contradistinction to sick building syndrome, symptoms are not associated with a single physical environment but can occur anywhere.

CLINICAL SYMPTOMS

Exposure to low levels of a wide variety of chemically unrelated substances elicits a myriad of complaints in people with multiple chemical sensitivity. Adults with this condition often can recall an initial sensitizing exposure to an overpowering chemical, often occurring in the workplace. Symptoms can involve any organ system and commonly include headache, fatigue, gastrointestinal problems, joint and muscle pains, skin problems, and upper respiratory tract complaints. Most patients have neurologic or neuropsychological effects (such as "mental fog" or impaired cognition, confusion, memory loss, paresthesias, irritability, and depression) as prominent features of the syndrome. Other features include malaise, dizziness, burning sensations, and breathlessness. In children and adolescents, hyperactivity and attention deficits have been cited by some as developmental consequences of multiple chemical sensitivity.[5]

Symptoms can wax and wane unpredictably over time; sensitivity expands from a single "inciting" chemical to a wide variety of unrelated substances. Pesticides, fragrances in perfumes, after shaves or other household products, copy machine emissions, latex, food dyes and additives, cigarette smoke, formaldehyde, nylon fabrics, rayon material, and gases released from new carpets are substances commonly implicated in multiple chemical sensitivity.[6] Some people complain of foul odors (cacosmia) from chemicals or perfumes as triggers for their symptoms. The olfactory nerve mediates odor perception, while branches of the trigeminal nerve perceive irritation and pungency for taste and smell. Odor seems to be a prominent factor in precipitating the symptoms and serves as an important warning for the presence of toxic exposures. Most investigators agree that an explanation of the role of odor is a necessary component of any model of the causes of multiple chemical sensitivity.

Reportedly, symptoms also can migrate from one target organ system to another over time (switching). The progressive nature of symptoms, experienced after smaller and smaller doses of precipitants, the olfactory warning of offending odors, and the progressive restrictions on the patient's activities and habitable environments all characterize this condition.

EPIDEMIOLOGY

One major difficulty in studying the epidemiology of multiple chemical sensitivity is the lack of a case definition agreed on by the medical and scientific community. Many published reports consist of case series or the clinical experiences of referral practices; none describe affected children. Small surveys have estimated the prevalence rates of self-reported multiple chemical sensitivity among adults to be approximately 12%,[7,8] although one subspecialty-based study (allergy, otolaryngology, occupational medicine) found an overall prevalence rate ranging from 5% to 27% of referrals.[9] None of these studies included children. The prevalence of food additive intolerance in children and adolescents 5 to 16 years of age has been estimated at 1% to 2%,[10] and it is much lower for immune-mediated allergy to food additives.

HISTORICAL BACKGROUND

The late Theron Randolph, an allergist from Chicago, first described multiple chemical sensitivity during the 1950s.[11] He believed that traditional allergists defined "sensitivity" too narrowly by limiting it exclusively to antibody-antigen reactions. He hypothesized that foods and chemicals might cause other derangements of the immune system. Increasing exposure to petroleum products, pesticides, synthetic textiles, and food additives in modern life were identified as responsible for his patients' health problems, which included mental and behavioral disturbances, as well as rhinitis, headache, and asthma. A group of physicians, often called "clinical ecologists," who supported Dr Randolph's concept of environmental illness, founded the American Academy of Environmental Medicine.

In several position papers, traditional medical organizations have questioned the scientific basis of this syndrome. The American Academy of Allergy, Asthma and Immunology asserted that there were no adequate studies to support the theories of the clinical ecologists and, in 1986, issued a position statement stating that the diagnostic and therapeutic principles of clinical ecology were based on unproven methods.[12] Similarly, the American College of Physicians in 1989 and the American Medical Association in 1992 criticized clinical ecology.[13,14] A position statement by the American College of Occupational and Environmental Medicine in 1999 called for more research into the "phenomenon" of multiple chemical sensitivity.[15]

PROPOSED CAUSATIVE MECHANISMS

A number of different models have been proposed to explain multiple chemical sensitivity. A model of immunologic dysfunction postulates that chemicals may damage the immune system so that it no longer functions normally. However, no clinical laboratory, other than those associated with clinical ecologists, has found consistent immune abnormalities in patients with multiple chemical sensitivity.[16]

Some have proposed that altered activity of receptors, such as the vanilloid and/or N-methyl-D-aspartate receptors, in the central and peripheral nervous systems underlie the reactions to xenobiotics experienced by individuals with multiple chemical sensitivity.[17] Another theory of causation involves the impaired metabolism of toxic chemicals, such that altered biotransformations lead to idiosyncratic toxic effects of common substances. One study found genotypic differences in a group of women with multiple chemical sensitivity versus controls in homozygous active CYP2D6 and rapid NAT2 enzyme systems. Gene-gene interactions between both enzymes predicted a substantially elevated risk in group membership.[18]

Investigators also have proposed a classic conditioned response to odor as an explanation for multiple chemical sensitivity. After an initial traumatic exposure to a strong-smelling odor, subsequent exposure may cause a conditioned response to much lower concentrations of the chemical. This conditioned response may be accompanied by varying degrees of "stimulus generalization" to the development of symptoms in response to other strong odors. Some researchers have suggested that an extreme form of this response be called an "odor-triggered panic attack."[19]

Affective disorders, somatoform disorders, and anxiety are the most frequent psychological conditions used to explain multiple chemical sensitivity.[20] People in whom multiple chemical sensitivity develops have a high degree of preexisting psychiatric morbidity and a tendency toward somatization.[21] These findings suggest that psychological factors, although not necessarily causative, may predispose some people to develop a generalized chemical sensitivity. Comorbidities, such as post-traumatic stress disorder or childhood physical or sexual abuse, also may have roles as underlying determinants of vulnerability to the later development of multiple chemical sensitivity.[22]

The limbic-olfactory model provides a speculative biological explanation for affective and cognitive symptoms. The model depends on the anatomic links between the olfactory nerve, the limbic system, and other regions of the brain. Subconvulsive kindling (the ability of a subthreshold electrical or chemical stimulus to cause a response) and time-dependent sensitization are central nervous system constructs that provide a mechanism by which low-level chemical exposures can be amplified and produce symptoms referable to multiple organ systems.[23] Other proposed causes, such as "neuropathic" porphyria[24] or hypersensitization to yeast, have been discredited.

CLINICAL EVALUATION OF A CHILD BELIEVED TO HAVE CHEMICAL SENSITIVITY

The pediatrician should approach the evaluation of a child whose parents believe that multiple chemical sensitivity is the cause of the child's symptoms in the same manner as any other problem: with a thorough history, a physical examination, and a methodical workup. Table 55.1 offers some diagnostic criteria that, although not studied systematically, may be applicable to children and adolescents. By using the history and selecting appropriate clinical tests, the pediatrician should first rule in or rule out conditions that are part of the differential diagnosis. Other diseases to consider are those with symptoms that are nonspecific and inconstant, including Lyme disease, Munchausen by proxy, or psychosocial problems such as school phobia. The assessment should be directed towards the inclusion or exclusion of other diagnoses, such as asthma, migraine, allergies, or an autoimmune disease. Specific environmental causes of systemic illness should be considered. Carbon monoxide poisoning, for example, can produce generalized complaints, such as headache, fatigue, dizziness, nausea, and lethargy and confusion. Chronic poisoning with heavy metals such as mercury, arsenic, or lead can sometimes result in behavioral symptoms and appetite disturbances.

Table 55.1: Diagnostic Elements of Multiple Chemical Sensitivity Syndrome in Children*

Nature of Incitants Provoking a Response

■ Responses to offending environmental toxicants occur at levels of exposure below the 2.5th percentile for responses in the general population.

■ Child responds to multiple substances that are unrelated chemically. The symptoms are not confined to one environment (eg, only "sick" buildings).

Biological Plausibility, Identifiable Exposure

■ Symptoms are reproducible with exposure with reasonable consistency.

■ Symptoms resolve after removal of incitant exposures.

■ An identifiable exposure preceded the onset of the problem.

Characteristics of Responses

■ Adverse responses affect more than one body system.

■ Primary complaints include neuropsychological symptoms.

■ The child exhibits altered sensitivity to odor.

■ The disorder is chronic.

Diagnosis

■ No single, accepted test of physiological function correlates with the symptoms.

Subjective Responses and Ameliorative Actions of Affected Children

■ The caregivers and/or child perceive the child's response as unpleasant.

■ The family has sought professional advice.

■ The individual's caregivers believe he or she has a disorder.

■ The family takes action to avoid exposures to symptom-inducing chemicals.

*Modified from Nethercott JR, Davidoff LL, Curbow B, Abbey H.[25]

Chronic or seasonal upper respiratory tract symptoms and wheezing suggest the possibility that the child has allergies and asthma, respectively. Although rhinorrhea, nasal obstruction, and sneezing would suggest an allergic etiology, children and adolescents may present with fatigue and irritability because of sleep disorders, perhaps induced by upper airway obstruction. Allergic stigmata found on physical examination, supported with appropriate laboratory studies, skin testing, and in cases of suspected reactive airway disease, pulmonary function tests, will suggest a diagnosis. Headache and dizziness, common complaints in multiple chemical sensitivity, are sometimes seen in children and adolescents with sinus disease.

Psychiatric disorders in parents and/or children, dysfunctional family dynamics, or child abuse and neglect must be considered in the evaluation of children or adolescents presenting for assessment of multiple chemical sensitivity syndrome.

A positive family history for psychiatric diagnoses and treatment may be common in these patients. For some families, the illness may serve as a coping strategy or a more socially acceptable medical condition within which to express depressive symptoms. Children or adolescents may be attracted to the attention they gain when they are in the dependency role of patient.

DIAGNOSTIC METHODS

No laboratory tests are diagnostic, although a number of unproven tests have been proposed. For example, the use of positron emission tomography and single photon emission computed tomography scans has not been standardized or validated and is not recommended. Diagnostic provocation-neutralization tests with different chemicals ("desensitization" routines of frequent injections or sublingual or dermal application of incitants), advocated by clinical ecologists, have been repudiated as being without scientific basis or validity and may cause harm themselves. The American College of Physicians reviewed 15 studies of provocation-neutralization testing performed by clinical ecologists and criticized the introduction of bias, lack of controls, and their uniformly poor methodologic designs.[13]

Testing of hair, blood, urine, or other tissues to screen for environmental chemicals generally is not helpful. When appropriate, laboratory testing to rule in or rule out other diagnoses or underlying medical conditions should be performed. Testing should be performed only at laboratories that adhere to the guidelines for quality control and laboratory operations established by the Clinical Laboratory Improvement Amendments (CLIA) of 1988.

TREATMENT

The demands of adult patients with multiple chemical sensitivity on health care professionals, their high use of health care resources, and their dissatisfaction with proffered advice, especially if that advice suggests psychological counseling as a management option, are frustrating for patient and practitioner. Patients with multiple chemical sensitivity are high-frequency users of medical facilities and suffer a considerable amount of functional disability because of their complaints and the strategies they must use to get through the day. Parental overuse of care services can be challenging to pediatricians, who must nevertheless continue to offer their availability and support in the best interests of the child.

Proposed therapies include restricted, rotating diets, provocation-neutralization, and the use of saunas for chemical detoxification. Patients with multiple chemical sensitivity seek out a variety of treatments, not only from physicians but also clinical ecologists, naturopaths, homeopaths, and other practitioners. Clinical ecologists and others may recommend herbs, oxygen, oral nystatin, and minerals to treat their patients by improving their "tolerance" of the environment, although a scientific basis for such treatments is lacking. Some postulate that sufferers of multiple chemical sensitivity have deficits of essential cofactors or enzymes necessary for chemical "detoxification"; they prescribe dietary supplements, herbs, antioxidants, and vitamins to repair such theoretical deficiencies.

Some therapies used hold special risks for children and adolescents, and their use should be discouraged. Parents should be warned against potentially harmful and expensive remedies, such as chelation, gamma globulin injections, catharsis, or "sweat therapies," because there is little scientific evidence that these are effective for treatment. Chelation can cause death from hypocalcemia, neurologic damage, and other adverse events (see Chapter 46). Severely restricted diets may not supply the essential protein, minerals, vitamins, and other nutrients needed for a growing body. Desensitization remedies and products containing multiple herbs, dietary supplements, and/or megavitamins may be especially harmful to children and adolescents who are still developing. Children may have limited capacity to detoxify certain herbs, minerals, hormones, and dietary supplements through the liver and kidneys, with a consequent higher risk of toxic reactions. They may experience allergic reactions to such substances as well as those used in "desensitization" routines.

Many patients restrict their activities and reconstruct their habitats so that they can avoid those environmental agents causing symptoms, essentially living in a relatively chemical-free environment. There are known sensitizing chemicals in some household products, such as paraphenylenediamine found in hair dyes and henna-based temporary tattoos,[26,27] colors (eg, tartrazine, azo dyes, amaranth), flavorings (eg, ethylvanilline, monosodium glutamate), antioxidants (eg, butylated hydroxytoluene) and other preservatives (eg, benzoic acid, sodium benzoate, sulphites) in foods,[2,10] and some common chemicals used as fragrances in a range of products from detergents to toothpaste to moisturizers. Avoidance of such compounds when purchasing household items is an important strategy pursued by affected families. A word of caution: some "fragrance-free" home products actually contain chemicals to mask the natural odor of the shampoo or sunscreen; other "fragrance free" products still use preservatives, such as benzyl alcohol.[28]

Some adults use barrier clothing such as special masks, gloves, coveralls, and even self-contained breathing apparatus in the attempt to avoid chemical triggers. The disability in adults is such that they often isolate themselves from others socially and cannot hold a job. Children and adolescents who cannot attend school or develop normal peer relationships because of multiple chemical sensitivity would be similarly disabled. These children should be managed in consultation with a social worker or other mental health professional.

Newer inventories show promise for standardizing the diagnosis and measuring the impact and severity of multiple chemical sensitivity.[29] Biopsychological modalities of management, including biofeedback, electrophysiological monitoring, coping strategies, cognitive-behavioral therapy, family-centered therapy, and behavioral modification (psychological deconditioning) techniques are worth investigating in children.[30] Addressing directly any parental mistrust and hostility to allopathic medicine is important. Offering to work with families should extend to collaboration with school systems, social services, and other community-based agencies in helping families cope with the condition.

CONCLUSIONS

Examining a child purported to have multiple chemical sensitivity is a challenge for the pediatrician who is faced with treating the child's health as it fits into the family's belief system. Exploring the basis for the beliefs and keeping an open mind to the different values that underlie them will allow effective and compassionate use of the pediatrician's medical knowledge and skills.

Frequently Asked Questions

Q   *I have been told that my child has a short attention span and that he frequently is inattentive in class. The teacher has suggested psychological testing. My child is fine at home. Could these problems be related to chemical exposure at school?*

A   A thorough evaluation of the child's difficulty and appropriate testing are initial steps in dealing with this problem. Sources of potential environmental contamination cited in schools include cleaning agents, art supplies (eg, glues, markers, and aerosol sprays), pesticides, and diesel exhaust fumes from school buses. Dust and molds also are sources of indoor air pollution. Symptoms in one setting only (the school) may suggest an environmental etiology. While performing such a thorough evaluation, pediatricians also should keep in mind that parental anxieties about learning and behavior problems might be displaced toward concerns about chemical exposures in the school.

Q   *My child is being made sick by the chemicals that she is exposed to in school. Can you, as my pediatrician, intervene and help me decrease my child's exposure to chemicals in the school?*

A   Parents often ask pediatricians to write a letter supporting the child's withdrawal from some activity or area in the school. In these instances, the pediatrician should be open-minded but careful about fostering negative associations between the child and the child's environment. A thorough history and physical examination of the child, with attention to finding or excluding other medical diagnoses, is an essential first step. Another issue raised by this question is less obvious but of crucial importance in considering the problem of chemical sensitivity in children. It usually is the parent who attributes the child's symptoms to chemical exposures in various environments, and the parent may have fixed beliefs about the causal relationship in their advocacy for their child. Although there might sometimes be a temporal relationship between the exposure and symptoms, the association may or may not be causal. The pediatrician can be proactive in working closely with both the parents and school officials toward an assessment of the school environment and an educational solution that serves the best interests of the child. A regional pediatric environmental health specialty unit and local and/or state health department officials may be of assistance as additional resources to the pediatrician, the school, and the family.

Q *What do I need to do to my home to prevent my child from being exposed to chemicals that might be toxic?*

A It is important for parents to understand that their child's exposure to chemicals is cumulative: the sum of inhalation, ingestion, and dermal exposures. Parents should be encouraged to consider all activities and situations in which their child might be exposed. The home may be a source of environmental exposures (Chapter 4). The school environment may be a source of additional exposures to chemicals (see Chapter 11). One common environmental exposure is to secondhand tobacco smoke—thus, one of the most important things parents can do is to eliminate their child's exposure to secondhand tobacco smoke. Parents should also know that "thirdhand" tobacco smoke[31]—the smoke residue remaining on items such as clothing and furniture—may be irritating. Smoking should be prohibited inside the home and smokers should change their clothes and wash their hands before interacting with a child. The substitution of environmentally friendly alternatives for household solvents, cleaners, pesticides, and other chemicals are prudent measures that all families can adopt.

References

1. Woolf A. A 4-year-old girl with manifestations of multiple chemical sensitivities. *Environ Health Perspect.* 2000;108(12):1219–1223
2. Inomata N. Multiple chemical sensitivities following intolerance to azo dye in sweets in a 5-year-old girl. *Allergol Int.* 2006;55(2):203-205
3. Cullen MR. The worker with multiple chemical sensitivities: an overview. *Occup Med.* 1987;2(4):655–661
4. Multiple chemical sensitivity: a 1999 consensus. *Arch Environ Health.* 1999;54(3):147–149
5. Kidd PM. Attention deficit/hyperactivity disorder (ADHD) in children: rationale for its integrative management. *Altern Med Rev.* 2000;5(5):402–428
6. Hu H, Stern A, Rotnitzky A, Schlesinger L, Proctor S, Wolfe J. Development of a brief questionnaire for screening for multiple chemical sensitivity syndrome. *Toxicol Ind Health.* 1999;15(6):582–588
7. Kreutzer R, Neutra RR, Lashuay N. Prevalence of people reporting sensitivities to chemicals in a population-based survey. *Am J Epidemiol.* 1999;150(1):1–12
8. Meggs WJ, Dunn KA, Bloch RM, Goodman PE, Davidoff AL. Prevalence and nature of allergy and chemical sensitivity in a general population. *Arch Environ Health.* 1996;51(4):275–282

9. Kutsogiannis DJ, Davidoff AL. A multiple center study of multiple chemical sensitivity syndrome. *Arch Environ Health.* 2001;56(3):196–207

10. Madsen C. Prevalence of food additive intolerance. *Hum Exp Toxicol.* 1994;13(6):393-399

11. Randolph TG. Sensitivity to petroleum including its derivatives and antecedents. *J Lab Clin Med.* 1952;40:931–932

12. Executive Committee of the American Academy of Allergy and Immunology. Clinical ecology. *J Allergy Clin Immunol.* 1986;78(2):269–271

13. American College of Physicians. Clinical ecology. *Ann Intern Med.* 1989;111(2):168–178

14. Council on Scientific Affairs, American Medical Association. Clinical ecology. *JAMA.* 1992;268(24):3465–3467

15. American College of Occupational and Environmental Medicine. ACOEM position statement. Multiple chemical sensitivities: idiopathic environmental intolerance. *J Occup Environ Med.* 1999;41(11):940–942

16. Simon GE, Daniell W, Stockbridge H, Claypoole K, Rosenstock L. Immunologic, psychological, and neuropsychological factors in multiple chemical sensitivity. A controlled study. *Ann Intern Med.* 1993;119(2):97–103

17. Pall ML, Anderson JH. The vanilloid receptor as a putative target of diverse chemicals in multiple chemical sensitivity. *Arch Environ Heal.* 2004;59(7):363-369

18. McKeown-Eyssen G. Case-control study of genotypes in multiple chemical sensitivity: CYP2D6, NAT1, NAT2, PON1, PON2 and MTHFR. *Int J Epidemiol.* 2004;33(5):971-978

19. Staudenmayer H. Multiple chemical sensitivities or idiopathic environmental intolerances: psychophysiologic foundation of knowledge for a psychogenic explanation. *J Allergy Clin Immunol.* 1997;99(4):434–437

20. Terr AI. Environmental illness. A clinical review of 50 cases. *Arch Intern Med.* 1986;146(1): 145–149

21. Black DW, Rathe A, Goldstein RB. Environmental illness. A controlled study of 26 subjects with "20th century disease." *JAMA.* 1990;264(24):3166–3170

22. Black DW, Okiishi C, Gable J, Schlosser S. Psychiatric illness in the first-degree relatives of persons reporting multiple chemical sensitivities. *Toxicol Ind Health.* 1999;15(3-4):410–414

23. Ross PM, Whyser J, Covello VT, et al. Olfaction and symptoms in the multiple chemical sensitivities syndrome. *Prev Med.* 1999;28(5):467–480

24. Ellefson RD, Ford RE. The porphyrias: characteristics and laboratory tests. *Regul Toxicol Pharmacol.* 1996;24(1 Pt 2):S119–S125

25. Nethercott JR, Davidoff LL, Curbow B, Abbey H. Multiple chemical sensitivities syndrome: toward a working case definition. *Arch Environ Health.* 1993;48(1):19–26

26. Sosted H, Johansen JD, Andersen KE, Menne T. Severe allergic hair dye reactions in 8 children. *Contact Dermatitis.* 2006;54(2):87-91

27. Marcoux D, Couture-Trudel PM, Riboulet-Delmas G, Sasseville D. Sensitization to parapheylenediamine from a streetside temporary tattoo. *Pediatr Dermatol.* 2002;19(6):498-502

28. Scheinman PL. The foul-side of fragrance-free products: what every clinician should know about managing patients with fragrance allergy. *J Am Acad Dermatol.* 1999;41(6):1020-1024

29. Miller CS, Prihoda TJ. The Environmental Exposure and Sensitivity Inventory (EESI): a standardized approach for measuring chemical intolerances for research and clinical applications. *Toxicol Ind Health.* 1999;15(3-4):370–385

30. Spyker DA. Multiple chemical sensitivities—syndrome and solution. *J Toxicol Clin Toxicol.* 1995;33(2):95–99

31. Winickoff JP, Friebely J, Tanski SE, et al. Beliefs about the health effects of "thirdhand" smoke and home smoking bans. *Pediatrics.* 2009;123(1):e74-e79

Chapter 56

Nontherapeutic Use of Antibiotics in Animal Agriculture

■ ■ ■ ■ ■ ■

Agricultural antibiotics, including ones used for nontherapeutic purposes, create environmental reservoirs in which bacteria are exposed to antibiotics, contributing significantly to the development and dissemination of antibiotic resistance. Over time, many strains of bacteria have evolved resistance to antibiotics; resistant bacteria are "selected" and survive. Antibiotic resistance in many pediatric pathogens is widespread, including infectious agents encountered in community-acquired (eg, *Campylobacter* species, *Salmonella* species) and hospital-acquired (eg, *Enterococcus* species, *Staphylococcus aureus*) infections. Overuse or misuse of antibiotics in veterinary and human medicine is responsible for much of the resistance. Infants and children are at increased risk of morbidity and mortality from infection with antibiotic-resistant foodborne organisms as well as from bacteria acquiring resistance indirectly from environmental reservoirs related to food-animal production.[1]

According to data collected for the first time by the Food and Drug Administration (FDA) in 2009, nearly 29 million lb (13.1 million kg) of antimicrobials are used annually in animal agriculture.[2] The vast majority are given as routine additives to animal feed for broiler chickens, turkeys, beef cattle, pigs and other food animals. These official data largely confirm the decade-old estimate by the Union of Concerned Scientists that more than 70% of all US antimicrobials are added at subtherapeutic levels to the feed or drinking water of healthy animals over prolonged periods to promote growth, increase feed efficiency, and prevent disease. Feed additives approved by the Food and Drug Administration include antibacterials (antibiotics) as well as antiparasitics.

ANTIBIOTIC USE IN FOOD ANIMAL PRODUCTION

As in human medicine, therapeutic use of antimicrobials in clinically ill animals involves use of curative doses of antibiotics for relatively short periods. A wide variety of antibiotics are approved for therapeutic use in animals. Many of the antibiotics are identical or substantially similar to those used in human medicine.[1] Only some of these approved antibiotics require a veterinarian's prescription. In contrast to human medicine, therapeutic agents may be delivered to entire herds or flocks, rather than to individual animals, depending on the disease, type of food animal, and production facility. The typical poultry shed contains around 25 000 birds.[3]

When a sick animal is discovered, the entire population is considered at risk and treated by placing antibiotics in the drinking water. Animals receive variable doses of antibiotic depending on water intake, and environmental contamination from spilled and discarded water is inevitable.

In 1995, the FDA first approved fluoroquinolone antibiotics for use in drinking water, to treat flocks for respiratory disease identified in some of the birds.[4] As critics had warned, resistant human infections rapidly followed. By 1999, the Centers for Disease Control and Prevention (CDC) reported that 1 in 6 human *Campylobacter* infections was resistant to fluoroquinolone, and the FDA concluded that use of fluoroquinolones in poultry had been "not shown to be safe."[5] In July 2005, nearly 5 years after first proposing it, the FDA withdrew approval for the sale of fluoroquinolone poultry products.[6]

The other 2 categories of antibiotic use in animal production—disease prevention (prophylaxis) and growth promotion/feed efficiency—involve the addition of subtherapeutic doses of antibiotics to the feed of healthy animals over long portions of their life cycle. Because both practices generate similar selective pressure on microbial populations, these uses will be discussed under the common term "nontherapeutic use." Use of antibiotics for these nontherapeutic indications does not require a veterinarian's prescription. With release of the 2009 FDA data, there now can be no dispute that most antimicrobial use in the United States involves these latter, nontherapeutic uses.

Growth promotion/feed efficiency refers to the ability to grow animals larger and faster on less food by adding small amounts of antibiotics to feed and has been practiced since the mid-1950s or earlier.[7] Administration of most growth promoters is accomplished by adding the drug to the feed or water over much of the life cycle. The biological basis for this acceleration of growth is unknown, but one theory is that subclinical infections are treated before becoming overt illness, animal health is preserved, and growth is enhanced. Of 22 antibiotics approved as growth promoters in the United States, more than half are closely related or identical to important human-use compounds.[8,9] Others, such as the ionophores (molecules that disrupt transmembrane ion concentration gradients required for

Table 56.1: Major Antibiotic Classes Approved for Use in Animals*

ANTIBIOTIC CLASS	SPECIES	PROPHYLAXIS	GROWTH PROMOTION
Aminoglycosides	Beef cattle, goats, poultry, sheep, swine	Yes	No
Penicillins	Beef cattle, dairy cows, fowl, poultry, sheep, swine	Yes	Yes
Ionophores	Beef cattle, dairy cows, fowl, goats, poultry, rabbits, sheep	Yes	Yes
Lincosamides	Poultry, swine	Yes	Yes
Macrolides	Beef cattle, poultry, sheep, swine	Yes	Yes
Polypeptides	Beef cattle, fowl, poultry, swine	Yes	Yes
Streptogramins	Beef cattle, poultry, swine	Yes	Yes
Sulfonamides	Beef cattle, fowl, poultry, swine	Yes	Yes
Tetracyclines	Beef cattle, dairy cows, fowl, honey bees, poultry, sheep, swine	Yes	Yes
Other Antibiotics			
Bambermycin	Beef cattle, poultry, swine	Yes	Yes
Carbadox	Swine	Yes	Yes
Novobiocin	Fowl, poultry	Yes	No
Spectinomycin	Poultry, swine	Yes	No

* US General Accounting Office.[9] Code of Federal Regulations, Title 21, Chapter 1, Subpart E (Animal Drugs, Feeds and Related Products), updated May 21, 2009.

functioning and survival of microorganisms, therefore having antibiotic properties), are not considered to be of human importance, although there is at least a hypothetical concern that their use may also select for bacterial resistance. A number of antibiotics also are used routinely to prevent high-prevalence diseases in food animals. Table 56.1 gives a list by drug class of several of these nontherapeutic uses.

ANTIBIOTIC RESISTANCE RESULTING FROM AGRICULTURAL ANTIBIOTIC USE

Bacteria exposed to various concentrations of antibiotics select for resistance. In agriculture, the widespread use of antibiotics contributes to antimicrobial resistance transmitted to humans.[10-12]

More specifically, the routine, nontherapeutic use of antibiotic feed additives for healthy animals is known to produce reservoirs of resistant organisms, which ultimately reach humans and can cause disease.[13,14] Additionally, although the FDA process for granting approval for antimicrobials in animal feed is applied to just 1 antimicrobial at a time, manufacturers can and typically do sell feed additives that are compound products, consisting of multiple agents. A common poultry feed additive, for example, might include an antibacterial of human importance, an ionophore, and a growth-promoting arsenic compound. In its current process, the FDA does not consider the potential for these antimicrobial combinations to enhance selection for resistance or to select for multidrug resistance.

When animals become colonized with resistant organisms, these organisms can reach humans through the food chain, via direct contact, or through contamination of water or crops by excreta.[15] Increasingly, food animals are raised in large numbers under close confinement, transported in large groups to slaughter, and processed very rapidly.[16] These stressful conditions cause increased bacterial shedding and inevitable contamination of hide, carcass,[17] and meat[18] with fecal bacteria. Dissemination of resistant pathogens via the food chain is further facilitated by centralized food processing and packaging, particularly of ground meat products, and broad distribution through food wholesalers and retail chains.[19] Farmers, farm workers, and farm families[14] as well as casual visitors[20] are at documented increased risk of infection with resistant organisms. Recent data from the Netherlands and North America implicate food animal use of antibiotics with the common finding of an agricultural strain of methicillin-resistant *Staphylococcus aureus* (MRSA) in these animals as well as in farmers, in veterinarians, and on some retail meats.[21-30]

Under optimal conditions, resistance can develop from a new mutation within hours or days.[13,31] Most resistance genes, however, are acquired from other bacteria via horizontal gene transfer.[32] Resistance genes frequently are located on extrachromosomal plasmids containing 10 or more different resistance genes and can be transmitted between bacteria of the same or different species. This permits the selection of multidrug resistance as a response to the presence of a single antimicrobial agent. The diverse and efficient mechanisms whereby bacteria share genetic material have caused experts to go beyond consideration of movement of resistant bacterial cells to studies of the ecology and movement of resistance genes in reservoirs where bacteria and antibiotics coexist.[33] Important reservoirs include the rumen and/or gut of food animals eating feed containing antibiotics and the gut of humans exposed to antibiotics.[34] Increasing numbers of studies document resistance gene movement between commensal bacteria and pathogens, and transfer of these genes among animal species, including humans.[35]

Environmental reservoirs are important contributors to the movement of resistance genes. Antibiotics have been measured in water near animal waste lagoons,[36] surface waters, and river sediments.[37] Investigators have found resistance genes identical to those found in swine waste lagoons in groundwater and soil microbes hundreds of meters downstream.[38] Multiple environmental and animal reservoirs involved in dissemination of resistance genes may ultimately be found.

A number of studies have attempted to document the effects of agricultural use of antibiotics on human health. Advances in molecular epidemiology over the past 2 decades have enabled investigators to document direct links between antibiotic use in animals and resistant infection in humans. For example, the dissemination of antibiotic-resistant *Salmonella* infections throughout the food chain is well documented. A 6-state outbreak of plasmid-mediated, multidrug-resistant *Salmonella newport* infections was traced through the food chain to a feedlot using nontherapeutic doses of chlortetracycline as a growth promoter in feed.[39] This study found an elevated risk of illness with resistant versus sensitive strains occurring among patients taking antibiotics for other infections (odds ratio, 51.3; P = .001), suggesting that asymptomatic carriage of the epidemic strain was converted to symptomatic infection by the use of antibiotics. Two of 3 children younger than 10 years in the outbreak had received antibiotics before the onset of symptoms.

Infants and young children are vulnerable to infections with resistant foodborne pathogens by indirect exposures as well. Bezanson and coworkers[40] described a plasmid-mediated, 6-drug–resistant strain of *Salmonella typhimurium* infection acquired asymptomatically by a pregnant woman from raw milk and passed to her infant at birth and secondarily to several other babies in the newborn nursery. (Pasteurization would almost certainly have prevented this.) In another newborn nursery outbreak, multidrug-resistant *Salmonella heidelberg* caused bloody diarrhea in 3 infants.[41] The index case was a term infant delivered by Cesarean section after 18 hours of ruptured membranes; until delivery, the mother had been working with calves from a herd containing several sick animals. Child care settings, because of staff members caring for large numbers of young children who are not yet toilet trained, provide another unique pediatric environment in which foodborne pathogens may be easily transmitted.[42]

Antibiotic resistance is an increasing and serious problem. Consumers, pediatricians, and public health and federal agencies should take steps to institute universal judicious use of antibiotics, promote better infection control, improve animal husbandry, and eliminate all unnecessary use of antibiotics in humans as well as animals to preserve efficacy and delay antibiotic resistance, thus providing increased time for development of new preventive and therapeutic strategies.

Frequently Asked Questions

Q *If the use of antibiotic growth promoters is eliminated, will meat and poultry become very expensive?*

A No. Best estimates are that the cost to the consumer would increase at most by no more than a few pennies per pound.

Q *Can animals be successfully raised and brought to slaughter without the use of antibiotics to prevent illness?*

A Yes. European countries that have banned nontherapeutic use of antibiotics in food animal production have found that by improving animal husbandry practices and hygiene, animals can be raised successfully without requiring routine prophylactic antibiotics while reducing total antibiotic use by significant amounts. In addition, US Department of Agriculture-certified organic producers in the United States use no antibiotics, as a condition of their certification.

Q *Do the antibiotics added to animal feed stay in the animals and eventually reach humans who consume meat and poultry?*

A The greater health concern is not for antibiotic residues in food, but rather for the creation of agricultural reservoirs of resistance that may reach humans. With respect to residues, there are regulations requiring specific "washout" periods. Antibiotics must be stopped for a prescribed number of days or weeks, depending on the drug, prior to slaughter of animals or collection of dairy products. These restrictions are designed to prevent animal proteins from containing unsafe levels of antibiotics at the time of slaughter or harvest. The success of these regulations depends on the compliance of food animal producers and the adequacy of enforcement and inspection programs.

Q *What can pediatricians do to discourage use of unnecessary antibiotics in animals?*

A Pediatricians should educate patients on appropriate use of antibiotics in the clinical setting and consistently practice the judicious use of antibiotics in their therapeutic interventions. By advocating for food produced without routine or unnecessary antibiotics, pediatricians can help leverage the purchasing power of schools, supermarkets, and hospitals to aid the transition of American agriculture away from routine and nontherapeutic antibiotic use. One effort, Health Care Without Harm (www. HealthyFoodinHealthcare.org), is working with hospitals and the entities that contract with them to preferentially purchase and serve meat from animals raised without routine or unnecessary antibiotics. Pediatricians in farm states can advocate for reducing or eliminating use of nontherapeutic antibiotics in local animal agriculture through letters to the editor, communication with state legislators and regulators, and discussions with the media.

Q *What can parents do to discourage use of unnecessary antibiotics in animals?*

A Through their own purchases, parents can support individual producers who do not use nontherapeutic antibiotics in their animal husbandry practices. These producers can be identified directly, such as via state and federal programs highlighting community supported agriculture, or in the retail setting by looking for animal-based foods labeled with the "USDA Organic" seal indicating that animals have been raised without nontherapeutic antibiotics. Meat from livestock carrying the (2007) USDA-approved "grass fed" label are raised on forage, not grain, and therefore are unlikely to have been given feed antibiotics.

References

1. Shea KM; American Academy of Pediatrics, Committee on Environmental Health, Committee on Infectious Diseases. Nontherapeutic use of antimicrobial agents in animal agriculture: implications for pediatrics. *Pediatrics*. 2004;114(3):862-868

2. US Food and Drug Administration. *CVM Reports on Antimicrobials Sold or Distributed for Food-Producing Animals*. Available at: http://www.fda.gov/AnimalVeterinary/NewsEvents/CVMUpdates/ucm236143.htm. Accessed 29 Mar 2011

3. Doye D, Freking B, Payne J. *Broiler Production: Considerations for Potential Growers.* Oklahoma Cooperative Extension Factsheet 1992. Available at http://www.ansci.umn.edu/poultry/resources/F-202-broilerproduction.pdf. Accessed 30 March 2011.

4. Food and Drug Administration. Enrofloxacin for Poultry: Opportunity For Hearing. *Federal Register.* 2000;65:64954

5. Food and Drug Administration. Enrofloxacin for Poultry: Opportunity for Hearing: Correction. *Federal Register*. 2001;66:6623

6. Food and Drug Administration. Enrofloxacin for Poultry: Final Decision on Withdrawal of New Animal Drug Application Following Formal Evidentiary Public Hearing: Availability. *Federal Register*. 2005;70:44105

7. Dibner JJ, Richards, JD. Antibiotic growth promoters in agriculture: history and mode of action. *Poultry Science.* 2005;84:634-643. Available at http://www.google.com/search?q=History+of+antibiotic+growth+promotion&rls=com.microsoft:en-us&ie=UTF-8&oe=UTF-8&startIndex=&startPage=1. Accessed March 30, 2011

8. US Department of Agriculture, Center for Veterinary Medicine. *Green Book On-Line.* Available at: http://www.fda.gov/AnimalVeterinary/Products/ApprovedAnimalDrugProducts/ucm042847.htm. Accessed October 18, 2010

9. US General Accounting Office. *Report to the Honorable Tom Harkin, Ranking Minority Member, Committee on Agriculture, Nutrition, and Forestry, US Senate: Food Safety: The Agricultural Use of Antibiotics and Its Implications for Human Health.* Washington, DC: US General Accounting Office; 1999. Publication GAO/RCED-99-74

10. Institute of Medicine, Board on Global Health. *Microbial Threats to Health: Emergence, Detection, and Response.* Washington, DC: National Academies Press; 2003. Available at: http://books.nap.edu/books/030908864X/html/R1.html#pagetop. Accessed October 18, 2010

11. World Health Organization, Food and Agriculture Organization of the United Nations, and World Organization for Animal Health. WHO/FAO/OIE Expert Workshop on Non-human Antimicrobial Usage and Antimicrobial Resistance, Executive Summary. Geneva, Switzerland; December 1–5, 2003. Available at: http://www.who.int/foodsafety/publications/micro/en/exec_sum.pdf. Accessed October 18, 2010

12. Alliance for Prudent Use of Antibiotics. The need to improve antimicrobial use in agriculture: ecological and human health consequences. *Clin Infect Dis.* 2002;34(Suppl 3):S71-S144. Available at: http://www.journals.uchicago.edu/CID/journal/contents/v34nS3.html. Accessed October 18, 2010

13. Khachatourians GG. Agricultural use of antibiotics and the evolution and transfer of antibiotic-resistant bacteria. *CMAJ.* 1998;159(9):1129–1136

14. Levy SB, FitzGerald GB, Macone AB. Changes in intestinal flora of farm personnel after introduction of a tetracycline-supplemented feed on the farm. *N Engl J Med.* 1976;295(11): 583–588

15. Witte W. Medical consequences of antibiotic use in agriculture. *Science.* 1998;279(5353): 996–997

16. Center for Science in the Public Interest, Environmental Defense Fund, Food Animal Concerns Trust, Public Citizen's Health Research Group, Union of Concerned Citizens. *Petition to Rescind Approvals for the Subtherapeutic Use of Antibiotics in Livestock Used in (or Related to Those Used in) Human Medicine.* Available at: http://www.cspinet.org/ar/petition_3_99.html. Accessed October 18, 2010

17. Barkocy-Gallagher GA, Arthur TM, Siragusa GR, et al. Genotypic analyses of *Escherichia coli* O157:H7 and O157 nonmotile isolate recovered from beef cattle and carcasses at processing plants in the Midwestern states of the United States. *Appl Environ Microbiol.* 2001;67(9): 3810–3818

18. Millemann Y, Gaubert S, Remy D, Colmin C. Evaluation of IS200-PCR and comparison with other molecular markers to trace *Salmonella enterica* subsp *enterica* serotype *typhimurium* bovine isolates from farm to meat. *J Clin Microbiol.* 2000;38(6):2204–2209

19. Tauxe RV, Holmberg SD, Cohen ML. The epidemiology of gene transfer in the environment. In: Levy SB, Miller RV, eds. *Gene Transfer in the Environment.* New York, NY: McGraw-Hill; 1989:377–403

20. Centers for Disease Control and Prevention. Outbreaks of *Escherichia coli* O157:H7 infections among children associated with farm visits—Pennsylvania and Washington, 2000. *MMWR Morb Mortal Wkly Rep.* 2001;50(15):293–297

21. van Duijkeren E, Ikawaty R, Broekhuizen-Stins MJ, et al. Transmission of methicillin-resistant *Staphylococcus aureus* strains between different kinds of pig farms. *Vet Microbiol.* 2008;126(4): 383-389

22. Wulf MW, Markestein A, van der Linden FT, Voss A, Klaassen C, Verduin CM. 2008. First outbreak of methicillin-resistant *Staphylococcus aureus* ST398 in a Dutch hospital, June 2007. *Euro Surveill.* 2008;13(9)8051

23. Rigen V, Lucia MM, van Keulen PH, Kluytmans JA. Increase in a Dutch hospital of methicillin-resistant *Staphylococcus aureus* related to animal farming. *Clin Infect Dis.* 2008;46(2):261-263

24. de Neeling AJ, an den Broek MJ, Spalburg EC, et al. 2007. High prevalence of methicillin-resistant *Staphylococcus aureus* in pigs. *Vet Microbiol.* 2007;122(3-4):366–372

25. Huijsdens XW, van Dijke BJ, Spalburg E, et al. Community-acquired MRSA and pig farming. *Ann Clin Microbiol Antimicrob.* 2006;5:26–29

26. Voss A, Loeffen F, Bakker J, Klaassen C, Wulf M. Methicillin-resistant *Staphylococcus aureus* in pig farming. *Emerg Infect Dis.* 2005;11(12):1965–1966

27. Graveland H, Wagenaar J, Broekhuizen-Stins M, et al. *Staphylococcus aureus* (MRSA) in Veal Calf Farmers and Veal Calves in The Netherlands. Poster presented at: ASM Conference on Antimicrobial Resistance in Zoonotic Bacteria and Food-borne Pathogens; Copenhagen, Denmark; June 16-18, 2008

28. De Boer E, Zwartkruis-Nahuis JT, Wit B, et al. Prevalence of methicillin-resistant *Staphylococcus aureus* in meat. *Int J Food Microbiol*. 2008;134(1-2):52-56

29. Khanna T, Friendship R, Dewey C, Weese JS. Methicillin-resistant *Staphylococcus aureus* colonization in pigs and pig farmers. *Vet Microbiol*. 2007;128(3-4):298-303

30. Smith TC, Male MJ, Harper AL, et al. Methicillin-resistant *Staphylococcus aureus* (MRSA) strain ST398 is present in midwestern U.S. swine and swine workers. *PLoS ONE*. 2009;4(1):e4258

31. American Society of Microbiology. *Antimicrobial Resistance: An Ecological Perspective*. Available at: http://academy.asm.org/images/stories/documents/antimicrobialresistance.pdf. Accessed October 18, 2010

32. Levy SB, Marshal BM. Genetic transfer in the natural environment. In: Sussman M, Collins GH, Skinner FA, Stewart-Tall DE, eds. *Release of Genetically-engineered Micro-organisms*. London, England: Academic Press; 1988:61–76

33. Mazel D, Davies J. Antibiotic resistance in microbes. *Cell Mol Life Sci*. 1999;56(9-10):742–754

34. Shoemaker NB, Wang GR, Salyers AA. Evidence of natural transfer of a tetracycline resistance gene between bacteria from the human colon and bacteria from the bovine rumen. *Appl Environ Microbiol*. 1992;58(4):1313–1320

35. Hummel R, Tschape H, Witte W. Spread of plasmid-mediated nourseothricin resistance due to antibiotic use in animal husbandry. *J Basic Microbiol*. 1986;26(8):461–466

36. Meyer MT, Kolpin DW, Bumgarner JE, Varns JL, Daughtridge JV. Occurrence of antibiotics in surface and ground water near confined animal feeding operations and waste water treatment plants using radioimmunoassay and liquid chromatography/electrospray mass spectrometry. Presented at: 219th Meeting of the American Chemical Society; March 26–30, 2000; San Francisco, CA

37. Halling-Sorensen B, Nors Nielsen S, Lanzky PF, et al. Occurrence, fate and effects of pharmaceutical substances in the environment—a review. *Chemosphere*. 1998;36(2):357–393

38. Chee-Sanford JC, Aminov RI, Krapac IJ, Garrigues-Jeanjean N, Mackie RI. Occurrence and diversity of tetracycline resistance genes in lagoons and groundwater underlying two swine production facilities. *Appl Environ Microbiol*. 2001;67(4):1494–1502

39. Holmberg SD, Osterholm MT, Senger KA, Cohen ML. Drug-resistant *Salmonella* from animals fed antimicrobials. *N Engl J Med*. 1984;311(10):617–622

40. Bezanson GS, Khakhria R, Bollegraaf E. Nosocomial outbreak caused by antibiotic-resistant strain of *Salmonella typhimurium* acquired from dairy cattle. *Can Med Assoc J*. 1983;128(4):426–427

41. Lyons RW, Samples CL, DeSilvan HN, Ross KA, Julian EM, Checko PJ. An epidemic of resistant *Salmonella* in a nursery. Animal-to-human spread. *JAMA*. 1980;243(6):546–547

42. Holmes SJ, Morrow AL, Pickering LK. Child-care practices: effects of social change on the epidemiology of infectious diseases and antibiotic resistance. *Epidemiol Rev*. 1996;18(1):10–28

Chapter 57

Precautionary Principle

■ ■ ■ ■ ■ ■

INTRODUCTION

One of the central challenges in environmental health is determining how best to set environmental and chemical management policies and standards that protect health in the constantly changing context of complexity, incomplete information, and scientific uncertainty. The more science probes the health effects of interactions between genes and environmental exposures,[a] the more complex, interdependent and subtle becomes our understanding of the cause and effect relationships of disease (and health). Reductionist, one cause-one effect models of disease—reinforced by the development of germ theory—break down. The traditional approach to setting an environmental standard for a particular chemical has been to identify a limit of exposure below which the statistical likelihood of specific adverse health outcomes is minimized. In such analyses, the chemical is examined individually—that is, without consideration of exposures to other chemicals that may potentiate or reduce effects of exposures.

For some well-understood environmental health threats (eg, mercury, dioxins, radon), traditional quantitative human health risk assessment (see Chapter 58) is a powerful tool that can successfully protect health. For most environmental exposures, however, the level of knowledge of toxicology, human exposure, and interactions is insufficient to permit definitive decision making to protect health. The rapidly changing organ systems of the growing and developing child further challenge this inherently resource-intensive approach to controlling

---

[a] Environmental exposures in this context can be biological, chemical and/or physical, internal and/or external.

Table 57.1: Some International Agreements Invoking Precaution[3]
Montreal Protocol on Substances that Deplete the Ozone Layer, 1987
Third North Sea Conference, 1990
The Rio Declaration on Environment and Development, 1992
Framework Convention on Climate Change, 1992
Treaty of European Union (Maastricht Treaty), 1992
Cartagena Protocol on Biosafety, 2000
Stockholm Convention on Persistent Organic Pollutants, 2001

environmental health risks. In response to this, a broader approach, sometimes called the "Precautionary Principle" (also known as the "precautionary approach" or "precaution"), has been increasingly invoked as an alternative.

PRECAUTION: BACKGROUND AND DEFINITIONS

Precaution is an old weapon of public health. When Dr. John Snow removed the handle to the Broad Street pump in 1854 and stopped the cholera epidemic in London without identifying the causal organism, this was a precautionary action, albeit taking place after significant exposures and consequences had been demonstrated. When the US Congress inserted the Delaney Clause into the Food, Drug and Cosmetics Act in 1957, banning animal carcinogens from the human food chain, this was a precautionary action.[1] Precaution is also a core component of both preventive medicine and disease management. In public health, precaution is analogous to primary prevention (eg, neonatal screening and childhood immunizations). In clinical medicine, it is reflected in the classical medical maxim, "First, do no harm."

The concept of precaution was first incorporated into environmental law as the *Vorsorgeprinzip* (foresight or precautionary principle) in the German Clean Air Act of 1974. Since then, it has been specified in numerous international agreements, treaties, and laws (Table 57.1). This principle, applicable to the environment, was most famously articulated in Principle 15 of the 1992 Rio Declaration on Environment and Development: "In order to protect the environment, the precautionary approach shall be widely applied by States according to their capabilities. Where there are threats of serious or irreversible damage, lack of full scientific certainty shall not be used as a reason for postponing cost-effective measures to prevent environmental degradation."[2] Since the Rio Declaration, environmental health professionals and advocates have increasingly sought to integrate precaution into policy. Although no specific definition has been universally accepted, a good working definition has been proposed by the European Environment Agency (EEA):

> The Precautionary Principle provides justification for public policy actions in situations of scientific complexity, uncertainty and ignorance, where there may be a need to act in order to avoid, or reduce, potentially serious or irreversible threats to health or the environment, using an appropriate level of scientific evidence, and taking into account the likely pros and cons of action or inaction.[3]

This working definition importantly identifies that public policy action to protect health and/or the environment is the purpose of applying precaution, that the setting requiring precaution is one of imperfect information, and that the consequences of both action and inaction should be considered. In other words, when there is scientific evidence of potential serious harm from environmental exposure(s), preventive or protective action should not need to await acquisition of knowledge that is comprehensive, detailed and/or mechanistic (ie, based on scientific evidence of the precise mechanism that causes harm). Instead, the Precautionary Principle is a process that takes preventive action in the face of incomplete information, shifting the burden of proof to those desiring to take a risky action, exploring a wide range of alternative actions to achieve given goals, and broadening the discussion to include the public and not just regulatory agencies and the industries being regulated. The concept is logical, but the application is controversial.[4,5]

One major cause of controversy involves conflicting opinions about the stage at which the Precautionary Principle should be applied in the risk assessment, risk management, risk communication continuum (see Chapter 58). Some experts advocate applying it throughout the process, but others insist that it should only be used in risk management after risk is calculated using strict, quantitative procedures. A second category of disagreement is whether the Precautionary Principle can or does represent a reproducible, standardized process of decision making; a general approach and process; or more properly, a philosophical stance that determines how risk is evaluated and decisions are made. Finally, some experts tend to consider standard risk assessment apart from and in opposition to the Precautionary Principle in philosophy and approach, and others consider them as a unified approach, applicable differently depending on the question or risk under consideration and the quality and quantity of the evidence available.[6] These debates are the subject of scores of scholarly articles and numerous books, the details of which are beyond the scope of this chapter. Discussed below is a brief outline of 2 extreme positions to introduce some dimensions of the debate. This is followed by a discussion of how and why the

Precautionary Principle is inherently important to children's health using the historical example of leaded gasoline.

QUANTITATIVE RISK ASSESSMENT

US federal agencies have commonly applied a quantitative approach to risk assessment using a standardized 4-stage system including hazard identification, dose-response assessment, exposure assessment, and risk characterization. The outcome of this process is a probability statement of what proportion of a specified population will be expected to develop an adverse health condition from a specific level of exposure. This estimate then forms the basis for decisions made by risk managers and policy makers to determine public environmental health policy, often on the narrow question of how much exposure to a specific agent or stressor can be tolerated without excess illness. This approach has been criticized as being generally conducted with little public input, requiring great amounts of data, being built on default assumptions that may not be accurate, placing the burden of proof of harm on the regulatory agencies, and inadequately dealing with uncertainty, data gaps, and ignorance.

CONTRASTING POLICY APPROACHES

A common oversimplification of the contrasting approaches is summed up as follows: risk assessment assumes a stressor, chemical or technology is "innocent until proven guilty" whereas the Precautionary Principle assumes it is "guilty until proven innocent." Barrett and Raffensperger[7] compare dimensions of 2 idealized models that correspond to the strict separation of quantitative risk assessment (based in mechanistic science) and the Precautionary Principle (based in precautionary science). Two of these dimensions, Error and Authority, are reviewed here to help illustrate the contrasting positions.

The contrasting approaches to error (ie, assumptions used in statistical calculations, leading to overregulation or underregulation, that are retrospectively shown to be incorrect) differ in the trade-off between type I (false-positive) and type II (false-negative) errors.[8] Standard risk assessment methods tend to minimize type I errors, whereas the precautionary approach seeks to minimize type II errors. Rarely can both types of errors be minimized simultaneously. Traditionally, scientific research seeks to minimize type I errors. Because scientific knowledge builds iteratively, identifying a false positive as a true positive and building more research on an incorrect assumption would lead to both faulty science and wasted resources. In the context of medicine, however, it is often desirable to accept more false positives to avoid false negatives. For example, given that a safe, inexpensive and reliable screening test is available to identify a curable but potentially fatal disease at a preclinical stage, most would agree that it is better to err in the direction of overidentifying individuals who potentially have the disease (increase type I errors) so as not to miss people who may die without treatment (minimize type II errors). Strong proponents of standard environmental health risk assessment would argue that it is preferable to avoid false positives. Strong proponents of precaution would argue in favor of minimizing false negatives.

A second dimension often used to separate the 2 approaches is differing definitions of authority. Authority refers to who is qualified or entrusted to determine risk. Under the strict definition of risk assessment, it is an applied, quantitative scientific method conducted by scientists and validated by independent scientific review. The approach seeks to eliminate social or ethical considerations, avoid bias, and produce an objective, value-free, quantitative prediction of risk usually with a quantitative expression of statistical uncertainty. The questions and processes are defined and specified by scientists and are usually narrow in scope as is consistent with best scientific practices. Under the precautionary approach, open-ended dialogue, multidisciplinary participation, qualitative and quantitative inputs, and public review are used to incorporate the larger social and ethical context and definitions of risk. The expression of risk may be qualitative, narrative, and/or quantitative.

PRECAUTIONARY PRINCIPLE AND RISK ASSESSMENT INTEGRATED

Rather than viewing standard risk assessment and the Precautionary Principle as distinct and at odds, they can be seen as parts of an integrated strategy available to describe and minimize risks from environmental stressors.[9] Depending on the conditions and questions, one approach might be more appropriate than the other (Table 57.2). Almost always, information about basic questions of toxicity and exposure will be incomplete and imperfect. Ideally, environmental health policy makers would utilize the full spectrum of tools and inputs to develop the most health protective laws and regulations using a unified approach that is flexible, iterative, and inclusive of quantitative and qualitative inputs.

CHILDREN'S ENVIRONMENTAL HEALTH ISSUES AND PRECAUTION

For many children's environmental health issues, policy emphasizing a precautionary approach is most logical.[10,11] The traditional quantitative risk assessment approach is inherently time- and data-intensive, especially so for the many life stages of children's exposures and vulnerabilities (see Chapter 3). Information on developmental, reproductive, and transgenerational toxicity is incomplete or absent for many environmental exposures. Traditional dose-response analysis fails to adequately consider exposures during critical periods of development. These issues create large data gaps and uncertainties in the inputs required for traditional quantitative human health risk assessment. In addition, children's exposures are, in general, involuntary, and children will inherit the environmental,

Table 57.2: Characteristics of Hazards and Preferred Regulatory Approach	
EMPHASIZE PRECAUTIONARY PRINCIPLE	**EMPHASIZE QUANTITATIVE RISK ASSESSMENT**
Manmade	Naturally occurring
Novel/not yet introduced	Established/already in the environment
Serious toxicity	Minor toxicity
Irreversible toxicity	Reversible toxicity
Very potent	Less potent
Dispersible (ubiquitous distribution)	Nondispersible (finite distribution)
Persistent	Transient
Bioaccumulative	Does not bioaccumulate
Nonessential use	Critical use
No threshold of toxicity	Threshold of toxicity
Large scale (eg, global)	Small scale (eg, occupational)
Harmful to immature systems	Not harmful to immature systems
Transgenerational effects	No transgenerational effects
Alternatives exist	No alternatives exist
Large uncertainty in data	Small uncertainty in data

health, and social consequences of decisions made during their minorities. Inclusion of a precautionary approach to controlling environmental health risks is ideal for protecting their future well-being and that of future generations.

HISTORICAL CASE STUDY—TETRAETHYL LEAD IN GASOLINE

The history of childhood lead poisoning offers clear illustrations of what can happen when precaution is ignored.[12-14] In the 1920s, tetraethyl lead was identified as a cheap and effective antiknock agent for internal combustion engines and added to gasoline. Unlike the lead oxides used in paints, tetraethyl lead is absorbed through the skin. After a series of fatal incidents with researchers and production workers, the Surgeon General of the United States Public Health Service declared a moratorium on "ethyl" production in 1925 and convened a group of experts to assess the situation. The ethyl producers argued for lifting the moratorium to maintain industrial progress, but doctors and public advocates articulated a precautionary message. In response, the Surgeon General appointed an advisory panel of 7 physicians and scientists and gave them 7 months to conduct research and report their findings. The panel completed a single case-control study of 252 gas station employees and chauffeurs that failed to find a statistically significant correlation between use of ethyl gas additives and elevation of blood and stool lead concentrations. The panel stressed that this study was not definitive and that longer experience and differing populations were needed in the evaluation.[12] Disregarding this warning, the Surgeon General lifted the moratorium, and leaded gas became ubiquitous, resulting in inhalational lead exposure of the entire population, including infants and children.

From 1950 to 1990, information about the dangers of lead poisoning in children exploded. Data began to accumulate on the long-term morbidity of acute lead poisoning in children. The "threshold" level for public health action fell as the special vulnerabilities of children were more precisely documented.[15] The differences in absorption, distribution, and metabolism of lead in infants and children compared with adults were identified, and the long-term, chronic toxicities, particularly to the central nervous system, were described. Even during this period, however, there were loud voices arguing that lead exposure without acute poisoning was of no significance, and lead continued to be used in many products. A growing body of evidence, however, documents the adverse neurodevelopmental effects of even low lead levels. Lead finally fell to regulation and was banned from gasoline because of the cumulative impact of studies of its effects and the need to comply with the Clean Air Act of 1970, which required manufacturers to apply catalytic converters to automobile internal combustion engines to reduce the toxicity of emissions. Phasing out lead in gasoline resulted in dramatic declines in population lead concentrations.[16] It took almost a century to develop the comprehensive data on childhood lead toxicity; earlier application of the Precautionary Principle could have prevented exposure and damage to generations of children.

APPLYING THE PRECAUTIONARY PRINCIPLE

Despite the increasing endorsement of the Precautionary Principle in international treaties and national and state laws, there remains a lack of clarity on how it should be applied.[17] There is general agreement on 4 central components[18]:

- taking preventive action in the context of scientific uncertainty;
- shifting the burden of proof of safety to those advocating a potentially risky action;
- exploring a comprehensive set of alternative actions to achieve desired goals; and
- enlarging the decision-making process to include the public and other stakeholders.

Tools of precaution include but are not limited to development of clean production processes that eliminate use of toxic materials and creation of toxic waste, substitution of nontoxic or less toxic materials and/or components, regulatory reform and overhaul incorporating strong principles of precaution, restricting or minimizing use of toxic substances, and total bans. Critical to the transition to precaution is reframing the questions asked about environmental exposures. For example, rather than asking how much exposure to a potentially toxic substance is tolerable, precaution would ask how exposures can be prevented through application of alternative technologies.

Large initiatives in precaution are underway in the European Union under the Registration, Evaluation, Authorisation and Restriction of Chemicals (REACH) program and in states such as California and Massachusetts with their recent strict toxic chemical laws. These initiatives and others, along with the widening dialogue on precaution involving multiple stakeholders, are the kinds of processes that will help to clarify and develop consensus regarding the practical application of the Precautionary Principle in environment and health policy into the future.

Frequently Asked Questions

Q *Does the Precautionary Principle stifle innovation?*

A Because the Precautionary Principle explicitly requires exploration of alternative technologies and solutions by both experts and the public, it can enhance innovation. For example, developing renewable, clean energy to satisfy increased energy demands would be preferred over creating more coal-fired power plants. Using biodegradable, nontoxic, non-heavy metal-containing pigments would be preferred over older pigments containing known carcinogens and heavy metals.

Q *Isn't the Precautionary Principle "anti-scientific?"*

A Seen as an overall, broad approach to risk characterization and risk management, the precautionary approach encompasses all of traditional quantitative risk assessment and also explicitly recognizes uncertainty, knowledge gaps, ignorance, and alternatives. This can be interpreted as being more scientifically rigorous, because unknown factors are highlighted and analysis of these unknown factors is part of the decision process, development of ongoing research questions and a search for additional solutions.

Q *Why do pediatricians need to know about the Precautionary Principle?*

A Children's special vulnerabilities to environmental harm make application of the Precautionary Principle particularly important. Pediatricians have a tradition of child health advocacy, and the Precautionary Principle is an important preventive tool.

Q   *Will applying the Precautionary Principle always result in bans?*

A   There are many precautionary tools available, including bans and restricted use, substitution, redesign, improved materials management, etc. Some bans, such as banning lead from gasoline, paint, and children's toys and jewelry, are appropriate. In other situations, restrictions or substitutions may be sufficient.

References

1. Harrendoes P, Gee D, MacGarvin M, et al, eds. *Late Lessons from Early Warnings: The Precautionary Principle 1986-2000.* Environmental Issue Report No 22. Luxembourg: European Environment Agency, Office of Official Publications for the European Communities; 2001

2. United Nations Environment Program. Rio Declaration on Environment and Development. Available at: http://www.unep.org/Documents.Multilingual/Default.asp?DocumentID=78&ArticleID=1163. Accessed October 18, 2010

3. Gee D. Late lessons from early warnings; toward realism and precaution with endocrine-disrupting substances. *Environ Health Perspect.* 2006;114(Suppl 1):152-160

4. Stirling A. Risk, precaution and science: towards a more productive policy debate. *EMBO Reports.* 2007;8(4):308-315

5. Peterson M. The Precautionary Principle should not be used as a basis for decision-making. *EMBO Rep.* 2007;8(4):305-308

6. Silbergeld EK. Commentary: the role of toxicology in prevention and precaution. *Int J Occcup Med Environ Health.* 2004;17(1):91-102

7. Barrett K, Raffensperger C. Precautionary Science. In: Raffensperger C, ed. *Protecting Public Health and the Environment: Implementing the Precautionary Principle.* Covelo, CA: Island Press; 1999:51-70

8. Gee D. Establishing evidence for early action: the prevention of reproductive and developmental harm. *Basic Clin Pharm Toxicol.* 2008;102(2):257-266

9. Stirling A. Risk, precaution and science: towards a more productive policy debate. *EMBO Rep.* 2007;8(4):308-315

10. Tickner JA, Hoppin P. Children's environmental health: a case study in implementing the Precautionary Principle. *Int J Occup Environ Health.* 2000;6(4):281-288

11. Jaronsinska D, Gee D. Children's environmental health and the precautionary principle. *Int J Hyg Environ Health.* 2007;210(5):541-546

12. Warren C. *Brush with Death: A Social History of Lead Poisoning.* Baltimore, MD: The Johns Hopkins University Press; 2000

13. English PC. Old Paint: *A Medical History of Childhood Lead-Paint Poisoning in the United States to 1980.* New Brunswick, NJ: Rutgers University Press; 2001

14. Berney B. Round and round it goes: the epidemiology of childhood lead poisoning, 1950-1990. In: Kroll-Smith S, Brown P, Gunter VJ, eds. *Illness and the Environment: A Reader in Contested Medicine.* New York, NY: New York University Press; 2000:215-257

15. ATSDR Case Studies in Environmental Medicine. Lead Toxicity. Available at: http://www.atsdr.cdc.gov/csem/lead/pbcover_page2.html. Accessed March 28, 2011

16. Centers for Disease Control and Prevention. Update: blood lead levels—United States, 1991-1994. *MMWR Morb Mortal Wkly Rep.* 1997;46(7):141-144

17. Lokke S. The Precautionary Principle and chemical regulation: past achievements and future possibilities. *Environ Sci Pollut Res.* 2006;13(15):342-349

18. Kriebel D, Tickner J, Epstein P, et al. The Precautionary Principle in environmental science. *Environ Health Perspect.* 2001;109(9):871-876

Chapter 58

Risk Assessment, Risk Management, and Risk Communication

■ ■ ■ ■ ■ ■

It is useful for pediatricians and other health care professionals to be familiar with risk assessment, risk management, and risk communication approaches applicable to environmental contaminants. Although these 3 activities do not always occur together, they frequently occur sequentially when individuals first identify risks, then establish policies to minimize risks and maximize benefit, and ultimately communicate and exchange information with the recipient. Over time, this tripartite process is iterative, providing effective adaptation to new information or changing evidence. Pediatricians may be involved in these activities as community advisors, advocates, and practitioners.

Clinicians are usually well versed in addressing health risks for individual patients. Characterizing the nature and extent of particular health risks for a patient, developing approaches for managing those risks, and counseling about risk are part of routine clinical practice. For example, a pediatrician may inquire about a child's exposure to secondhand tobacco smoke. After taking a medical history, the clinician can determine the magnitude, extent, and conditions of exposure—this is risk assessment. The family may then be advised about the potential health risks in a general sense as well as in the context of the particular child. For example, there is often greater risk if the child has asthma—this is risk communication. Tailored and relevant anticipatory guidance and counseling to engage the family in reducing or eliminating secondhand smoke exposure—risk management—is the final step of this process.

Legislative and administrative mandates (eg, regulations and policies) have shaped formal processes for assessing and managing environmental exposures of concern at the population level. This decision making relies on scientific evidence found in toxicologic and epidemiologic research data bases. The characteristics of the population served often help to determine how this tripartite process can be accomplished most effectively. This chapter discusses the concepts of risk assessment, risk management, and risk communication as applied to health hazards that children encounter in their environment as well as some tools available for the task.

Historically, governmental mandates to regulate environmental hazards possess defined procedures for the conduct of risk assessment, management, and communication and have focused on known or suspected toxic substances (eg, those with potential for carcinogenicity). Most have emphasized chemical exposures, but other environmental exposures (such as allergens, ultraviolet radiation, and violence) present health risks to children and can be evaluated using a risk paradigm. For some of these, such as nanotechnology, few health and safety data exist.

RISK ASSESSMENT

The first step in risk assessment is defining the question to be answered. This includes identifying potentially relevant exposures and establishing their sources in the child's environment. Once defined, further information regarding exposure and the potential for adverse health effects should be sought. Public health and regulatory bodies with responsibility for evaluating environmental health risks often follow established protocols designed to study a particular type of substance or condition. In 1983, The National Research Council proposed a 4-step risk assessment paradigm, which consists of (1) hazard identification; (2) dose-response assessment; (3) exposure assessment; and (4) risk characterization.[1] These concepts continue to be employed in modern regulatory and nonregulatory settings. This model was designed primarily to evaluate chemicals. It relies on scientific studies to identify health outcomes (often referred to as "endpoints"), evaluate dose-response relationships, characterize exposures, and determine population level risks associated with these exposures. The broader potential of this model will also be discussed in this chapter.

Risk assessors, in general, examine the effects of chemical toxicants/carcinogens on populations using quantitative methods and statistical paradigms to apply or establish governmental regulations and guidelines. Clinicians may use this process in a less formal way for environmental agents, chemical and nonchemical. Clinicians usually focus on risks to individuals or small groups using a qualitative approach, applying a "best fit" diagnosis for many different environmental hazards. Table 58.1 compares and contrasts the formal process and the process as it may be practiced by clinicians.

Table 58.1: Risk Assessment as Performed by Risk Assessors and Clinicians		
RISK ASSESSMENT STEP	**QUESTIONS ASKED BY RISK ASSESSOR**	**QUESTIONS ASKED BY CLINICIAN**
Hazard assessment	What are the chemicals of concern, and what kind of harm are they known or suspected to cause? Which chemicals will we focus on?	What information do we have about an environmental problem, what chemicals or other agents were involved, and what sources of information are there?
Dose-response assessment	What effects are seen in animals or humans at different exposure levels? What are the doses at which cancerous and non-cancerous effects occur? Is there a threshold below which no effect is expected?	What information is available from a literature review, consultation with experts? How do the levels at which effects have been demonstrated compare with levels in the patient or community? Are these levels higher than regulatory limits?
Exposure assessment	What are the sources and duration of exposures? How many people are exposed? What does our monitoring or modeling data predict about the range of doses in the population?	Is there a chance that the patient may be coming in contact with (breathing, touching, ingesting, etc) this exposure source? How often and for how long? Is the source highly contaminated or only slightly contaminated?
Risk characterization	Given the above, what are the human impacts of current exposures? What is the population risk? Are there sensitive subpopulations? How confident are we in this analysis?	Are regulations based on effects in the fetus or child? Is there reason to be concerned that this patient or children in general may be at greater risk from exposure to this chemical or agent than adults may?
Risk communication	Is the information relevant to the audience and understandable? Does it respond to public concerns? What are the limitations in this assessment?	Have I listened to the concerns presented, responded with compassion, and helped identify information needed and credible sources for obtaining it? What additional steps are needed?

Modified from: Miller and Solomon.[2]

Step 1: Hazard Identification

Hazard identification is a qualitative step that involves identifying and reviewing data to help elucidate health concerns and endpoints that may be associated with exposure to a substance. To determine causality between exposures and health effects, the US Environmental Protection Agency (EPA) and other authoritative health and regulatory bodies employ "weight of evidence" classification schemes based on their reviews of existing evidence.[3] The standard scheme assigns highest confidence to epidemiologic studies followed (in descending order) by studies of laboratory animals, in vitro studies, and structure-activity relationships (predicting a chemical's possible activity on the basis of knowledge of its chemical structure).

Step 2: Dose-Response Assessment

Dose-response assessment seeks to determine the relationship between the magnitude of the dose and the occurrence or lack of occurrence of health effects. Dose-response information for chemicals is usually derived from experimental studies of toxicity in animals. Epidemiologic studies may also provide information on the relationship between exposure variations and health outcomes. In regulatory settings, to generate a useful dose-response curve, sophisticated toxicologic studies, extrapolation schemes, and pharmacokinetic modeling are used with the goal of finding the maximal safe exposure of an individual to a specific chemical. Study designs and interpretation of data vary according to the health endpoint of concern. For example, carcinogens are considered to be "nonthreshold" hazards. That is, there is no exposure level below which a carcinogen is considered "safe." Therefore, rather than seeking a threshold effect, researchers expose groups of animals to several high doses of the toxicant, and the resulting data are fit into a simple linear model extrapolated to zero. The assumption of a linear relationship is believed to be conservative and protective of human health. This model or its variations can be applied to nonchemical environmental exposures and their outcomes, such as allergen exposure and the risk of developing asthma.

Step 3: Exposure Assessment

Exposure assessment is used to determine the likely human exposures to the hazard identified. To be most informative, it must accurately characterize all important sources of a particular toxicant or other substance in the environment (eg, groundwater, surface water, air, soil, food, human milk), and quantify exposures (eg, μg/L in drinking water, μg/g in soil). Realistic exposure scenarios must be considered to identify at-risk populations or subpopulations, duration of exposure, routes of exposure, timing of exposure, types of substances, etc. In recent years, efforts to improve exposure assessment for children have been increasing, given that children's physiological and behavioral characteristics greatly influence their exposures compared with those of adults.[3] Understanding these differences is key to accurately evaluate the hazards to children from environmental pollutants or conditions. Biomarkers, such as urinary or blood concentrations of substances or their metabolites, have been increasingly used to more accurately determine exposure. Biomarkers in exposed populations complement exposure assessment on the basis of measurements in environmental media.[2]

Step 4: Risk Characterization

The last step of risk assessment—risk characterization—involves the synthesis of the dose-response and exposure assessments. Results are often expressed as the maximum acceptable exposure that ensures that the health of an exposed population is protected, or as the number of people likely to be affected at a certain level of exposure.

For carcinogens, risk is typically characterized as the number of excess cancers that may occur in a population following continuous, low-dose exposure at a specific average level over a 70-year lifetime. Risk is generally considered to be acceptable if the exposure results in an increase of less than 1 excess cancer per 1 million (10^{-6}) people exposed over a lifetime. Because of children's increased biological vulnerability, the EPA recently established guidelines that weigh exposures during infancy, childhood, or adolescence more heavily when data specific to these age groups are not available.[4]

Noncarcinogens with presumed thresholds for adverse health effects are evaluated by comparing the estimated exposure, on the basis of exposure assessment, to the acceptable exposure level defined by the dose-response data. In general, extrapolation from testing of toxicity in animals is required to determine a reference dose (used by EPA) or an acceptable daily intake (used by the Food and Drug Administration). If these values are not exceeded over a lifetime, there should be no unacceptable effects in exposed humans. To determine what level of exposure to a chemical is likely to be safe in humans, risk assessors use the most reliable animal or human data at which no adverse effects were observed (NOAEL) or the lowest level at which adverse effects were observed (LOAEL). These values are then divided by uncertainty or safety factors to account for the various extrapolations required (Table 58.2). Safety or uncertainty factors usually are multiples of 10, an arbitrary multiplier, but may be applied as some fraction of 10 depending on the quality of data available. Use of an additional safety factor has been considered in recent years to account for the potential increased susceptibility of children when data on early life exposures are inadequate.

The formal output of this 4-step risk assessment process is an expression of risk, most commonly quantified as the proportion (or probability) of a specific

Table 58.2: Extrapolation From Animal Toxicity Data to Reference Dose (RfD)*

$$RfD^* = \frac{NOAEL \text{ or } LOAEL}{UF_1 \times UF_{2...}}$$

EXAMPLES OF UNCERTAINTY FACTORS	
10 X	Human variability
10 X	Extrapolation from animals to humans
10 X	Use of LOAEL instead of NOAEL
10 X	Increased child susceptibility
0.1–10 X	Modifying factor

Adapted from National Library of Medicine.[5]
RfD indicates reference dose; NOAEL, no observed adverse effect level; LOAEL, lowest observed adverse effect level; UF, uncertainty factor.
*Reference doses are calculated by the EPA. Similar measures include Acceptable Daily Intake (used by the Food and Drug Administration; the same calculation is performed, but modifying factors are not used) and Minimal Risk Levels (calculated by the Agency for Toxic Substances and Disease Registry for noncancer endpoints).

population (or populations) exposed to a toxicant at a particular level that will express a particular health effect related to that exposure. The less formal application of these concepts by clinicians can provide a method for addressing environmental health concerns of their patients or communities.

After more than 2 decades of experience with the process of risk assessment of chemicals by the EPA, several shortcomings have been revealed. In 2008, the National Academy of Sciences published *Science and Decisions, Advancing Risk Assessment,*[3] a report that evaluated the current process of risk assessment and the causes for extensive gridlock. The National Academy of Sciences' recommendations to the EPA focused on enhancing collaborative involvement throughout the EPA risk assessment process, further defining the scope of risk assessment, providing guidelines for use when data are lacking, and expanding application of the process to nonchemical agents and stressors.

While regulators grapple with the formal processes, the core concepts remain a useful framework for clinicians. Better characterization of the environmental sources of concern can be obtained by reviewing the scientific and medical literature and investigating the child's environment, either from the health history or from on-site investigation by trained environmental assessors. Governmental agencies such as the federal EPA, regional EPA offices, the Agency for Toxic Substances and Disease Registry, the Consumer Product Safety Commission, the Centers for Disease Control and Prevention, the Food Safety and Inspection Service, and others may also have relevant information. For well-characterized exposures, dose-response relationships may be relatively well defined, permitting crude exposure estimates using estimations based on established facts about the exposure, the environmental history, and the medical history. This information can then be compiled, and a determination of potential risks versus benefits of continued exposure versus mitigation can be developed. At times, the appropriate therapeutic and mitigation decisions will be obvious, such as removing all sources of lead from the environment of a child with elevated blood lead levels.[6] At other times, however, the answer may not be clear cut—for example, recommending removal of carpeting in the bedroom of a child with dust mite sensitivity and asthma when the father has just lost his job and the family cannot afford to pay for the removal.

RISK MANAGEMENT

Public agencies (federal, state, and local) responsible for minimizing environmental health risks review the results of commissioned risk assessments and, when possible, enact and amend regulations to reduce such health risks through an ongoing iterative process. Examples include banning hazardous substances from products and tightening controls on levels of emissions allowed. Considering scientific uncertainties, risk-benefit relationships and cost-benefit relationships are part of this process. A pediatrician can play a role in risk management for organizations and communities as well as for individual patients. A pediatrician may help to set policies for hospital and outpatient care on the basis of risk assessment data collected in-house or by public agencies. One example is the mandated use of soap and water and alcohol-based hand sanitizers for hand cleansing to reduce the risk of spreading highly infectious or aggressive microbial agents, such as methicillin-resistant *Staphylococcus aureus* (MRSA). A number of schools have taken action in their cafeterias to manage the availability of foods high in fat and calories to combat obesity in their students. Pediatricians may play important roles as advocates for changes in policies such as these.

When pediatricians and others address concerns about environmental factors, they may find that the evidence base that informs risk characterization for children is inadequate.[7] Taking precautionary measures when there is an environmental threat is welcomed by many individuals and communities, especially when adequate data are not available. The Precautionary Principle is discussed in greater detail in Chapter 57.

RISK COMMUNICATION

Risk communication can be defined as the exchange of information about the nature, magnitude, significance, and control of a risk. The exchange goes both ways. Parents frequently ask questions about the potential health effects of environmental exposures. Pediatricians often need to discuss environmental health risks and interventions with patients or parents and sometimes with representatives of the family, such as attorneys. At other times, they may need to address larger audiences, such as parent groups, colleagues, and governmental agencies. Communities and environmental advocacy groups are often in need of physicians with a clinical background to advise them about the potential health implications of various situations and exposures and identify paths of action. Clinicians generally hold positions of trust and high credibility within their communities and, thus, may serve as knowledgeable intermediaries between affected communities and other parties.

Risk communication is not a "one size fits all" procedure. The characteristics of the audience, the nature of the environmental hazard, the qualifications of the presenter, the social context of the risk, and other factors determine the risk message perceived ("risk perception") by the audience (Table 58.3). Two additional factors may affect risk communication[7]: (1) the need to build trust; and (2) the concept of cognitive attenuation.

When people are highly concerned, anxious, or fearful, they want to know that the person they are speaking with cares about them. Trust develops by demonstrating 4 qualities:

- Care and empathy;
- Honesty and openness;
- Dedication and commitment; and
- Competence and expertise.

Active listening, removing physical barriers between the clinician and the audience, mirroring (identifying similarities between clinician and audience), and residing in the neighborhood enhance trustworthiness. Cognitive attenuation refers to the "mental noise" that interferes with the ability to process information. This can be accentuated by fear, anxiety, or high levels of concern.

Effective communication addresses the needs of the various components of the audience. The audience may be composed of people from different backgrounds. The clinician should aim to know and involve the audience in the decision-making process. The process can begin by assessing the answers to these questions: What are the personal characteristics of audience members? What are their concerns? What are the relevant social and ethical factors? It is important for the clinician to know about the nature of the hazard being discussed. Is it natural or man-made? Catastrophic or not? Adults or children affected? When possible, it is advisable to develop alternatives to public hearings

Table 58.3: Some Factors Related to Decreased or Increased Perception of Risk[2]	
DECREASES PERCEIVED RISK	**INCREASES PERCEIVED RISK**
Hazard factors	
Familiar	Unfamiliar
Not catastrophic	Catastrophic or catastrophic potential
Natural	Synthetic
Adults affected	Fetuses or children affected
Nondreaded effect	Dreaded effect (cancer, birth defects)
Voluntary	Involuntary
Personal factors	
Male gender	Female gender
White race	Nonwhite race
Scientist	Nonscientist
Employed by industry or government	Employed by academic institutions
Social and ethical factors	
Trust in the risk communicator	Mistrust
Trust in the risk imposer (polluter)	Mistrust
Equal distribution of risk and benefits	Unfair or unequal distribution of risks and benefits
No perception of preexisting problem	Perception of unfair burden of cumulative risk in the community

through meetings with smaller numbers of people that are more conducive to an effective exchange of information. Awareness of how these factors influence the audience's perception of the risk and addressing those that can be addressed ultimately will determine the success or failure of the risk communication.

Developing the Message

Suggestions for developing a message for communicating risk have been published.[7] Sticking to the "rule of 3" is important, because people can only process 2 or 3 bits of information at a time, and they have a natural ability to remember triplets. In practical terms, this means developing no more than 3 key messages, with

3 supporting facts for each key message and 3 facts supporting each of these. It is also important to avoid "negative amplification," the concept whereby people give greater weight and attend more to negative information than positive. Presenting more positive information than negative can be effective, as is avoiding sentences with negative words, such as "no," "not," and "never." Lastly, keeping the message simple and using straightforward language and terms will help the audience to more clearly understand messages. Face-to-face communication is always preferred.

A Pediatrician's Role in Addressing Risk

Pediatricians may have many opportunities to apply risk principles when addressing environmental health concerns from patients and their communities. These are extensions of routine pediatric practice. For example, when evaluating a child with asthma, the components of risk assessment can be used: (1) defining the question—are there environmental factors that are making the patient's asthma worse? (2) understanding the scientific evidence base that links environmental triggers with asthma status and control; (3) taking an environmental history to identify the presence and extent of environmental triggers in the child's everyday environments; (4) developing a management plan that includes reducing exposure to relevant environmental triggers and possibly desensitizing the child to these triggers; and (5) educating the patient and family regarding the role of these factors in the child's asthma. All of this can be delivered in a dialogue engaging the parent and using terminology and a level of language that parent and child (if appropriate) can understand.

Beyond interacting with individual patients and families, it is likely that a pediatrician will have numerous opportunities to use the 7 cardinal rules of risk communication (Table 58.4) and other communication skills discussed in this chapter. Interacting with media, public health, and environmental agencies; contributing to health care policy; and providing community education are opportunities to assess, manage, and communicate risk in different ways.

For the community, the media is critical in getting the story out. The pediatrician should be proactive in contacting the media with accurate health information, correcting misinformation, promoting appropriate caution, and allaying fears.[9] These activities involve media skills that can be learned.

SUMMARY

Faced with an environmental or health risk, the process of risk assessment, risk management, and risk communication can be used as a unit or as individual components to evaluate, manage, and share knowledge and recommendations about the potential risk at the level of an individual patient encounter or in a larger public health context, such as a community. Although this process is most

Table 58.4: Seven Cardinal Rules of Risk Communication[8]

1. Accept and involve the public as a partner—your goal is an exchange of information, not to diffuse public concerns or convince the public of your point of view.

2. Plan carefully and evaluate your efforts—conform your interaction to the nature of subject matter, the nature of the audience, and your goals.

3. Listen to the public's specific concerns—trust, credibility, competence, fairness, and empathy are more important to your audience than statistics and detail.

4. Be honest, frank, and open—it is hard to regain credibility and trust once they have been lost.

5. Work with other credible sources—conflicts and disagreements among risk communicators create problems communicating with the audience.

6. Meet the needs of the media—they are usually more interested in politics, simplicity, and danger than risk, complexity, and safety.

7. Speak clearly and with compassion—don't forget to acknowledge the tragedy of human injury or environmental contamination. People can understand risk information but may not agree with you.

often associated with the evaluation of chemicals, it lends itself well to many other environmental agents, conditions, and stressors.

Risk management, as a regulatory and policy tool, aims to eliminate or at least control sources of exposures. The same approach to eliminating or mitigating sources of exposures of concern can be applied in environmental risk management for individual patients and families.

Risk communication should be based on the needs, beliefs, and knowledge base of the audience. The venue for delivering the message should be as appropriate as possible to be certain that 2-way communication is achieved and all parties understand one another. Careful consideration should be given to the social context in which the public perceives the risk, because this can distort the public's perception.

References

1. Committee on the Institutional Means for Assessment of Risks to Public Health and National Research Council, Commission on Life Sciences. *Risk Assessment in the Federal Government: Managing the Process.* Washington, DC: National Academies Press; 1983

2. Miller M, Solomon G. Environmental risk communication for the clinician. *Pediatrics.* 2003;112:211-217

3. Committee on Improving Risk Analysis Approaches Used by the US Environmental Protection Agency, National Research Council. *Science and Decisions: Advancing Risk Assessment.* Washington, DC: National Academies Press; 2008

4. US Environmental Protection Agency. *Child-Specific Exposure Factors Handbook.* Washington, DC: US Environmental Protection Agency; 2008

5. National Library of Medicine. Risk assessment. In: *Toxicology Tutor I. Basic Principles.* Washington, DC: US Department of Health and Human Services; Available at: http://sis.nlm. nih.gov/enviro/toxtutor/Tox1.html. Accessed June 14, 2011

6. State of California Environmental Protection Agency, Air Resources Board. *Lead Risk Management Activities.* Available at: http://www.arb.ca.gov/toxics/lead/lead.htm. Accessed April 6, 2011

7. Anderson ME, Kirkland KH, Guidotti TL, Rose C. A case study of tire crumb use on playgrounds: risk analysis and communication when major clinical knowledge gaps exist. *Environ Health Perspect.* 2006;114(1):1-3

8. Covello V, Allen F. *Seven Cardinal Rules of Risk Communication.* Washington, DC: US Environmental Protection Agency, Office of Policy Analysis; 1992

9. Galvez MP, Peters R, Graber N, Forman J. Effective risk communication in children's environmental health: lessons learned from 9/11. *Pediatr Clin North Am.* 2007;54(1):33-46

Chapter 59

Environmental Health Advocacy

■ ■ ■ ■ ■ ■

"It is not enough, however, to work at the individual bedside in the hospital. In the near or dim future, the pediatrician is to sit in and control school boards, health departments, and legislatures. He is a legitimate advisor to the judge and jury, and a seat for the physician in the councils of the republic is what the people have a right to demand." — Abraham Jacobi, MD

A pediatrician's role in protecting children from environmental hazards does not end at the office door. Advocacy work at all levels is an essential component of pediatric environmental health promotion and is critical to the reduction and prevention of children's exposure to environmental hazards. By nature of their training and expertise, pediatricians are uniquely qualified to provide greater context and meaning to debates over pressing environmental issues, and their input is critical to ensuring that the needs of children are met when critical policy decisions are made. This chapter outlines the need for pediatricians to advocate about environmental health issues; the kinds of advocacy work in which pediatricians can engage to achieve successful changes in public policy; the importance of consistent, coordinated messages about environmental health issues; and key tools and resources that are available for effective advocacy work.

Environmental health issues are particularly in need of enthusiastic engagement by pediatricians. Not only are children uniquely vulnerable to environmental harms reviewed throughout this handbook, but these harms affect potentially every aspect of a child's present and future health and well-being. Since the 1970s,[1] landmark legislation has been passed and renewed addressing clean air, clean water, chemicals, pesticides, product safety, and many other key environmental health issues. The development and application of this patchwork quilt of laws and regulations often require policy makers to seek technical and complex guidance from stakeholder groups. Pediatricians possess the knowledge and first-hand experience that may help to close the gaps in environmental policies that allow toxic exposures to continue. As a group with a common mission, pediatricians are powerful advocates on behalf of children's health and must lend their expertise to policy makers when environmental health policy decisions that affect children are being made.

Advocacy and the practice of pediatrics have always been intrinsically connected.[2,3] Advocacy is such an integral part of pediatric practice that it is included as a component of pediatric residency training. Advocacy also is central to the mission of many nongovernmental organizations and professional organizations, such as the American Academy of Pediatrics (AAP).

LEVELS OF PEDIATRIC ADVOCACY

Four levels of pediatric advocacy work have been identified.[4] *Individual advocacy* involves direct care and resources provided to patients and families every day. An example of individual advocacy is calling an insurance company or contacting a social service agency about abating a health hazard in the home that is exacerbating a child's asthma. Although pediatricians routinely engage in individual advocacy efforts, individual advocacy is often is the first step in broader efforts on the community, state, and federal levels.

Community advocacy builds on and reaches beyond individual advocacy in that it affects children within the community. A "community" can be defined geographically (as in a neighborhood, school district, or city) or culturally (as an ethnic or racial group or religious cluster). Community advocacy takes into consideration the environmental and social factors influencing child health and addresses ways in which pediatricians can work with community partners to address issues that negatively affect their patients.

State advocacy efforts by pediatricians focus primarily on the state legislative process. State legislatures play an increasingly important role in health policy and are a prolific source of new laws and regulations—as a whole, the nation's approximately 7380 state legislators consider more than 150 000 bills every year.[5] Although state legislatures are the primary focus of advocacy on the state level, there are also opportunities for advocacy with the state executive branch through the governor's office, with state agencies and regulatory activities, through the budget process, and through the judicial branch. Working through their AAP chapters and in coalitions with other advocacy groups, pediatricians have had major effects on environmental health issues in their states. Issues include improving indoor air quality by eliminating secondhand smoke exposure, improving outdoor air quality by limiting emissions of pollutants, promoting screening for lead poisoning, and many others.

Federal advocacy involves national environmental health issues. For dozens of years, pediatricians have advocated on the federal level about issues such as food safety, toxic chemicals in children's products, global climate change, and other environmental issues that affect children's health.[6] The AAP Washington Office provides technical and strategic assistance for pediatricians to testify at congressional hearings and coordinates national advocacy efforts. The testimony given by pediatricians during congressional hearings, their briefings for members of Congress, their comments regarding proposed federal regulations, and their engagement in related activities are critical to the success of these efforts in Washington, DC.

A pediatrician may feel that to become involved in advocacy, he or she must know everything about an issue and about the political or legislative process. The clinical skills a clinician already possesses, however, are similar to those needed to be an effective advocate—the ability to translate complex scientific and medical concepts into simple language, to diagnose a problem, and to outline a course of treatment. Advocacy may begin as soon as a particular problem is identified. The next step is to bring awareness of the issue to decision makers and others who can help to generate a solution. Although one does need a basic understanding of the legislative and policy process (which can be obtained through resources available from the AAP[3]), 2 of the most important attributes needed for success are enthusiasm and a willingness to speak out on behalf of children.

Coordination is key to the success of any advocacy effort. By working with and through their AAP chapters, pediatricians can take full advantage of the resources and information available from the AAP, the state chapter, and its coalition partners.

Broadening support, either through gaining the participation of other pediatricians in efforts or by seeking the partnership of other organizations that share similar goals and priorities, is critical to a successful effort. This broad base of support will demonstrate to community leaders and elected officials that there are many people who care about environmental health issues and that those people are taking action to create change.

Pediatricians often use media to promote their advocacy efforts. The 4 types of advocacy can be enhanced by using media to spotlight the issues through such activities as letters to the editor, op-ed pieces, calling attention to the issue through news stories, or getting editorial support. Enhancing understanding of the issue using social media can result in a magnifying effect. Pediatricians may know that having the media on one's side when talking with legislators can make all the difference in ensuring a successful outcome. Conversely, media opposition can make advocacy an uphill struggle.

When working on issues as important as pediatric environmental health, it may be hard to imagine that others would not support a pediatrician's efforts, or even oppose them. However, pediatricians' advocacy priorities will nearly always compete with those of other groups over resources and funding or reflect different points of view. It is often helpful to bring several pediatricians to the table to underscore the importance of the particular issue to decision makers as they consider positions of differing interests.

The success of pediatric environmental advocacy ultimately rests with the volunteer efforts of individual pediatricians. The AAP, along with many of its state chapters, has lobbyists and other public policy staff who help to shape laws and regulations on behalf of children. However, the work of professional lobbying staff alone is not enough. The unique perspective and credibility of pediatricians propel these issues forward in a way that a lobbyist alone cannot. The pediatrician's voice is critical in helping create the social and political change needed to make lasting advancements in environmental health policy.[7]

For more information on advocacy by pediatricians and how pediatricians can have an effect on child health policy, please see the *AAP Advocacy Guide*.

Resources

American Academy of Pediatrics

Department of Federal Affairs
www.aap.org/advocacy/washing/mainpage.htm

Division of State Government Affairs
www.aap.org/advocacy/stgov.htm

Chapter and District Information
www.aap.org/member/chapters/chapserv.htm

AAP Member Center
www.aap.org/moc

State

Council of State Governments
www.csg.org

National Association of Counties
www.naco.org

National Conference of State Legislatures
www.ncsl.org

National Governors Association
www.nga.org

National Association of State and Territorial Health Officials
www.astho.org

National Association of County and City Health Officials
www.naccho.org

State Environmental Agencies
www.epa.gov/epahome/state.htm

Federal
White House
www.whitehouse.gov

Official Web Portal of the Federal Government
www.usa.gov

Regulations issued by Federal Agencies
www.regulations.gov

Congressional
Thomas: Legislative Information on the Internet
thomas.loc.gov

US House of Representatives
www.house.gov

US Senate
www.senate.gov

References

1. US Environmental Protection Agency. EPA Accomplishments. Available at: http://www.epa.gov/history/accomplishments.htm. Accessed April 6, 2011
2. Gruen RL, Campbell EG, Blumenthal D. Public roles of US physicians: community participation, political involvement, and collective advocacy. *JAMA.* 2006;296(20):2467-2475.
3. Rushton FE Jr, American Academy of Pediatrics, Committee on Community Health Services. The pediatrician's role in community pediatrics. *Pediatrics.* 2005;115(4):1092-1094
4. American Academy of Pediatrics. *AAP Advocacy Guide.* Available at: www.aap.org/moc/advocacyguide. Accessed April 6, 2011
5. Council of State Governments. *The Book of the States 2010.* Lexington, KY: Council of State Governments; 2010
6. Goldman L, Falk H, Landrigan PJ, Balk SJ, Reigart JR, Etzel RA. Environmental pediatrics and its impact on government health policy. *Pediatrics.* 2004;113(4 Suppl):1146-1157
7. American Academy of Pediatrics, Council on Community Pediatrics and Committee on Native American Child Health. Policy statement—health equity and children's rights. *Pediatrics.* 2010;125(4):838-849

Appendix A

Resources for Pediatric Environmental Health

■ ■ ■ ■ ■ ■

The American Academy of Pediatrics has not reviewed the material on these Web sites. Inclusion in this list does not imply endorsement.

Organization	Contact Information
GOVERNMENT	
US FEDERAL & STATE GOVERNMENTS	
Agency for Toxic Substances and Disease Registry (ATSDR) US Department of Health and Human Services (DHHS) 1600 Clifton Rd NE; Mail Stop E-28 Atlanta, GA 30333	Web: http://www.atsdr.cdc.gov Information Center Clearinghouse: Phone: 404-639-6360 Fax: 404-639-0744 Emergency Response Branch Phone: 404-639-0615
— ATSDR GATHER (Geographic Analysis Tool for Health and Environmental Research)	Web: http://gis.cdc.gov
— ATSDR Toxicological Profiles	Web: http://www.atsdr.cdc.gov/toxprofiles/index.asp
— ATSDR Regional Offices	Web: http://www.atsdr.cdc.gov/dro
California Environmnetal Protection Agency 1001 I Street P.O. Box 2815 Sacramento, CA 95812-2815	Web: http://www.calepa.ca.gov 1001 I Street P.O. Box 2815 Sacramento, CA 95812-2815

Organization	Contact Information
GOVERNMENT	
US FEDERAL & STATE GOVERNMENTS	
California Electric and Magnetic Fields (EMF) Program 1515 Clay St, Suite 1700 Oakland, CA 94612	Web: http://www.dhs.ca.gov/ehib/emf
National Center for Environmental Health (NCEH) Centers for Disease Control & Prevention (CDC) 4770 Buford Hwy, NE Mail Stop F-28 Atlanta, GA 30341-3724	Web: http://www.cdc.gov/nceh E-mail: ncehinfo@cdc.gov NCEH Health Line: 888-232-6789
— NCEH Asthma Program	Web: http://www.cdc.gov/asthma
— NCEH Lead Poisoning Prevention Program	Web: http://www.cdc.gov/nceh/lead
— National Report on Human Exposure to Environmental Chemicals	Web: http://www.cdc.gov/exposurereport
National Institute for Occupational Safety and Health (NIOSH)	Web: http://www.cdc.gov/niosh/homepage.html E-mail: cdcinfo@cdc.gov Phone: 800-35-NIOSH (800-356-4674)
— NIOSH Young Worker Safety and Health	http://www.cdc.gov/niosh/topics/youth
Consumer Product Safety Commission (CPSC) 4340 East West Hwy Bethesda, MD 20814	Web: http://www.cpsc.gov Phone: 800-638-2772 Fax: 301-504-0124
US Environmental Protection Agency (EPA) 1200 Pennsylvania Ave NW Washington, DC 20460	Web: http://www.epa.gov Administrative Phone: 202-272-0167
— EPA Office of Children's Health Protection	Web: http://yosemite.epa.gov/ochp/ochpweb.nsf/content/homepage.htm Office of Child Health Protection Phone: 202-564-2188
— EPA Office of Pesticide Programs	Web: http://www.epa.gov/pesticides Office of Pesticide Programs Phone: 703-305-5017 National Pesticides Hotline: 800-222-1222

Organization	Contact Information
GOVERNMENT	
US FEDERAL & STATE GOVERNMENTS	
— EPA Office of Air and Radiation	Office main Web : http://www.epa.gov/oar Indoor air Web : http://www.epa.gov/iaq Indoor Air Quality Information Clearinghouse Phone: 800-438-4318 Tools for Schools Program Web: http://www.epa.gov/iaq/schools/index.html Air Now–ground-level ozone Web: http://www.epa.gov/airnow The Healthy School Environments Assessment Tool (HealthySEATv2) http://www.epa.gov/schools/healthyseat/index.html
— EPA Endocrine Disruptor Screening Program	Web: http://www.epa.gov/scipoly/oscpendo
— EPA Children's Environmental Health Research Centers	Web: http://www.epa.gov/ncer/childrenscenters/newsroom/archive.html Health Research Initiative
— EPA Chemical Emergency Preparedness and Prevention	Web: http://www.epa.gov/region5superfund/cepps Chemical Spills Emergency Hotline: 800-424-8802 Hazardous Waste/Community Right to Know Hotline: 800-424-9346
— EPA Office of Water	Web: http://www.epa.gov/water/index.html Safe Drinking Water Hotline: 800-426-4791 Drinking Water Advisories Web: http://www.epa.gov/waterscience/drinking Fish Consumption Advisories Web: http://www.epa.gov/ost/fish
— EPA Office of Pollution Prevention & Toxics	Web: http://www.epa.gov/opptintr/index.html Toxic Substances Control Act (TSCA) Information Line: 202-554-1404
— EPA Toxics Release Inventory Program	Web: http://www.epa.gov/tri
— EPA Children's Environmental Health Resource, Toxicity and Exposure Assessment for Children's Health (TEACH)	http://www.epa.gov/teach

Organization	Contact Information
GOVERNMENT	
US FEDERAL & STATE GOVERNMENTS	
— EPA–America's Children & the Environment	http://www.epa.gov/economics/children
— EPA Sunwise Program	http://www.epa.gov/sunwise
Center for Food Safety and Applied Nutrition (CFSAN) Food and Drug Administration (FDA) 5100 Paint Branch Parkway College Park, MD 20740-3835	Web: http://www.cfsan.fda.gov Phone: 888-SAFEFOOD
Food Safety: Gateway to Government Food Safety Information	Web: http://www.FoodSafety.gov
Food Safety and Inspection Service Food Safety Education Office 1400 Independence Ave, SW Washington, DC 20250	Web: http://www.fsis.usda.gov E-mail: fsis.webmaster@usda.gov Phone: 301-504-9605 Fax: 301-504-0203
National Institute of Environmental Health Sciences (NIEHS) US DHHS PO Box 12233 Research Triangle Park, NC 27709	Web: http://www.niehs.nih.gov Phone: 919-541-1919 Fax: 919-541-3592
— The Environmental Genome Project	Web: http://www.niehs.nih.gov/research/supported/programs/egp
— NIEHS Children's Environmental Health Research Initiative	Web: http://www.niehs.nih.gov/research/supported/centers/prevention/index.cfm
— The National Toxicology Program (NTP)	Web: http://ntp-server.niehs.nih.gov
— Center for the Evaluation of Risks to Human Reproduction	Web: http://cerhr.niehs.nih.gov
— Environmental Health Perspectives	Web: http://ehp03.niehs.nih.gov/home.action
National Cancer Institute (NCI) US Department of Health and Human Services National Institutes of Health (NIH) 9000 Rockville Pike Bethesda, MD 20892	Web: http://www.nci.nih.gov Surveillance, Epidemiology and End Results (SEER) Program Web: http://seer.cancer.gov Phone: 800-4-CANCER

Organization	Contact Information
GOVERNMENT	
US FEDERAL & STATE GOVERNMENTS	
National Library of Medicine, Environmental Health & Toxicology	Web: http://sis.nlm.nih.gov/enviro.html
— TOXNET	Web: http://toxnet.nlm.nih.gov
— Drugs and Lactation Database (LactMed)	Web: http://toxnet.nlm.nih.gov/cgi-bin/sis/htmlgen?LACT
National Children's Study (NCS) Longitudinal Cohort Study of Environmental Effects on Child Health and Development	http://www.nationalchildrensstudy.gov
Office of Healthy Homes and Lead Hazard Control US Department of Housing & Urban Development 451 7th St SW Washington, DC 20410	Web: http://www.hud.gov/offices/lead
US Global Change Research Program Suite 250 1717 Pennsylvania Ave, NW Washington, DC 20006	Web: http://www.climatescience.gov Phone 202-223-6262
1-800-QUIT-NOW	Web: http://1800quitnow.cancer.gov Phone: 1-800-QUIT-NOW
NON-US GOVERNMENT	
European Union information on Environmental Health	http://europa.eu/pol/env/index_en.htm
Registration, Evaluation, Authorization and Restriction of Chemicals (REACH)	http://ec.europa.eu/environment/chemicals/reach/reach_intro.htm
Nongovernmental Organizations	
Alliance for Health Homes 50 F St, NW Suite 300 Washington, DC 20002	Web: http://www.afhh.org/index.htm E-mail: afhh@afhh.org Phone: 202-347-7610
American Academy of Pediatrics Julius B. Richmond Center of Excellence 141 Northwest Point Blvd Elk Grove Village, IL 60007	Web: http://aap.org/richmondcenter Phone: 847-434-4264

Organization	Contact Information
Nongovernmental Organizations	
American Association of Poison Control Centers 3201 New Mexico Ave NW Suite 310 Washington, DC 20016	Web: http://www.aapcc.org Phone: 202-362-7217
American Cancer Society 1599 Clifton Rd NE Atlanta, GA 30329	Web: http://www.cancer.org Phone: 404-320-3333 or 800-ACS-2345 Fax: 404-329-7530
American Lung Association 61 Broadway 6th Floor New York, NY 10016	Web: http://www.lungusa.org Phone: 800-LUNG-USA
American Public Health Association 800 I St NW Washington, DC 20001	Web: www.apha.org Phone: 202-777-2742
Association of Occupational and Environmental Clinics (AOEC) Pediatric Environmental Health Specialty Units	Web: http://www.aoec.org http://www.aoec.org/PEHSU
Association of State and Territorial Health Officials (ASTHO)	Web: http://www.astho. org/?template=environment.html
Asthma and Allergy Foundation of America 1233 20th St NW Suite 402 Washington, DC 20005	Web: http://www.aafa.org Phone: 202-466-7643 Fax: 202-466-8940
Beyond Pesticides 701 E St SE, #200 Washington DC 20003	Web: http://www.beyondpesticides.org E-mail: info@beyondpesticides.org Phone: 202-543-5450 Fax: 202-543-4791
Canadian Association of Physicians for the Environment 208-145 Spruce St Ottawa, ON K1R 6P1 Canada	Web: www.cape.ca/children.html E-mail: info@cape.ca Phone: 613-235-2273 Fax: 613-233-9028
Canadian Institute of Child Health 384 Bank St, Suite 300 Ottawa, ON K2P 1Y4 Canada	Web: http://www.cich.ca E-mail: cich@cich.ca Phone: 613-230-8838 Fax: 613-230-6654
The Canadian Partnership for Children's Health and Environment (CPCHE) 215 Spadina Avenue, Suite 130 Toronto, Ontario, Canada M5T 2C7	Web: http://www. healthyenvironmentforkids.ca/english Phone: 819-458-3750 E-mail: info@healthyenvironmentforkids.ca

Organization	Contact Information
Nongovernmental Organizations	
Center for Health, Environment and Justice (CHEJ) PO Box 6806 Falls Church, VA 22040	Web: http://www.chej.org E-mail: chej@chej.org Phone: 703-237-2249
Child Proofing Our Communities Campaign	Web: www.childproofing.org E-mail: childproofing@chej.org Phone: 703-237-2249, ext 21 Fax: 703-237-8389
Children's Environmental Health Network 110 Maryland Ave NE, Suite 511 Washington, DC 20002	Web: http://www.cehn.org E-mail: cehn@cehn.org Phone: 202-543-4033 Fax: 202-543-8797
Children's Health Environmental Coalition PO Box 1540 Princeton, NJ 08542	Web: http://www.checnet.org
Children's Environmental Health Institute (CEHI) PO Box 50342 Austin, TX 78763 – 0342	Web: http://www.cehi.org E-mail: janie.fields@cehi.org Phone: 512-567-7405
North American Commission for Environmental Cooperation (CEC) 393, rue St-Jacques Ouest Bureau 200 Montréal, QC H2Y 1N9 Canada	Web: http://www.cec.org/Page.asp?PageID=1115&AA_SiteLanguageID=1 E-mail: info@ccemtl.org Phone: 514-350-4300 Fax: 514-350-4314
Commonweal PO Box 316 Bolinas, CA 94924	Web:http://www.commonweal.org E-mail: commonweal@commonweal.org Phone: 415-868-0970 Fax: 415-868-2230
Earth Portal	Web: http://www.earthportal.org
Encyclopedia of the Earth	Web: http://www.eoearth.org
EMR Network PO Box 5 Charlotte, VT 05445	Web: http://www.emrnetwork.org/index.htm E-mail: info@emrnetwork.org Phone: 978-371-3035
Environmental Defense 257 Park Ave S New York, NY 10010	Web: http://www.environmentaldefense.org Phone: 212-505-2100 Fax: 212-505-2375
Scorecard	Web: http://scorecard.org

Organization	Contact Information
Nongovernmental Organizations	
Environmental Justice Resource Center at Clark Atlanta University 223 James P Brawley Dr SW Atlanta, GA 30314	Web: http://www.ejrc.cau.edu Phone: 404-880-6911 Fax: 404-880-6909
Environmental Working Group (EWG) 1436 U St NW Suite 100 Washington, DC 20009	Web: http://www.ewg.org
FoodNews	Web: http://www.foodnews.org
EXTOXNET InfoBase	Web: http://ace.ace.orst.edu/info/extoxnet
Farm*A*Syst 303 Hiram Smith Hall 1545 Observatory Dr Madison, WI 53706-1289	Web: http://www.uwex.edu/farmasyst Phone: 608-262-0024 E-mail: farmasys@uwex.edu
Health Care Without Harm 1755 S St, NW, Suite 6B Washington DC 20009	Web: http://www.noharm.org E-mail: info@hcwh.org Phone: 202-234-0091
Healthy Schools Network, Inc. 773 Madison Ave Albany, NY 12208	Web: http://www.healthyschools.org E-mail: info@healthyschools.org Phone: 518-462-0632 Fax: 518-462-0433
Home*A*Syst Program 303 Hiram Smith Hall 1545 Observatory Dr Madison, WI 53706	Web: http://www.uwex.edu/homeasyst E-mail: homeasys@uwex.edu Phone: 608-262-0024 Fax: 608-265-2775
Institute for Agriculture and Trade Policy 2105 1st Ave S Minneapolis, MN 55404	Web: http://www.iatp.org Phone: 612-870-0453 Fax: 612-870-4846
Institute for Children's Environmental Health 1646 Dow Rd Freeland, WA 98249	Web: www.iceh.org and www.partnersforchildren.org Phone: 360-331-7904 E-mail: emiller@iceh.org Fax: 360-331-7908
International Research and Information Network for Children's Health, Environment and Safety (INCHES)	Web: http://www.inchesnetwork.org/index.html
Learning Disabilities Association of America 4156 Library Rd Pittsburgh, PA 15234-1349	Web: http://www.ldanatl.org E-mail: info@ldaamerica.org Phone: 412-341-1515; 412-341-8077 Fax: 412-344-0224

Organization	Contact Information
Nongovernmental Organizations	
March of Dimes Birth Defects Foundation 1275 Mamaroneck Ave White Plains, NY 10605	Web: http://www.modimes.org Phone: 914-428-7100 Fax: 914-428-8203
Allergy & Asthma Network Mothers of Asthmatics 2751 Prosperity Ave, Suite 150 Fairfax, VA 22031	Web: http://www.aanma.org Phone: 800-878-4403 Fax: 703-573-7794
National Association of County and City Health Officials (NACCHO) 1100 17th St, 2nd Floor Washington, DC 20036	Web: http://www.naccho.org Phone: 202-783-5550 Fax: 202-783-1583
National Center for Healthy Housing 10227 Wincopin Circle, Suite 100 Columbia, MD 21044	Web: http://www.centerforhealthyhousing. org/index.htm Phone: 410-992-0712 Fax: 410-715-2310
National Council on Skin Cancer Prevention	Web: http://www.skincancerprevention.org
National Environmental Education Foundation 4301 Connecticut Avenue NW, Suite 160 Washington, DC 20008	Web: http://www.neefusa.org Phone: 202-833-2933 Fax: 202-261-6464
National Lead Information Center 422 S Clinton Ave Rochester, NY 14620	Web: http://www.epa.gov/lead/nlic.htm Phone: 800-424-LEAD (5323)
National Pesticide Information Center (NPIC)	Web: http://npic.orst.edu
National Safety Council, Environmental Health and Safety 1025 Connecticut Ave NW; Suite 1200 Washington, DC 20036	Web: http://www.nsc.org/ safety_home/Resources/Pages/ EnvironmentalHealthandSafety.aspx
National Safety Council (NSC), Environmental Health Center, Indoor Air Quality	Web: http://www.nsc.org/news_resources/ Resources/Documents/Indoor_Air_ Quality.pdf
Natural Resources Defense Council 40 West 20th St New York, NY 10011	Web: http://www.nrdc.org E-mail: nrdcinfo@nrdc.org Phone: 212-727-2700 Fax: 212-727-1773
Organization of Teratology Information Specialists	Web: http://www.otispregnancy.org

Organization	Contact Information
Nongovernmental Organizations	
Our Stolen Future	Web: http://www.ourstolenfuture.org/index.htm
Pediatric Environmental Health Specialty Units (PEHSUs)	Web: http://www.aoec.org/pesu.htm www.pehsu.net (includes links to all PEHSUs)
— Pediatric Environmental Health Center at Children's Hospital/ Occupational & EnvironmentalHealth Center at Cambridge Hospital	Web: www.childrenshospital.org/pehc Phone: 888-CHILD 14 (888-244-5314) or 617-355-8177
— Pediatric Environmental Health Specialty Unit Mount Sinai School of Medicine	Web: http://www.mssm.edu/research/programs/pediatric-environmental-health-specialty-unit Phone: 866-265-6201 (toll-free) or 212-241-0938
— Mid-Atlantic Center for Children's Health and the Environment (MACCHE)	Web: http://www.health-e-kids.org Phone: 866-MACCHE1 (866-622-2431) or 202-994-1166
— Pediatric Environmental Health Specialty Unit, Southeast Region	Web: http://www.sph.emory.edu/PEHSU Phone: 877-33PEHSU (877-337-3478) (toll-free) or 770-956-9636
— Great Lakes Center for Children's Environmental Health	Web: http://www.uic.edu/sph/glakes/kids Phone: 800-672-3113 (toll-free) or 312-633-5310
— Southwest Center for Pediatric Environmental Health	Web: http://www.swcpeh.org/ E-mail: swcpeh@uthct.edu Phone: 888-901-5665 (toll-free) or 903-531-0830 (local) Fax: 903-877-7982
— Mid-AmericaPediatric Environmental Health Specialty Unit	www.childrensmercy.org/mapehsu Phone: (913) 588-6638 Toll Free (800) 421-9916 E-mail mapehsu@cmh.edu
— Rocky Mountain Regional Pediatric Environmental Health Specialty Unit	Web: www.rmrpehsu.org Phone: 877-800-5554 (toll-free)
— Pediatric Environmental Health Specialty Unit University of California San Francisco & University of California Irvine	Web: www.ucsf.edu/ucpehsu Phone: 866-UC-PEHSU (866-827-3478) (same toll-free phone for both sites—San Francisco and Irvine), 415-206-4320 (local San Francisco), or 949-824-8961 (local Irvine)

Organization	Contact Information
Nongovernmental Organizations	
— Northwest Pediatric Environmental Health Specialty Unit 325 9th Ave Mail Stop 359739 Seattle, WA 98104-2499	Web: http://depts.washington.edu/pehsu Phone: 877-KID-CHEM (877-543-2436) (restricted to west of the Mississippi River)
— Pediatric Environmental Health Clinic Misericordia Child Health Centre Edmonton, AB Canada	E-mail occdoc@connect.ab.ca Phone: 780-930-5731
— Unidad Pediatrica Ambiental–Mexico Pediatric Environmental Health Specialty Unit (UPA-PEHSU) Cuernavaca, Morelos Mexico	E-mail ecifuent@correo.insp.mx Phone: 800-001-7777, 52-777-102-1259 (outside of Mexico)
Physicians for Social Responsibility 1875 Connecticut Ave NW, Suite 1012 Washington, DC, 20009	Web: http://www.psr.org E-mail: psrnatl@psr.org Phone: 202-667-4260 Fax: 202-667-4201
— Pediatric Environmental Health Toolkit	http://www.psr.org/resources/pediatric-toolkit.html
School Integrated Pest Management	Web: http://schoolipm.ifas.ufl.edu
Smoke Free Homes	Web: http://www.kidslivesmokefree.org
Teratology Society 1821 Michael Faraday Dr Suite 300 Reston, VA 20190	Web: http://www.teratology.org E-mail: tshq@teratology.org Phone: 703-438-3104
Tulane/Xavier Center for Bioenvironmental Research 1430 Tulane Ave, SL-3 New Orleans, LA 70112	Web: http://www.cbr.tulane.edu E-mail: cbr@tulane.edu Phone: 504-585-6910 Fax: 504-585-6428
University of Minnesota Environmental Health & Safety Program W-140 Bayton Health Service 410 Church St SE Minneapolis, MN 55455x	Web: http://www.dehs.umn.edu E-mail: dehs@tc.umn.edu
Centers for Children's Environmental Health & Disease Prevention Research	http://www.niehs.nih.gov/research/supported/centers/prevention/grantees/index.cfm
— Columbia University Mailman School of Public Health	Web: http://cpmcnet.columbia.edu/dept/sph/ccceh/index.html

Organization	Contact Information
Nongovernmental Organizations	
— University of Washington Center for Child Environmental Health Risk Research	Web: http://depts.washington.edu/chc
— Johns Hopkins University Center for Childhood Asthma in the Urban Environment	Web: http://www.epa.gov/ncer/childrenscenters/hopkins.html
— University of California, Davis Environmental Factors in the Etiology of Autism	Web: http://www.vetmed.ucdavis.edu/cceh
— University of California at Berkeley Exposure & Health of Farm Worker Children in California	Web: http://ehs.sph.berkeley.edu/chamacos
— University of Illinois, Urbana-Champaign FRIENDS Children's Environmental Health Center	Web: http://www.epa.gov/ncerqa/childrenscenters/illinois.html
— Mount Sinai School of Medicine Inner City Toxicants, Child Growth & Development	Web: http://www.mssm.edu/research/programs/childrens-environmental-health-and-disease-prevention-research-center
— Children's Environmental Health and Disease Prevention Center at Dartmouth	Web: http://www.dartmouth.edu/~childrenshealth/index.html
— University of Southern California Respiratory Disease & Prevention	Web: http://www.usc.edu/schools/medicine/departments/preventive_medicine/divisions/occupational/occ_environmental/cehc
— Children's Hospital Medical Center University of Cincinnati Children's Environmental health Center	Web: http://www.cincinnatichildrens.org/research/project/enviro/default.htm
World Health Organization (WHO) Public Health and Environment	Web: http://www.who.int/phe/en
— WHO Environmental Health Information	Web: http://www.who.int/topics/environmental_health/en
— Healthy Environments for Children Alliance (HECA)	Web: http://www.who.int/heca/en
— Global Initiative on Children's Environmental Health Indicators	Web: http://www.who.int/ceh/indicators/en
— Children's Environmental Health	Web: http://www.who.int/ceh/en
— Children's Environment and Health Action Plan for Europe	Web: http://www.euro.who.int/__data/assets/pdf_file/0006/78639/E83338.pdf

Organization	Contact Information
Nongovernmental Organizations	
— WHO water specific information	Web: http://www.who.int/water_sanitation_health
— WHO chemical specific information	Web: http://www.who.int/pcs
— WHO information about ionizing radiation	Web: http://www.who.int/ionizing_radiation/en
— WHO information about air quality and health	Web: http://www.who.int/mediacentre/factsheets/fs313/en
— WHO information about ultraviolet radiation	Web: http://www.who.int/peh-uv
— WHO information about electro-magnetic fields	Web: http://www.who.int/peh-emf/en
— WHO information about occupational health	Web: http://www.who.int/oeh/index.html
— Intergovernmental Panel on Climate Change (IPCC)	Web: http://www.ipcc.ch/index.htm

Curricula for Environmental Education and Environmental Health Science Education in Primary and Secondary Schools

■ ■ ■ ■ ■ ■

Environmental education is defined as "an active process that increases awareness, knowledge, and skills that result in understanding, commitment, informed decisions, and constructive action that ensure stewardship of all interdependent parts of the earth's environment" (North Carolina Environmental Education Plan, April 1995). Environmental education should begin early and continue through high school. Children who receive environmental education may be able to prevent environmental exposures through personal health choices and through community involvement. As adults, these children should be well prepared to participate in the political process as informed and environmentally literate citizens. A number of excellent environmental education curricula have been developed. The development and selection of environmental education materials is based on the Environmental Education Materials: Guidelines for Excellence published in 1996 and revised in 2004. More than 1000 practitioners and scholars developed the Guidelines through a critique and consensus process (http://www.naaee.org/programs-and-initiatives/guidelines-for-excellence/materials-guidelines/materials-guidelines).

Environmental health science education has been an emerging area of study and curriculum development since the mid 1990s. Within the school system, environmental health can play a valuable role in bridging the gap between traditional environmental education and health education. Too often, students see environmental health as health of the environment and may not consider how the environment can affect their health. To address this educational need and to incorporate health into the environment picture, many novel and engaging environmental health education curricular materials have been created to align with the National Science Education Standards (http://www.nap.edu/catalog. php?record_id=4962). Most recently, on the basis of findings of the Environment as an Integrative Context (EIC) Model developed by the State Education and Environment Roundtable (SEER) in 1997, problem-based and integrated environmental health curricula have been created, implemented and evaluated (http://www.niehs.nih.gov/health/scied/integrated/index.cfm). Preliminary research shows a variety of positive outcomes for teachers who implement and for students who are exposed to problem-based and integrated curricula (http:// www.niehs.nih.gov/research/supported/programs/ehsic/highlights.cfm).

As evidenced by various projects, the most successful environmental and environmental health science education programs result from combining excellent curricula with the efforts of enthusiastic individuals (teachers, parents, and administrators) at the local level. These programs can provide primary and secondary school students with sufficient knowledge to participate in activities that will help to improve the environmental health knowledge and overall health of their communities, including their families. Curricula relevant to communities might include topics such as global climate change and its effects on children's health, sun safety, drinking water contaminants, the causes and effects of outdoor air pollution, and the importance of avoiding secondhand smoke.

Health care professionals can stimulate and strengthen environmental health education efforts in schools through volunteer activities in the classroom, school health programs, and technical partnerships with local school boards and state departments of education. Classroom volunteer work can include assisting teachers in designing and executing hands-on environmental science and environmental health activities that actively link human health to the state of the physical environment. Within the tradition of school health is the concept of the "healthy school environment." Clinicians can help local schools identify ways in which the school environment can be made healthier. A first step might involve evaluating the school facility for any environmental, health, and safety issues. On the basis of that evaluation, a school might choose to address a specific agent or toxicant. For example, a clinician could help to develop a plan for the school to reduce pesticide use, or work with students and faculty to ensure that the school is in compliance with state and federal health and safety regulations. Health care professionals can participate in PTA activities and teacher training on environmental health issues pertinent to their community, drawing examples from their practices. Health care professionals located at universities might approach their education departments to learn about ongoing or planned work in the area of

Appendix B: Curricula for Environmental Education and Environmental
Health Science Education in Primary and Secondary Schools

881

environmental health science education and determine whether partnership opportunities exist. Finally, they can work with the district or state department of education to help introduce environmental health education systemically. Increasingly, states are creating offices of environmental education within departments of education to stimulate preservice and in-service teacher training as well as to include environmental sciences in K–12 curricula. Health care professionals can add insight and expertise to this process by stimulating discussion about the links between the environment and human health.

Environmental Education Curricula and Resources

General Environmental Education

1. Project Learning Tree, 1111 19th St NW, Suite 780, Washington, DC 20036, phone: 202-463-2462, Internet: http://www.plt.org. Project Learning Tree uses the forest and trees as a "window on the world" to increase students' understanding of our complex environment, stimulate critical and creative thinking, develop the ability to make informed decisions on environmental issues, and instill the confidence and commitment to take responsible action on behalf of the environment (K–12).

2. Project WILD, 5555 Morningside Dr, Suite 212, Houston, TX 77005, phone: 713-520-1936, Internet: http://www.projectwild.org. The *Project WILD K–12 Activity Guide* focuses on wildlife and habitat, and the *Project WILD Aquatic Education Activity Guide* emphasizes aquatic wildlife and aquatic ecosystems. The guides are organized thematically and are designed for integration into existing courses of study.

3. Project WET, 1001 West Oak, Suite 210, Bozeman, MT 59715, phone: 406-585-2236 or toll-free at 866-337-5486, Internet: http://www.projectwet.org. The goal of Project WET is to promote awareness, appreciation, knowledge, and stewardship of water resources through the development and dissemination of classroom-ready teaching aids and the establishment of state and internationally sponsored programs (K–12).

4. North American Association for Environmental Education, 2000 P St, NW, Suite 540, Washington, DC 20036, phone: 202-419-0412, Internet: http://www.naaee.org. NAAEE is an association that represents professional environmental educators. Two projects are noteworthy regarding curricula. First, the *EE-Link* web site provides an array of information about teaching and curricula resources (http://eelink.net). Second, the *National Project for Excellence in Environmental Education (NPEEE)* has developed national guidelines for materials, K-12 students, educators, and nonformal programs

(http://www.naaee.org/programs-and-initiatives/guidelines-for-excellence). Of particular importance are the Environmental Education Materials: Guidelines for Excellence and the Excellence in Environmental Education: Guidelines for Learning (K-12). The Materials Guidelines are a set of recommendations for developing and selecting environmental education materials to ensure quality. The Learner Guidelines set a standard for high-quality environmental education based on what an environmentally literate person should know and be able to do in grades K-12.

5. US Environmental Protection Agency, Office of Children's Health Protection and Environmental Education, Environmental Education Division, 1200 Pennsylvania Avenue, NW, Room 1426, Washington, DC, 20460, phone: 202-564-0443, Internet: http://www.epa.gov/enviroed. The Division implements the National Environmental Education Act of 1990. One program funded by this office is the Environmental Education and Training Partnership, which provides training and support to teachers and other education professionals (http://www.eetap.org). EETAP has developed many resources for educators such as "Meeting Standards Naturally"—a CD/ROM which includes curriculum activities that demonstrate how environmental lessons can support grade level education standards. Other EPA environmental education resources include Web sites designed for children (http://www.epa.gov/kids), middle school students (http://www.epa.gov/students), high school students (http://www.epa.gov/highschool), and teachers (http://www.epa.gov/teachers).

6. National Environmental Education Foundation, 4301 Connecticut Avenue, NW, Suite 160, Washington, DC, 20008, Internet: http://www.neefusa.org. NEEF is a private, nonprofit organization chartered by Congress under the National Environmental Education Act of 1990 to advance environmental knowledge. NEEF's National Environmental Education Week program provides references to environmental education and environmental health education curricula as well as resources and tools for health care providers.

7. California Department of Education, Office of Environmental Education, 1430 N St, Sacramento, CA 95814, Internet: http://www.cde.ca.gov/pd/ca/sc/oeeintrod.asp. This office has reviewed and rated hundreds of environmental education curricula (K–12) and published them in a compendium.

Environmental Health Science Education

1. National Institute of Environmental Health Sciences (NIEHS), Division of Extramural Research and Training. PO Box 12233 (MD-EC21), Research Triangle Park, NC 27709, phone: 919-541-7733. Education outreach

Appendix B: Curricula for Environmental Education and Environmental
Health Science Education in Primary and Secondary Schools

883

is a key mechanism for achieving the mission of the National Institute
of Environmental Health Sciences. The Environmental Health Science
Education Web site provides educators, students and scientists with easy
access to reliable tools, resources, and classroom materials. It invests in the
future of environmental health science by increasing awareness of the link
between the environment and human health (http://www.niehs.nih.gov/
health/scied/index.cfm).

NIEHS also supported the development of standards-based curricular
materials that integrate environmental health sciences within a variety of
subject areas (eg, biology, geography, history, math, civics, art). More than 81
materials were created by 9 projects. These materials can be found at: http://
www.niehs.nih.gov/health/scied/integrated/index.cfm.

2. University of Medicine & Dentistry of New Jersey School of Public Health.
    ToxRAP and SUC2ES2 (Students Understanding Critical Connections
    between the Environment, Society and Self): http://www.niehs.nih.gov/
    research/supported/programs/ehsic/grantees/umdnjsph.cfm. Using a
    curriculum development model, teachers, scientists, and education specialists
    worked collaboratively to develop 3 curriculum guides. In this innovative,
    3-part curricular series, students become health hazard detectives to coopera-
    tively investigate environmental health hazards and their impact on human
    health. By applying an environmental health risk assessment framework,
    students learn how to state a health problem, investigate hazards and people
    who may be exposed, and identify hazard-control methods. A detective
    theme helps students to study air contaminants and learn the principles of
    toxicology and the process of risk assessment.

3. Baylor College of Medicine Center for Educational Outreach. My World
    and My World and Me. Developed by teams of educators, scientists, and
    health specialists at Baylor College of Medicine, My World (http://www.
    ccitonline.org/ceo/content.cfm?menu_id=103) and My World and Me
    (http://www.ccitonline.org/ceo/content.cfm?menu_id=104) educational
    materials provide students and teachers with knowledge of the environment
    and its relationship to human health.

    BioEd Online: http://www.bioedonline.org/. BioEd Online is an online
    educational resource for educators, students, and parents, sponsored by the
    Baylor College of Medicine. BioEd Online utilizes state-of-the-art technol-
    ogy to give instant access to reliable, cutting-edge information and educa-
    tional tools for biology and related subjects. The goal is to provide useful,

accurate, and current information and materials that build on and enhance the skills and knowledge of science educators. Developed under the guidance of an expert editorial board, BioEd Online offers high-quality resources.

4. Bowling Green State University, Project EXCITE: Environmental Health Science Exploration Through Cross-Disciplinary & Investigative Team Experiences: http://www.bgsu.edu/colleges/edhd/programs/excite. Project EXCITE engages students in valuable learning experiences across disciplinary areas using locally relevant environmental health science topics. The project reflects current thinking about effective teaching and learning and is aligned with national and state education goals. Project EXCITE emphasizes critical thinking and problem solving skills, interdisciplinary connections, collaborative learning, and the use of technology. Students investigate local environmental health science issues, explain fundamental understandings of concepts, and apply the knowledge and skills generated to improve performance on standardized achievement tests.

5. Maryland Public Television. EnviroHealth Connections: http://www.thinkport.org/classroom/connections/default.tp. The curricular materials developed for this project include lesson plans, videos, and online interactive activities. They are disseminated to teachers throughout Maryland and beyond on the EnviroHealth Connections (http://envirohealth.thinkport.org). The Connections Web site hosts more than 60 classroom-tested lesson plans aligned to state standards. Additional materials include a teacher discussion board, PowerPoint presentations by researchers at the Johns Hopkins Bloomberg School of Public Health, and links to other high-quality resources. Also accessible through the Web site is Meet the Experts: Environmental Health, an interactive question and answer activity that features 13 professionals whose careers center on environmental health. Students learn what these individuals studied in school; how and why they began their careers; and how their environmental health work affects our lives.

6. Oregon State University. Hydroville Curriculum Project: http://www.hydroville.org. The Hydroville Curriculum Project (HCP) has created problem-based curricula for high school students focusing on environmental health science. The problems occur in the fictitious town of Hydroville, which has to contend with 1 of 3 environmental health scenarios: a pesticide spill, a problem with air quality at a local middle school, and a water quality problem. The Hydroville curricula are based on real-life case studies and use real data. The town of Hydroville could be a town anywhere in America. Students work in teams to solve environmental health problems. This

integrated curriculum promotes teamwork, critical thinking, subject integration, and problem-solving. Oregon State University provides additional environmental health science education resources for K-12 Education at http://ehsc.oregonstate.edu.

7. Texas A&M University System. Partnership for Environmental Education and Rural Health (PEER): http://peer.tamu.edu. The Partnership for Environmental Education and Rural Health is a program for rural middle school students and teachers. The program aims to improve student enthusiasm for learning, increase overall academic performance of students, and encourage teachers throughout the state across all subject areas to use environmental health science topics to motivate students and help them relate science instruction to real-world situations.

8. University of Miami Coral Gables. Atmospheric and Marine-Based Interdisciplinary Environmental Health Training (AMBIENT): http://www.rsmas.miami.edu/groups/niehs/ambient. The AMBIENT Project is a systemic approach to environmental health science education. Focused around the 4 themes of air, water, soil and food, a health-science problem-based learning approach is delivered by trained educators to the ethnically diverse population of high school students in Miami-Dade County. The AMBIENT curriculum modules consist of a number of segments. Some can be taught independently and others are meant to be used together in a certain order. All modules begin with a Teacher's Guide, which contains the basic information necessary to knowledgeably lead class discussions and guide students' research efforts.

9. University of Rochester. My Environment, My Health, My Choices: http://www2.envmed.rochester.edu/envmed/ehsc/outreach/index.html. My Environment, My Health, My Choices is an environmental health curriculum development project sponsored by the University of Rochester's Environmental Health Sciences Center. The project involves teachers from the greater Rochester, New York area (as well as throughout New York State) who create environmental health curriculum units with the support of University of Rochester faculty. The curriculum units focus on specific environmental health questions or problems that are of local, regional, or national concern. Such problems include, for example, water pollution due to farm runoff, links between air pollution and asthma, and the health effects linked to pesticides.

10. University of Washington, Integrated Environmental Health Middle School Project: http://www.iehms.com/online and http://hsc.unm.edu/pharmacy/ iehms/about.shtml. The Integrated Environmental Health Middle School Project (IEHMSP) introduces middle school teachers and students in Washington State and New Mexico to the field of environmental health sciences and facilitates interdisciplinary teaching across the middle school curriculum. The IEHMSP has developed a multitiered model of integrated and contextualized learning. Project materials have been used by school districts across Washington State and in New Mexico. Additional resources are offered for K-12 Classroom Outreach at http://depts.washington.edu/ ceeh/Outreach/k12.html.

Healthy School Environments Resources

1. US Environmental Protection Agency, Indoor Environments Division, Office of Air and Radiation, 1200 Pennsylvania Avenue, NW, MC 6609J, Washington, DC, 20460, phone: 202-343-9315, Internet: http://www. epa.gov/schools/. The EPA has developed a 1-stop location for information and links to school environmental health issues. EPA and non-EPA on-line resources are available to assist facility managers, school administrators, architects, design engineers, school nurses, parents, teachers, and staff in addressing environmental health issues in schools. The Healthy School Environments Assessment Tool (HealthySEAT) is a unique software tool designed to help school districts evaluate and manage their school facilities for key environmental, safety, and health issues (http://www.epa.gov/schools/ healthyseat/index.html).

Appendix C

AAP Policy Statements, Technical Reports, and Clinical Reports Authored by the Council on Environmental Health

■ ■ ■ ■ ■ ■

Please visit the American Academy of Pediatrics (AAP) public online policy site for updated information and access to AAP policy documents: http://www.aappolicy.org.

CURRENT STATEMENTS

Chemical-Management Policy: Prioritizing Children's Health
PEDIATRICS, Vol. 127, No. 5, 983-990, May 2011

Ultraviolet Radiation: A Hazard to Children and Adolescents
(Policy Statement)
PEDIATRICS, Vol. 127, No. 3, 588-597, March 2011

Ultraviolet Radiation: A Hazard to Children and Adolescents
(Technical Report)
PEDIATRICS, Vol. 127, No. 3, e791-e817, March 2011

Tobacco Use: A Pediatric Disease
PEDIATRICS, Vol. 124, No. 5, 1474-1487, November 2009

Secondhand and Prenatal Tobacco Smoke Exposure
PEDIATRICS, Vol. 124, No. 5, e1017-e1044, November 2009

Drinking Water From Private Wells and Risks to Children
(Policy Statement)
PEDIATRICS, Vol. 123, No. 6, 1599-1605, June 2009

Drinking Water From Private Wells and Risks to Children
(Technical Report)
PEDIATRICS, Vol. 123, No. 6, e1123-e1137, June 2009

The Built Environment: Designing Communities to Promote Physical Activity in Children
PEDIATRICS, Vol. 123, No. 6, 1591-1598, June 2009

Global Climate Change and Children's Health
(Policy Statement)
PEDIATRICS, Vol. 120, No. 5, 1149-1152, November 2007

Global Climate Change and Children's Health
(Technical Report)
PEDIATRICS, Vol. 120, No. 5, e1359-e1367, November 2007

Spectrum of Noninfectious Health Effects From Molds
(Policy Statement)
PEDIATRICS, Vol. 118, No. 6, 2582-2586, December 2006

Spectrum of Noninfectious Health Effects From Molds
(Technical Report)
PEDIATRICS, Vol. 118, No. 6, e1909-e1926, December 2006

Chemical-Biological Terrorism and Its Impact on Children
PEDIATRICS, Vol. 118, No. 3, 1267-1278, September 2006

Infant Methemoglobinemia: The Role of Dietary Nitrate in Food and Water
PEDIATRICS, Vol. 116, No. 3, 784-786, September 2005

Lead Exposure in Children: Prevention, Detection, and Management
PEDIATRICS, Vol. 116, No. 4, 1036-1046, October 2005

Ambient Air Pollution: Health Hazards to Children
PEDIATRICS, Vol. 114, No. 6, 1699-1707, December 2004

Nontherapeutic Use of Antimicrobial Agents in Animal Agriculture: Implications for Pediatrics
PEDIATRICS, Vol. 114, No. 3, 862-868, September 2004

Appendix C: AAP Policy Statements, Technical Reports, and Clinical Reports Authored by the Council on Environmental Health

889

Radiation Disasters and Children
PEDIATRICS, Vol. 111, No. 6, 1455–1466, June 2003

Mercury in the Environment: Implications for Pediatricians
PEDIATRICS, Vol. 108, No. 1, 197–205, July 2001

RETIRED STATEMENTS

Pediatric Exposure and Potential Toxicity of Phthalate Plasticizers
PEDIATRICS, Vol. 111, No. 6, 1467–1474, June 2003
Retired January 2011

Irradiation of Food
PEDIATRICS, Vol. 106, No. 6, 1505–1510, December 2000
Retired October 2004

**Chemical-Biological Terrorism and Its Impact on Children:
A Subject Review**
PEDIATRICS, Vol. 105, No. 3, 662–670, March 2000
Retired September 2006

Thimerosal in Vaccines—An Interim Report to Clinicians
PEDIATRICS, Vol. 104, No. 3, 570–574, September 1999
Retired November 2002

Ultraviolet Light: A Hazard to Children
PEDIATRICS, Vol. 104, No. 2, 328–333, August 1999
Retired March 2011

Screening for Elevated Blood Lead Levels
PEDIATRICS, Vol. 101, No. 6, 1072–1078, June 1998
Retired October 2005

Risk of Ionizing Radiation Exposure to Children: A Subject Review
PEDIATRICS, Vol. 101, No. 4, 717–719, April 1998
Retired April 2002

Toxic Effects of Indoor Molds
PEDIATRICS, Vol. 101, No. 4, 712–714, April 1998
Retired December 2006

Noise: A Hazard to the Fetus and Newborn
PEDIATRICS, Vol. 100, No. 4, 724–727, October 1997
Retired April 2006

Environmental Tobacco Smoke: A Hazard to Children
PEDIATRICS, Vol. 99, No. 4, 639–642, April 1997
Retired November 2009

Hazards of Child Labor
PEDIATRICS, Vol. 95, No. 2, 311–313, February 1995
Retired January 2005

PCBs in Breast Milk
PEDIATRICS, Vol. 94, No. 1, 122–123, July 1994
Retired February 2001

Use of Chloral Hydrate for Sedation in Children
PEDIATRICS, Vol. 92, No. 3, 471–473, September 1993
Retired February 2000

Lead Poisoning: From Screening to Primary Prevention
PEDIATRICS, Vol. 92, No. 1, 176–183, July 1993
Retired June 1998

Ambient Air Pollution: Respiratory Hazards to Children
PEDIATRICS, Vol. 91, No. 6, 1210–1213, June 1993
Retired December 2004

Radon Exposure: A Hazard to Children
PEDIATRICS, Vol. 83, No. 5, 799–802, May 1989
Retired February 2001

Childhood Lead Poisoning
PEDIATRICS, Vol. 79, No. 3, 457–465, March 1987
Retired October 1993

Asbestos Exposure in Schools
PEDIATRICS, Vol. 79, No. 2, 301–305, February 1987
Retired February 2001

Involuntary Smoking: A Hazard to Children
PEDIATRICS, Vol. 77, No. 5, 755–757, May 1986
Retired April 1997

Smokeless Tobacco — A Carcinogenic Hazard to Children
PEDIATRICS, Vol. 76, No. 6, 1009–1011, December 1985
Retired February 2001

Appendix C: AAP Policy Statements, Technical Reports, and Clinical
Reports Authored by the Council on Environmental Health

891

Special Susceptibility of Children to Radiation Effects
PEDIATRICS, Vol. 72, No. 6, 809, December 1983
Retired April 1998

**Environmental Consequences of Tobacco Smoking: Implications
for Public Policies that Affect the Health of Children**
PEDIATRICS, Vol. 70, No. 2, 314–315, August 1982
Retired February 1987

National Standard for Airborne Lead
PEDIATRICS, Vol. 62, No. 6, 1070–1071, December 1978
Retired February 1987

PCBs in Breast Milk
PEDIATRICS, Vol. 62, No. 3, 407, September 1978
Retired September 1994

Infant Radiant Warmers
PEDIATRICS, Vol. 61, No. 1, 113–114, January 1978
Retired June 1995

Hyperthermia from Malfunctioning Radiant Heaters
PEDIATRICS, Vol. 59, No. 6, 1041–1042, June 1977
Retired February 1987

Carcinogens in Drinking Water
PEDIATRICS, Vol. 57, No. 4, 462–464, April 1976
Retired February 1987

Effects of Cigarette Smoking on the Fetus and Child
PEDIATRICS, Vol. 57, No. 3, 411–413, March 1976
Retired September 1994

Noise Pollution: Neonatal Aspects
PEDIATRICS, Vol. 54, No. 4, 476–478, October 1974
Retired October 1997

Animal Feedlots
PEDIATRICS, Vol. 51, No. 3, 582–592, March 1973
Retired September 1994

Lead Content of Paint Applied to Surfaces Accessible to Young Children
PEDIATRICS, Vol. 49, No. 6, 918–921, June 1972
Retired February 1987

Pediatric Problems Related to Deteriorated Housing
PEDIATRICS, Vol. 49, No. 4, 627, April 1972
Retired February 1987

Earthenware Containers: A Potential Source of Acute Lead Poisoning
Newsletter, Vol. 22, No. 13, 4, August 15, 1971
Retired February 1987

Neurotoxicity from Hexachlorophene
Newsletter, Vol. 22, No. 7, 4, May 1971
Retired February 1987

Acute and Chronic Childhood Lead Poisoning
PEDIATRICS, Vol. 47, No. 5, 950–951, May 1971
Retired November 1986

Pediatric Aspects of Air Pollution
PEDIATRICS, Vol. 46, No. 4, 637–639, October 1970
Retired February 1987

More on Radioactive Fallout
Newsletter Supplement, Vol. 21, No. 8, April 15, 1970
Retired February 1987

Smoking and Children: A Pediatric Viewpoint
PEDIATRICS, Vol. 44, No. 5, Part 1, 757–759, November 1969
Retired February 1987

Present Status of Water Pollution Control
PEDIATRICS, Vol. 34, No. 3, 431–440, September 1964
Retired February 1987

Hazards of Radioactive Fallout
PEDIATRICS, Vol. 29, No. 5, 845–847, May 1962
Retired February 1995

Statement on the Use of Diagnostic X-Ray
PEDIATRICS, Vol. 28, No. 4, 676–677, October 1961
Retired February 1987

Appendix C: AAP Policy Statements, Technical Reports, and Clinical
Reports Authored by the Council on Environmental Health

893

PEDIATRICS SUPPLEMENTS

A Partnership to Establish an Environmental Safety Net for Children
Supplement to PEDIATRICS, Vol. 112, No. 1, Part II, July 2003

The Susceptibility of the Fetus and Child to Chemical Pollutants
Supplement to PEDIATRICS, Vol. 53, No. 5, Part II, May 1974

Conference on the Pediatric Significance of Peacetime Radioactive Fallout
Supplement to PEDIATRICS, Vol. 41, No. 1, Part II, January 1968

AAP Patient Education Materials Related to Environmental Health Issues

■ ■ ■ ■ ■ ■

Following is a list of patient education materials from the American Academy of Pediatrics relating to environmental health issues. Many titles are available in brochure format, sold in packs of 50. All titles are available in 8 ½" x 11" handout format to subscribers of Patient Education Online at www.patiented. aap.org. Contact the AAP bookstore at 888-227-1770 or visit the bookstore online at www.aap.org/bookstore to place an order or for more information.

- Acute Ear Infections and Your Child
- Allergies in Children
- Anemia and Your Young Child
- Asthma and Your Child
- Dangers of Secondhand Smoke
- Fun in the Sun: Keep Your Family Safe
- Lead Is a Poison: What You Need to Know
- Middle Ear Fluid and Your Child
- The Risks of Tobacco Use
- Smokeless Tobacco: What You Need to Know
- Tobacco: Straight Talk for Teens
- Your Child and the Environment

Parents can access information on AAP's parenting Web site HealthyChildren.org.

Chairs of the AAP Council on Environmental Health

■ ■ ■ ■ ■ ■

Committee on Radiation Hazards and Epidemiology of Malformations

Robert A. Aldrich, MD; 1957–1961

> In 1961, the committee was split in 2: a short-lived Committee on Malformations and the Committee on Environmental Hazards.

Committee on Environmental Hazards

Lee E. Farr, MD; 1961–1967
Paul F. Wehrle, MD; 1967–1973
Robert W. Miller, MD, DrPH; 1973–1979
Laurence Finberg, MD; 1979–1980

> In 1979, the AAP established the Committee on Genetics with Charles Scriver, MD, as chair. In 1980, the AAP combined this committee with the Committee on Environmental Hazards to form the:

Committee on Genetics & Environmental Hazards

Laurence Finberg, MD; Cochair, 1980–1983
Charles Scriver, MD; Cochair, 1980–1983

> In 1983, the 2 committees were separated again.

Committee on Environmental Hazards

Philip J. Landrigan, MD, MSc; 1983–1987
Richard J. Jackson, MD, MPH; 1987–1991

> In 1991, the committee was renamed the Committee on Environmental Health.

Committee on Environmental Health

J. Routt Reigart, MD; 1991–1995

Ruth A. Etzel, MD, PhD; 1995–1999

Sophie J. Balk, MD; 1999–2003

Michael W. Shannon, MD, MPH; 2003–2007

In 2009, the committee adopted the AAP's "Council" format.

Council on Environmental Health

Helen J. Binns, MD, MPH; 2007–2011

Jerome A. Paulson, MD; 2011–

Selected Abbreviations

■ ■ ■ ■ ■ ■

2,4-D	2,4-dichlorophenoxyacetic acid
2-PAM	Pralidoxime
4-MBC	4-methyl-benzylidene camphor
ACE	angiotensin-converting enzyme
AChE	acetylcholinesterase
AAP	American Academy of Pediatrics
ALARA	as low as reasonably achievable
AP	Approved Product
ACMI	Art & Creative Materials Institute
ACS	American Cancer Society
ADHD	attention deficit/hyperactivity disorder
AHERA	Asbestos Hazard Emergency Response Act
AI	adequate intake
AQI	Air Quality Index
ASD	autism spectrum disorders
ASTM D4236	American Society for Testing and Materials Standard (art materials)
AT	ataxia-telangiectasia
ATSDR	Agency for Toxic Substances and Disease Registry
BAL	British anti-lewisite (2,3-dimercatopropanol, dimercaprol)
BBP	butyl benzyl phthalate
BLL	blood lead level

BP-3	benzophenone-3
BPA	bisphenol A
c-decaBDE	*c*-decabrominated diphenyl ether
c-octaBDE	*c*-octabrominated diphenyl ether
c-pentaBDE	*c*-pentabrominated diphenyl ether
CaNa$_2$EDTA	edentate disodium calcium
CCA	chromated copper arsenate
CDC	Centers for Disease Control and Prevention
CEHAPE	Children's Environment and Health Action Plan for Europe
CERCLA	Comprehensive Environmental Response, Compensation, and Liability Act
CFC	chlorofluorocarbon
CFL	compact fluorescent light
CFOI	Census of Fatal Occupational Injuries
CFR	Code of Federal Regulations
CFU	colony forming unit
CHEERS	Children's Health Environmental Exposure Research Study
CLIA	Clinical Laboratory Improvement Amendments
ClO$_4^-$	perchlorate
CO	carbon monoxide
CO$_2$	carbon dioxide
COHb	carboxyhemoglobin
CNS	central nervous system
CP	Certified Product
CPSC	Consumer Product Safety Commission
CPT	Current Procedural Terminology
CT	computed tomography
DALY	disability-adjusted life year
dB	decibel
dBA	decibels weighted by the A scale
DBP	dibutyl phthalate
DDE	dichlorodiphenyldichloroethylene
DDT	dichlorodiphenyltrichloroethane
DEET	*N,N*-diethyl-m-toluamide, also known as *N,N*-diethyl-3-methyl-benzamide
DEHP	di(2-ethylhexyl) phthalate

DEP	diethyl phthalate
DES	diethylstibestrol
DHA	dihydroxyacetone
DHA	docosahexaenoic acid
DHHS	Department of Health and Human Services
DIDP	di-isodecyl phthalate
DINP	di-isononyl phthalate
DMP	dimethyl phthalate
DMPS	2,3-dimercaptopropane-1-sulfonate (dimaval)
DMSA	dimercaptosuccinic acid (succimer)
DnBP	di-n-butyl phthalate
DNL	day-night average sound level
DnOP	di-n-octylphthalate
DOP	dioctyl phthalate
DSHEA	Dietary Supplement Health and Education Act
DSM-IV-TR	*Diagnostic and Statistical Manual of Mental Disorders, Fourth Edition, Text Revision*
ED	emergency department
EEA	European Environment Agency
EEG	electroencephalogram
EHR	electronic health record
EMF	electric and magnetic fields
EMLAP	Environmental Microbiology Laboratory Accreditation Program
EPA	eicosapentaenoic acid
EPA	Environmental Protection Agency
eV	electron volts
FEMA	Federal Emergency Management Agency
FEV_1	forced expiratory volume in 1 second
FLSA	Fair Labor Standards Act
FDA	Food and Drug Administration
FQPA	Food Quality Protection Act
FSIS	Food Safety and Inspection System
GABA	gamma-aminobutyric acid
GIS	geographic information systems
Gy	gray

G6PD	glucose-6-phosphate dehydrogenase
HBV	hepatitis B virus
HDL	high-density lipoprotein
HDPE	high-density polyethylene
HEPA	high-efficiency particulate air
HL	Health Label (Non-Toxic)
HONC	Hooked on Nicotine Checklist
HPV	high production volume
HPV	human papilloma virus
HUD	Department of Housing and Urban Development
HVAC	heating, ventilation, and air conditioning
Hz	hertz
IAQ	indoor air quality
IARC	International Agency for Research on Cancer
ICD-9-CM	International Classification of Diseases, Ninth Revision, Clinical Modification
IFCS	International Forum on Chemical Safety
Ig	immunoglobulin
IPCC	Intergovernmental Panel on Climate Change
IPM	integrated pest management
IRB	institutional review board
J	joule
kGy	kilogray
KI	potassium iodide
kV	kilovolt
Leq24	24-hour equivalent noise exposure
LOAEL	lowest observable adverse effect level
MCV	mean corpuscular volume
MCL	maximum contaminant level
MEHP	mono(2-ethylhexyl) phthalate
MERV	minimum efficiency reporting value
MHz	megahertz
MMA	methyl methacrylate
MMR	measles-mumps-rubella
MMT	methylcyclopentadienyl manganese tricarbonyl
MRA/MRI	magnetic resonance angiogram/magnetic resonance imaging

mrem	millirem
MRSA	methicillin-resistant *Staphylococcus aureus*
MSDS	Material Safety Data Sheet
MSG	monosodium glutamate
mSv	millisievert
MTBE	methyl tertiary butyl ether
Na_2EDTA	edentate disodium
NAAQS	National Ambient Air Quality Standards
NAS	National Academy of Sciences
NCI	National Cancer Institute
NEISS-Work	National Electronic Injury Surveillance System occupational supplement
NHANES	National Health and Nutrition Examination Survey
NIEHS	National Institute of Environmental Health Sciences
NIHL	noise-induced hearing loss
NIOSH	National Institute for Occupational Safety and Health
NITS	noise-induced threshold shift
nm	nanometer
NMP	N-methyl-2-pyrrolidone
NMSC	nonmelanoma skin cancer
NO_2	nitrogen dioxide
NO_3-N	nitrate-nitrogen
NOAEL	no observable adverse effect level
NOC	*N*-nitroso compound
NPL	National Priorities List
NRC	National Research Council
NRC	Nuclear Regulatory Commission
NSAID	nonsteroidal anti-inflammatory drug
NTD	neural tube defect
NTP	National Toxicology Program
OEHHA	California Office of Environmental Health Hazard Assessment
OMC	octyl methoxycinnamate
OSHA	Occupational Safety and Health Administration
Pa	pascal
PABA	para amino benzoic acid

PAH	polycyclic aromatic hydrocarbon
PBB	polybrominated biphenyl
PBDE	polybrominated diphenyl ether
PC	polycarbonate
PCB	polychlorinated biphenyl
PCDD	polychlorinated dibenzodioxin
PCDF	polychlorinated dibenzofuran
pCi	picocurie
PDD	pervasive developmental disorder
PEHSU	Pediatric Environmental Health Specialty Unit
PFC	polyfluoroalkyl chemical
PFOA	perfluorooctanoic acid
PFOS	perfluorooctane sulfonate
PKU	phenylketonuria
PM_{10}	particles with aerodynamic diameter smaller than 10 μm
$PM_{2.5}$	particles with aerodynamic diameter smaller than 2.5 μm
PM_1	particles with aerodynamic diameter smaller than 1 μm
POP	persistent organic pollutant
PP	polypropylene
ppb	parts per billion
ppm	parts per million
ppt	parts per trillion
PTS	persistent toxic substance
PVC	polyvinyl chloride
rad	radiation absorbed dose
RAST	radioallergosorbent test
REACH	Registration, Evaluation, Authorization and Restriction of Chemical substances
RBE	relative biological effectiveness
RCRA	Resource Conservation and Recovery Act
RDW	red cell distribution width
rem	roentgen equivalent man
RfD	reference dose
SAICM	Strategic Approach to International Chemicals Management
SAMSHA	Substance Abuse and Mental Health Services Administration
SARA	Superfund Amendments and Reauthorization Act

SARS	severe acute respiratory syndrome
SIDS	sudden infant death syndrome
SHS	secondhand smoke
SO_2	sulfur dioxide
SPF	sun protection factor
SPL	sound pressure level
H_2SO_4	sulfuric acid
Sv	sievert
T-2	trichothecene mycotoxin
T_4	thyroxine
TCDD	2,3,7,8 tetrachlorodibenzo-p-dioxin
TEQ	toxic equivalent
TSH	thyroid stimulating hormone
TNF-a	tumor necrosis factor-alpha
TRI	Toxics Release Inventory
TSCA	Toxic Substances Control Act
UL	Underwriters Laboratories
UN	United Nations
UNEP	United Nations Environment Programme
UPF	ultraviolet protection factor
USDA	US Department of Agriculture
UVA	ultraviolet A
UVB	ultraviolet B
UVC	ultraviolet C
UVR	ultraviolet radiation
VEE	Venezuelan equine encephalitis
VOC	volatile organic compound
WHO	World Health Organization
WTO	World Trade Organization
XRF	x-ray fluorescence
YRBSS	Youth Risk Behavior Surveillance System
YTS	Youth Tobacco Survey

Index